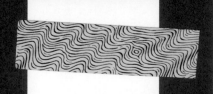

# Fluid, Electrolyte, and Acid—Base Physiology

FIFTH EDITION

# Fluid, Electrolyte, and Acid–Base Physiology

## A Problem-Based Approach

*Kamel S. Kamel,* MD, FRCPC

ST. MICHAEL'S HOSPITAL
UNIVERSITY OF TORONTO
TORONTO, ONTARIO, CANADA

*Mitchell L. Halperin,* MD, FRCPC

ST. MICHAEL'S HOSPITAL
UNIVERSITY OF TORONTO
TORONTO, ONTARIO, CANADA

ELSEVIER

# ELSEVIER

1600 John F. Kennedy Blvd.
Ste 1800
Philadelphia, PA 19103-2899

FLUID, ELECTROLYTE, AND ACID–BASE PHYSIOLOGY:
A PROBLEM-BASED APPROACH, 5TH EDITION                    ISBN: 978-0-323-35515-5

---

### Notices

Knowledge and best practice in this field are constantly changing. As new research and experience broaden our understanding, changes in research methods, professional practices, or medical treatment may become necessary.

Practitioners and researchers must always rely on their own experience and knowledge in evaluating and using any information, methods, compounds, or experiments described herein. In using such information or methods they should be mindful of their own safety and the safety of others, including parties for whom they have a professional responsibility.

With respect to any drug or pharmaceutical products identified, readers are advised to check the most current information provided (i) on procedures featured or (ii) by the manufacturer of each product to be administered, to verify the recommended dose or formula, the method and duration of administration, and contraindications. It is the responsibility of practitioners, relying on their own experience and knowledge of their patients, to make diagnoses, to determine dosages and the best treatment for each individual patient, and to take all appropriate safety precautions.

To the fullest extent of the law, neither the Publisher nor the authors, contributors, or editors, assume any liability for any injury and/or damage to persons or property as a matter of products liability, negligence or otherwise, or from any use or operation of any methods, products, instructions, or ideas contained in the material herein.

---

**Library of Congress Cataloging-in-Publication Data**

Names: Halperin, M. L. (Mitchell L.), author. | Kamel, Kamel S., author.
Title: Fluid, electrolyte, and acid-base physiology : a problem-based
    approach / Kamel S. Kamel, Mitchell L. Halperin.
Description: 5th edition. | Philadelphia, PA : Elsevier, [2017] | Author's
    names reversed on previous edition. | Includes bibliographical references
    and index.
Identifiers: LCCN 2016037933 | ISBN 9780323355155 (hardcover : alk. paper)
Subjects: | MESH: Water-Electrolyte Imbalance--physiopathology | Acid-Base
    Imbalance--physiopathology | Water-Electrolyte Imbalance--diagnosis |
    Acid-Base Imbalance--diagnosis | Potassium--metabolism
Classification: LCC RC630 | NLM WD 220 | DDC 616.3/992--dc23 LC record
available at https://lccn.loc.gov/2016037933

*Content Strategist:* Maureen Iannuzzi
*Senior Content Development Specialist:* Joan Ryan
*Publishing Services Manager:* Catherine Jackson
*Project Manager:* Kate Mannix
*Design Direction:* Ryan Cook

*To Marylin and Brenda:*
*We are indeed extremely*
*grateful for your patience*
*and your strong,*
*unwavering support.*

# Acknowledgment

We are extremely grateful to our friend and colleague Professor Martin Schreiber for his critical review of the entire book and the several insightful comments he provided. Martin, you are truly a good man.

# Preface

About 6 years have passed between this, the fifth edition of *Fluid, Electrolyte, and Acid–Base Physiology*, and the fourth edition. For this edition, Professor Kamel S. Kamel has taken the role of lead author, while Professor Marc Goldstein, because of other commitments and time constraints, has decided not to participate.

Our initial intention with this edition was to provide limited updates of a few chapters. We ended up, however, extensively revising the book, so that it is almost entirely rewritten. Although the effort was substantial and the time commitment was much more than we anticipated, we could not be more proud of the product. In this fifth edition of *Fluid, Electrolyte, and Acid–Base Physiology*, we have tried to provide a comprehensive, go-to guide to the diagnosis and management of fluid-electrolyte and acid–base disorders. The book aims to move from basic physiology to pathophysiology to practical clinical guidance, taking into account new discoveries and new insights into fluid-electrolyte and acid–base physiology, as well as new options available for treatment. We emphasize principles of metabolic regulation and biochemistry to promote an in-depth understanding of metabolic acid–base disorders. We also emphasize integrative, whole-body physiology to provide a more in-depth understanding of the pathophysiology of fluid, electrolyte, and acid–base disorders. The style of the book, which we believe has been appealing to readers, has not changed. As in previous editions, we have attempted to provide information in an easy-to-understand way, with emphasis on how to apply the information to clinical practice, supported by numerous diagrams, flow charts, and tables. To engage and challenge the reader, we have included several clinical cases and questions throughout each of the chapters in the book.

We believe that this fifth edition of *Fluid, Electrolyte, and Acid–Base Physiology* will provide a useful resource to learners at different levels, from medical students to postgraduate trainees, and to practitioners such as general internists and specialists with an interest in the area of fluid-electrolyte and acid–base disorders.

# Interconversion of Units

Because some readers will be more familiar with the International System of Units (SI units) and others will prefer the conventional units used in the United States, we provide the following conversion table. To convert units, multiply the reported value by the appropriate conversion factor.

| PARAMETER | CONVENTIONAL TO SI UNITS | SI TO CONVENTIONAL UNITS |
|---|---|---|
| Sodium | × 1 = mmol/L | × 1 = mEq/L |
| Potassium | × 1 = mmol/L | × 1 = mEq/L |
| Chloride | × 1 = mmol/L | × 1 = mEq/L |
| Bicarbonate | × 1 = mmol/L | × 1 = mEq/L |
| Calcium | × 0.25 = mmol/L | × 4.0 = mg/dL |
| Urea | × 0.36 = mmol/L | × 2.8 = mg/dL |
| Creatinine | × 88.4 = µmol/L | × 0.0113 = mg/dL |
| Glucose | × 0.055 = mmol/L | × 18 = mg/dL |
| Albumin | × 10 = g/L | × 0.1 = mg/dL |

# Contents

# List of Cases

# List of Flow Charts

# section one
# Acid—Base

Acid-Base

# Principles of Acid–Base Physiology

# Introduction

**DEFINITIONS**

- *Acids* are compounds that are capable of donating H⁺ ions; when an acid (HA) dissociates, it yields an H⁺ ion and its conjugate base or anion (A⁻).
- *Bases* are compounds that are capable of accepting H⁺ ions.
- *Valence* is the net electrical charge on a compound or an element.

$$HA \rightleftharpoons H^+ + A^-$$

**ACIDEMIA VERSUS ACIDOSIS**

- *Acidemia* describes an increased concentration of H⁺ ions in plasma.
- *Acidosis* is a process in which there is an addition of H⁺ ions to the body; this may or may not cause acidemia.

**ACID–BASE TERMS**

- *Concentration of H⁺ ions:* The normal value in plasma is 40±2 nmol/L, which is 0.000040 mmol/L.
- *pH* is the negative logarithm of the [H⁺] in mol/L, its normal value in plasma is 7.40±0.02.
- $HCO_3^-$ *ions:* the conjugate base of carbonic acid is the "H⁺ ion remover" of the BBS; its concentration in plasma is close to 25 mmol/L, but there are large fluctuations throughout the day (22 to 31 mmol/L).
- $PCO_2$: The major carbon waste product of fuel oxidation is carbon dioxide. Its concentration is reflected by its partial pressure ($PCO_2$). The normal arterial $PCO_2$ is 40±2 mm Hg. The $PCO_2$ in blood-draining skeletal muscles is ~6 mm Hg greater than the arterial $PCO_2$ at rest.

Our goal in this chapter is to describe the physiology of hydrogen ions (H⁺) and how acid–base balance is achieved. From a chemical perspective, H⁺ is the smallest ion (atomic weight 1) and its concentration in body fluids is tiny (a million-fold lower than that of its major partner, $HCO_3^-$). Nevertheless, H⁺ ions are extremely powerful because they are intimately involved in the capture of energy from oxidation of fuels by driving regeneration of adenosine triphosphate ($ATP^{4-}$). In this context, the electrical charge on the protons is far more important than their chemical concentration.

The concentration of H⁺ ions in body fluids must be maintained in a very narrow range. If their concentration rises, H⁺ ions will bind to intracellular proteins, and this changes their charge, shape, and possibly their functions, with possible dire consequences. Hence, a system is needed to remove H⁺ ions, even if their concentration is not appreciably elevated. This function is achieved by the bicarbonate buffer system (BBS). The special feature that allows the BBS to function as an effective buffer is that a low $PCO_2$ drives the reaction of H⁺ ions with $HCO_3^-$ anions (see Eqn 1). Because a small increase in H⁺ ion concentration in plasma stimulates the respiratory center and causes hyperventilation, the concentration of $CO_2$ in each liter of alveolar air and hence in the arterial blood will be lower. Nevertheless, as we stress throughout this chapter, because the bulk of the BBS is in the intracellular fluid and the interstitial space of skeletal muscles, a low $PCO_2$ in their capillary blood is required to ensure the safe removal of H⁺ ions.

Removal of H⁺ ions by the BBS leads to a deficit of $HCO_3^-$ ions. Accordingly, one must have another system that adds new $HCO_3^-$ ions to the body as long as acidemia persists. This task is achieved by the kidneys, in the metabolic process of excretion of ammonium ions ($NH_4^+$) in the urine.

A high rate of excretion of $NH_4^+$ ions must be achieved while maintaining a urine pH that is close to 6.0 to avoid precipitation of uric acid. Base balance is maintained by excreting an alkali load in the urine as a family of organic anions rather than $HCO_3^-$ ions. This avoids having a high urine pH and the risk of precipitation of calcium phosphate in the luminal fluid.

$$H^+ + HCO_3^- \rightleftharpoons CO_2 + H_2O \qquad (1)$$

## OBJECTIVES

■ To describe the major processes that lead to acid and base balance.

### ACID BALANCE

1. *Production of acids*: H⁺ ions are produced in a metabolic process when all of their products have a greater anionic charge than all of their substrates.
2. *Buffering of H⁺ ions*: This should minimize H⁺ ion binding to proteins in vital organs (i.e., the brain and the heart). To do so, H⁺ ions must react with $HCO_3^-$ ions. The vast majority of $HCO_3^-$ ions in the body is in the interstitial and intracellular compartments of skeletal muscle. The key to achieving this function is to have a low $PCO_2$ in the capillaries of skeletal muscle.
3. *Kidneys add new $HCO_3^-$ ions to the body*: This occurs primarily when $NH_4^+$ ions are excreted in the urine.

### BASE BALANCE

1. *Input of alkali*: This occurs primarily when fruit and vegetables are ingested because they contain the K⁺ salts of organic acids that are metabolized to yield $HCO_3^-$ anions.
2. *Elimination of alkali*: This is achieved in a two-step process: (1) the alkali load stimulates the production of endogenous organic

acids (e.g., citric acid), the H$^+$ ions of which eliminate HCO$_3^-$ anions, and (2) the kidneys excrete organic anions (e.g., citrate anions) with K$^+$ ions in the urine.

■ To emphasize that acid–base balance is achieved while maintaining the urine pH close to 6.0. This minimizes the risk of forming uric acid precipitate if the urine pH were acidic (pK = 5.3), or calcium phosphate precipitate if the urine pH were alkaline (pK = 6.8). In addition, eliminating alkali via the excretion of organic anions (e.g., citrate anions) lowers the concentration of ionized calcium in the urine.

# PART A
# CHEMISTRY OF H$^+$ IONS

## H$^+$ IONS AND THE REGENERATION OF ATP

Three important steps constitute the metabolic process for the regeneration of ATP (called *coupled oxidative phosphorylation*); this involves H$^+$ ions in a major way. First, the energy needed to perform biological work in the cytosol of cells (e,g., ion pumping by Na-K-ATPase) is provided when the terminal high-energy phosphate bond in ATP$^{4-}$ is hydrolyzed. This converts ATP$^{4-}$ to adenosine diphosphate (ADP$^{3-}$), divalent inorganic phosphate (HPO$_4^{2-}$) ions, and H$^+$ ion. Second, ADP enters the mitochondria on the adenine nucleotide translocator, while ATP exits. HPO$_4^{2-}$ ions and H$^+$ ions enter mitochondria by a symporter. Third, oxidation of the reduced form nicotinamide adenine dinucleotide (NADH, H$^+$) produces nicotinamide adenine dinucleotide (NAD$^+$) and two electrons. This represents the first step in the electron transport chain. Flow of these electrons through coenzyme Q and ultimately cytochrome C releases the energy that is used to pump H$^+$ ions from the mitochondrial matrix through the inner mitochondrial membrane. This creates a very large electrical driving force (~150 mV) and a smaller chemical driving force for H$^+$ ion re-entry. This

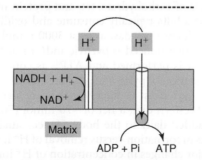

**Figure 1-1  H$^+$ Ions and the Regeneration of ATP.** The horizontal structure represents the inner mitochondrial membrane with its inner and outer bilayers. The dashed line at the top represents the outer mitochondrial membrane. Oxidation of the reduced form of nicotinamide adenine dinucleotide (*NADH, H$^+$*) produces *NAD$^+$* and two electrons. Flow of these electrons through the electron transport chain releases the energy that is used to pump H$^+$ ions from the mitochondrial matrix through the inner mitochondrial membrane. This creates a very large electricochemical driving force for H$^+$ ion re-entry. This energy is recaptured as H$^+$ ions flow through the H$^+$ ion channel portion of the H$^+$-adenosine triphosphate (*ATP*) synthase in the inner mitochondrial membrane, which is coupled to ATP regeneration from ADP and inorganic phosphate (*Pi*). *ADP*, Adenosine diphosphate.

energy is recaptured as $H^+$ ions flow through the $H^+$ ion channel portion of the $H^+$-ATP synthase in the inner mitochondrial membrane, which is coupled (linked) to $ATP^{4-}$ regeneration provided that $ADP^{3-}$ and $HPO_4^{2-}$ are available inside these mitochondria (Figure 1-1). Hence, availability of ADP in the mitochondria sets an upper limit on the rate of coupled oxidative phosphorylation (see margin note).

### UNCOUPLING OF OXIDATIVE PHOSPHORYLATION

This limitation by availability of $ADP^{3-}$ (rate of biological work) on the rate of fuel oxidation can be bypassed if oxidation of more fuel than what is needed to regenerate $ATP^{4-}$ is advantageous. This is achieved by uncoupling of oxidative phosphorylation. In this process, $H^+$ ions re-enter the mitochondrial matrix by a different $H^+$ ion channel, one that is not linked to the conversion of $ADP^{3-}$ to $ATP^{4-}$.

## CONCENTRATION OF H⁺ IONS

The concentration of $H^+$ ions in all body compartments must be maintained at a very low level. This is because $H^+$ ions bind very avidly to histidine residues in proteins. Binding of $H^+$ ions to proteins changes their charge to a more positive valence, which might alter their shape, and possibly their functions. Because most proteins are enzymes, transporters, contractile elements, and structural compounds, a change in their functions could pose a major threat to survival. Nevertheless, there are examples when this binding of $H^+$ ions to proteins has important biologic functions (see margin note).

The concentration of $H^+$ ions in body fluids is exceedingly tiny (in the nmol/L range) and, moreover, is maintained within a very narrow range. In the extracellular fluid (ECF) compartment, the concentration of $H^+$ ions is $40 \pm 2$ nmol/L, while in the ICF compartment, the concentration of $H^+$ ions is ~80 nmol/L. In fact, the concentration of their partner, $HCO_3^-$ ions, in the ECF compartment (~25 mmol/L), is almost one million-fold higher than that of $H^+$ ions.

This is impressive because an enormous quantity of $H^+$ ions is produced and removed by metabolism each day relative to the amount of $H^+$ ions in the body (see margin note). In more detail, acids are obligatory intermediates of carbohydrate, fat, and protein metabolism. For example, because adults typically consume and oxidize about 270 g (1500 mmol) of glucose per day, at least 3000 mmol (3,000,000,000 nmol) of $H^+$ ions are produced as pyruvic and/or L-lactic acids in glycolysis when work is performed and $ATP^{4-}$ is converted to $ADP^{3-}$. The complete oxidation of pyruvate/L-lactate anions to $CO_2$ and $H_2O$ removes the $H^+$ ions almost as quickly as they are formed. In an adult eating a typical Western diet, a net of ~70 mmol (70,000,000 nmol) of $H^+$ ions are added daily to the body. Hence, small discrepancies between the rates of formation versus removal of $H^+$ ions, if sustained, can result in major changes in concentration of $H^+$ ions. This implies that there are very effective control mechanisms that minimize fluctuations in concentration of $H^+$ ions in body fluids.

### ATP/ADP TURNOVER

- It is important to appreciate that the actual concentration of ATP in cells is small (~5 mmol/L) and that of ADP is extremely tiny (~0.02 mmol/L), but their rate of *turnover* is enormous.
- The weight of ATP in the brain is just a few grams (concentration of ATP 0.005 mol/L, molecular weight ~700 g/mol, brain weight in adult of about 1.5 kg— 80% of which is intracellular fluid [ICF]).
- The brain consumes close to 3 mmol of $O_2$ per minute or 4.5 mol of $O_2$ per day. Because ~6 mol of ATP are formed per mole of $O_2$ consumed, the brain regenerates 27 mol of ATP per day (4.5 mol of $O_2 \times 6$ ATP/$O_2$). Hence, the daily turnover of ATP in the brain is almost 20 kg (27 mol × mol wt ~700 g/1000 = 18.9 kg).

### BENEFIT OF H⁺ ION BINDING TO HEMOGLOBIN

- When $H^+$ ions bind to hemoglobin in systemic capillaries, hemoglobin can off load oxygen ($O_2$) at a higher $PO_2$, which improves the diffusion of $O_2$ into cells.
- In contrast, when $H^+$ ions dissociate from hemoglobin in the capillaries in the lungs (driven by a higher $PO_2$), this leads to a greater uptake of $O_2$ from alveolar air for a given alveolar $PO_2$.

### AMOUNT OF H⁺ IONS IN THE BODY

- ECF: 15 L × 40 nmol/L = 600 nmol
- ICF: 30 L × 80 nmol/L = 2400 nmol

---

## QUESTIONS

(See Part C for discussion of questions)

1-1 *In certain locations in the body, $H^+$ ions remain free and are not bound. What is the advantage in having such a high concentration of $H^+$ ions?*

1-2 *What is the rationale for the statement, "In biology only weak acids kill"?*

# PART B
# DAILY BALANCE OF H⁺ IONS

## PRODUCTION AND REMOVAL OF H⁺ IONS

- *$H^+$ ion production*: $H^+$ ions are produced when neutral compounds are converted to anions.
- *$H^+$ ion removal*: $H^+$ ions are removed when anions are converted to neutral products.

To determine whether $H^+$ ions are produced or removed during metabolism, we use a "metabolic process" analysis. A metabolic process is made up of a series of metabolic pathways that carry out a specific function; these pathways may be located in more than one organ. To establish the balance for $H^+$ ions in a metabolic process, one needs only examine the valences of all of its substrates and products, while ignoring all intermediates (see Chapter 5 for more details). If the sum of all of these valences is equal, there is no net production or removal of $H^+$ ions. When the products of a metabolic process have a greater anionic charge than its substrates, $H^+$ ions are produced (e.g., incomplete oxidation of the major energy fuels, carbohydrates, and fats). Conversely, when the products of a metabolic process have a lesser anionic charge than its substrates, $H^+$ ions are removed.

About 85% of kilocalories consumed, in a typical Western diet, are in the form of carbohydrates and fat. There is no net production of $H^+$ ions when glucose and triglycerides are completely oxidized to $CO_2 + H_2O$ because the substrates and the end products of these metabolic processes are neutral compounds. There is a *net* $H^+$ ion load, however, when complete oxidation of these fuels does not occur. L-Lactic acid accumulates during hypoxia, because its rate of production from glycolysis far exceeds its rate of removal via oxidation and/or gluconeogenesis. Ketoacids are produced during states of a net lack of insulin if their rate of production from metabolism of free fatty acids (triglycerides) in the liver exceeds their rate of removal by the brain and the kidneys.

The metabolism of certain dietary constituents leads to the addition of $H^+$ ions (e.g., proteins) or $HCO_3^-$ ions (e.g., fruit and vegetables) to the body. A general overview of the components of the daily turnover of $H^+$ ions is illustrated in Figure 1-2. Overall, one must examine balances for both acids and bases to have a true assessment of $H^+$ ion balance.

### ACID BALANCE

Oxidation of two classes of amino acids (cationic amino acids [e.g., lysine, arginine] and sulfur-containing amino acids [e.g., cysteine, methionine]) yields an $H^+$ ion load (Table 1-1). In contrast, $H^+$ ions are removed during the oxidation of anionic amino acids (e.g., glutamate, aspartate), because all the products of their oxidation are neutral compounds (urea, glucose, or $CO_2 + H_2O$). Because the number of cationic and anionic amino acids is nearly equal in the amino acid mixture in beefsteak, the $H^+$ ion load that causes a deficit of $HCO_3^-$ ions is mainly from the metabolism of sulfur-containing amino acids that yield sulfuric acid ($H_2SO_4$).

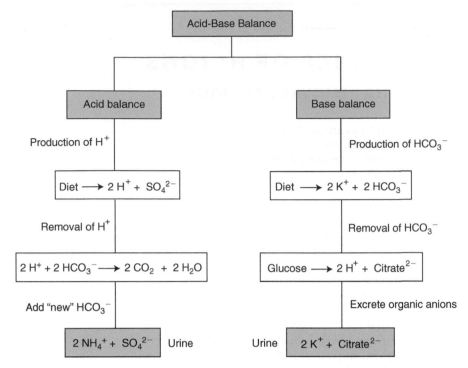

**Figure 1-2 Overview of the Daily Turnover of H⁺ Ions.** Acid balance is shown on the *left*, and base balance is shown on the *right*. There are three components to acid balance: (1) production of H⁺ ions, (2) $HCO_3^-$ ions remove this H⁺ ion load, and (3) the kidneys add new $HCO_3^-$ ions to the body when $NH_4^+$ ions are excreted in the urine. There are also three components to base balance: (1) the alkali load of the diet is converted to $HCO_3^-$ ions in the liver, (2) organic acids are formed in the liver and their H⁺ ions remove $HCO_3^-$ ions, and (3) excretion of these new organic anions along with the potassium (K⁺) ions from the diet in the urine.

---

TABLE 1-1    **H⁺ ION FORMATION OR REMOVAL IN METABOLIC REACTIONS**

---

**Reactions that yield H⁺ ions (more net negative charge in products than in substrates)**

Glucose→L-lactate⁻+H⁺ (new L-lactate anions)

$C_{16}$ fatty acid→4 ketoacid anions⁻+4H⁺ (new ketoacid anions)

Cysteine →urea+$CO_2$+$H_2O$+2H⁺+$SO_4^{2-}$ (new $SO_4^{2-}$ anions)

Lysine⁺→urea+$CO_2$+$H_2O$+H⁺ (loss of cationic charge in lysine)

**Reactions that remove H⁺ ions (more net positive charge in products than in substrates)**
L-Lactate⁻+H⁺→glucose (L-lactate anion removed)

Glutamate⁻→urea+$CO_2$+$H_2O$

Citrate³⁻+3H⁺→$CO_2$+$H_2O$ (citrate anion removed)

**H⁺ are neither produced nor removed in the following reactions**
Glucose→glycogen or $CO_2$+$H_2O$ (neutrals to neutrals)

Triglyceride→$CO_2$+$H_2O$ (neutrals to neutrals)

Alanine→urea+glucose or $CO_2$+$H_2O$ (neutrals to neutrals)

---

## $H_2SO_4$

H⁺ ions cannot be eliminated by metabolism of $SO_4^{2-}$ anions to neutral end products (because no such pathway exists) or by being excreted bound to $SO_4^{2-}$ anions in the urine (because of the low affinity of $SO_4^{2-}$ anions for H⁺ ions). Hence, these H⁺ ions must be titrated initially with $HCO_3^-$ ions and, as a result, $CO_2$ is formed. Acid balance is restored when these $SO_4^{2-}$ anions are excreted in the urine with an equivalent amount of $NH_4^+$ ions because new $HCO_3^-$ ions are generated in this process (Figure 1-3).

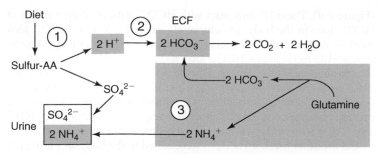

**Figure 1-3  H⁺ Ion Balance during the Metabolism of Sulfur-Containing Amino Acids.** Renal events are represented in the *large shaded area*. When sulfur-containing amino acids are converted to $SO_4^{2-}$ anions, H⁺ ions are produced (*site 1*). H⁺ ions react with $HCO_3^-$ ions, and this produces a deficit of $HCO_3^-$ ions in the body (*site 2*). To achieve H⁺ ion balance, new $HCO_3^-$ ions must be regenerated. Metabolism of the amino acid glutamine in cells of proximal tubules produces $NH_4^+$ ions and dicarboxylate anions. $HCO_3^-$ ions are added to the body when these anions are metabolized to a neutral end product and $NH_4^+$ ions are excreted in the urine with $SO_4^{2-}$ anions (*site 3*). *ECF*, Extracellular fluid.

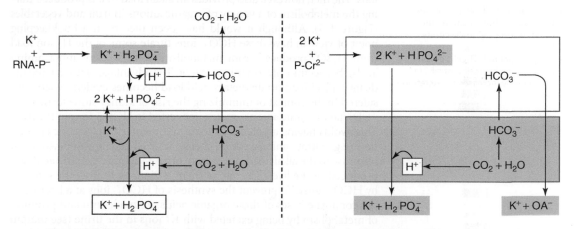

**Figure 1-4  H⁺ Ion Balance during the Metabolism of Organic Phosphates.** The upper rectangle represents the body, the lower, large shaded rectangle represents events in the kidney, the small shaded rectangle represents excretion in the urine. The acid–base impact of the metabolic process involving phosphate depends on whether their metabolism resulted in the addition of the monovalent inorganic phosphate ($H_2PO_4^-$) or the divalent inorganic phosphate ($HPO_4^{2-}$) to the body. As shown in the *left panel of the figure*, if $H_2PO_4^-$ were added to the body and then excreted in the urine as $H_2PO_4^-$, there is no net loss or gain of $HCO_3^-$ ions in this process. On the other hand, if $HPO_4^{2-}$ were added to the body, at a urine pH of ~6 it will be excreted as $H_2PO_4^-$. Hence, a new $HCO_3^-$ ion is generated in this process (*right panel of the figure*). To maintain acid–base balance in response to this alkali load, there is increased production of endogenous organic acids. Their H⁺ ions remove these $HCO_3^-$ ions, while their conjugate bases (organic anions [OA⁻]) are excreted in the urine as K⁺ salts. *P-Cr²⁻*, Phosphocreatine ²⁻; *RNA-P*, ribonucliec acid.

## Dietary phosphate

The source of phosphate in the diet consists primarily of intracellular organic phosphates (including energy storage compounds e.g., ATP⁴⁻ and phosphocreatine²⁻ in beefsteak, and nucleic acids [RNA, DNA]) and phospholipids, which are primarily in organ meat (e.g., liver). The accompanying cation for both forms of intracellular organic phosphates is primarily potassium (K⁺) ions. The acid–base impact of the metabolic process involving phosphate depends on whether their metabolism resulted in the addition of the monovalent inorganic phosphate $\left(H_2PO_4^-\right)$ or the divalent inorganic phosphate $\left(HPO_4^{2-}\right)$ to the body. In more detail, if $H_2PO_4^-$ were added, because it has a pK of 6.8, close to one bound H⁺ ion per $H_2PO_4^-$ is released in the body at normal blood pH values (7.40)

### RENAL HANDLING OF ORGANIC ANIONS

- Approximately 360 mEq of organic anions are filtered daily (glomerular filtration rate [GFR] of 180 L/day, concentration of OA⁻ in plasma ~2 mEq/L). Of these anions, 90% are reabsorbed and only ~10% are excreted.
- An alkali load diminishes the reabsorption of organic anions such as citrate in the PCT, and hence increases their excretion in the urine to achieve base balance.

### URINE CITRATE AS A WINDOW ON pH OF THE PROXIMAL TUBULE CELL

- A low pH in PCT cells increases the reabsorption of citrate; the urine becomes virtually citrate free.
- A higher pH in PCT cells diminishes the reabsorption of citrate and thereby increases its excretion rate.

(Figure 1-4). These $H^+$ ions react with $HCO_3^-$ ions, creating a deficit of $HCO_3^-$ ions in the body. To achieve $H^+$ ion balance, new $HCO_3^-$ ions must be regenerated. This occurs in two steps: (1) the kidney converts $CO_2 + H_2O$ to $H^+$ ions $+ HCO_3^-$ ions and (2) these $H^+$ are secreted and bind to filtered $HPO_4^{2-}$ anions. Thus, $H_2PO_4^-$ is excreted when the urine pH is in the usual range (i.e., ~6), while $HCO_3^-$ ions are added to the body. Hence, elimination of $H^+$ ions produced during the metabolism of organic phosphates to $H_2PO_4^-$ does not require the excretion of $NH_4^+$ ions. There is no net loss or gain of $HCO_3^-$ ions in this process.

On the other hand, if $HPO_4^{2-}$ were added to the body, at a urine pH of ~6, it will be excreted as $H_2PO_4^-$. Hence, new $HCO_3^-$ ions are generated in this process. To maintain acid–base balance, one possible mechanism is increased production of endogenous organic acids in response to this alkali load. Their $H^+$ ions remove this $HCO_3^-$ ion load, while their conjugate bases are excreted in the urine as $K^+$ salts (see Figure 1-4).

## BASE BALANCE

All the emphasis so far has been on the production and removal of $H^+$ ions. The diet, however, also provides an alkali load that is produced during the metabolism of a variety of organic anions in fruit and vegetables (Figure 1-5). Although it would have been nice from a bookkeeping point of view to have these $HCO_3^-$ ions titrate some of the $H^+$ ion load from $H_2SO_4$ produced from metabolism of sulfur-containing amino acids, this occurs only to a minor extent. The advantage of not having the dietary alkali load titrate dietary acid load becomes evident when considered in the context of minimizing the risk of kidney stone formation.

Dietary organic anions are first converted to $HCO_3^-$ ions in the liver. This avoids having a potentially toxic anion enter the systemic circulation (e.g., citrate anions, which chelate ionized calcium in plasma). In response to the alkali load, a variety of organic acids (e.g., citric acid) are produced in the liver. The fate of their $H^+$ ions is similar: the removal by $HCO_3^-$ ions. To prevent the synthesis of $HCO_3^-$ ions at a later time, the conjugate bases of these organic acids are made into end products of metabolism by being excreted with $K^+$ ions in the urine (see margin note), and hence base balance is achieved. As discussed later, the pH of cells of the proximal convoluted tubule (PCT) plays an important role in determining the rate of excretion of citrate and other organic anions in the urine. In fact, the rate of excretion of citrate in the urine is thought to provide a window on pH in the cells of PCT (see margin note).

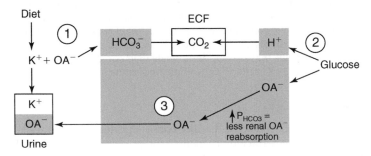

**Figure 1-5 Overview of Base Balance.** Base balance is achieved in three steps. The first is the production of $HCO_3^-$ ions from dietary $K^+$ salts of organic anions in the liver (*site 1*). This is followed by the production of organic acids in the liver; their $H^+$ ions titrate these $HCO_3^-$ ions (*site 2*). The renal component of the process is shown in the *large shaded area* (*site 3*). The organic anions are filtered and only partially reabsorbed by the kidney; hence, they are made into end products of metabolism by being excreted in the urine. *ECF*, Extracellular fluid.

From an integrative physiology point of view, the elimination of dietary alkali in the form of organic anions has a number of advantages in terms of minimizing the risk of kidney stone formation. In more detail, it avoids the excretion of $HCO_3^-$ ions, and hence the likelihood of kidney stones that form when the urine pH is too high (e.g., $CaHPO_4$). In addition, the elimination of this dietary alkali in the form of citrate anions lessens the likelihood of forming calcium-containing kidney stones because citrate anions chelate ionized calcium in the urine.

---

## QUESTION

(See Part C for discussion of questions)

1-3 *Does consumption of citrus fruit, which contains a large quantity of citric acid and its $K^+$ salt, cause a net acid or a net alkali load?*

## BUFFERING OF H⁺ IONS

- The most important goal of buffering is to minimize the binding of $H^+$ ions to intracellular proteins in vital organs (e.g., the brain and the heart)

The traditional view of the buffering of $H^+$ ions during metabolic acidosis is "*proton*-centered" (i.e., it focuses solely on diminishing the concentration of $H^+$ ions). It is based on the premise that $H^+$ ions are very dangerous; therefore, anything that minimizes a rise in their concentration is beneficial. An argument to support this view is that a high concentration of $H^+$ ions may depress myocardial contractility. The evidence for this effect, however, is from experimental studies in animals or isolated perfused hearts preparations. Furthermore, it is not consistent with the very high cardiac output observed during a sprint when the blood pH may be below 7.0. In addition, this view of buffering of $H^+$ ions does not take into consideration the price to pay to achieve this goal. In more detail, binding of $H^+$ ions to proteins will change their "ideal or native" valence (protein⁰) to become more cationic or less anionic (protein⁺) (see Eqn 2). This may alter their shape and possibly their functions (as enzymes, transporters, contractile elements, or structural compounds), which may have deleterious effects.

$$H^+ + Protein^0 \rightarrow H \cdot Protein^+ \tag{2}$$

We emphasize a different way to analyze buffering of an $H^+$ ion load and suggest that a "*brain protein*-centered" view of buffering of $H^+$ ions in the patient with metabolic acidosis may offer a better way to understand the pathophysiology, which has important implications for therapy. The major tenet of this view is that the role of buffering is not simply to lower the concentration of $H^+$ ions but to minimize the binding of $H^+$ ions to proteins in cells of vital organs (e.g., the brain and the heart).

### BICARBONATE BUFFER SYSTEM

- $H^+$ ions must by removed by the BBS to avoid their binding to intracellular proteins.
- A low $PCO_2$ is a prerequisite for optimal function of the BBS.

Even though at plasma pH of 7.4, the BBS is very far displaced from its pK (pH ~6.1) and hence is not an ideal chemical buffer,

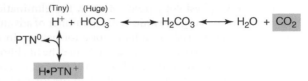

(Tiny)   (Huge)

$$H^+ + HCO_3^- \longleftrightarrow H_2CO_3 \longleftrightarrow H_2O + CO_2$$

$PTN^0$

$H \cdot PTN^+$

**Figure 1-6 Buffer Systems.** Proteins in cells have an "ideal charge" (depicted as $PTN^0$). Binding of $H^+$ ions to these proteins increases their net positive charge ($H \cdot PTN^+$) and may compromise their functions. Hence, the key principle is that new $H^+$ ions must be removed by binding to $HCO_3^-$ ions so that very few $H^+$ ions can bind to proteins ($PTN^0$) in cells. To force $H^+$ ions to bind to $HCO_3^-$ ions, the $PCO_2$ must fall in cells despite the fact that cells produce an enormous quantity of $CO_2$.

**QUANTITY OF BICARBONATE IONS IN THE BODY**

ECF compartment:
25 mmol/L × 15 L = 375 mmol
ICF compartment:
12.5 mmol/L × 30 L = 375 mmol

nevertheless it is the most important physiologic buffer. This is caused by the fact that it can remove $H^+$ ions without requiring a high $H^+$ ion concentration. As shown in Eqn 1, a *low* $PCO_2$ "pulls" the BBS reaction to the right. As a result, the concentration of $H^+$ ions falls, which decreases the binding of $H^+$ ions to proteins (Figure 1-6). In addition, the BBS is capable of removing a large quantity of $H^+$ ions because there is a large amount of $HCO_3^-$ ions in the body, ≈750 mmol in a 70 kg adult (see margin note).

### Which $PCO_2$ is important for the bicarbonate buffer system to function optimally?

- The arterial $PCO_2$ reflects, but is not equal to, the $PCO_2$ in brain cells; it sets a minimum value for the $PCO_2$ in capillaries of all other organs in the body.
- The bulk of the BBS is in the interstitial space and in cells of skeletal muscle, hence $PCO_2$ in muscle capillary blood reflects the effectiveness of the BBS in removing an $H^+$ ion load.

The process to lower the $PCO_2$ begins with stimulation of the respiratory center in the brain. This is a most appropriate response because it ensures that the brain will always have an "ideal" $PCO_2$ in its ECF and ICF compartments. In more detail, hyperventilation results in a lower arterial $PCO_2$. Because the rate of production of $CO_2$ in the brain is relatively constant (i.e., its oxygen consumption does not vary appreciably and its blood flow is autoregulated), a lower arterial $PCO_2$ will predictably result in a lower $PCO_2$ in the ECF and ICF compartments of the brain. Therefore, there is only a minimal binding of $H^+$ ions to intracellular proteins in the brain during metabolic acidosis, which decreases the possible detrimental effects on neuronal function. Accordingly, the arterial $PCO_2$ reflects the $PCO_2$ in brain cells in the absence of a marked degree of contraction of the effective arterial blood volume (EABV) during which the brain fails to autoregulate its rate of blood flow.

**ABBREVIATIONS**

EABV, effective arterial blood volume

The question, however, is whether a low arterial $PCO_2$ is sufficient to ensure optimal function of the BBS in other organs. Because $CO_2$ diffuses rapidly, distances are short, and time is not a limiting factor, the $PCO_2$ in capillaries is virtually identical to the $PCO_2$ in cells and in the interstitial compartment of the ECF in a given region. Therefore, it is the capillary $PCO_2$ (rather than the arterial $PCO_2$) that reveals whether the BBS has operated efficiently in removing a load of $H^+$ ions (Table 1-2). Notwithstanding, the arterial $PCO_2$ sets the lower limit for the $PCO_2$ in capillaries.

TABLE 1-2     **THE BLOOD PCO$_2$ AND ITS IMPLICATIONS FOR BRAIN PROTEIN-CENTERED BUFFERING OF H$^+$**

| SITE OF SAMPLING | BBS BUFFERING | FUNCTIONAL IMPLICATIONS |
|---|---|---|
| • Arterial PCO$_2$ | • Reflects the PCO$_2$ in brain if the blood flow rate is autoregulated | • Assesses alveolar ventilation<br>• Sets the lower limit for the capillary PCO$_2$ |
| • Mixed venous PCO$_2$ | • Not really able to define site of H$^+$ ion buffering | • Cannot tell if H$^+$ ions are bound to brain proteins |
| • Brachial vein PCO$_2$ | • Reflects the PCO$_2$ in skeletal muscle cells and their interstitial compartment | • A low venous PCO$_2$ is needed to force H$^+$ ions to be buffered by HCO$_3^-$ ions in muscle cells<br>• A high PCO$_2$ suggests that the BBS in muscle is not functioning optimally; as a result, H$^+$ ions may bind to brain proteins. |

*BBS,* Bicarbonate buffer system.

The capillary PCO$_2$ is higher than the arterial PCO$_2$ because cells consume O$_2$ and add CO$_2$ to their capillary blood. The capillary PCO$_2$ is influenced by the value of the arterial PCO$_2$ and the rate of addition of CO$_2$ to capillary blood in individual organs. For instance, if most of the oxygen in each liter of blood delivered to a certain area is consumed, the PCO$_2$ in its capillary blood will rise appreciably. There are two conditions in which most of the O$_2$ delivered in a liter of blood is consumed: (1) a rise in the rate of metabolism without a change in the rate of blood flow, or (2) a decrease in the rate of blood flow with no change in the rate of O$_2$ consumption.

Although the capillary PCO$_2$ reveals whether the BBS has operated efficiently, one cannot measure it directly. The venous PCO$_2$, however, closely reflects the capillary PCO$_2$ in its drainage bed. There is one caveat—if an appreciable quantity of blood shunts from the arterial to the venous circulation and bypasses cells, this venous PCO$_2$ does not reflect the PCO$_2$ in the interstitial space and in cells in its drainage bed.

The question now is which venous PCO$_2$ should be measured to assess the effectiveness of the BBS. Because of its size, skeletal muscle has the largest content of HCO$_3^-$ ions in the body in its cells and interstitial space. Therefore, in patients with metabolic acidosis, the PCO$_2$ should be measured in free-flowing brachial venous blood to assess the effectiveness of the BBS.

### Failure of the bicarbonate buffer system

The main cause of failure of the BBS in skeletal muscle is a very marked decline in its blood supply—this is the case when metabolic acidosis is accompanied by a contracted EABV. Hence, while the arterial PCO$_2$ may be low due to stimulation of the respiratory center by acidemia, the PCO$_2$ in intracellular fluid and interstitial space in muscle may not be low enough for effective buffering of H$^+$ ions by the BBS (Figure 1-7). As a result, the degree of acidemia may become more pronounced and more H$^+$ ions may bind to proteins in the extracellular and intracellular fluids in other organs, including the brain. Notwithstanding, because of autoregulation of cerebral blood flow, it is likely that the PCO$_2$ in brain capillary blood

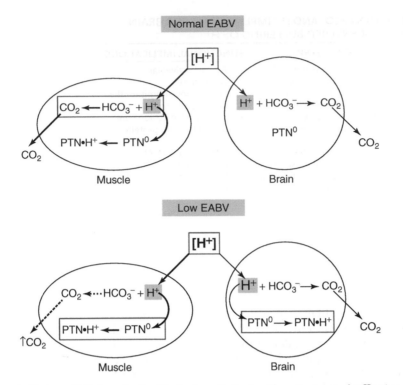

**Figure 1-7 Buffering of H⁺ Ions in the Brain in a Patient with a Contracted Effective Arterial Blood Volume (EABV).** Buffering of H⁺ ions in a patient with a normal effective arterial blood volume and thereby a low venous $PCO_2$ is depicted in the *top portion of the figure*. The vast majority of H⁺ ion removal occurs by bicarbonate buffer system (BBS) in the interstitial space and in cells of skeletal muscles. Buffering of an H⁺ ion load in a patient with a contracted EABV and thereby a high venous $PCO_2$ is depicted in the *bottom portion of the figure*. A high $PCO_2$ prevents H⁺ ion removal by the BBS in muscles. As a result, the circulating H⁺ ion concentration rises, which increases the H⁺ ion burden for brain cells. Unless there is a severe degree of contraction of the EABV and failure of auto-regulation of cerebral blood flow, the BBS in the brain will continue to titrate much of this large H⁺ ion load. Because of the limited content of $HCO_3^-$ ions in the brain and because the brain receives a relatively larger proportion of blood flow, there is a risk that more H⁺ ions will bind to proteins in the brain cells.

will change minimally unless there is a severe degree of contraction of the EABV and failure of autoregulation of cerebral blood flow. Hence, the BBS in the brain will continue to titrate much of this large H⁺ ion load. Considering, however, the limited content of $HCO_3^-$ ions in the brain, and that the brain receives a relatively larger proportion of the cardiac output, there is a risk that more H⁺ ions will bind to proteins in the brain cells, further compromising their functions.

In summary, patients with metabolic acidosis and a contracted EABV have a high $PCO_2$ in venous blood draining skeletal muscle, and therefore they fail to titrate an H⁺ load with their BBS in skeletal muscle. Hence, there is a much higher H⁺ ion burden in their brain cells, with possible detrimental effects. At usual rates of blood flow and metabolic work at rest, brachial venous $PCO_2$ is about 46 mm Hg, which is ~6 mm Hg greater than the arterial $PCO_2$. If the blood flow rate to the skeletal muscles declines because of a low EABV, the brachial venous $PCO_2$ will be increased to greater than 6 mm Hg higher than the arterial $PCO_2$. Based on this analysis, it follows that in patients with metabolic acidosis, the clinician should administer enough saline to increase the blood flow rate to muscle to restore the usual brachial venous minus arterial $PCO_2$ difference, i.e., back to ~6 mm Hg.

(See Part C for discussion of questions)

1-4 *Why is the L-lactic acidosis that occurs during cardiogenic shock so much more devastating than the L-lactic acidosis that occurs during a sprint if the $P_{L\text{-}lactate}$, arterial pH, and $P_{HCO_3}$ are identical?*

1-5 *The heart extracts close to 70% of the oxygen from each liter of coronary artery blood. What conclusions can you draw about buffering of $H^+$ ions in the heart? Might there be advantages because of this high extraction of $O_2$ per liter of blood flow?*

## ROLE OF THE KIDNEY IN ACID–BASE BALANCE

The kidneys must perform two tasks to maintain acid balance. First, the kidney must reabsorb virtually 100% of the filtered $HCO_3^-$ ions; this is achieved primarily by $H^+$ ion secretion in the PCT. Second, the kidneys must add new $HCO_3^-$ ions to the body to replace what is lost in buffering of an added acid load; this is achieved principally in the metabolic process that ends by excreting $NH_4^+$ ions in the urine.

### Reabsorption of Filtered $HCO_3^-$ Ions

- The kidneys must prevent the excretion of the very large quantity of filtered $HCO_3^-$ ions. In this process there is no addition of new $HCO_3^-$ ions to the body.

It is important to recognize that a huge amount of $HCO_3^-$ is filtered and reabsorbed each day (GFR of 180 $L/day \times P_{HCO_3}$ 25 mmol/L = 4500 mmol). The bulk of filtered $HCO_3^-$ ions (approximately 80% [~3600 mmol/day] [see margin note]) is reabsorbed by the PCT.

#### Reabsorption of NaHCO₃ in the proximal convoluted tubule

Reabsorption of $HCO_3^-$ ions in PCT occurs in an indirect fashion via $H^+$ ion secretion. In this process, the PCT reclaims the vast majority of filtered $HCO_3^-$ ions, but there is no generation of new $HCO_3^-$ ions. Nevertheless, if this process were to fail, there will be a loss of $NaHCO_3$ in the urine and the development of metabolic acidosis (this disorder is called *proximal renal tubular acidosis*; it is discussed in Chapter 4).

The process of $HCO_3^-$ ion reabsorption in PCT has four interconnected steps (Figure 1-8):

1. *$H^+$ ion secretion into the luminal fluid.*
   This is largely mediated by the $Na^+/H^+$ exchanger-3 (NHE-3) in the apical membrane of PCT cells. This is an electroneutral exchanger because for every $Na^+$ ion reabsorbed, one $H^+$ ion is secreted into its lumen. The driving force to reabsorb $Na^+$ ions by NHE-3 is provided by the very low concentration of $Na^+$ ions inside PCT cells, because of the active transport of $Na^+$ ions out of cells by Na-K-ATPase in their basolateral membrane.

2. *Secreted $H^+$ ions combine with $HCO_3^-$ ions in the lumen to form $H_2CO_3$.*
   $H_2CO_3$ dissociates into $CO_2$ and $H_2O$. This dissociation reaction occurs virtually as soon as $H_2CO_3$ is formed because it is catalyzed by the enzyme carbonic anhydrase IV ($CA_{IV}$), an isoform of carbonic anhydrase that is bound to the brush boarder of PCT cells. $CO_2$ that is formed in the lumen crosses the apical membrane and enters the PCT cells (see margin note).

**ABBREVIATIONS**

NBCe1, electrogenic Na-bicarbonate cotransporter 1
mTAL, medullary thick ascending limb
MCD, medullary collecting duct

**PERCENT OF FILTERED $HCO_3^-$ REABSORBED IN PCT**

- This is a minimum estimate of the percent of the filtered $HCO_3^-$ ions that is reabsorbed in PCT. This is because it is based on data from micropuncture studies in rats. The site of micropuncture, the last accessible part of the PCT on the surface pf the cortex, is, however, not the end of the PCT.

**ENTRY OF $CO_2$ INTO PCT CELLS**

- This was thought to occur by diffusion of $CO_2$ through the lipid bilayer of the apical membrane of PCT cells.
- There are data to suggest that entry of $CO_2$ is via the luminal water channel, AQP1, which can also behave as a gas channel.

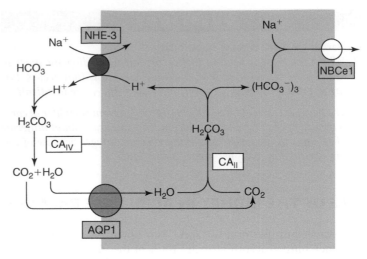

**Figure 1-8 Reabsorption of NaHCO₃ in the Proximal Convoluted Tubule.** The components of the process of indirect reabsorption of NaHCO₃ are shown in the figure. H⁺ ion secretion is largely via Na⁺/H⁺ exchanger 3 (NHE-3). HCO₃⁻ ions exit the cell via an electrogenic Na-bicarbonate cotransporter (NBCe1). This process requires a luminal carbonic anhydrase (CA)$_{IV}$ and intracellular CA$_{II}$. CO₂ that is formed in the lumen enters the cell likely via a luminal aquaporin 1 water channel (AQP1).

**3.** *Inside the cell, CO₂ and H₂O recombine to form H₂CO₃.*

Another isoform of carbonic anhydrase, carbonic anhydrase II (CA$_{II}$) is present inside cells; it accelerates the dissociation of H₂CO₃ into H⁺ ions and HCO₃⁻ ions. While H⁺ ions are secreted into the luminal fluid, HCO₃⁻ ions exit the cell across the basolateral membrane, completing the process of indirect reabsorption of HCO₃⁻ ions.

**4.** *HCO₃⁻ ions exit from PCT cells.*

HCO₃⁻ ions are transported out of PCT cells at the basolateral membrane via a sodium coupled, electrogenic bicarbonate cotransporter, NBCe1. This transporter permits an ion complex of one Na⁺ ion and the equivalent of three HCO₃⁻ ions to exit as a divalent anion, $Na(HCO_3^-)_3^{2-}$.

### Regulation of proximal tubular reabsorption of bicarbonate ions

*Luminal HCO₃⁻ ion concentration*

HCO₃⁻ reabsorption is increased as luminal HCO₃⁻ ion concentration rises because there are more H⁺ ion acceptors in the luminal fluid. The opposite is also true: HCO₃⁻ ion reabsorption is decreased with a fall in luminal HCO₃⁻ ion concentration.

*Luminal H⁺ ion concentration*

A higher concentration of H⁺ ions in the lumen of the PCT inhibits H⁺ ion secretion. This scenario occurs, for example, when a patient is given acetazolamide, a drug that inhibits luminal carbonic anhydrase. In this setting, H⁺ ion secretion is diminished because of the rise in the concentration of carbonic acid (H₂CO₃) and thereby of H⁺ ions in the lumen; hence, a smaller amount of filtered HCO₃⁻ ions is reclaimed.

### Concentration of H⁺ ions in PCT cells

A rise in the concentration of H⁺ ions in PCT cells stimulates the secretion of H⁺ ions because of the binding of H⁺ ions to a modifier site on NHE-3, which activates this cation exchanger. Intracellular acidosis also increases NBCe1 activity. These effects, however, are not very important during metabolic acidosis because of the smaller filtered load of $HCO_3^-$ ions.

Changes in intracellular H⁺ ion concentration may explain the effect of K⁺ ions to modulate the reabsorption of $HCO_3^-$ ions in the PCT. Hypokalemia is associated with intracellular acidosis, enhanced reabsorption of $HCO_3^-$ ions (together with stimulation of ammoniagenesis), and the development of metabolic alkalosis. In contrast, hyperkalemia is associated with a fall in H⁺ ion concentration in PCT cells, diminished reabsorption of $HCO_3^-$ ions (together with decreased ammoniagenesis), and the development of hyperchloremic metabolic acidosis.

### Peritubular HCO₃⁻ ion concentration

An increase in the peritubular concentration $HCO_3^-$ ions decreases $HCO_3^-$ ion reabsorption in the PCT.

### Peritubular PCO₂

A high peritubular $PCO_2$ stimulates the reabsorption of $NaHCO_3$ by the PCT (see margin note). The $P_{HCO_3}$ is elevated in patients with chronic respiratory acidosis.

### Angiotensin II

Angiotensin II, which is released in response to a decreased EABV, is the most important regulator of reabsorption of $NaHCO_3$ in the PCT. Angiotensin II stimulates $NaHCO_3$ reabsorption by activating protein kinase C, which in turn phosphorylates and activates NHE-3. As discussed in Chapter 10, activating NHE-3 and the reabsorption of $NaHCO_3$ in the PCT leads to an increased reabsorption of NaCl in this nephron segment.

### Parathyroid hormone

Acting through adenylyl cyclase and production of cyclic adenosine monophosphate (cAMP), parathyroid hormone has a small effect to inhibit the reabsorption of $HCO_3^-$ ions in the PCT.

To illustrate the interplay of the different factors that affect reabsorption of $HCO_3^-$ ions in PCT, consider this example of a patient who was given a diuretic and developed hypokalemia. $P_{HCO_3}$ will rise initially because of a decreased ECF volume (contraction alkalosis). In addition, hypokalemia is associated with intracellular acidosis, which stimulates ammoniagenesis and hence the addition of new $HCO_3^-$ ions to the ECF compartment. Factors that stimulate the reabsorption of $HCO_3^-$ ions in the PCT include a higher luminal concentration of $HCO_3^-$ ions, the effect of angiotensin II (released in response to a lower EABV) to activate NHE-3, the effect of intracellular acidosis (associated with hypokalemia) to activate NHE-3 and NBCe1, and the higher peritubular $PCO_2$ (metabolic alkalemia suppresses ventilation, leading to a compensatory rise in the arterial $PCO_2$). On the other hand, the rise in the peritubular

**EFFECT OF PERITUBULAR HCO₃⁻ ION CONCENTRATION, PERITUBULAR PCO₂**

- To separate the effects of peritubular $HCO_3^-$ ion concentration versus peritubular $PCO_2$ and/or peritubular pH on $HCO_3^-$ ion reabsorption in PCT, a technique to generate "out of equilibrium" $HCO_3^-$ ion solution was developed. Its premise is that the reaction of $CO_2$ and $H_2O$ to generate $H_2CO_3$ occurs relatively slowly, whereas the reaction of dissociation of $H_2CO_3$ to H⁺ ions and $HCO_3^-$ ions occurs rapidly. Hence, methods were developed to rapidly mix two solutions with different compositions and use the resulting solution before it comes to equilibrium.
- Studies using this technique showed that altering the peritubular pH at fixed $HCO_3^-$ and $PCO_2$ did not change the reabsorption of $HCO_3^-$ ions by the PCT. It was then suggested that the basolateral membrane contains proteins that function as $HCO_3^-$ ion and/or $CO_2$ sensors to mediate the effects of peritubular $HCO_3^-$ and peritubular $PCO_2$ on $HCO_3^-$ ion reabsorption in the PCT.

$HCO_3^-$ ion concentration will diminish the reabsorption of $HCO_3^-$ ions in PCT cells. A new steady state $P_{HCO_3}$ will be achieved, reflecting the balance of these opposing forces.

### Renal threshold for reabsorption of $HCO_3^-$ ions

It is important to recognize that a renal threshold for the reabsorption of $NaHCO_3$ was demonstrated in experiments in animals and humans during the infusion of $NaHCO_3$. This, however, expands the EABV because of the load of $Na^+$ ions, which lowers angiotensin II levels and thereby depresses the reabsorption of the extra $NaHCO_3$ in the PCT. In addition, the rise in peritubular $HCO_3^-$ ion concentration diminishes the reabsorption of $HCO_3^-$ ions in the PCT. Because this does not represent a physiologic setting in which the $P_{HCO_3}$ is increased, this experimental setting may not define normal physiology. In fact, no renal threshold for the reabsorption of $NaHCO_3$ was demonstrated in an experiment in rats when the $P_{HCO_3}$ was raised without expanding the EABV (Figure 1-9).

The best example of a rise in $P_{HCO_3}$ without expansion of the EABV in normal physiology is the rise in $P_{HCO_3}$ that occurs during alkaline tide because of secretion of HCl into the lumen of the stomach. Electroneutrality is maintained because there is an exchange of $Cl^-$ ions for $HCO_3^-$ ions in the ECF compartment with a 1:1 stoichiometry. The $P_{HCO_3}$ rises to about 30 mmol/L, but the urine contains very little $HCO_3^-$ ions. This is because subjects on a typical Western diet have an EABV that leads to levels of angiotensin II that are sufficient to stimulate $H^+$ ion secretion in PCT cells and the reabsorption of $HCO_3^-$ ions

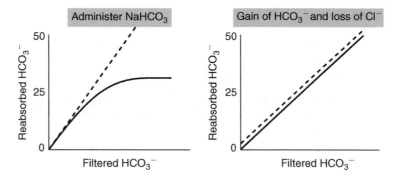

**Figure 1-9 Apparent Threshold for the Reabsorption of NaHCO₃ in the Proximal Convoluted Tubule.** The quantity of $HCO_3^-$ ions filtered (glomerular filtration rate [GFR] $\times P_{HCO_3}$) is depicted on the *x*-axis, and the quantity of $HCO_3^-$ ions reabsorbed at this same GFR is depicted on the *y*-axis. The *dashed line* represents equality between filtered and reabsorbed $HCO_3^-$ ions. When the $P_{HCO_3}$ is below the normal value, all the filtered $HCO_3^-$ ions are reabsorbed and there is no bicarbonaturia. As shown in the *left portion of the figure*, when the $P_{HCO_3}$ is increased above 25 to 30 mmol/L *and* the effective arterial blood volume is expanded (e.g., administration of $NaHCO_3$), virtually all of the extra filtered $HCO_3^-$ ions escape reabsorption in the proximal convoluted tubule and are excreted in the urine. In contrast, as shown in the *right portion of the figure*, when the $P_{HCO_3}$ is increased *without* expanding the effective arterial blood volume (e.g., inducing a deficit of HCl), virtually all of the extra filtered $HCO_3^-$ ions are reabsorbed in the proximal convoluted tubule and there is no bicarbonaturia despite a very high $P_{HCO_3}$. Hence, there is an apparent threshold for the reabsorption of $NaHCO_3$ in the proximal convoluted tubule only when the effective arterial blood volume is expanded.

despite the presence of a higher peritubular $HCO_3^-$ ion concentration. Avoiding bicarbonaturia during alkaline tide has several advantages. These include preventing the loss of $Na^+$ and $K^+$ ions that would accompany $HCO_3^-$ ions in the urine, preventing an alkaline urine pH and the risk of precipitation of $CaHPO_4$ stones, and also perhaps avoiding the need for a higher rate of ammoniagenesis to generate new $HCO_3^-$ ions to replace the $HCO_3^-$ ions that were lost in the urine.

### Reabsorption of $NaHCO_3$ in the loop of Henle

It is not clear how much $HCO_3^-$ ions are reabsorbed in the thick ascending limb of the loop of Henle. Extrapolating from micropuncture data in rats, if about 80% of the filtered load of $HCO_3^-$ ions is reabsorbed in the portion of the PCT prior to the site of micropuncture, then close to 900 mmol of $HCO_3^-$ ions per day escape reabsorption in this portion of the PCT. Micropuncture data in rats show that only a small amount of $HCO_3^-$ ions is delivered to the distal convoluted tubule. Therefore, almost 900 mmol of $HCO_3^-$ ions are reabsorbed in the pars recta portion of PCT and/or the thick ascending limb of the loop of Henle. Hence, close to 800 mmol of $HCO_3^-$ are removed either in the pars recta segment of the PCT and/or in the thick ascending limb of the loop of Henle. The general scheme for the mechanism for $HCO_3^-$ ion reabsorption in the thick ascending limb of the loop of Henle is similar to that in PCT. $H^+$ secretion is via an NHE-3, whereas $HCO_3^-$ exit, however, is likely via a basolateral $Cl^-/HCO_3^-$ anion exchanger (AE).

### Reabsorption of $NaHCO_3$ in the distal nephron

A small quantity of $HCO_3^-$ ions is delivered to the distal nephron in normal physiology. Reabsorption of $HCO_3^-$ ions occurs in the α-intercalated cells. $H^+$ ions—derived from the dissociation of $H_2O$—are secreted via an $H^+$-ATPase in the luminal membrane. $OH^-$ ions are removed instantaneously by combining with $CO_2$ to form $HCO_3^-$ ions; the process is catalyzed by carbonic anhydrase II. $HCO_3^-$ ions exit via a $Cl^-/HCO_3^-$ anion exchanger in the basolateral membrane.

## EXCRETION OF AMMONIUM IONS

- For every $NH_4^+$ ion excreted in the urine, one new $HCO_3^-$ ion is added to the body.
- Because the overall function of this metabolic process is to add *new* $HCO_3^-$ to the body when there is a deficit of $HCO_3^-$ ions, it is activated when there is a chronic $H^+$ ion load.

The metabolic process that leads to acid balance is described in Figure 1-10. Oxidation of sulfur-containing amino acids in proteins results in an $H^+$ ion load. These $H^+$ ions are eliminated after reacting with $HCO_3^-$ ions in the body. The kidneys must replace this deficit of $HCO_3^-$ ions by forming new $HCO_3^-$ ions and $NH_4^+$ ions in a 1:1 stoichiometry and excreting the $NH_4^+$ ions in the urine to make them an end product of metabolism (Figure 1-11).

The usual rate of excretion of $NH_4^+$ ions is 20 to 40 mmol/day. In response to a chronic acid load, however, the kidney can excrete close to 3 mmol of $NH_4^+$ ions/kg body weight/day in children and close to 200 mmol/day in adults.

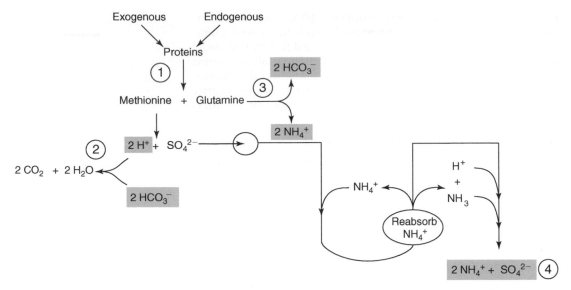

**Figure 1-10  Overview of Acid Balance: Focus on Ammonium.** Sulfur-containing amino acids (e.g., methionine) are converted to H+ ions and $SO_4^{2-}$ anions (*site 1*). A deficit of $HCO_3^-$ ions is created when these new H+ ions react with $HCO_3^-$ ions (*site 2*). Glutamine is converted to $NH_4^+$ ions and $HCO_3^-$ ions in cells of the proximal convoluted tubule; the new $HCO_3^-$ ions are added to the body to replace the deficit of $HCO_3^-$ ions (*site 3*). $NH_4^+$ ions are made into an end product of this metabolic process by being excreted in the urine with equivalent amounts to $SO_4^{2-}$ anions (*site 4*).

## Production of $NH_4^+$ ions

$NH_4^+$ ions are produced from metabolism of the amino acid glutamine in the cells of the PCT. Glutamine is the most abundant amino acid in proteins, and it can also be made in the liver and skeletal muscle. Therefore, its availability is not likely to limit renal ammoniagenesis except perhaps in severely malnourished patients. In chronic metabolic acidosis, in addition to apical uptake of glutamine, there is also increased basolateral uptake of glutamine in cells of the PCT, and in its entry into mitochondria. In the mitochondria, glutamine is metabolized to glutamate via the enzyme phosphate-dependent glutaminase (PDG), producing one $NH_4^+$ ion. Metabolism of glutamate in the enzymatic reaction involving glutamate dehydrogenase (GDH) produces the anion α-ketoglutarate$^{2-}$ and another $NH_4^+$ ion. Conversion of α-ketoglutarate$^{2-}$ to neutral end products, $CO_2$ or glucose, results in the formation of two new $HCO_3^-$ ions. The activity of the enzymes PDG, GDH, and phosphoenolpyruvate carboxykinase, which is a key enzyme in the gluconeogenesis pathway, are all increased in chronic metabolic acidosis and in hypokalemia (see margin note on next page). Thus, the net products of this metabolism of glutamine are 2 $NH_4^+$ ions and 2 $HCO_3^-$ ions. The new $HCO_3^-$ ions are added to the renal venous blood. To maintain this gain of new $HCO_3^-$ ions, $NH_4^+$ ions must be excreted in the urine. If not excreted in the urine, $NH_4^+$ ions will be returned into the systemic circulation via the renal vein. Metabolism of one $NH_4^+$ ion in the liver to produce urea consumes one $HCO_3^-$ ion, hence there is no net gain of $HCO_3^-$ ions (see Figure 1-11).

There is a lag period before glutamine is selected as the fuel for oxidation in PCT cells; hence $NH_4^+$ ion production does not rise appreciably during acute and transient acidemia. For example, when there is a large H+ ion load caused by the overproduction of L-lactic acid during a sprint, there is no need to augment the oxidation of glutamine to

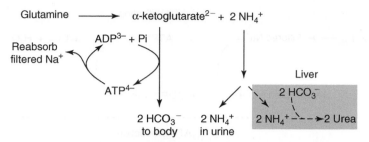

**FORMATION OF UREA**

- Each urea molecule has 2 nitrogen atoms. One nitrogen atom comes from $NH_4^+$ ions, the other comes from the amino acid aspartate.

**Figure 1-11 Biochemical Features in the Conversion of Glutamine to $HCO_3^-$ Ions and $NH_4^+$ Ions.** The metabolism of glutamine occurs in mitochondria of proximal convoluted tubule cells. Initially, glutamine is converted to α-ketoglutarate²⁻ anion plus 2 $NH_4^+$ ions. Two new $HCO_3^-$ ions are generated and added to the body after the α-ketoglutarate²⁻ anion is converted to neutral end products. To complete the process of $HCO_3^-$ ion gain, $NH_4^+$ ions must be excreted in the urine; this prevents the conversion of $NH_4^+$ ions and $HCO_3^-$ ions to urea in the liver (*shaded rectangle*). *ADP*, Adenosine diphosphate; *ATP*, adenosine triphosphate; *Pi*, inorganic phosphate.

eliminate this $H^+$ ion load because the L-lactate⁻ anion will be metabolized and $HCO_3^-$ ions will be produced in a relatively short period of time. Hence, PCT cells continue to oxidize fuels of carbohydrate (L-lactate⁻ anions) or fat origin (fatty acids) in this setting. This lag period offers a biologic advantage because it avoids catabolism of lean body mass to provide glutamine, the substrate for ammoniagenesis, when it may not be needed.

- Availability of ADP in PCT cells is diminished when less work is performed in these cells (i.e., less reabsorption of filtered $Na^+$ ions); this leads to a decrease in the rate of production of $NH_4^+$ ions.

There is an upper limit on the rate of $NH_4^+$ production in cells of the PCT set by the rate of regeneration of $ATP^{4-}$ in these cells. In more detail, in the process of glutamine metabolism to $CO_2$ or glucose, $NAD^+$ is reduced to $NADH + H^+$. To continue glutamine oxidation requires that $NADH + H^+$ be converted back to $NAD^+$. This occurs during coupled oxidative phosphorylation, in which $ATP^{4-}$ is regenerated from $ADP^{3-}$ and inorganic phosphate (Pi). $ADP^{3-}$, in turn, is produced from hydrolysis of $ATP^{4-}$ when biological work is performed. Although several fuels may be oxidized to convert $ADP^{3-}$ back to $ATP^{4-}$ in the process of oxidative phosphorylation, glutamine is "selected" when a sustained acid load has caused a higher concentration of $H^+$ ions in PCT cells. In this context, the oxidation of glutamine occurs almost exclusively in mitochondria in PCT cells because this nephron segment reabsorbs close to four-fifths of the filtered load of $Na^+$ ions (~22,500 mmol/day) and thereby generates enough $ADP^{3-}$ to permit a high rate of production of $NH_4^+$ ions when needed. As the GFR falls, a smaller amount of $Na^+$ ions is filtered and therefore, a smaller amount of $Na^+$ ions is reabsorbed by PCT cells. Because the work in these cells is diminished, there is a lower rate of utilization of $ATP^{4-}$ (Figure 1-12). This may account for the low rate of excretion of $NH_4^+$ ions in patients with advanced renal insufficiency, even in the presence of metabolic acidemia. The rate of production of $NH_4^+$ ions could be lower than expected if there is a high availability of an alternate fuel competing with glutamine for this limited amount of $ADP^{3-}$. An example is the ketoacidosis of prolonged fasting, in which oxidation of some of the reabsorbed ketoacid anions in the PCT

**POTASSIUM DISORDERS AND RENAL AMMONIAGENESIS**

- Hypokalemia is associated with a low pH in the cells of PCT, which augments renal ammoniagenesis.
- The converse is also true: hyperkalemia is associated a lower $H^+$ ion concentration (higher pH) in cells of the PCT. Hyperkalemia is the most common cause of hyperchloremic metabolic acidosis caused by a diminished rate of production of $NH_4^+$ ions.

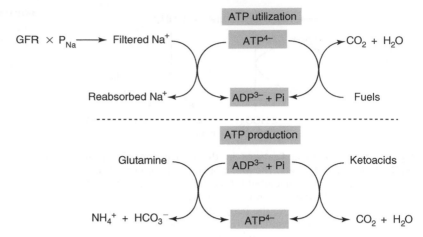

**Figure 1-12 Setting the Maximum Rate of Production of $NH_4^+$ Ions.** The utilization of adenosine triphosphate ($ATP^{4-}$) in the proximal convoluted tubule cells are depicted in the *top portion of the figure*; $ATP^{4-}$ is used primarily to reabsorb filtered $Na^+$ ions. This generates the adenosine diphosphate ($ADP^{3-}$) and inorganic phosphate (Pi) needed to permit the oxidation of glutamine to form $NH_4^+$ ions and new $HCO_3^-$ ions, which is depicted in the *bottom portion of the figure*. Fuels compete for the available $ADP^{3-}$; glutamine is selected in the presence of chronic metabolic acidemia and $NH_4^+$ ion production is increased, providing that there is enough filtered $Na^+$ ions to have high rates of $ADP^{3-}$ generation. In contrast, in the presence of high filtered loads of ketoacids, less glutamine can be oxidized in PCT cells because ketoacids are reabsorbed in cells of the PCT and their oxidation limits the amount of $ADP^{3-}$ available for oxidation of glutamine.

cells diminishes the rate of oxidation of glutamine and production of $NH_4^+$ ions. Of note, an identical amount of $ADP^{3-}$ is required for the oxidation of 1 mmol of β-hydroxybutyrate and 1 mmol of glutamine (see Figure 1-12). Nevertheless, from an acid balance point of view, oxidation of β-hydroxybutyrate⁻ anions (which yields $HCO_3^-$ ions), or their excretion in the urine with $NH_4^+$ ions, are equal.

## Transport of $NH_4^+$ ions

### Proximal convoluted tubule

$NH_4^+$ ions produced in the PCT cells are preferentially secreted into the lumen; a small amount is transported across the basolateral membrane and exits the kidney via the renal vein. The major mechanism for the entry of $NH_4^+$ ions into the lumen of the PCT is by $NH_4^+$ ions replacing $H^+$ ions on NHE-3, thus making it a $Na^+/NH_4^+$ cation exchanger.

### Loop of Henle

This segment of the process to excrete $NH_4^+$ ions begins with the reabsorption of $NH_4^+$ ions in the medullary thick ascending limb (mTAL) of the loop of Henle. This is achieved by having $NH_4^+$ ions replace $K^+$ ions on the luminal $Na^+$, $K^+$, 2 $Cl^-$-cotransporter (NKCC-2). $NH_4^+$ ions exit across the basolateral membrane is likely by replacing $H^+$ ions on another $Na^+/H^+$ cation exchanger, NHE-4. This provides the "single effect" for a countercurrent exchange of $NH_4^+$ ions in the loop of Henle, in which $NH_3/NH_4^+$ ions move from the medullary interstitial compartment, where their concentration is high, to the thin descending limb of the loop of Henle, where their concentration is low. The net effect of this process of medullary recycling of $NH_4^+$ ions

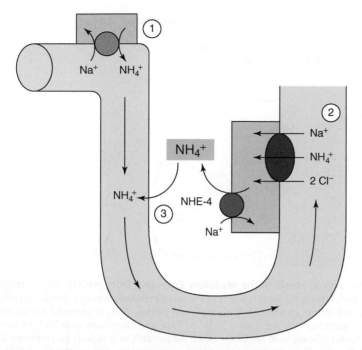

**Figure 1-13 Generation of a High NH$_4^+$ Ion Concentration in the Medullary Interstitial Compartment.** The *U-shaped structure* is the loop of Henle. The first step in the process that raises the concentration of NH$_4^+$ ions in the medullary interstitial compartment is NH$_4^+$ ion production in the proximal convoluted tubule; NH$_4^+$ ions enter the lumen on the Na$^+$/H$^+$ exchanger (*site 1*). The second step is the reabsorption of NH$_4^+$ ions via the Na$^+$, K$^+$, 2 Cl$^-$ cotransporter (NKCC-2) in the medullary thick ascending limb of the loop of Henle (*site 2*). NH$_4^+$ ions exit across the basolateral membrane is likely by replacing H$^+$ ions on another Na$^+$/H$^+$ exchanger, NHE-4. The third step is the entry of NH$_4^+$ ions into the descending limb of the loop of Henle, completing a countercurrent exchange of NH$_4^+$ ions (*site 3*).

is to raise the concentrations of NH$_4^+$ ions deep in the medullary interstitial compartment (Figure 1-13) to aid the transport of NH$_3$ into the lumen of the medullary collecting duct.

### Collecting duct

The mechanism of NH$_4^+$ ion secretion involves parallel NH$_3$ and H$^+$ ion secretion into the lumen of the collecting duct (see margin note).

### NH$_3$ secretion

Transport of NH$_3$ into the lumen of the MCD was thought of as a process of "diffusion trapping." In essence, distal H$^+$ ion secretion lowers the luminal fluid pH, which should decrease the NH$_3$ concentration in the lumen of the MCD to permit more NH$_3$ to diffuse from the interstitial compartment to the lumen of the MCD, where it is trapped as NH$_4^+$ ions. This mechanism has been largely discarded because its two requirements are not achieved (see margin note).

The current model is that NH$_3$ is transported from the interstitial fluid into the lumen of the collecting duct via nonerythroid Rh glycoproteins, Rhbg and Rhcg, that function as gas channels (Figure 1-14). NH$_3$ is transported across the basolateral membrane of the collecting duct, predominantly by Rhcg, but also partly by Rhbg. NH$_3$ transport across the luminal membrane of collecting duct cells is via Rhcg. NH$_4^+$ ions enter these channels, where they

## SITE OF NH$_4^+$ ION ADDITION IN THE COLLECTING DUCT

- Experimental studies in rats with chronic metabolic acidosis using the microcatheterization technique indicated that most of the NH$_4^+$ ions that were excreted in the urine were added between the PCT and the earliest and terminal segments of the cortical distal nephron.
- It is not clear that this is also the case in humans. A major difference between rats and humans in terms of NH$_4^+$ ion excretion is that rats do not require high rates of excretion of NH$_4^+$ ions because the diet of the rat supplies 10-fold more alkali than acid. Therefore, faced with an acid load, rats achieve acid balance by decreasing the rate of excretion of organic anions in the urine rather than by increasing the rate of excretion of NH$_4^+$ ions.
- The addition of a large amount of NH$_4^+$ ions to the luminal fluid in the cortical collecting duct requires a high concentration of NH$_4^+$ ions in the peritubular interstitial fluid. This may be difficult to achieve because of the high blood flow in the cortex. Furthermore, there may be a risk if a large amount of NH$_4^+$ ions were to enter the systemic circulation.
- In addition, humans with diseases that cause medullary interstitial damage have a low rate of excretion of NH$_4^+$ ions and develop metabolic acidosis on this basis. This suggests that an important site for addition of NH$_4^+$ ions in humans is the medullary collecting duct (MCD).

## DIFFUSION TRAPPING

- Because of its high pK (approximately 9.15) in biological fluids, the vast majority of ammonia (NH$_4^+$ + NH$_3$) will be present as NH$_4^+$. Hence, the concentration of NH$_3$ in the renal medullary interstitial compartment is too low to support rapid rates of diffusion. At a luminal fluid pH of 6.5, 0.2% of the total ammonium will be in the form of NH$_3$. This ratio of NH$_3$ to total ammonia will drop to 0.07% at luminal fluid pH of 6.0 and to 0.02 at luminal fluid pH of 5.5. Therefore, lowering luminal fluid pH even to a value of 5.5 does not result in a large concentration difference for NH$_3$ between the medullary interstitial fluid and the luminal fluid to augment the driving force for NH$_3$ diffusion by an appreciable amount.
- Because NH$_3$ is a small and uncharged molecule, it was thought to be highly permeable across lipid membranes. This, however, is not the case because evidence shows that NH$_3$ has very limited permeability across cell membranes.

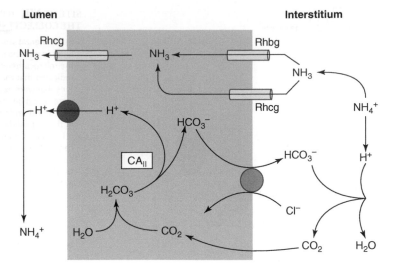

**Figure 1-14 Transfer of NH$_4^+$ from the Loop of Henle to the Medullary Collecting Duct (MCD).** The *rectangle* represents a medullary collecting duct cell. NH$_3$ is transported across the basolateral membrane, predominantly via Rh C glycoprotein (*Rhcg*), and to some extent also via Rh B glycoprotein (*Rhbg*). NH$_3$ is secreted across the apical membrane via Rhcg. H$^+$ ions are secreted into the lumen by H$^+$ ATPase and combines with NH$_3$ to form NH$_4^+$ ions. Inside the cell, CO$_2$ + H$_2$O form carbonic acid (H$_2$CO$_3$), which dissociates very rapidly (accelerated by intracellular carbonic anhydrase II [CA$_{II}$]), into H$^+$ and HCO$_3^-$ ions. HCO$_3^-$ ions exit the cell via the Cl$^-$/HCO$_3^-$ anion exchanger at the basolateral membrane. HCO$_3^-$ ions combine with H$^+$ ions that are released from NH$_4^+$ ions to form H$_2$CO$_3$, which dissociates into CO$_2$ + H$_2$O. CO$_2$ enters the cell and is used to produce H$^+$ ions inside cells.

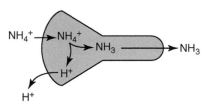

**Figure 1-15 A Closer Look at the NH$_3$ Channel.** The funnel shaped structure represents an Rh glycoprotein, which functions as an NH$_3$ channel. The lipophilic environment at the mouth of the channel lowers the pK of NH$_4^+$ ion and hence NH$_4^+$ ions are converted to NH$_3$ + H$^+$ ions. This raises the local concentration of NH$_3$ close to 1000-fold and permits NH$_3$ to diffuse through the channel.

### NH$_4^+$ ION TRANSPORT IN THE INNER MEDULLARY COLLECTING DUCT

- There is almost no Rh glycoprotein expression in the inner MCD.
- There are data to suggest that the major mechanism for NH$_4^+$ uptake is via NH$_4^+$ replacing K$^+$ on the basolateral Na-K-ATPase. While apical transport is likely with NH$_3$, the specific mechanism has not been clarified.

### H$^+$/K$^+$-ATPase

The main function of the H$^+$/K$^+$-ATPase is to reabsorb K$^+$ ions in conditions of K$^+$ ion depletion. This reabsorption of K$^+$ ions and secretion of H$^+$ ions requires that there be H$^+$ ion acceptors available in the lumen of the distal nephron. These luminal H$^+$ ion acceptors are HCO$_3^-$ ions and NH$_3$ because virtually all the HPO$_4^{2-}$ anions have already been converted to H$_2$PO$_4^-$ anions in upstream nephron segments.

are converted to NH$_3$ + H$^+$ ions in the lipophilic environment at the mouth of the channel, which lowers the pK of NH$_4^+$ ion. This raises the local concentration of NH$_3$ close to 1000-fold and permits NH$_3$ to diffuse through the channel (Figure 1-15) (see margin note).

### H$^+$ ion secretion

H$^+$ pumps are located primarily in the luminal membranes of the mitochondria-rich α-intercalated cells. There are two major H$^+$ pumps in this segment, an H$^+$-ATPase and an H$^+$/K$^+$-ATPase, the former is particularly important from an acid–base perspective (see margin note).

## NET ACID EXCRETION

The formula of net acid excretion (NAE) is thought to describe the renal contribution to maintain acid–base balance (Eqn 3), with the excretion of NH$_4^+$ ions and titratable acids as the processes that generate $HCO_3^-$ ions minus the amount of $HCO_3^-$ ions that are lost in the urine.

$$NAE = (U_{NH_4} + U_{TA}) - U_{HCO_3} \qquad (3)$$

There are, however, two major issues with this calculation that should be pointed out.

### Titratable acids

The major titratable acid in the urine is the monovalent organic phosphate $(H_2PO_4^-)$. Nevertheless, not all the phosphate excreted in the urine as $H_2PO_4^-$ represents a gain of $HCO_3^-$ ions (see Figure 1-4). Only if phosphate has entered the body as divalent organic phosphate $(HPO_4^{2-})$ does its excretion in the urine as $H_2PO_4^-$ lead to a net gain of $HCO_3^-$ ions. In contrast, if phosphate entered the body as $H_2PO_4^-$, which is then excreted in the urine as $H_2PO_4^-$, there is no net gain of $HCO_3^-$ ions in this process.

### Alkali loss

The NAE formula describes the alkali loss as the excretion of $HCO_3^-$ ions. Because the urine pH is usually close to 6 for most of the 24-hour period, there is no bicarbonaturia. Hence, it was suggested to revise the formula of NAE to include the excretion of organic anions. Not all the excreted organic anions in the urine, however, represent a loss of $HCO_3^-$ ions. In more detail, if endogenous organic acids were produced to titrate an alkali load, with subsequent excretion of their anions with $K^+$ or $Na^+$ ions in the urine, there is no net loss or gain of $HCO_3^-$ ions in this process. On the other hand, if, for example, ketoacids were produced and their anions were excreted in the urine with $K^+$ or $Na^+$ ions, this represents a loss of alkali because these anions could have been metabolized to produce $HCO_3^-$ ions. Hence, their excretion in the urine represents the loss of potential $HCO_3^-$ ions.

## URINE pH AND KIDNEY STONE FORMATION

- The elimination of an acid load via the excretion of $NH_4^+$ ions and of an alkali load via the excretion of organic anions ensures that the urine pH can be maintained close to 6.0.

Acid and base balances must be achieved while maintaining an ideal composition of the urine to prevent the precipitation of solutes and minimize the risk of forming kidney stones. The central factors are the pH of the urine (Figure 1-16) and the concentration of poorly soluble constituents in the urine. The safe range for the urine pH is one that is close to 6.0 for most of the day.

### Low Urine pH and Uric Acid Stones

The pK of uric acid in the urine is close to 5.3. Therefore, at a urine pH of 5.3, half of the amount of the total urate in the urine will be in the form of uric acid, which is poorly soluble in water (solubility 0.6 mmol/L). A low urine pH is the most important risk factor for formation of uric acid stones. The medullary shunt for $NH_3$ minimizes the likelihood of having a low urine pH because it provides the $H^+$ ion acceptor, $NH_3$, to adjust the urine pH to a value close to 6.0 when $H^+$ ion secretion in the distal nephron is stimulated by acidemia. In

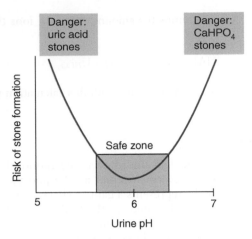

**Figure 1-16  Urine pH and the Risk of Kidney Stone Formation.** The ideal range (safe zone) for the urine pH is a value close to 6.0. When the urine pH is significantly less than 6.0, there is an increased risk of forming uric acid stones. When the urine pH is significantly greater than 6.0, there is an increased risk of forming calcium phosphate ($CaHPO_4$) stones.

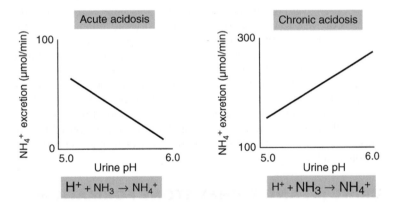

**Figure 1-17  Urine pH and the Excretion of $NH_4^+$ Ions.** In acute acidosis (shown on the *left*), distal $H^+$ ion secretion is stimulated, but there is a lag period before a high rate of ammoniagenesis is achieved. The urine pH is low (temporarily), and there is only a *modest* rise in the rate of $NH_4^+$ ion excretion. In chronic metabolic acidosis (shown on the *right*), both the $H^+$ ion secretory rate and the $NH_3$ availability are greatly increased. The increase in $NH_3$ availability is relatively larger than the increment in $H^+$ ion secretion. Therefore, a high rate of excretion of $NH_4^+$ ions is achieved, whereas the urine pH is close to 6.0.

fact, high rates of excretion of $NH_4^+$ ions are achieved during chronic metabolic acidosis, where the urine pH is close to 6.0 (Figure 1-17).

### High Urine pH and $CaHPO_4$ Kidney Stones

The excretion of dietary alkali in the form of organic anions minimizes the likelihood of having bicarbonaturia and a urine pH that is in the high 6 range. The concentration of $HPO_4^{2-}$ in the urine, which precipitates with ionized calcium, increases as the urine becomes more alkaline (pK is 6.8). Of greater importance, one of these urinary organic anions (i.e., citrate) chelates ionized calcium in the urine, which minimizes the risk of precipitation of $CaHPO_4$.

# PART C
# INTEGRATIVE PHYSIOLOGY

## WHY IS THE NORMAL BLOOD pH 7.40?

Because there are three parameters in the BBS equation—the pH, $PCO_2$, and $P_{HCO_3}$—once two of them have been set, the third must follow. To select the one to examine first, we decided to turn to the most important element for survival; the continued regeneration of $ATP^{4-}$. To improve our analysis, we examined this process under conditions of maximum stress. $ATP^{4-}$ must be regenerated at extremely high rates during the "fight or flight" response. Thus, our focus is on the need to supply $O_2$ at maximum rates. Because $CO_2$ is formed when $O_2$ is consumed, it seemed logical to start with the arterial $PCO_2$.

### WHY IS THE ARTERIAL PCO₂ 40 mm Hg?

The content of $O_2$ in air is directly proportional to its $PO_2$ because there are no bound forms of $O_2$ in air. $O_2$ is poorly soluble in water, so it is transported in a bound form in blood (i.e., bound to hemoglobin in red blood cells). Hemoglobin in blood will be fully saturated with $O_2$ when the $PO_2$ in blood is 100 mm Hg. Therefore, the $PO_2$ in alveolar air should be very close to 100 mm Hg at all times. The $PO_2$ of humidified air is 150 mm Hg. Hence, no more than one-third of the $O_2$ from each liter of inspired air should be extracted. If more than one-third of the $O_2$ is extracted in the lungs, the $PO_2$ in alveolar air falls and thus each liter of arterial blood carries less $O_2$ because $PO_2$ in arterial blood will be lower. Therefore, when the rate of consumption of $O_2$ rises, many more liters of air must be inspired per minute to ensure that the $PO_2$ in alveoli remains close to 100 mm Hg. In fact, the capacity to breathe must greatly exceed the maximum cardiac output.

$CO_2$ is formed when $O_2$ is consumed. The ratio of $CO_2$ production to oxygen consumption is called the *respiratory quotient (RQ)*. When a typical Western diet is consumed, the RQ is close to 0.8 (see margin note). Thus, the rise in the $PCO_2$ in the alveolar air is 0.8 times the fall in its $PO_2$. When one-third of the content of oxygen in alveolar air is extracted, the $PCO_2$ in alveolar air rises to 40 mm Hg (RQ of $0.8 \times 50$ mm Hg). This means that the $PCO_2$ in arterial blood is 40 mm Hg.

One can anticipate that it is necessary to have control mechanisms to ensure that the $PCO_2$ in arterial blood remains very close to 40 mm Hg—this is achieved because the arterial $PCO_2$ is a regulator of alveolar ventilation.

The controls described so far do not indicate how to regulate the blood pH, but two variables remain to be examined. Either the pH or the $P_{HCO_3}$ must be regulated to determine the value of the third parameter in the BBS. We cannot determine with certainty which one it is, but we choose to examine the $P_{HCO_3}$.

### WHAT IS AN IDEAL P_HCO₃?

The following issues are important to select the ideal $P_{HCO_3}$. The $P_{HCO_3}$ should be as high as possible to remove the $H^+$ ion load during the recovery period of vigorous exercise (e.g., hunting in Paleolithic times). The $P_{HCO_3}$ should not, however, be too high because this will increase the concentration of carbonate $\left(CO_3^{2-}\right)$ ions and lead to a lower concentration of ionized $Ca^{2+}$ because of precipitation of calcium carbonate

**RESPIRATORY QUOTIENT**

The ratio of $CO_2$ produced to $O_2$ consumed is called the RQ.
- When carbohydrates are oxidized, the RQ is 1.0.

  $C_6H_{12}O_6 + 6\,O_2 \rightarrow 6\,CO_2 + 6\,H_2O$

- When fatty acids are oxidized, the RQ is 0.7.

  $C_{16}H_{32}O_2 + 23\,O_2 \rightarrow 16\,CO_2 + 16\,H_2O$

- When a typical Western diet is consumed, the RQ is close to 0.8 because of the mixture of fat and carbohydrate in the diet.
- Because the brain oxidizes glucose as its primary fuel, its RQ is 1.0.

($CaCO_3$) in the ECF compartment. Meanwhile, for optimal bone turnover, it is advantageous to have near-equal concentrations of ionized $Ca^{2+}$ and divalent inorganic phosphate ($HPO_4^{2-}$) in the ECF compartment.

At a pH of 7.40 in the ECF compartment, four-fifths of total inorganic phosphate in the ECF compartment is in the form of $HPO_4^{2-}$. Because the concentration of total inorganic phosphate in plasma is close to 1.5 mmol/L, at a pH of 7.40, the concentration of $HPO_4^{2-}$ will be 1.2 mmol/L. Hence, the concentration of ionized $Ca^{2+}$ will need to be close to 1.2 mmol/L.

Therefore, it seems that a $P_{HCO_3}$ of 25 mmol/L (which sets the plasma pH at 7.40 when the $PCO_2$ is 40 mm Hg) is an ideal value because the product of the concentrations of ionized $Ca^{2+}$ and $CO_3^{2-}$ ions does not exceed their solubility product constant ($K_{sp}$).

### What Conclusions Can Be Drawn?

The normal values for the concentrations of $H^+$ ions (pH), $PCO_2$, and $P_{HCO_3}$ are 40 nmol/L (7.40), 40 mm Hg, and 25 mmol/L, respectively, and this has several advantages. The $PCO_2$ is likely dictated by considerations related to $O_2$ transport. To have a high concentration of $HCO_3^-$ ions to remove a large $H^+$ ion load, and also one that produces the ideal $HPO_4^{2-}$ ions and thereby ionized $Ca^{2+}$ ion concentration in the ECF compartment, without exceeding the $K_{sp}$ for $CaCO_3$, the $P_{HCO_3}$ should be close to 25 mmol/L. Accordingly, the concentration of $H^+$ ions will be 40 nmol/L (pH 7.40).

## METABOLIC BUFFERING OF H⁺ IONS DURING A SPRINT

Skeletal muscle cells must deal with large inputs and outputs of $H^+$ ions during a sprint without compromising the functions of other organs in the body, especially those that are essential for survival (e.g., the brain and the heart).

### An Overview of the Acid–Base Changes During a Sprint

The following sequence of events leads to changes in $H^+$ ion production and removal in skeletal muscle during a sprint.

There is an initial small production of $H^+$ ions when work begins, as $ATP^{4-}$ (5 mmol/kg of skeletal muscle) is hydrolyzed, which produces $ADP^{3-} + HPO_4^{2-} + H^+$.

There are two processes, however, that lead to a large removal of $H^+$ ions early during a sprint. First, the accumulation of $ADP^{3-}$ results in a large removal of $H^+$ ions when $ADP^{3-}$ reacts with phosphocreatine$^{2-}$ and is converted back to $ATP^{4-}$. This reaction is catalyzed by creatine kinase, a single enzyme that has a very high activity, which allows its substrates and products to be interconverted at an extremely rapid rate. Hence, as soon as the concentration of $ADP^{3-}$ rises (and it rises enormously because the concentration of $ADP^{3-}$ is so low in cells), phosphocreatine$^{2-}$ is converted to $ATP^{4-}$ plus creatine$^0$ (see margin note on the next page). Because the substrates of this reaction have a greater negative valence than its products, $H^+$ ions are consumed (see Eqns 4 and 5). Second, because the quantity of phosphocreatine$^{2-}$ is very large (25 mmol/kg of skeletal muscle), there is an enormous production of $HPO_4^{2-}$. Because the cell pH is close to the pK for the phosphate buffer system, around half of the $HPO_4^{2-}$ formed from phosphocreatine$^{2-}$ will be converted to $H_2PO_4^-$, and hence there is net removal of H$^+$ ions (i.e., a gain of alkali) in cells. For this to occur, a large source of H$^+$ ions is needed, and this comes from nonbicarbonate buffers in cells because they donate their H$^+$ ions when the concentration of H$^+$ ions declines. The major donor of H$^+$ ions is histidines in proteins and in carnosine (see margin note).

$$ATP^{4-} \rightarrow ADP^{3-} + HPO_4^{2-} + H^+ \qquad (4)$$

$$ADP^{3-} + phosphocreatine^{2-} + H^+ \rightarrow ATP^{4-} + creatine^0 \quad (5)$$

As work is performed, hydrolysis of existing and newly formed ATP$^{4-}$ in skeletal muscle continues at a rapid rate. Accumulation of ADP$^{3-}$ drives glycolysis and eventually a large number of H$^+$ ions are produced during the sprint (see margin note).

The BBS of skeletal muscle cannot remove many H$^+$ ions at this time because virtually all of the O$_2$ in each liter of blood in skeletal muscle capillaries is converted to CO$_2$, and this results in a high PCO$_2$ in skeletal muscle cells and in its interstitial fluid, which prevents H$^+$ ion removal by the BBS. Therefore, as H$^+$ ion concentration in skeletal muscle cells rises, these H$^+$ ions bind quickly to histidines in proteins and carnosines that had donated their H$^+$ ions, and therefore provide "parking spots" for these newly formed H$^+$ ions. Nevertheless, because glycolysis continues to occur at a very rapid rate, eventually, however, the concentration of H$^+$ ions will rise dramatically, and this forces H$^+$ ions to bind to intracellular proteins, which may have deleterious effects (e.g., inhibition of phosphofructokinase-1, thereby diminishing the flux in glycolysis and the regeneration of ATP$^{4-}$). Therefore, the subject is forced to stop running.

## RECOVERY FROM THE SPRINT

During the recovery from vigorous exercise, a sudden, large H$^+$ ion load is produced during the regeneration of phosphocreatine$^{2-}$ because the other reactant is creatine$^0$ (the reverse of the reaction shown in Eqn 5). Of great importance, however, is that the BBS can now operate effectively in skeletal muscle cells and in its interstitial fluid to remove enough of these H$^+$ ions to avoid cell damage by this very large H$^+$ ion load. The key here is the large fall in PCO$_2$ in capillaries of skeletal muscle. This occurs because there is still a large blood flow rate to muscle, and, moreover, the sprinter is hyperventilating because of the acidemia and the continued adrenergic drive.

---

### QUESTION

1-6  *What is the major function of phosphocreatine in aerobic exercise?*

---

### DISCUSSION OF QUESTIONS

1-1  *In certain locations in the body, H$^+$ ions remain free and are not bound. What is the advantage in having such a high concentration of H$^+$ ions?*

A high concentration of H$^+$ ions causes a large number of H$^+$ ions to bind to proteins, which change their charge and shape. Although this is generally undesirable because it may lead to a change in function, it has certain biologic advantages. For example, this binding of H$^+$ ions to dietary proteins in the lumen of the stomach changes their shape so that pepsin can gain access to sites that permit hydrolysis of these proteins. Accordingly, the anion secreted by the stomach along with

---

**FUNCTIONS OF PHOSPHOCRE-ATINE**

- In anaerobic exercise, its major function is as an energy reserve. There is a very high concentration of phosphocreatine in muscle cells (~25 mmol/L).
- In aerobic exercise, the major function of phosphocreatine is in energy transfer in muscle cells (see discussion of Question 1-6).

**CARNOSINE**

- Carnosine is a dipeptide of β-alanine and histidine, which is particularly abundant in skeletal muscle (~25 mmol/kg).

**SITE AT WHICH H$^+$ ARE PRO-DUCED IN GLYCOLYSIS**

- Contrary to common belief, glycolysis is not a metabolic pathway that causes net production of H$^+$ ions.
- Rather, if one analyzes the metabolic process (and counts the valences in Eqns 6 and 7), one can see that the initial step is work; hydrolysis of ATP$^{4-}$ and production of ADP$^{3-}$+ HPO$_4^{2-}$ is the step that produces the H$^+$ ions (Eqn 6) and not the second step, where glucose is converted to two L-lactate$^-$ anions (Eqn 7).

$$Work + 2ATP^{4-} \rightarrow 2ADP^{3-} + 2H^+ + 2HPO_4^{2-} \qquad (6)$$

$$Glucose + 2(ADP^{3-} + HPO_4^{2-}) \rightarrow 2(ATP^{4-} + L\text{-lactate}^-) \quad (7)$$

$H^+$ ions is $Cl^-$ ions because $Cl^-$ ions do not bind $H^+$ ions until the pH is very low. HCl dissociates completely in aqueous solutions, and because there are no major buffers in gastric fluid, the $H^+$ ion concentration is high and $H^+$ ions bind avidly to dietary proteins and denature them.

A second example of when it is beneficial to have a high $H^+$ ion concentration in certain locations involves "stripping" of hormones from their protein receptors. This happens when the receptor plus its bound hormone complex is gathered into a sac (called an *endosome* [*endo-* means *in* and *-some* means *body*]) where its membrane secretes $H^+$ ions using an $H^+$-ATPase, raising the concentration of $H^+$ ions in this local environment. As a result, this makes the protein receptor and the hormone itself more positively charged, which alters their shape, and decreases the affinity of binding of the receptor to that hormone. The hormone is then sent to a site where there are proteolytic enzymes that destroy it (proteasome), while the receptor recycles back to the cell membrane. This diminishes the need for continuing resynthesis of receptor proteins (e.g., this recycling of receptors in cell membranes occurs almost 180 times in the lifetime of the insulin receptor).

1-2  *What is the rationale for the statement, "In biology only weak acids kill"?*

Chemistry books classify acids as strong or weak based on their dissociation constants (or pK, the pH at which the acid is 50% dissociated); strong acids have a much lower pK. This difference is of little importance in biology because the dissociation of virtually all weak and strong acids is much greater than 99% at pH values of close to 7. In addition, most acids encountered in physiology are weak acids (e.g., L-lactic acid, ketoacids).

1-3  *Does consumption of citrus fruit, which contains a large quantity of citric acid and its $K^+$ salt, cause a net acid or a net alkali load?*

The addition of citric acid will initially result in an $H^+$ load because citric acid dissociates into $H^+$ ions and citrate anions. This $H^+$ ion load will be removed when citrate anions are metabolized to neutral end products because this will produce $HCO_3^-$ anions. Metabolism of citrate anions that were added as $K^+$ ion salts (not with $H^+$ ions) will lead to a gain of $HCO_3^-$ ions. Therefore, there is a net gain of alkali with the consumption of citrus fruit.

1-4  *Why is the L-lactic acidosis that occurs during cardiogenic shock so much more devastating than the L-lactic acidosis that occurs during a sprint if the $P_{L\text{-}lactate}$, arterial pH, and $P_{HCO3}$ are identical?*

There are two components to the answer. First, cells in vital organs in the patient with cardiogenic shock suffer from a lack of $ATP^{4-}$ because they are deprived of oxygen. In contrast, the brain and the heart are not undergoing anaerobic metabolism during a sprint. Hence, only skeletal muscle has a very large demand for anaerobic conversion of $ADP^{3-}$ to $ATP^{4-}$ to enable the performance of work. Second, there is also a major difference with respect to buffering of $H^+$ ions. Only the patient with poor cardiac function has a very slow blood flow rate to vital organs. As a result, the $PCO_2$ in brain cells rises markedly, and $H^+$ ions cannot be eliminated by their BBS. Accordingly, more $H^+$ ions bind to intracellular proteins and, as a result, these vital organs fail to function in an optimal fashion.

1-5  *The heart extracts close to 70% of the oxygen from each liter of coronary artery blood. What conclusions can you draw about buffering of $H^+$ ions in the heart? Might there be advantages because of this high extraction of $O_2$ per liter of blood flow?*

Because so much $O_2$ is extracted from each liter of blood delivered to the heart, cardiac myocytes add a large amount of $CO_2$ to each liter of coronary sinus blood. Accordingly, the venous $PO_2$ is low and the venous $PCO_2$ is high—each has potentially important effects.

## Low Venous $PO_2$

There are two opposing factors to consider.
- *Risk*
  A low capillary $PO_2$ slows the rate of diffusion of $O_2$ and thus its rate of delivery to cardiac mitochondria. On the other hand, beating of the heart "stirs" its interstitial fluid, which accelerates diffusion.
- *Benefits*
  First, a low interstitial $PO_2$ is advantageous if it leads to new blood vessel formation and thus the formation of collaterals with interweaving connections. Second, in conjunction with the high $PCO_2$, a low $PO_2$ produces a vasodilatory ambiance that leads to an ability of the arterioles of the heart to vasodilate in response to less robust stimuli that accompany a need for increased cardiac work.

## High Venous $PCO_2$

There are two opposing factors to consider.
- *Risk*
  A high venous and cellular $PCO_2$ reduces the effectiveness of the BBS of the heart. This should not be a problem as long as the heart maintains its aerobic state because in this setting, the rate of $H^+$ ion removal will be equal to the rate of $H^+$ ion formation.
- *Benefits*
  First, a high capillary $PCO_2$ in the heart causes a rightward shift in the $O_2$/hemoglobin dissociation curve; this improves the diffusion of $O_2$ into cardiac myocytes. Second, the high interstitial $PCO_2$ enhances the response of arterioles of the heart to vasodilatory stimuli that are released in response to increased cardiac work (e.g., adenosine).

### 1-6 *What is the major function of phosphocreatine in aerobic exercise?*

There is no net change in the concentrations of phosphocreatine$^{2-}$ or creatine$^0$ in skeletal muscle during vigorous *aerobic* exercise. Hence, it may appear that there is no role for this phosphocreatine$^{2-}$/creatine$^0$ system as an energy reserve at this time. This is not the case, however: the absence of change in their concentrations reflects that hydrolysis and resynthesis of phosphocreatine$^{2-}$ occurs at equal and very rapid rates.

Creatine$^0$ and phosphocreatine$^{2-}$ are used as an "energy shuttle" between contractile elements and mitochondria in muscle cells during aerobic exercise. During heavy aerobic exercise, ATP$^{4-}$ is converted to ADP$^{3-}$ at very rapid rates in the vicinity of muscle contractile elements. Notwithstanding, the site where ADP$^{3-}$ is converted back to ATP$^{4-}$ is in mitochondria, and this is a large distance for diffusion. Diffusion is slow when concentration differences in absolute terms are low or if distances are large. Because the concentration of free ADP$^{3-}$ is extremely tiny (0.025 mmol/L) and the distance in skeletal muscle cells is large, there would be a very low rate of ATP$^{4-}$ synthesis relative to the enormous amount of ATP$^{4-}$ required for vigorous exercise, unless this diffusion step could be accelerated or bypassed. Nature's solution is to use

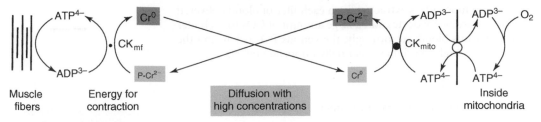

**Figure 1-18 Phosphocreatine Energy Shuttle.** Events are located in skeletal muscle (and heart) cells. To overcome the need for diffusion of adenosine diphosphate ($ADP^{3-}$), the conversion of $ADP^{3-}$ to adenosine triphosphate ($ADP^{4-}$) near muscle contractile elements (shown to the *left*) leads to the conversion of phosphocreatine$^{2-}$ ($P-Cr^{2-}$) to creatine$^0$. Because the sum of the concentrations of these latter compounds is close to 25 mmol/L, they can diffuse instead of $ADP^{3-}$ between these contractile elements and mitochondria (shown to the *right*). For emphasis, the sites where concentrations are higher are indicated by the *larger* and *darker red rectangles*. *CK,* Creatine kinase; $CK_{mf}$, creatine kinase near muscle fibers; $CK_{mito}$, creatine kinase near mitochondria.

a "bypass strategy"—to have creatine$^0$ and/or phosphocreatine$^{2-}$ diffuse instead of $ADP^{3-}$ and $ATP^{4-}$ because the concentrations of the former pair are more than 1000-fold higher than that of $ADP^{3-}$ (Figure 1-18). To achieve these effects, there are two different creatine kinase enzymes. Hydrolysis of phosphocreatine$^{2-}$ occurs in one area of skeletal muscle cells: the region where the contractile elements exist. Resynthesis of phosphocreatine$^{2-}$ occurs near the mitochondria. Hydrolysis and resynthesis of phosphocreatine$^{2-}$ occur at very rapid rates. This way of accelerating diffusion is absolutely necessary during vigorous exercise. In fact, mice that lack these creatine kinase enzymes in their hearts are fine at rest but are unable to perform even modest exercise.

# chapter 2

# Tools to Use to Diagnose Acid–Base Disorders

# Introduction

There are four primary acid–base disturbances, two metabolic and two respiratory. Each of these disorders has an expected compensatory response, which is aimed at minimizing the change in $H^+$ ion concentration. These expected responses, unfortunately, must be memorized. Knowing these expected responses helps identify mixed acid–base disorders.

As was emphasized in Chapter 1, the role of buffering in patients with metabolic acidosis is not simply to lower the concentration of $H^+$ ions but, of even greater importance, to minimize the binding of $H^+$ ions to proteins in cells of vital organs (e.g., the brain and the heart). This "safe" removal of $H^+$ ions occurs via the bicarbonate buffer system (BBS), the bulk of which is in the intracellular fluid and the interstitial space of skeletal muscle. Free-flowing brachial venous partial pressure of carbon dioxide ($PCO_2$), which reflects the capillary blood $PCO_2$ in skeletal muscles, should be measured in patients with metabolic acidosis to assess the effectiveness of BBS in removing the $H^+$ ion load.

The role of the kidney in chronic metabolic acidosis is to generate new bicarbonate ions ($HCO_3^-$) by increasing the rate of excretion of ammonium ($NH_4^+$) ions.

Metabolic alkalosis is an electrolyte disorder accompanied by an elevated concentration of $HCO_3^-$ ions in plasma ($P_{HCO_3}$) and a rise in plasma pH. Most patients with metabolic alkalosis have a deficit of NaCl, KCl, and/or HCl, each of which leads to a higher $P_{HCO_3}$. The expected physiologic response in patients with metabolic alkalosis is hypoventilation and hence an increase in the arterial $PCO_2$.

In patients with respiratory acid–base disorders, the expected change in $P_{HCO_3}$ differs depending on whether the disorder is acute or chronic.

We emphasize that one must integrate all the information from the medical history and the physical examination together with the laboratory data to make an acid–base diagnosis.

## ABBREVIATIONS

BBS, bicarbonate buffer system
$HCO_3^-$, bicarbonate ions
$P_{HCO_3}$, concentration of $HCO_3^-$ ions in plasma
ECF, extracellular fluid
$P_{Anion\ gap}$, anion gap in plasma
$P_{Albumin}$, concentration of albumin in plasma
[$H^+$], concentration of hydrogen ions
ICF, intracellular fluid
EABV, effective arterial blood volume
PCT, proximal convoluted tubule
$P_K$, concentration of potassium ($K^+$) ions in plasma
$P_{Na}$, concentration of sodium ($Na^+$) ions in plasma
$P_{Cl}$, concentration of chloride ($Cl^-$) ions in plasma

---

## OBJECTIVES

■ To illustrate the tools needed to identify whether there is an acid–base disorder and why it is present. Our emphasis will be on metabolic acidosis.

■ To illustrate how to obtain a quantitative estimate of the extracellular fluid (ECF) volume to assess the content of $HCO_3^-$ ions in the ECF compartment to determine if metabolic acidosis is present in a patient with significantly contracted ECF volume.

■ To illustrate how to determine whether metabolic acidosis is due to the overproduction of acids or the loss of sodium bicarbonate ($NaHCO_3$).

■ To illustrate how to assess whether $H^+$ ions were removed appropriately by the BBS in a patient with metabolic acidosis.

■ To illustrate how to assess the rate of excretion of $NH_4^+$ ions in the urine in a patient with metabolic acidosis, and to illustrate the urine tests that may help to identify the cause of a low rate of excretion of $NH_4^+$ ions.

### CASE 2-1: DOES THIS MAN REALLY HAVE METABOLIC ACIDOSIS?

A 25-year-old man was perfectly healthy until 24 hours ago, when he developed severe, watery diarrhea. He had no intake of food or water. He noted that he had very little urine output over the last several hours. His blood pressure is 90/60 mm Hg, pulse rate is 110 beats per minute, and his jugular venous pressure is low. Acid–base measurements in arterial blood reveal a pH 7.39, $P_{HCO_3}$ 24 mmol/L, and $PCO_2$ 39 mm Hg. His $P_{Anion\ gap}$ is 24 mEq/L. His diarrhea volume is estimated to be ~5 L, and the concentration of $HCO_3^-$ ions in a sample of his diarrhea fluid is 40 mmol/L. His hematocrit on admission is 0.60, and his $P_{Albumin}$ is 8.0 g/dL (80 g/L).

### Questions

Does this patient have a significant degree of metabolic acidosis? What is the basis for the high $P_{Anion\ gap}$?

### CASE 2-2: LOLA KAYE NEEDS YOUR HELP

Lola Kaye, an 18-year-old woman, is brought to the emergency department because of severe weakness. Her blood pressure is low (80/50 mm Hg), and her pulse rate is high (124 beats per minute). Her respiratory rate is not low (20 breaths per minute). Her jugular venous pressure is low. The only laboratory values available at this time are from arterial blood gas measurements: pH 6.90 ([H$^+$] = 125 nmol/L), $PCO_2$ = 30 mm Hg. She does not have a history of diabetes mellitus and denies ingestion of methanol or ethylene glycol.

### Question

What is/are the major acid–base diagnosis/diagnoses in this patient?

---

# PART A
# DIAGNOSTIC ISSUES

## DISORDERS OF ACID–BASE BALANCE

Before the discussion of each of the acid–base disorders, there are two points that are not included in the traditional approach to acid–base disorders and require emphasis.

### THE $P_{HCO_3}$ IS INFLUENCED BY CHANGES IN THE ECF VOLUME

Concentration terms can be altered by changes in their numerator and/or their denominator. The concentration of $HCO_3^-$ in the ECF compartment can be influenced by changes in the amount of $HCO_3^-$ in the ECF compartment and/or changes in the ECF volume. Therefore, a patient may have metabolic acidosis with a near normal $P_{HCO_3}$ and hence no appreciable acidemia, if the ECF volume is very contracted. Hence, a quantitative assessment of ECF volume is required to estimate the amount of $HCO_3^-$ ions in the ECF compartment and determine if metabolic acidosis is present (see the discussion of Case 2-1).

### MEASUREMENT OF BRACHIAL VENOUS $PCO_2$ TO ASSESS BUFFERING OF AN H$^+$ ION LOAD BY BBS

In Chapter 1, we emphasized that H$^+$ ions must be removed by the BBS to minimize their binding to proteins in cells of vital organs (e.g., the brain and the heart). A low $PCO_2$ in the interstitial fluid compartment of the ECF of muscles and in muscle cells, where the bulk of the BBS

**NORMAL ACID–BASE VALUES IN PLASMA**

- pH: 7.40±0.02
- [H$^+$]: 40±2 nmol/L
- $P_{HCO_3}$: 25±2 mmol/L
- Arterial $PCO_2$: 40±2 mm Hg
- Venous $PCO_2$: At usual rates of blood flow and metabolic work at rest, brachial venous $PCO_2$ is about 46 mm Hg (~6 mm Hg greater than the arterial $PCO_2$)

**DEFINITIONS**
- Acidemia is a low pH or a high concentration of H+ ions in plasma.
- Acidosis is a process that adds H+ ions to or removes $HCO_3^-$ ions from the body.

**pH VERSUS [H+]**
- The authors prefer to think in terms of the [H+] rather than the pH, but the principles are the same: a low [H+] is a high pH, and vice versa.

exists, is a prerequisite to achieve this safe removal of H+ ions. The traditional approach to acid–base disorders focuses only on the arterial $PCO_2$, which is influenced predominantly by regulation of ventilation. Having a low arterial $PCO_2$ does not ensure that the $PCO_2$ is low in the interstitial fluid compartment of the ECF of muscles and in muscle cells, because that $PCO_2$ is also influenced by both the rate of production of $CO_2$ and the blood flow rate to muscles. Patients with metabolic acidosis and a contracted effective arterial blood volume (EABV) have a high $PCO_2$ in the interstitial fluid of skeletal muscles and skeletal muscle cells (reflected by a high $PCO_2$ in their venous blood), and therefore may fail to titrate an H+ ion load with the BBS in their skeletal muscle. As a result, the degree of acidemia may become more pronounced, and more H+ ions may bind to proteins in the extracellular and intracellular fluids in other organs, including the brain. Notwithstanding, because of autoregulation of cerebral blood flow, it is likely that there will be only minimal changes in the $PCO_2$ in brain capillary blood unless there is a severe degree of contraction of the EABV with failure of autoregulation of cerebral blood flow. Therefore, the BBS in the brain will continue to titrate much of this large H+ ion load. Considering the limited content of $HCO_3^-$ ions in the brain and that the brain receives a relatively larger proportion of the cardiac output, there is a risk that more H+ ions will bind to proteins in brain cells, further compromising their functions. At usual rates of blood flow and metabolic work at rest, brachial venous $PCO_2$ is about 46 mm Hg, which is ~6 mm Hg greater than the arterial $PCO_2$. If the blood flow rate to the skeletal muscles declines owing to a low EABV, the brachial venous $PCO_2$ will be more than 6 mm Hg higher than the arterial $PCO_2$. Based on this analysis, and although experimental evidence to support this view is lacking, we recommend that in patients with metabolic acidosis, enough saline should be administered to increase the blood flow rate to muscle to restore the difference between the brachial venous $PCO_2$ and the arterial $PCO_2$ to its usual value of ~6 mm Hg.

## DISORDERS WITH A HIGH CONCENTRATION OF H+ IONS IN PLASMA

- There are two types of acid–base disorders (Flow Chart 2-1):
  - Metabolic acid–base disorders: the primary change is in the $P_{HCO_3}$
  - Respiratory acid–base disorders: the primary change is in the arterial $PCO_2$

If the concentration of H+ ions in plasma is higher (pH is lower) than normal values, the patient has acidemia. There are two potential primary disorders: metabolic acidosis or respiratory acidosis.

### Metabolic acidosis

Metabolic acidosis is a process that adds H+ ions to or removes $HCO_3^-$ ions from the body, which will lead to a decrease in the content of $HCO_3^-$ ions in the ECF compartment. An expected physiologic response to acidemia of metabolic origin is hyperventilation, which leads to a lower arterial $PCO_2$. The $P_{HCO_3}$ may be close to normal if there is a very contracted ECF volume, and hence there may be no changes in the arterial pH and $PCO_2$. Free-flowing brachial venous $PCO_2$, which best reflects the capillary blood $PCO_2$ in skeletal muscles, should be measured in patients with metabolic acidosis to assess the effectiveness of the BBS in removing the H+ ion load.

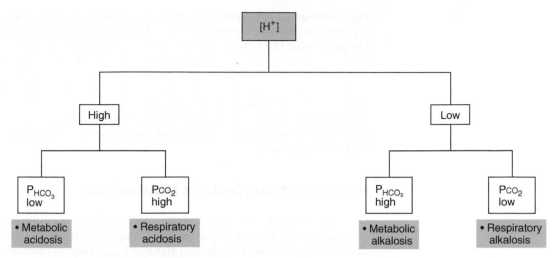

**Flow Chart 2-1  Initial Diagnosis of Acid–Base Disorders.** Start with the plasma [H⁺]. The final diagnoses are shown as statements headed by bullets below the boxes. However, if the ECF volume
is very contracted, a patient may have metabolic acidosis with a near normal $P_{HCO_3}$ and therefore
no appreciable acidemia.

## Respiratory acidosis

Respiratory acidosis is caused by impaired ventilation, and is characterized by a high arterial blood $PCO_2$ and [H⁺]. The expected physiologic response is an increase in $P_{HCO_3}$. The increase in $P_{HCO_3}$ is tiny
in patients with acute respiratory acidosis, because it reflects a shift
to the left in the bicarbonate buffer reaction (see Eqn 1). In patients
with chronic respiratory acidosis, there is a much larger increase in
$P_{HCO_3}$ due to the effect of associated intracellular acidosis in cells of
the proximal convoluted tubule (PCT) to stimulate ammoniagenesis,
which adds more $HCO_3^-$ ions to the body, and the effect of the high
peritubular $PCO_2$ to enhance $HCO_3^-$ ion reabsorption by the PCT.

$$H^+ + HCO_3^- \rightleftharpoons CO_2 + H_2O \qquad (1)$$

## DISORDERS WITH A LOW CONCENTRATION OF H⁺ IONS IN PLASMA

If the concentration of H⁺ in plasma is lower (pH is higher) than normal, the patient has alkalemia. Again, there are two potential primary
disorders: metabolic alkalosis or respiratory alkalosis.

## Metabolic alkalosis

This is a process that raises the $P_{HCO_3}$ and lowers the concentration of
H⁺ ions in the ECF compartment. The expected physiologic response
is hypoventilation and hence an increase in the arterial $PCO_2$; the rise
in $PCO_2$, however, is usually modest because of the effect of the resultant hypoxemia to stimulate ventilation.

## Respiratory alkalosis

Respiratory alkalosis is due to hyperventilation and is characterized by
low arterial $PCO_2$ and plasma [H⁺]. The expected physiologic response
is a reduction in the $P_{HCO_3}$. As in respiratory acidosis, this response
is modest in patients with acute respiratory alkalosis; it reflects the
effect of the low $PCO_2$ to shift the bicarbonate buffer reaction to the

right (see Eqn 1). In patients with chronic respiratory alkalosis, there is a more appreciable decrease in $P_{HCO_3}$ because of the effect of the low peritubular $PCO_2$ to decrease the reabsorption of $HCO_3^-$ ions by the PCT. However, the concentration of $H^+$ ions in plasma may not change appreciably if the patients has an acid-base disorder that tends to increase the concentration of $H^+$ ions in plasma, and a concomitant acid-base disorder, but one that tends to decrease the concentration of $H^+$ ions in plasma (e.g., chronic respiratory acidosis due to chronic obstructive airway disease and metabolic alkalosis due to the administration of diuretics).

## MAKING AN ACID–BASE DIAGNOSIS

One must integrate the clinical picture and the laboratory data to make a proper acid–base diagnosis. For example, the finding of acidemia, a high arterial $PCO_2$, and an elevated $P_{HCO_3}$ does not indicate that chronic respiratory acidosis is present if that patient does not have a chronic problem with ventilation; rather, the patient may have a metabolic alkalosis with an acute respiratory acidosis.

In addition to the parameters mentioned above commonly used in making an acid–base diagnosis, we use the hematocrit and/or total protein concentration in plasma to obtain a quantitative estimate of the ECF volume and calculate its content of $HCO_3^-$ ions, and the brachial venous $PCO_2$ to assess the effectiveness of the BBS in a patient with metabolic acidosis.

## LABORATORY TESTS USED IN A PATIENT WITH METABOLIC ACIDOSIS

In this section we provide the rationale for some of the laboratory tests that are used in the clinical approach to the patient with metabolic acidosis (Table 2-1). The specific questions to be addressed are shown in the table; the importance of each will become clear when the specific disorders are discussed in the following chapters.

### QUESTIONS TO ASK IN THE CLINICAL APPROACH TO THE PATIENT WITH METABOLIC ACIDOSIS

### Is the Content of $HCO_3^-$ Ions in the ECF Compartment Low?

Calculate the content of $HCO_3^-$ ions in the ECF compartment ($P_{HCO_3} \times$ ECF volume) if the ECF volume is appreciably low. The hematocrit or the concentration of total proteins in plasma are useful to obtain a quantitative estimate of the ECF volume (see margin note).

### Is There an Overproduction of Acids?

Overproduction of acids is detected by the appearance of new anions. The presence of new anions in plasma can be detected by a rise in the $P_{Anion\,gap}$. The presence of new anions in the urine can be detected by calculating the anion gap in the urine (see margin note); for this calculation, the concentration of $NH_4^+$ ions in the urine ($U_{NH_4}$) should be estimated using the calculations of the urine osmolal gap ($U_{Osmolal\,gap}$).

### Is the Metabolic Acidosis due to the Ingestion of Alcohols?

This is detected by calculation of the osmolal gap in plasma ($P_{Osmolal\,gap}$). A high $P_{Osmolal\,gap}$ indicates the presence of an unmeasured, uncharged

---

**USE OF THE HEMATOCRIT TO ESTIMATE THE ECF VOLUME**

- Blood volume in an adult subject is ~70 mL/kg body weight. Therefore, in a 70 kg subject, blood volume is close to 5 L, with a RBC volume of 2 L and a plasma volume of 3 L. The hematocrit (the ratio of RBC volume to blood volume) is 0.40. When the hematocrit is 0.50, and assuming no change in RBC volume, the new plasma volume can be calculated as follows:

   $0.50 =$ RBC (2 L)/blood volume (X L)

   $X = 4$ L

   $\therefore$ Plasma volume = blood volume (4 L) – RBC volume (2 L) = 2 L

- Therefore, the plasma volume is reduced by one-third. Ignoring changes in Starling forces for simplicity (see following margin note), the ECF volume has decreased to approximately two-thirds of its normal volume.

**STARLING FORCES**

Starling forces determine the distribution of volume between the intravascular and the extravascular or interstitial compartment of the ECF volume. The higher colloid osmotic pressure in plasma helps defend the plasma volume at the expense of the interstitial fluid volume. Hence, the degree of ECF volume contraction is even higher than that estimated from the calculated reduction in plasma volume.

**URINE ANION GAP**

To detect new anions in the urine, we use the formula:
$U_{Na} + U_K + U_{NH_4} - U_{Cl}$

TABLE 2-1   **TOOLS USED IN THE CLINICAL APPROACH TO PATIENTS WITH METABOLIC ACIDOSIS**

| QUESTION | PARAMETER ASSESSED | TOOLS TO USE |
|---|---|---|
| • Is the content of $HCO_3^-$ ions low in the ECF? | • ECF volume | • Hematocrit or total plasma proteins |
| • Is metabolic acidosis due to overproduction of acids? <br> • Is metabolic acidosis due to ingestion of alcohol? | • Appearance of new anions in the body or the urine <br> • Detect alcohols as unmeasured osmoles | • $P_{Anion\ gap}$ <br> • Urine anion gap <br> • $P_{Osmolal\ gap}$ |
| • Is buffering of $H^+$ ions by BBS in skeletal muscle? | • Buffering of $H^+$ ions by $HCO_3^-$ ions in muscle interstitial fluid and in its intracellular fluid compartment | • Brachial venous $PCO_2$ |
| • Is the renal response to chronic acidemia adequate? | • Examine the rate of excretion of $NH_4^+$ ions in the urine | • $U_{Osmolal\ gap}$ |
| • If $NH_4^+$ ion excretion is high, which anion is excreted with $NH_4^+$ ions? | • Gastrointestinal loss of $NaHCO_3$ <br> • Acid added, but the anions are excreted in the urine with $NH_4^+$ ions | • Urine $Cl^-$ <br> • Urine anion gap |
| • What is the basis for a low excretion of $NH_4^+$ ions? | • Low distal $H^+$ ion secretion <br> • Low $NH_3$ availability <br> • Both defects | • Urine pH > 7.0 <br> • Urine pH ~ 5.0 <br> • Urine pH ~ 6.0 |
| • Where is the defect in $H^+$ ion secretion? | • Distal $H^+$ ion secretion <br> • Proximal $H^+$ ion secretion | • $PCO_2$ in alkaline urine <br> • $FE_{HCO_3}$, $U_{Citrate}$ |

compound in plasma. In clinical practice, this calculation is helpful to detect the presence of alcohols (e.g., ethanol, ethylene glycol, methanol, isopropyl alcohol) in plasma.

### Is Buffering of the $H^+$ Ion Load by BBS in Skeletal Muscle?

To make this assessment, we measure the brachial venous $PCO_2$. A value that is more than 6 mm Hg higher than the arterial $PCO_2$ indicates that the $PCO_2$ in the interstitial space and cells of skeletal muscle is high, and therefore the BBS in skeletal muscle is ineffective in removing the $H^+$ ion load.

### In a Patient with Chronic Hyperchloremic Metabolic Acidosis (HCMA), Is the Rate of Excretion of $NH_4^+$ Ions High Enough So That the Kidneys Are Not the Sole Cause of Acidosis?

The $U_{Osmolal\ gap}$ is the best indirect test to estimate the $U_{NH_4}$. To convert the $U_{NH_4}$ in a spot urine sample into a 24-hour excretion rate, divide $U_{NH4}$ by the concentration of creatinine in the urine ($U_{Creatinine}$) and multiply the $U_{NH_4}/U_{Creatinine}$ ratio by an estimate of the rate of creatinine excretion over a 24-hour period (20 mg or 0.2 mmol per kg body weight). A low rate of excretion of $NH_4^+$ ions is the hallmark of a group of diseases called renal tubular acidosis.

### If the Rate of Excretion of $NH_4^+$ Ions Is High, What Is the Anion Excreted with $NH_4^+$ Ions in the Urine?

If the anion is $Cl^-$ ions, the cause of the metabolic acidosis is usually loss of $NaHCO_3$ via the gastrointestinal tract (e.g., diarrhea). In contrast, if the anion is not Cl ions, the cause of metabolic acidosis is overproduction of an organic acid with a high rate of excretion of its anion in the urine (e.g., hippuric acid in the patient with glue sniffing; see Chapter 3).

### If the Rate of Excretion of $NH_4^+$ Ions Is Low, What Is the Basis for the Low $NH_4^+$ Ion Excretion Rate?

The urine pH is helpful to identify the pathophysiology of the low rate of excretion of $NH_4^+$ ions. If the urine pH is greater than 6.5, the low rate of excretion of $NH_4^+$ ions is due to a reduced net rate of $H^+$ ion

**ABBREVIATIONS**

HCMA, hyperchloremic metabolic acidosis

$FE_{HCO_3}$, fractional excretion of $HCO_3^-$ ions

$U_{Citrate}$, concentration of citrate in the urine

$P_{Osmolal\ gap}$, osmolal gap in plasma

$P_{Osm}$, plasma osmolality

$U_{NH_4}$, concentration of $NH_4^+$ ions in the urine

$U_{Na}$, concentration of sodium ions in the urine

$U_K$, concentration of potassium ions in the urine

$U_{Cl}$, concentration of chloride ions in the urine

$U_{Osm}$, urine osmolality

$U_{Osmolal\ gap}$, osmolal gap in the urine

$U_{Creatinine}$, concentration of creatinine in the urine

secretion in the distal nephron. To determine the basis of this lesion, measure the $PCO_2$ in alkaline urine. If the urine pH is close to 5, the low rate of excretion of $NH_4^+$ ions is usually due to a disease leading to a diminished production of $NH_4^+$ ions. On the other hand, if urine pH is close to 6, that diminishes the availability of both $H^+$ ions and $NH_3$ in the lumen of the distal nephron (see Chapter 4 for further discussion).

### Is There a Defect in $H^+$ Ion Secretion in the Proximal Tubule?

A fractional excretion of $HCO_3^-$ ($FE_{HCO3}$) that is greater than 15% after giving an $NaHCO_3$ load that raises the $P_{HCO_3}$ to close to 24 mmol/L indicates a defect in $H^+$ ion secretion in the PCT.

A high rate of excretion of citrate anions in these patients could be due to an alkaline PCT cell pH (see Chapter 4 for further discussion) or a component of a generalized PCT cell dysfunction (i.e., Fanconi syndrome).

## LABORATORY TESTS

### 1. The anion gap in plasma

- The anion gap in plasma ($P_{Anion\ gap}$), calculated as ($P_{Na} - [P_{Cl} + P_{HCO_3}]$), is helpful to detect metabolic acidosis because of the gain of acids if the anion of the added acid is largely retained in plasma.
- Because of differences in laboratory measurements, there is a large difference among laboratories in the normal mean value of $P_{Anion\ gap}$. In addition, there is a wide range in what is considered normal $P_{Anion\ gap}$.
- The $P_{Anion\ gap}$ reflects the net anionic valence on plasma albumin. Hence, the normal baseline value should be adjusted for the concentration of albumin in plasma ($P_{Albumin}$).

Accumulation of acids ($H^+ + A^-$) in the ECF compartment will result in the loss of $HCO_3^-$ ions and the gain of new anions ($A^-$). These new anions can be detected by their electrical presence, because electroneutrality must be maintained, and hence the sum of all cations and the sum of all anions in plasma must be equal. For convenience, however, one does not need to measure the concentrations of all the cations and all the anions in plasma but rather that of the major cation in plasma—sodium ($Na^+$) ions—and the major anions in plasma— chloride ($Cl^-$) and $HCO_3^-$ ions. Although other cations and anions in plasma are ignored in this calculation, this does not pose a problem for clinical purposes, either because their concentrations are relatively low (e.g., $Ca^{2+}$, $Mg^{2+}$, $HPO_4^{2-}$, $SO_4^{2-}$ ions) or do not vary substantially (e.g., $K^+$ ions).

The term $P_{Anion\ gap}$ is used for the difference between the plasma concentration of $Na^+$ ions and the concentrations of $Cl^-$ and $HCO_3^-$ ions in plasma, which reflect the usual excess of the other unmeasured anions in plasma over that of the other unmeasured cations in plasma. This difference is largely due to the net anionic valence on plasma proteins, principally plasma albumin. If the difference is larger than the normal value of $P_{Anion\ gap}$, then other anions are present in plasma. Of note, however, because of differences in laboratory methods (e.g., measurement of $P_{Cl}$), there is a large difference in the mean value for the $P_{Anion\ gap}$ reported by clinical laboratories. Furthermore, regardless of the laboratory method used, there is a wide range within the normal values of the $P_{Anion\ gap}$. Although it is imperative that the clinician knows the normal values of the $P_{Anion\ gap}$ for his/her clinical laboratory, it would be difficult to know what is the individual patient baseline $P_{Anion\ gap}$ within the wide range of normal values (see margin note).

**NORMAL VALUE OF PLASMA ANION GAP**

• We will use a normal value of $P_{Anion\ gap}$ of 12 mEq/L for illustrative purposes.

### An example

Consider the following example, in which 10 mmol of L-lactic acid is added to each liter of ECF volume. L-lactic acid dissociates into $H^+$ ions and L-lactate anions in the ECF compartment, and $H^+$ ions are removed virtually exclusively by reacting with $HCO_3^-$ ions, leaving L-lactate anions as the footprint of the L-lactic acid that was added to the ECF compartment. For simplicity, events in cells are ignored and we assume that there was no change in ECF volume (Figure 2-1).

| PLASMA (mEq/L) | $P_{Na}$ | $P_{Cl}$ | $P_{HCO_3}$ | $P_{Anion\ gap}$ |
|---|---|---|---|---|
| Normal | 140 | 103 | 25 | 12 |
| L-Lactic acid (10 mmol/L) | 140 | 103 | 15 (= 25 − 10) | 22 (= 12 + 10) |

The patient has a normal baseline value of the $P_{Anion\ gap}$ of 12 mEq/L $(140 - [103 + 25])$ at the start. With the addition of 10 mmol of L-lactic acid to each liter of ECF volume, $H^+$ ions react with $HCO_3^-$ anions; therefore, there is a decrease in $P_{HCO_3}$ from 25 mmol/L to 15 mmol/L. Meanwhile, because 10 mmol of L-lactate anions are added to each liter of the ECF volume, there is an increase in $P_{Anion\ gap}$ from its baseline value of 12 mEq/L to 22 mEq/L $(140 - [103 + 15])$. This is best thought of as the increment over the normal baseline $P_{Anion\ gap}$ (i.e., 12 + 10 mEq/L), because this forces one to think of the normal value for the $P_{Anion\ gap}$ and to ask whether there is any reason for the patient not to have a normal baseline $P_{Anion\ gap}$ (e.g., hypoalbuminemia).

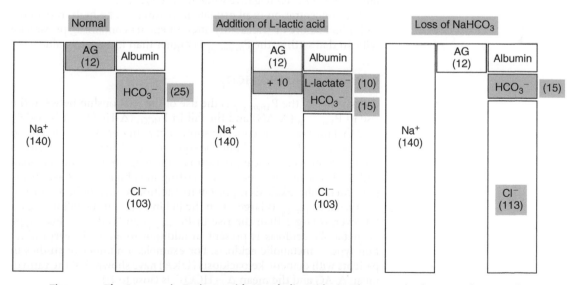

**Figure 2-1 The $P_{Anion\ gap}$ in Patients with Metabolic Acidosis.** The normal values are shown in the left portion of the figure; the $P_{Anion\ gap}$ is the shaded area between the cation (*left*) and the anions (*right*) columns. When L-lactic acid is added (*middle*), the $P_{HCO_3}$ falls, and the $HCO_3^-$ anions are replaced with the L-lactate$^-$ anions such that the rise in the $P_{Anion\ gap}$ equals the fall in the $P_{HCO_3}$. A loss of $NaHCO_3$ is depicted in the right portion of the figure. Note that the $P_{HCO_3}$ fell from 25 mmol/L to 15 mmol/L, but no new anions were added. The rise in the $P_{Cl}$ from 103 mmol/L to 113 mmol/L reflects how electroneutrality is achieved. *AG*, Anion gap.

If the increase in $P_{Anion\ gap}$ was the same as in the preceding example, but the concentration of L-lactate$^-$ anions in plasma was only 5 mmol/L, L-lactic acidosis would not be the sole cause of the metabolic acidosis: the patient must have also accumulated unmeasured anions of other acids (e.g., ketoacid anions).

### Pitfalls in the use of the plasma anion gap

#### Issues related to $P_{Albumin}$

There are two pitfalls related to the $P_{Albumin}$. First, in some clinical situations, the $P_{Albumin}$ can be low (e.g., cirrhosis of the liver, malnutrition, or the nephrotic syndrome), whereas in others, the $P_{Albumin}$ can be high (e.g., a patient with a very contracted ECF volume). Hence, the baseline value for the $P_{Anion\ gap}$ must be adjusted for the $P_{Albumin}$. A rough guide for correcting the baseline value of the $P_{Anion\ gap}$ for the $P_{Albumin}$ is that for every 1.0 g/dL (10-g/L) decrease in $P_{Albumin}$, the $P_{Anion\ gap}$ is lower by 2.5 mEq/L. The converse is true for a rise in the $P_{Albumin}$.

The second point is that the valence or net anionic charge on $P_{Albumin}$ (or total plasma proteins) is not constant. For example, when the EABV is low, the $P_{Anion\ gap}$ increases. This rise in the $P_{Anion\ gap}$ is not explained by a gain of new anions, a change in plasma pH, or a change in $P_{Albumin}$; rather, it appears that the valence on $P_{Albumin}$ becomes more negative (see margin note).

#### Issues related to other cations and anions

Some patients with multiple myeloma have cationic proteins present in plasma that cause the $P_{Anion\ gap}$ to be lower. Usually Cl$^-$ anions balance the valence of these unmeasured cations.

The $P_{Cl}$ is overestimated in patients with bromide ingestion, leading to a low or even negative value for the $P_{Anion\ gap}$.

The concentration of phosphate in plasma can be high in patients with renal failure or transiently after an enema containing phosphate salts. In that setting, the $P_{Anion\ gap}$ is higher than its normal value.

### Delta anion gap/delta $HCO_3^-$

A derivative of the $P_{Anion\ gap}$ is the use of the relationship between the rise in $P_{Anion\ gap}$ ($\Delta$-AG) and the fall in $P_{HCO_3}$ ($\Delta$-$HCO_3$). It is widely held that the rise in the concentration of new anions, as reflected by an increase in the $P_{Anion\ gap}$, should be equal to the fall in the $P_{HCO_3}$. This is thought to provide a means to estimate the magnitude of the acid load and to detect the presence of coexisting metabolic acid–base disorders. Metabolic alkalosis is present in addition to metabolic acidosis if the rise in $P_{Anion\ gap}$ is larger than the fall in $P_{HCO_3}$. If the fall in $P_{HCO_3}$, however, is larger than the rise in $P_{Anion\ gap}$, an "NaHCO$_3$ loss" type of metabolic acidosis is present in addition to an acid overproduction type of metabolic acidosis. For example, a number of studies in patients with diabetic ketoacidosis (DKA) have shown that the ratio of mean $\Delta$-AG and the mean $\Delta - HCO_3^-$ is close to 1:1.

In addition to the pitfalls mentioned above and because in many cases one does not know what the baseline value of the $P_{Anion\ gap}$ or $P_{HCO_3}$ is in a particular patient because of the wide range of normal values (between 22-30 mmol/L), another caveat in using the $\Delta\,AG/\,\Delta\,HCO_3^-$ to gauge the magnitude of the acid load is failure to adjust for changes in the ECF volume. Consider, for example, a patient with DKA who has a $P_{HCO_3}$ of 10 mmol/L, and the expected

TABLE 2-2    **QUANTITATIVE DESCRIPTION OF THE FALL IN THE $P_{HCO_3}$ AND RISE IN THE $P_{Anion\ gap}$ IN PATIENTS WITH DIABETIC KETOACIDOSIS (DKA)***

| CONDITION | ECF VOLUME | $HCO_3^-$ Ions | | Ketoacid Anions | |
|---|---|---|---|---|---|
| | | CONCENTRATION (mmol/L) | CONTENT (mmol) | CONCENTRATION (mmol/L) | CONTENT (mmol) |
| Normal | 10 L | 25 | 250 | 0 | 0 |
| DKA | 7 L | 10 | 70 | 15 | 105 |
| Balance | −3 L | | −180 | | +105 |

*For simplicity, we ignored changes in the $P_{Anion\ gap}$ due to changes in the $P_{Albumin}$ in these calculations.

1:1 relationship between the rise in $P_{Anion\ gap}$ and the fall in the $P_{HCO_3}$ (Table 2-2). The patient had a normal ECF volume of 10 L before he developed DKA, but as a result of the glucose-induced osmotic diuresis and natruresis, his current ECF volume is only 7 L. Although the fall in the $P_{HCO_3}$ and the rise in the concentration of ketoacid anions are equal, the deficit of $HCO_3^-$ ions and the amount of ketoacids added to the ECF compartment are not. The sum of the content of $HCO_3^-$ ions and ketoacid anions in the ECF compartment prior to the patient developing DKA is 250 mmol ((25 + 0 mmol/L) × 10 L). Their sum, however, in the ECF compartment after the patient developed DKA is only 175 mmol ((10 + 15 mmol/L) × 7 L). The deficit of $HCO_3^-$ ions in this example is 180 mmol, but the quantity of new anions in the ECF is only 105 mmol. This is because there was another component of the loss of $HCO_3^-$ ions that occurred when ketoacids were added and some of the ketoacid anions were excreted in the urine with $Na^+$ and/or $K^+$ ions: an indirect form of $NaHCO_3$ loss, which is not reflected as an increase in the $P_{Anion\ gap}$. Hence, the rise in the $P_{Anion\ gap}$ did not reveal the actual quantity of ketoacids added, and the fall in $P_{HCO_3}$ did not reflect the actual magnitude of the deficit of $HCO_3^-$ ions. With expansion of the ECF volume with the administration of saline, the degree of $HCO_3^-$ ion deficit will become evident, as the fall in the $P_{Anion\ gap}$ will not be matched by an equal rise in the $P_{HCO_3}$.

## 2. The osmolal gap in plasma

The osmotic pressure of a solution is directly related to the concentration of its dissolved solutes. Hence, a molecule of protein, glucose, or $Na^+$ ions makes a virtually equal contribution to the osmotic pressure of a solution even though they vary greatly in their molecular weight. Because $Na^+$ ions are the major cation in plasma and the number of cations and anions in plasma must be equal, the value of $2 \times P_{Na}$ accounts for the vast majority of the osmotic pressure because of cations plus anions in plasma. Glucose and urea are the two major nonionized molecules in plasma that are likely to change significantly in their concentrations. Hence, the calculated plasma osmolality is $2\,(P_{Na}) + P_{Glucose} + P_{Urea}$ (where $P_{Glucose}$ and $P_{Urea}$ are in mmol/L) (see Table 2-3 for conversion of concentrations in mg/dL to mmol/L). The difference between the measured and the calculated plasma osmolality is the $P_{Osmolal\ gap}$. A value of the $P_{Osmolal\ gap}$ of up to 10 mosmol/kg $H_2O$ is considered to be normal (see margin note).

A high $P_{Osmolal\ gap}$ indicates the presence of an unmeasured, uncharged compound in plasma. In clinical practice, this calculation is helpful to detect the presence of alcohols (e.g., ethanol, ethylene glycol, methanol, isopropyl alcohol) in plasma. Ingestion of alcohols causes a large increase in $P_{Osmolal\ gap}$ because they are uncharged compounds, their molecular weights are low, and usually a large amount is ingested.

**OFFSETTING ERRORS IN THE CALCULATION OF THE PLASMA OSMOLAL GAP**

- One should recognize that the calculation of plasma osmolality does not include the concentrations of $K^+$, $Ca^{2+}$, and $Mg^{2+}$ ions in plasma and their accompanying anions; therefore, it underestimates the $P_{Osm}$.
- When the $P_{Na}$ is multiplied by 2, an offsetting error is introduced because some of the anions are multivalent (e.g., the number of charges attributable to $P_{Albumin}$ is ~16 mEq/L, but it represents < 1 mosmol/L).
- The $P_{Osmolal\ gap}$ will be overestimated if there is a laboratory error with the measurement of $P_{Na}$ (e.g., pseudohyponatremia due to hyperlipidemia or hyperproteinemia if the method used to measure $Na^+$ requires dilution of plasma). Hence, the calculated $P_{Osm}$ will be lower than the measured $P_{Osm}$.

TABLE 2-3    **CONVERSION BETWEEN mg/dL AND mmol/L***

| CONSTITUENT | MOLECULAR WEIGHT | mg/dL | mmol/L |
|---|---|---|---|
| Glucose | 180 | 90 | 5 |
| Urea | 60 | 30 | 5 |
| Urea nitrogen | 28 ($2 \times 14$) | 14 | 5 |

*To convert mg/dL to mmol/L, multiply mg/dL by 10, and then divide by the molecular weight.

### 3. Tests used to estimate the rate of excretion of $NH_4^+$ ions

Because most clinical laboratories do not routinely measure $U_{NH_4}$, clinicians must use indirect tests to estimate its rate of excretion in a patient with metabolic acidosis. Although these tests provide only semiquantitative estimates of the rate of excretion of $NH_4^+$ ions, this is adequate in most clinical settings with metabolic acidosis. This is because the information needed in a patient with chronic metabolic acidosis is whether the rate of $NH_4^+$ ion excretion is low enough to be the sole cause of acidosis or it is sufficiently high that another cause of the metabolic acidosis should be sought. Normal subjects consuming a typical Western diet excrete 30 to 40 mmol of $NH_4^+$ ions per day, whereas normal subjects who are given a large acid load for several days increase their rate of excretion of $NH_4^+$ ions to greater than 200 mmol/day. Therefore, in a patient with chronic metabolic acidosis and normal renal function, the expected rate of $NH_4^+$ ion excretion is greater than 200 mmol/day. If a patient has chronic HCMA, and the rate of $NH_4^+$ ion excretion is less than 40 mmol/day, a defect in the process of renal excretion of $NH_4^+$ ions is likely to be the sole cause of the metabolic acidosis—that is, renal tubular acidosis (RTA) (Flow Chart 2-2). In contrast, if the rate of excretion of $NH_4^+$ ions is about 100 mmol/day, although there is a renal component to the metabolic acidosis because the rate of excretion of $NH_4^+$ ions is lower than expected, the renal defect is not the sole cause of acidosis. One must look for another cause for the metabolic acidosis, such as loss of $NaHCO_3$ via the gastrointestinal tract or the addition of an acid with the excretion of its accompanying anion in the urine (e.g., hippuric acid in the patient with glue sniffing, with excretion of the anion hippurate in the urine with $Na^+$ or $K^+$ ions).

### *The urine net charge*

The premise of this test is that if the $U_{Cl}$ is appreciably greater than the $U_{Na} + U_K$, there is a high concentration of another cation (i.e., $NH_4^+$ ions) in the urine.

There are two issues in using the urine net charge to estimate the rate of excretion of $NH_4^+$ ions that diminish its utility. First, the calculation of the urine net charge to detect $NH_4^+$ ions is correct only if the anion that accompanies $NH_4^+$ ions in the urine is $Cl^-$ ions. For example, in a patient with diarrhea and HCMA due to loss of $NaHCO_3$, $NH_4^+$ ions are excreted in the urine with $Cl^-$ anions. Second, as shown in Equation 2, this calculation is based on a difference between the concentrations of unmeasured anions and cations in the urine that is assumed to be a constant value of 80 mEq. Therefore, if $U_{Na} + U_K$ exceeds $U_{Cl}$, one assumes that $U_{NH_4}$ is greater than 80 mEq, and hence renal tubular acidosis is not the cause of the metabolic acidosis in this patient because this rate of excretion of $NH_4^+$ ions even exceeds its usual rate of excretion in subjects consuming a typical Western diet. This, however, is not necessarily true for two reasons. First, this constant of 80 mEq is based on a urine volume of 1 L/day. Second, the rate of excretion of these unmeasured anions varies considerably depending on dietary intake. Therefore, we do not rely on the calculation of the urine net charge to obtain a reliable estimate of the rate of excretion of $NH_4^+$.

$$U_{NH_4} = (U_{Na} + U_K) - (U_{Cl} + 80) \qquad (2)$$

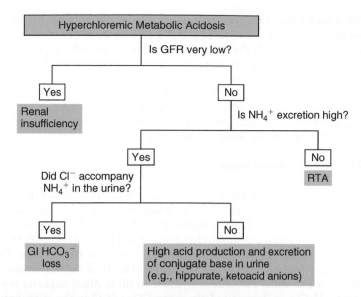

**Flow Chart 2-2 Steps in the Clinical Approach to Patients with Hyperchloremic Metabolic Acidosis Based on Evaluating the Rate of Excretion of $NH_4^+$ Ions.** We emphasize that this approach is used in patients with chronic hyperchloremic metabolic acidosis. The purpose of assessing the rate of excretion of $NH_4^+$ ions is to determine if it is high enough to suggest that a disorder of renal tubular acidosis is not the cause of acidosis. *GFR*, Glomerular filtration rate; *GI*, gastrointestinal; *RTA*, renal tubular acidosis.

### The urine osmolal gap

The $U_{Osmolal\ gap}$ is the best indirect test to assess the rate of excretion of $NH_4^+$ ions because it detects $NH_4^+$ ions in the urine regardless of the anion with which they are excreted. We emphasize that this calculation is used in patients with metabolic acidosis with the purpose of assessing if the rate of excretion of $NH_4^+$ ions is high enough to suggest that a disorder of renal tubular acidosis is not the sole cause of acidosis. The formula for the $U_{Osmolal\ gap}$ is shown in Equations 3 through 5; in these equations, all values are in mmol/L. The only difficulty in this calculation is that one must measure the concentration of urea and sometimes that of glucose in the urine. The test is unreliable to assess the rate of excretion of $NH_4^+$ ions if other osmoles, such as ethanol, methanol, ethylene glycol, or mannitol, are present in the urine. To estimate the concentration of $NH_4^+$ ions, divide the $U_{Osmolal\ gap}$ by 2, because the anions excreted in the urine with $NH_4^+$ ions are mainly monovalent. To estimate the rate of excretion of $NH_4^+$ ions, calculate the ratio of the $U_{NH_4}/U_{Creatinine}$, and multiply this ratio by the estimated rate of excretion of creatinine in this patient (see margin note).

$$U_{Osmolal\ gap} = \text{Measured } U_{Osm} - \text{Calculated } U_{Osm} \quad (3)$$

$$\text{Calculated } U_{Osm} = 2\ (U_{Na} + U_K) + U_{Glucose} + U_{Urea} \quad (4)$$

$$U_{NH4} = U_{Osmolal\ gap}\ /\ 2 \quad (5)$$

### 4. Tests used to evaluate the basis for a low rate of excretion of $NH_4^+$ ions

#### The urine pH

The urine pH is not a reliable indicator for the rate of excretion of $NH_4^+$ ions. For example, at a urine pH of 6.0, the $U_{NH_4}$ can be 20 or

**CREATININE EXCRETION**

- In normal subjects, this is approximately:
  - 20 mg/kg body weight/day
  - 0.2 mmol/kg body weight/day
- Body weight in this calculation is the lean body weight. Hence, this estimate of the rate of excretion of creatinine could have a large error in obese subjects or in cachectic patients with marked muscle wasting.

200 mmol/L (see Chapter 1, Fig. 1-17). On the other hand, the basis for the low rate of excretion of $NH_4^+$ ions may be deduced from the urine pH. A urine pH that is ~5 suggests that the basis for a low rate of excretion of $NH_4^+$ ions is primarily due to a decreased availability of $NH_3$ in the medullary interstitial compartment because of a low rate of production of $NH_4^+$ ions. On the other hand, urine pH that is > 7.0 suggests that $NH_4^+$ excretion is low because there is a defect in net $H^+$ ion secretion in the distal nephron. Both of these groups of disorders are discussed in more detail in Chapter 4.

### The $PCO_2$ in alkaline urine

The $PCO_2$ in alkaline urine is used to assess net $H^+$ ion secretion in the distal nephron in a patient with a low rate of $NH_4^+$ ion excretion and a urine pH > 7.0. The test begins after enough $NaHCO_3$ is administered to achieve a second-voided urine with a pH that is greater than 7.0 (see margin note). The secretion of $H^+$ ions (or $HCO_3^-$ ions) by the collecting duct leads to the formation of luminal $H_2CO_3$. Because there is no luminal carbonic anhydrase in these distal nephron segments, $H_2CO_3$ is dehydrated slowly to $CO_2 + H_2O$ in the medullary collecting duct and in the lower urinary collecting system. The result is a urine $PCO_2$ that is considerably greater than the blood $PCO_2$ (Figure 2-2).

The patient with normal secretion of $H^+$ ions in the collecting ducts should have a $PCO_2$ in alkaline urine that is close to 70 mm Hg. One caveat, however, is that the urine $PCO_2$ may be low despite a normal rate of distal secretion of $H^+$ ions if there is a major defect in renal concentrating ability. Patients with a defect in distal secretion of $H^+$ ions have a $PCO_2$ in alkaline urine that is close to that of their blood. In contrast, the $PCO_2$ in alkaline urine is high if there is back leak of $H^+$ ions in the distal nephron (e.g., because of drugs such as amphotericin B) or in patients with disorders in which $HCO_3^-$ ions are secreted in the distal nephron (e.g., some patients with Southeast Asian ovalocytosis; see margin note and Case 4-2 for further discussion).

**CAUTION**

- The patient with a low $P_K$ is at risk of developing a more severe degree of hypokalemia and perhaps a cardiac arrhythmia if given $NaHCO_3$. Hence, the $K^+$ ion deficit must be corrected before this test is performed.

**HIGH URINE $PCO_2$ IN PATIENTS WITH RTA BECAUSE OF DISTAL SECRETION OF $HCO_3^-$ IONS**

- When $HCO_3^-$ ions are secreted in the distal nephron, the luminal pH rises and $H^+$ ions are released from $H_2PO_4^-$ ions. Because these $H^+$ ions react with luminal $HCO_3^-$ ions, $CO_2$ is formed. Hence, $PCO_2$ in alkaline urine will be high.
- An example of this pathophysiology is some patients with Southeast Asian ovalocytosis who have a second mutation in the gene encoding for the $Cl^-/HCO_3^-$ anion exchanger that causes it to be mistargeted to the luminal membrane of intercalated cells in the collecting ducts.

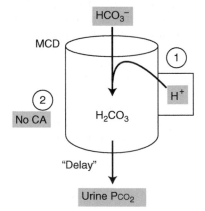

**Figure 2-2 The Basis for an Increased $PCO_2$ in Alkaline Urine.** When $NaHCO_3$ is given, there is a large delivery of $HCO_3^-$ ions to the distal nephron, which makes $HCO_3^-$ ions virtually the only $H^+$ ion acceptor in its lumen. Because there is no luminal carbonic anhydrase (CA), the $H_2CO_3$ formed is delivered downstream and forms $CO_2$ plus $H_2O$. Thus, if the urine $PCO_2$ is not appreciably higher than the plasma $PCO_2$, this provides evidence for impaired distal $H^+$ ion secretion. The urine $PCO_2$ can be high despite decreased net distal $H^+$ ion secretion if there is $H^+$ ion back-leak or secretion of $HCO_3^-$ ions in the distal nephron. *MCD*, Medullary collecting duct.

### The fractional excretion of $HCO_3^-$

The fractional excretion of $HCO_3^-$ ions is used to examine net $H^+$ ion secretion in PCT. In this test, $NaHCO_3$ is given to raise the $P_{HCO_3}$ to the normal range so that one can measure the rate of excretion of $HCO_3^-$ ions and compare it with the filtered load of $HCO_3^-$ ions (see Eqn 6; margin note). If more than 15% of filtered $HCO_3^-$ ions is excreted, there is a defect in proximal reabsorption of $HCO_3$ ions. This test is not usually needed in our opinion. These patients will be detected clinically by failure to correct their metabolic acidosis despite being given large amounts of $NaHCO_3$, as $HCO_3^-$ ions will be spilled in the urine, once the $P_{HCO_3}$ rises and the filtered load of $HCO_3^-$ ions exceeds the capacity for its reabsorption in PCT. Hypokalemia must be corrected first before the administration of $NaHCO_3$, because of the risk of worsening hypokalemia causing cardiac arrhythmia.

$$FE_{HCO_3} = (U_{HCO_3}/P_{HCO_3}) / (U_{creatinine}/P_{creatinine}) \times 100 \qquad (6)$$

### Rate of citrate excretion

The rate of excretion of citrate anions is a marker of pH in cells of the PCT. The daily rate of excretion of citrate anions in children and adults consuming their usual diet is ~400 mg/day (~2.1 mmol/day). The rate of excretion of citrate anions is very low in patients with metabolic acidosis. A notable exception, however, is patients with metabolic acidosis due to disorders causing an alkaline PCT cell pH, in whom the rate of excretion of citrate anions is not low (see Chapter 4).

**CALCULATION OF FRACTIONAL EXCRETION OF $HCO_3^-$**

- For this calculation, convert $P_{Creatinine}$ from mg/dL or μmol/L to mmol/L
- To convert $P_{Creatinine}$ from mg/dL to μmol/L, multiply by 88
- To convert $P_{Creatinine}$ from μmol/L to mmol/L, divide by 1000

# PART B
# IDENTIFYING MIXED ACID–BASE DISORDERS

## EXPECTED RESPONSES TO PRIMARY ACID–BASE DISORDERS

It has been observed that when a patient has one of the four primary acid–base disturbances, a predictable response occurs to return the plasma pH (($[H^+]$) in plasma) toward the normal range (Table 2-4). Only in chronic respiratory alkalosis might the plasma pH actually return to the normal range as a result of the expected renal response to lower the $P_{HCO_3}$. These expected values are largely empirical but are clinically helpful to determine whether more than one acid–base disorder is present in a patient, which may have both diagnostic and therapeutic implications. For example, if the $PCO_2$ is appreciably higher than expected in a patient with metabolic acidosis (i.e., the patient has a metabolic acidosis and concomitant respiratory acidosis), a cause of decreased ventilation (e.g., intake of drugs that suppress the respiratory center, respiratory muscle weakness due to hypokalemia) needs to be sought. Furthermore, the leverage in treatment, if severe acidemia is present, may be intubation and ventilation rather than the administration of alkali. On the other hand, if the arterial $PCO_2$ is appreciably lower than expected in a patient with metabolic acidosis (i.e., the patient has a metabolic acidosis and concomitant respiratory alkalosis), a cause of stimulation of ventilation (e.g., pneumonia, pulmonary embolism, aspirin overdose) must be sought. Clearly, making

TABLE 2-4   **EXPECTED RESPONSES TO PRIMARY ACID–BASE DISORDERS**

| DISORDER | EXPECTED CHANGE |
|---|---|
| **Metabolic acidosis** | For every mmol/L fall in $P_{HCO_3}$ from 25, the arterial $PCO_2$ falls by ~1 mm Hg from 40. |
| **Metabolic alkalosis** | For every mmol/L rise in $P_{HCO_3}$ from 25, the arterial $PCO_2$ rises by ~0.7 mm Hg from 40. |
| **Respiratory Acidosis** | |
| Acute | For every mm Hg rise in the arterial $PCO_2$ from 40, the plasma [$H^+$] rises by ~0.8 nmol/L from 40. |
| Chronic | For every mm Hg rise in arterial $PCO_2$ from 40, the plasma [$H^+$] rises by ~0.3 nmol/L from 40 and the $P_{HCO_3}$ rises by ~0.3 mmol/L from 25. |
| **Respiratory Alkalosis** | |
| Acute | For every mm Hg fall in arterial $PCO_2$ from 40, the plasma [$H^+$] falls by ~0.8 nmol/L from 40. |
| Chronic | For every mm Hg fall in arterial $PCO_2$ from 40, the $P_{HCO_3}$ falls by ~0.5 mmol/L from 25. |

such a diagnosis will have important implications for the management of these patients.

## HOW TO RECOGNIZE MIXED ACID–BASE DISORDERS

### EVALUATE THE ACCURACY OF THE LABORATORY DATA

There are two ways to detect laboratory errors in the measured values for acid–base parameters. The first way is to calculate the $P_{Anion\ gap}$. If it is very low or negative, there is probably an error in one of the electrolyte values, unless the patient has multiple myeloma (presence of a cationic paraprotein), has ingested bromide salts (bromide ions are measured as chloride by many laboratory methods, and furthermore, each bromide ion reacts as three or more chloride ions), has salicylate intoxication (high salicylate levels increase the permeability of certain ion selective electrodes used for measurement of $Cl^-$, resulting in falsely high $P_{Cl}$), or has a very low $P_{Albumin}$.

The second way to evaluate the laboratory results is to insert the arterial [$H^+$], $PCO_2$, and measured venous $P_{HCO_3}$ into the Henderson equation (see margin note). Of note, however, the $P_{HCO_3}$ measured in venous blood can be as much as 5 to 6 mmol/L higher than the arterial $P_{HCO_3}$. This may be the case, for example, under conditions of low cardiac output, when most of the oxygen delivered to an organ is extracted from its arterial blood; therefore, there is a large addition of $CO_2$ (and $HCO_3^-$ ions) to each liter of capillary blood. If the discrepancy is large enough to change the diagnosis, the test should be repeated and the error identified.

### CALCULATE THE $HCO_3^-$ ION CONTENT IN THE ECF VOLUME

This requires a quantitative assessment of the ECF volume. As discussed previously, we use the hematocrit or the concentration of total proteins in plasma for this purpose.

### EXAMINE THE ARTERIAL $PCO_2$ IN THE PATIENT WITH METABOLIC ACIDOSIS OR ALKALOSIS TO IDENTIFY THE PRESENCE OF A RESPIRATORY ACID–BASE DISTURBANCE DUE TO ALTERED VENTILATION

If the arterial $PCO_2$ is much higher than expected for the respiratory compensation for a metabolic acidosis or alkalosis (see Table 2-4),

**HENDERSON EQUATION**

- This equation has three parameters; if two are known, the third can be calculated. If all three are measured, the equation can be useful to detect whether there may be a laboratory error in the measurements.

$$[H^+]\ (nmol/L) = 24 \times PCO_2\ (mm\ Hg)/P_{HCO_3}$$

(To make the mathematics easier, one can use 24 or 25 as the constant in this equation.)

there is a coexistent primary respiratory acidosis. In contrast, if the arterial $PCO_2$ is much lower than expected for the respiratory compensation for a metabolic acidosis or alkalosis, primary respiratory alkalosis is also present.

## DETERMINE THE QUANTITATIVE RELATIONSHIP BETWEEN THE FALL IN $P_{HCO_3}$ AND THE RISE IN THE $P_{Anion\ gap}$

The relationship between the rise in $P_{Anion\ gap}$ ($\Delta$ AG) and the fall in $P_{HCO_3}$ ($\Delta$ $HCO_3$) is used to detect the presence of coexisting metabolic alkalosis (the rise in $P_{Anion\ gap}$ is larger than the fall in $P_{HCO_3}$) or the presence of both an acid overproduction type and an $NaHCO_3$ loss type of metabolic acidosis (the rise in $P_{Anion\ gap}$ is smaller than the fall in $P_{HCO_3}$). The difficulty with using this relationship is knowing what was the baseline value of the $P_{Anion\ gap}$ and $P_{HCO_3}$ in a particular patient, within the wide range of what is considered normal values. Hence, only large differences between the rise in $P_{Anion\ gap}$ and the fall in $P_{HCO_3}$ may be of clinical importance. The pitfalls in using this relationship in terms of failure to adjust for the net negative valence attributable to $P_{Albumin}$ and to account for changes in the ECF volume were discussed above.

## EXAMINE THE $P_{HCO_3}$ IN THE PATIENT WITH RESPIRATORY ACIDOSIS OR ALKALOSIS TO IDENTIFY THE PRESENCE OF A METABOLIC ACID–BASE DISTURBANCE

Decide whether the respiratory disorder is acute or chronic based on clinical grounds, not on the basis of laboratory tests. In acute respiratory acidosis or alkalosis, there should be only a slight change in $P_{HCO_3}$, whereas in chronic respiratory acidosis or alkalosis, the slope of [$H^+$] versus the arterial $PCO_2$ is much flatter because of a larger change in the $P_{HCO_3}$ (see Table 2-4).

In a patient with chronic respiratory acidosis, if the rise in $P_{HCO_3}$ is larger than what is expected for the renal compensation for the rise in $PCO_2$, there is a coexisting primary metabolic alkalosis. In contrast, in a patient with chronic respiratory alkalosis, if the fall in $P_{HCO_3}$ is larger than expected for the renal compensation for the fall in $PCO_2$, there is a coexisting primary metabolic acidosis.

## OTHER DIAGNOSTIC APPROACHES: THE STRONG ION DIFFERENCE

In 1981, Peter Stewart introduced a new approach to acid–base diagnoses based on physical concepts. The linchpin of this approach is that [$H^+$] in plasma is regulated by three independent variables: the strong ion difference (SID), the concentration of total weak acids ([$A_{TOT}$]), and the arterial $PCO_2$. $HCO_3^-$ ions are considered a dependent variable and hence are not directly involved in the regulation of [$H^+$]. Stewart constructed a polynomial formula with these three dependent variables to calculate [$H^+$] in a solution.

From a clinical point of view, the arterial pH and $PCO_2$ are measured and used to determine if a respiratory acid–base disorder is present. To understand how this approach is used to detect metabolic acid–base disorders, one needs to understand the concept of SID.

Because electroneutrality must be maintained, the SID in plasma must equal 0 and hence

$$(Na^+ + K^+ + Ca^{2+} + Mg^{2+}) - (Cl^- + lactate^- + other\ strong$$

$$anions) - (HCO_3^- + A^-) = 0 \qquad (7)$$

$A^-$ represents the bases of weak acids, primarily albumin and to a smaller extent phosphate (Eqn 7). Because the concentrations of lactate$^-$ and other strong anions are normally low, these can be ignored. The formula can be rearranged as follows (Eqn 8):

$$SID = (Na^+ + K^+ + Ca^{2+} + Mg^{2+}) - Cl^- = (HCO_3^- + A^-) \qquad (8)$$

If another anion is present in plasma, there will be a gap between the SID calculated as $(Na^+ + K^+ + Ca^{2+} + Mg^{2+}) - Cl^-$ (known as SID apparent [$SID_a$]) and the SID calculated as $(HCO_3^- + A^-)$ (known as SID effective [$SID_e$]). This difference between $SID_a$ and $SID_e$ is known as the *strong ion gap (SIG)*. Therefore, if the $SID_e$ is low, the patient has metabolic acidosis. If the $SID_e$ is low and there is a SIG, the metabolic acidosis is due to overproduction of acids. If the $SID_e$ is low and there is no SIG, the patient has HCMA. If the $SID_e$ is high, the patient has metabolic alkalosis.

For all its complexity, this approach provides a minor advantage over the traditional approach of using the $P_{Anion\ gap}$ in that it includes a measurement of $A^-$. This, however, can be overcome largely by adjusting the baseline value of the $P_{Anion\ Gap}$ for the $P_{Albumin}$.

Because $PCO_2$ is an independent variable in the regulation of $[H^+]$, the Stewart approach does not consider the expected changes in $PCO_2$ in patients with metabolic acid–base disorders as "compensatory" changes but rather as primary acid–base disorders. From a clinical point of view, this may imply the presence of another acid–base disorder, which may not be the case.

The Stewart approach introduces another category of acid–base disturbances that is caused by changes in the concentration of nonvolatile weak acids based on their calculation of $A_{TOT}$. Changes in $A_{TOT}$ are largely caused by changes in the $P_{Albumin}$. Hence, patients with high $P_{Albumin}$ have hyperalbuminemic acidosis, and those with a low $P_{Albumin}$ have hypoalbuminemic alkalosis. Although this may have a physicochemical basis, from a clinical point of view, this category does not seem to represent distinct acid–base disorders. Consider, for example, a patient with nephrotic syndrome and hypoalbuminemia who is given a diuretic, becomes hypokalemic, and develops metabolic alkalosis. Although the patient may have hypoalbuminemic alkalosis, there are many other factors (e.g., low EABV, hypokalemia) that could cause metabolic alkalosis in this patient. Furthermore, this label of hypoalbuminemic alkalosis does not provide useful insights into management of such a patient.

## DISCUSSION OF CASES

### Case 2-1: Does This Man Really Have Metabolic Acidosis?

**Does this patient have a significant degree of metabolic acidosis?**

There are several ways to decide whether metabolic acidosis is present, but not all of them yield the correct answer for the correct reasons.

*Laboratory data*

If one used a definition of metabolic acidosis that relies solely on concentration terms (pH = 7.39, $P_{HCO_3}$ = 24 mmol/L, and arterial $PCO_2$ = 39 mm Hg), the answer is no. On the other hand, because the $P_{Anion\ gap}$ is 24 mEq/L, one might conclude that this patient has two simultaneous acid-base disorders: a metabolic acidosis caused by added acids that resulted in a loss of $HCO_3^-$ ions, and a metabolic alkalosis that added $HCO_3^-$ ions back to the body; therefore, his $P_{HCO_3}$ was in the normal range.

### Clinical picture

The volume of fluid loss in diarrhea was estimated to be about 5 L; the concentration of $HCO_3^-$ in diarrheal fluid was 40 mmol/L. Therefore, there was a loss of ~200 mmol of $HCO_3^-$ ions (5 L×40 mmol/L). Hence, he does have a serious degree of metabolic acidosis even though he does not have acidemia. Moreover, there is no evidence of a gain of $HCO_3^-$ ions because he did not ingest $NaHCO_3$, there was no history of vomiting, and there was little excretion of $NH_4^+$ (little urine output). Recall that the concentration of $HCO_3^-$ ions is the quantity of $HCO_3^-$ ions in the ECF compartment divided by the ECF volume. Hence, we must determine whether there was an occult source of $HCO_3^-$ and/or a large decrease in the ECF volume.

### Correlating the clinical and laboratory information

One must distinguish between a process leading to a deficit of $HCO_3^-$ ions (as suggested from history and the $NaHCO_3$ loss in diarrhea fluid) and a process that caused the addition of acids (as suggested by the rise in $P_{Anion\ gap}$) because of different implications for therapy. To confirm that there is a deficit of $HCO_3^-$ ions, its content in the ECF compartment must be calculated. The hematocrit of 0.60 provides a quantitative, minimum estimate that his plasma volume was reduced from 3.0 to 1.3 L (i.e., by >50%). There was probably a greater reduction in his ECF volume than predicted from the decrease in his plasma volume. Therefore, if his ECF volume was 10 L before he became ill, his current ECF volume is 4 L. Therefore, we can conclude that he has metabolic acidosis with a large deficit of $HCO_3^-$ ions in his ECF compartment (24 mmol/L×4 L=96 mmol vs the usual 240 mmol [24 mmol/L×10 L]).

### What is the basis for the high $P_{Anion\ gap}$?

The high $P_{Anion\ gap}$ is mainly due to a very high $P_{Albumin}$ (because of the profoundly contracted ECF volume) rather than the addition of new acids. This is confirmed by the findings that there were only minor elevations in the concentrations of L-lactate, β-hydroxybutyrate, and D-lactate, which were each less than 1 mmol/L.

## CASE 2-2: LOLA KAYE NEEDS YOUR HELP

### What is/are the major acid–base diagnosis/diagnoses?

Lola has a very low blood pH (a high blood $[H^+]$) because of the following:

### Metabolic acidosis

Calculating the $P_{HCO_3}$ using the Henderson equation (see margin note) reveals that the $P_{HCO_3}$ is 6 mmol/L. Therefore, Lola has a severe degree of metabolic acidosis.

### Respiratory acidosis

With such a low $P_{HCO_3}$, the expected arterial $PCO_2$ should be less than 20 mm Hg. The effect of a $PCO_2$ of 30 versus 20 mm Hg on the

**HENDERSON EQUATION**

pH = 6.90, $[H^+]$ = 125 nmol/L

$[H^+] = 25 \times PCO_2/P_{HCO_3}$

$125 = 25 \times 30/P_{HCO_3}$

$P_{HCO_3} = 6$ mmol/L

**IMPACT OF A DIFFERENCE IN THE ARTERIAL PCO₂ ON THE DEGREE OF ACIDEMIA**

- $[H^+] = 24 \times PCO_2/P_{HCO_3}$
- If $PCO_2$ = 30 mm Hg
  $[H^+] = 24 \times 30 / 6 = 120$ nmol/L
- If $PCO_2$ = 20 mm Hg
  $[H^+] = 24 \times 20 / 6 = 80$ nml/L

$H^+$ concentration or pH in blood is very large (see margin note). Therefore, there is a second acid–base diagnosis: respiratory acidosis. Her brachial venous $PCO_2$ is 45 mm Hg. This is an important factor contributing to the danger of a high $H^+$ concentration because it reduces the ability to buffer most of the $H^+$ ion load by the BBS in skeletal muscle. Therefore, more of the $H^+$ ion load may bind to intracellular proteins in vital organs (e.g., brain cells).

## Additional Information about Case 2-2

On history, there was no evidence to suspect that Lola had chronic lung disease. On physical examination, she was conscious but somewhat obtunded. Her EABV appeared to be very low (blood pressure = 80/50 mm Hg, pulse rate = 124 beats per minute, her jugular venous pressure was flat). Of importance, her respiratory rate was 20 breaths per minute. On laboratory testing, she did not have elevated values for the $P_{Anion\ gap}$ or $P_{Osmolal\ gap}$. Her $P_K$ was 1.8 mmol/L, and there were prominent U waves on her EKG. Her $U_{Osm}$ was 400 mosmol/kg $H_2O$, $U_{Na}$ was 50 mmol/L, $U_K$ was 30 mmol/L, $U_{Cl}$ was 0, $U_{Urea}$ was 150 mmol/L, and $U_{Creatinine}$ was 3 mmol/L.

## Questions

What is the most likely basis for the metabolic acidosis?
What is the most likely basis for the respiratory acidosis?

## What Is the Most Likely Basis for the Metabolic Acidosis?

Because the $P_{Anion\ gap}$ and $P_{Osmolal\ gap}$ were not elevated, ketoacidosis, L-lactic acidosis, D-lactic acidosis, or the ingestion of methanol or ethylene glycol are unlikely causes of the metabolic acidosis. Therefore, the most likely basis for the metabolic acidosis is a deficit of $NaHCO_3$, which could be due to its loss in a direct or indirect form (see Chapter 4 for further discussion). Estimating the rate of excretion of $NH_4^+$ ions in the urine is needed to make a more specific diagnosis for the basis of the metabolic acidosis. The rate of excretion of $NH_4^+$ ions was estimated from the calculation of the $U_{Osmolal\ gap}$, and it was high (see margin note). The anion that accompanied $NH_4^+$ ions in the urine was not $Cl^-$ ions ($U_{Cl}$ = 0). Therefore, the metabolic acidosis was due to an overproduction of an acid, with a high rate of excretion of its anion in the urine. The patient was a glue sniffer. The pathophysiology of the metabolic acidosis due to glue sniffing is discussed in Chapter 3.

**CALCULATION OF THE URINE OSMOLAL GAP**

- Measured $U_{Osm}$ = 400
- Calculated $U_{Osm}$
  = 2 $(U_{Na} + U_K) + U_{Urea}$
  = 2 (50 + 30) + 150 = 310
- $U_{Osmolal\ gap}$ = 90
- $U_{NH_4}$ = 90/2 = 45 mmol/L
- $U_{NH_4} / U_{Creatinine}$ = 45/3 = 15
- Rate of excretion of creatinine in this patient was estimated to be 10 mmol/day.
- The rate of excretion of $NH_4^+$ ions = 150 mmol/day

## What Is the Most Likely Basis for the Respiratory Acidosis?

She has no evidence of chronic lung disease. Although she may have consumed drugs that caused depression of her central nervous system, the fact that her respiratory rate is not low led us to suspect that the depth of her breathing might be reduced owing to weakness of her respiratory muscles. The obvious cause of respiratory muscle weakness in this patient is profound hypokalemia ($P_K$ = 1.8 mmol/L; see margin note).

**CAUTION**

In this patient, do not give glucose or $NaHCO_3$ until her $P_K$ is brought up to a safe level of about 3.5 mmol/L, as their administration may lead to a shift of $K^+$ ions into cells, with the risk of worsening hypokalemia and the danger of cardiac arrhythmia.

chapter *3*

# Metabolic Acidosis:
# Clinical Approach

# Introduction

In this chapter, our goal is to provide a bedside approach to the patient with metabolic acidosis. This approach focuses not only on diagnosing the cause of metabolic acidosis but also (and importantly) on identifying and managing emergencies that are present and anticipating and preventing risks that are likely to arise during therapy.

An important component of our approach is to deduce whether there is a risk of excessive binding of $H^+$ ions to intracellular proteins in vital organs (e.g., the brain and the heart). We discuss how this may occur and how it can be reversed.

Metabolic acidosis can be caused by the gain of acids or the loss of sodium bicarbonate ($NaHCO_3$). We describe the clinical approach to determine the basis of metabolic acidosis by finding new anions in blood or the urine and examining the renal response to the presence of chronic metabolic acidemia by assessing the rate of excretion of $NH_4^+$ ions in the urine.

## OBJECTIVES

- To emphasize the following issues in the clinical approach to the patient with metabolic acidosis:
  1. Deal with emergencies first: Our first step is to recognize and manage threats to the patient's life and to anticipate and prevent risks that may arise during or because of therapy.
  2. Assess the effectiveness of the bicarbonate buffer system (BBS): Measurement of brachial venous $PCO_2$ provides a means to evaluate the effectiveness of the BBS in skeletal muscle, where the bulk of this buffer system exists, in removing the $H^+$ ion load.
  3. Determine whether the basis of the metabolic acidosis is the addition of acids and/or the loss of $NaHCO_3$: Look for the presence of new anions in plasma and urine, and assess the rate of excretion of $NH_4^+$ ions in the urine.

**ABBREVIATIONS**

BBS, bicarbonate buffer system
$NaHCO_3$, sodium bicarbonate
$P_{Glucose}$, concentration of glucose in plasma
$P_{Albumin}$, concentration of albumin in plasma

## CASE 3-1: STICK TO THE FACTS

A 28-year-old man with a known history of sniffing glue presented to the emergency room with profound muscle weakness and a very unsteady gait, which had become progressive over the last 3 days. On physical examination, his blood pressure was 100/60 mm Hg and his pulse rate was 110 beats per minute while lying flat. When he sat up, his blood pressure fell to 80/50 mm Hg and his pulse rate rose to 130 beats per minute. Neurological examination revealed severe muscle weakness but no other findings. His arterial blood pH was 7.20, $PCO_2$ was 25 mm Hg, and $P_{HCO_3}$ was 10 mmol/L. His $P_{Glucose}$ was 3.5 mmol/L (63 mg/dL), his $P_{Albumin}$ was 6.0 g/dL (60 g/L), and his hematocrit was 0.50. Other laboratory measurements in brachial venous blood and the urine are shown in the following table:

|  |  | VENOUS BLOOD | URINE |
|---|---|---|---|
| pH |  | 7.00 | 6.0 |
| $PCO_2$ | mm Hg | 60 | — |
| $HCO_3^-$ | mmol/L | 15 | <5 |
| $Na^+$ | mmol/L | 120 | 50 |
| $K^+$ | mmol/L | 2.3 | 30 |
| $Cl^-$ | mmol/L | 90 | 0 |
| Creatinine | mg/dL (μmol/L) | 1.7 (150) | 3.0 mmol/L |
| BUN (urea) | mg/dL (mmol/L) | 14 (5.0) | 150 mmol/L |
| Osmolality | mOsm/kg $H_2O$ | 250 | 400 |

## Questions

What dangers were present on admission?
What dangers should be anticipated during therapy?
What is the basis for the metabolic acidosis?

# PART A
# CLINICAL APPROACH

- The first step in the clinical approach to the patient with metabolic acidosis is to deal with emergencies on presentation and anticipate and prevent risks that may arise during therapy.
- The next two steps are: (1) Determine whether $H^+$ ions were buffered appropriately by the BBS. (2) Determine whether the basis of the metabolic acidosis is the addition of acids and/or the loss of $NaHCO_3$.

The initial steps in our approach to the patient with metabolic acidosis are illustrated in Flow Chart 3-1. The diagnosis of metabolic acidosis is based on one of the following criteria: (1) a low plasma pH and $P_{HCO_3}$ and (2) an appreciable decrease in the content of $HCO_3^-$ ions in the extracellular fluid (ECF) compartment in the patients who are ECF volume contracted. A quantitative estimate of the ECF volume is needed. Because one cannot obtain a quantitative estimate of the ECF volume with physical examination, we recommend using the

**ABBREVIATIONS**

ECF, extracellular fluid
ICF, intracellular fluid
EABV, effective arterial blood volume
GFR, glomerular filtration rate
GI, gastrointestinal
RTA, renal tubular acidosis
$P_{Anion\ gap}$, anion gap in plasma
$P_{Osmolal\ gap}$, osmolal gap in plasma
DKA, diabetic ketoacidosis
$P_K$, concentration of potassium ($K^+$) ions in plasma

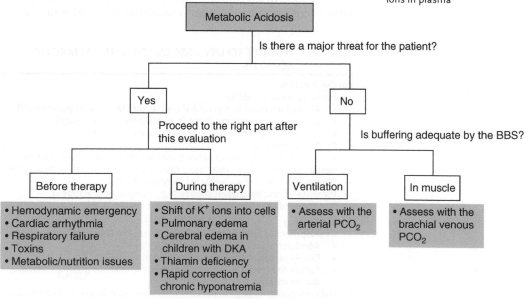

**Flow Chart 3-1 Initial Steps in the Evaluation of the Patient with Metabolic Acidosis.** One must use a definition of metabolic acidosis that is based not only on the $P_{HCO_3}$ but also on the content of $HCO_3^-$ ions in the extracellular fluid (ECF) compartment, if ECF volume is significantly contracted. The initial step is to deal with threats for the patient that may be present and anticipate those that may develop during therapy (*left side of the flow chart*). The next step is to assess buffering by the bicarbonate buffer system (BBS) in the interstitial space and cells of skeletal muscle to deduce whether more $H^+$ ions are likely to be bound to intracellular proteins in vital organs (e.g., the brain and the heart) (*right side of the flow chart*). DKA, Diabetic ketoacidosis.

hematocrit or the concentration of total protein in plasma to obtain this information (see the discussion of Case 2-1).

# EMERGENCIES IN THE PATIENT WITH METABOLIC ACIDOSIS

The common clinical practice is to begin the assessment of a patient with metabolic acidosis with an emphasis on diagnosis. We, however, recommend a different approach; our initial focus is to deal with threats to the patient's life that may be present, and to anticipate and prevent dangers that may arise during or because of therapy (Table 3-1). The diagnostic category of metabolic acidosis is made up of two major subgroups: one where the basis of the disorder is the addition of acids and the other where its basis is the loss of $NaHCO_3$. Although the emergencies may be different depending on the cause for the disorder, nevertheless, dealing with emergencies should take precedence over diagnostic issues.

## EMERGENCIES AT PRESENTATION

### Hemodynamic emergency

The most common example is the patient with L-lactic acidosis because of cardiogenic shock caused by a massive myocardial infarction. Survival in this setting depends on whether the cardiac output can be improved very quickly. In most of the other settings of metabolic acidosis caused by added acids, true hemodynamic emergencies are not common, with the exception of some patients with sepsis and others with DKA caused by the marked degree of decreased effective arterial blood volume (EABV) because of glucose-induced osmotic natriuresis and diuresis.

Patients with a significant degree of contraction of the EABV that causes hemodynamic instability require the urgent administration of a

TABLE 3-1 **THREATS TO LIFE ASSOCIATED WITH METABOLIC ACIDOSIS**

**On Presentation**
- Hemodynamic instability
  - Marked decrease in myocardial contractility (e.g., cardiogenic shock)
  - Very low intravascular volume (e.g., NaCl loss, hemorrhage)
  - Decreased peripheral vascular resistance (e.g., sepsis)
- Cardiac arrhythmia
  - Most frequently seen in patients with hyperkalemia or hypokalemia
- Respiratory failure (e.g., respiratory muscle weakness caused by hypokalemia)
- Presence of toxins (e.g., methanol, ethylene glycol)
- Presence of reactive oxygen species (e.g., pyroglutamic acidosis)
- Nutritional deficiency (especially of B vitamins)

**During Therapy**
- Development of cerebral edema during therapy of DKA in children
  - Administration of a bolus of insulin
  - Overly rapid or excessive administration of saline
  - Failure to prevent an appreciable fall in the effective plasma osmolality during therapy
- Pulmonary edema (e.g., in patients with severe diarrhea if the ECF volume is expanded and $NaHCO_3$ is not given)
- Too rapid a rise in the $P_{Na}$ in patients with chronic hyponatremia
- Development of a more severe degree of acidemia in a patient with metabolic acidosis
- Acute shift of $K^+$ into cells (e.g., administration of $NaHCO_3$ or glucose to patients with hypokalemia, administration of insulin to patients with DKA and hypokalemia)
- Wernicke's encephalopathy caused by failure to give thiamin (vitamin B₁) to a patient with chronic alcoholism and alcoholic ketoacidosis

large volume of isotonic saline. In contrast, if the patient is not hemo-dynamically compromised, aggressive infusion of isotonic saline is not warranted because this may lead to serious complications (see the following discussion).

### Cardiac arrhythmia

Patients with metabolic acidosis may develop a cardiac arrhythmia when there is a severe degree of hyperkalemia (e.g., patients with renal failure) or hypokalemia (e.g., certain patients with distal renal tubular acidosis [RTA], patients with metabolic acidosis caused by glue sniff-ing). In addition, hypokalemia may develop after therapy is initiated (see discussion of Case 3-1). The emergency treatment of hypokalemia and of hyperkalemia is discussed in Chapters 14 and 15, respectively.

### Failure of adequate ventilation

A severe degree of hypokalemia may lead to respiratory muscle weak-ness and respiratory failure. A more severe degree of acidemia devel-ops because of superimposed respiratory acidosis in a patient with metabolic acidosis. Enough KCl should be given to raise the concen-tration of potassium ($K^+$) ions in plasma ($P_K$) to 3.0 mmol/L in this setting; mechanical ventilation may be needed.

### Toxin-induced metabolic acidosis

Ingestion of methanol or ethylene glycol should always be suspected in a patient with metabolic acidosis, an elevated $P_{Anion\ gap}$, and no obvious cause for these findings, especially if the ECF volume is not signifi-cantly contracted (see Chapter 6). Failing to make this diagnosis can be devastating. If ingestion of these alcohols is suspected, one must cal-culate the $P_{Osmolal\ gap}$ (see Chapter 2). If the $P_{Osmolal\ gap}$ is considerably greater than 10 mosmol/kg $H_2O$, the diagnosis of ingestion of toxic alcohols should be confirmed by direct measurements of methanol and of ethylene glycol in plasma because the presence of ethanol in plasma also causes a high $P_{Osmolal\ gap}$. Because it is the products of the metab-olism of these alcohols that create the danger rather than the parent compounds, inhibition of their metabolism via the enzyme alcohol dehydroenase with the administration of ethanol (alcohol dehydroge-nase has a much higher affinity for ethanol than for methanol or eth-ylene glycol), or the administration of fomepizole (a direct inhibitor of alcohol dehydrogenase) is required until the facts become clear.

## DANGERS TO ANTICIPATE AFTER COMMENCING THERAPY

Several threats are anticipated during therapy in patients with meta-bolic acidosis.

### Dangers related to overly aggressive administration of saline

Although enough saline should be given if there is evident hemo-dynamic instability, several complications may arise from excessive administration of saline. In the absence of hemodynamic instability, we use the brachial venous $PCO_2$ as a guide to the amount of saline to be administered in the initial management of patients with metabolic acidosis (see the following). We also use the hematocrit to obtain a quantitative estimate of the ECF volume, and the $P_{Na}$ on presentation to get an estimate of the deficit of $Na^+$ ions and avoid the excessive administration of saline (see chapter 5 for further discussion).

### 1. A more severe degree of acidemia

A large fall in the $P_{HCO_3}$ may occur when a large volume of saline without $NaHCO_3$ is given to a patient who has metabolic acidosis caused by a large loss of $NaHCO_3$ and a severe degree of ECF volume contraction due to a large loss of NaCl (e.g., the patient with severe diarrhea). When saline is infused very rapidly, some of these patients may develop pulmonary edema. This occurs even though they have not been given enough saline to sufficiently re-expand their ECF volume. It is interesting to note that the pulmonary edema in these patients can be treated, and its occurrence can be prevented with the administration of $NaHCO_3$ (see discussion of Question 3-2). Therefore, the fluid that is administered to these patients to achieve ECF volume expansion should contain $NaHCO_3$ or anions that can be metabolized to produce $HCO_3^-$ anions (e.g., lactated Ringer's solution).

Three mechanisms may lead to a more severe degree of acidemia with the infusion of a large amount of saline in these patients.

#### i) Dilution of the concentration of $HCO_3^-$ in the ECF compartment

Because of a marked degree of ECF volume contraction, these patients may have a large deficit of $HCO_3^-$ ions in their ECF compartment that is not revealed by the fall in their $P_{HCO_3}$. Hence, the concentration of $HCO_3^-$ ions in the ECF compartment will fall when a large volume of saline is infused (same amount of $HCO_3^-$ ions in a larger ECF volume), and a more severe degree of acidemia will develop.

#### ii) Loss of more $NaHCO_3$ in diarrheal fluid

Re-expansion of the EABV increases the splanchnic blood flow and delivery of $Na^+$ and $Cl^-$ ions to the enterocytes. Therefore, a larger amount of $Na^+$ and $Cl^-$ ions may be secreted in the small intestine and then delivered to the colon. When a large volume of luminal fluid containing $Na^+$ and $Cl^-$ ions reaches the colon because the $Cl^-/HCO_3^-$ anion exchanger (AE) has a higher transport capacity than the $Na^+/H^+$ exchanger (NHE), a larger amount of $Cl^-$ ions is reabsorbed in exchange for $HCO_3^-$ ions relative to the amount of $Na^+$ ions that is reabsorbed in exchange for $H^+$ ions. Hence, the loss of $NaHCO_3$ in diarrheal fluid may rise markedly (see Fig. 4-3).

#### iii) Back-titration of $HCO_3^-$ ions by $H^+$ ions that were bound to intracellular proteins

Patients with a contracted EABV have a high $PCO_2$ in their skeletal muscle capillary blood because most of the $O_2$ delivered per liter of blood flow to muscle is consumed. Therefore, the BBS in skeletal muscle may fail to titrate an $H^+$ load, and hence $H^+$ ions bind to intracellular proteins. With expansion of the EABV, the blood flow rate to muscle rises. If the same amount of oxygen is consumed, the same amount of $CO_2$ will be produced and less $CO_2$ will be added to each liter of blood flow. Hence, the $PCO_2$ in muscle capillaries and in muscle cells will fall. This drives the BBS reaction to the right, causing a fall in $H^+$ ion concentration in muscle cells (see Eqn 1). As a result, many of the $H^+$ ions that are bound to proteins in muscle cells will be released. Some of these $H^+$ are exported out of muscle cells on the sodium-hydrogen exchanger-1 (NHE-1) because this cation exchanger is activated by a rise in the intracellular fluid (ICF) $H^+$ ion concentration. These $H^+$ ions titrate $HCO_3^-$ ions in the ECF compartment; therefore, the concentration of $HCO_3^-$ in the ECF compartment decreases and a more severe degree of acidemia develops (Figure 3-1).

$$H^+ + HCO_3^- \rightleftharpoons CO_2 + H_2O \qquad (1)$$

### 2. Cerebral edema in children with diabetic ketoacidosis

Children with DKA are at risk of developing cerebral edema during therapy (see Chapter 5 for more details). One of the factors that might predispose a patient to this dreaded complication is the administration of a large volume of saline. Although enough saline should be given to restore systemic hemodynamics, in the absence of hemodynamic instability, one should avoid giving too much saline or giving it too quickly. In this setting, we use the brachial venous $PCO_2$ as a guide to the amount of saline to be administered in the initial management (see the following). We also use the hematocrit and the $P_{Na}$ on presentation to obtain an estimate of the deficit of $Na^+$ ions and avoid the excessive administration of saline. Measures must also be taken

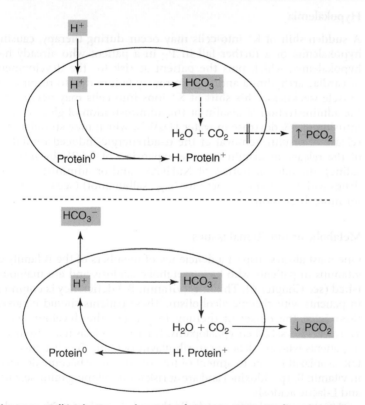

**Figure 3-1 Fall in the $P_{HCO_3}$ when Muscle Venous $PCO_2$ Declines in a Patient with Metabolic Acidosis.** The oval represents a muscle cell containing its $HCO_3^-$ and protein buffer systems. *Upper panel*: because of a contracted effective arterial blood volume (EABV), $PCO_2$ in muscle capillary blood will be high because most of the $O_2$ delivered per liter of blood flow to muscle is consumed. The bicarbonate buffer system (BBS) in skeletal muscle may fail to titrate an $H^+$ ion load, and therefore $H^+$ ions bind to intracellular proteins. *Lower panel*: with expansion of the EABV, the blood flow rate to muscle rises; therefore, the $PCO_2$ in muscle capillaries and in muscle cells falls. This drives the BBS reaction to the right, causing a fall in $H^+$ ions concentration in muscle cells. As a result, $H^+$ ions that are bound to proteins in muscle cells will be released, and titrate $HCO_3^-$ anions both in intracellular fluid and extracellular fluid compartments. $H^+$ ions are exported out of muscle cells on the sodium-hydrogen exchanger-1 (NHE-1) (not shown in the figure).

**PLASMA EFFECTIVE OSMOLALITY**

$= 2 P_{Na} + P_{Glucose}$, all in mmol/L

to prevent an appreciable fall in the plasma effective osmolality in the first 15 hours of therapy (see margin note) (see Chapter 5 for more details).

### 3. Rapid correction of chronic hyponatremia

Another important danger that may occur during therapy is a rapid and large rise in the $P_{Na}$ in a patient with chronic hyponatremia, which may lead to the development of osmotic demyelination syndrome. This is because a water diuresis may ensue as restoration of EABV removes the stimulus for the release of vasopressin and increases the delivery of filtrate to the distal nephron (see Chapter 10). The administration of desamino, D-arginine vasopressin (dDAVP) at the outset should be considered to prevent a water diuresis and minimize the risk of developing this devastating complication. After hemodynamic stability is restored, administration of a saline solution that is isotonic to the patient should be considered if further expansion of EABV is necessary.

### Hypokalemia

A sudden shift of $K^+$ into cells may occur during therapy, causing hypokalemia or a further fall in $P_K$ in a patient who already has hypokalemia, which puts the patient at risk for the development of cardiac arrhythmia and/or respiratory failure due to respiratory muscle weakness. This shift of $K^+$ ions into cells may occur with the administration of insulin or the administration of glucose (e.g., infusion of 5% dextrose in water [$D_5W$]), which may stimulate the release of insulin, removal of the α-adrenergic-induced inhibition of the release of insulin (e.g., re-expansion of EABV by infusing saline), the administration of $NaHCO_3$, and/or administration of drugs with $β_2$-adrenergic activity (e.g., salbutamol) (see Chapter 14 for more discussion).

### Metabolic or nutritional issues

One must always suspect a deficiency of members of the B family of vitamins in patients who have metabolic acidosis and are malnourished (see Chapter 6). Thiamin (vitamin $B_1$) deficiency is common in patients with chronic alcoholism. These patients should be given thiamin at the outset of therapy to prevent the development of Wernicke–Korsakoff encephalopathy. L-Lactic acidosis may also occur in patients who are deficient in riboflavin (vitamin $B_2$). Patients who take isoniazid for the treatment of tuberculosis may become deficient in vitamin $B_6$ (pyridoxine) and are at risk for developing mini-seizures and L-lactic acidosis.

Another example of a metabolic threat is in patients with pyroglutamic acidosis (see Chapter 6). In this disorder, the threat is caused by depletion of reduced glutathione and thereby compromised ability to detoxify reactive oxygen species.

## ASSESS THE EFFECTIVENESS OF THE BICARBONATE BUFFER SYSTEM

In Chapters 1 and 2, we emphasized that $H^+$ ions must be removed by the BBS to minimize their binding to proteins in cells of vital organs (e.g., the brain and the heart). A low $PCO_2$ in the interstitial fluid compartment of the ECF of muscles and in muscle cells, where the bulk of the BBS exists, is a prerequisite to achieve this safe removal of H⁺ ions. Acidemia stimulates the respiratory center, which leads to hyperventilation and a lower arterial $PCO_2$. Although the arterial $PCO_2$ may be low, the $PCO_2$ in intracellular fluid and interstitial space in muscle may not be low enough for effective buffering of H⁺ ions by the BBS because it is also influenced by both the rate of production of $CO_2$ and the blood flow rate to muscles. Patients with metabolic acidosis and a contracted EABV have a high $PCO_2$ in venous blood draining skeletal muscle (which reflects a high muscle capillary blood $PCO_2$, and therefore a high $PCO_2$ in the the interstitial fluid and cells of skeletal muscle) and therefore these patients may fail to titrate an H⁺ ion load with the BBS in skeletal muscle. As a result, the degree of acidemia may become more pronounced, and more H⁺ ions might bind to proteins in the extracellular and intracellular fluids in other organs, including the brain, with possible detrimental effects. At usual rates of blood flow and metabolic work at rest, brachial venous $PCO_2$ is ~46 mm Hg, which is ~6 mm Hg higher than the arterial $PCO_2$. If the blood flow rate to the skeletal muscles declines because of a low EABV, the brachial venous $PCO_2$ will be more than 6 mm Hg higher than the arterial $PCO_2$. Based on this analysis, and although experimental evidence to support this view is lacking, we recommend that in patients with metabolic acidosis, enough saline should be administered to increase the blood flow rate to muscle to restore the difference between the brachial venous $PCO_2$ and the arterial $PCO_2$ to its usual value of ~6 mm Hg to ensure that the BBS in muscle is operating effectively to remove the H⁺ ion load and therefore diminish binding of H⁺ ions to intracellular proteins in in vital organs (e.g., the brain and the heart).

## DETERMINE THE BASIS OF METABOLIC ACIDOSIS

The basis of metabolic acidosis could be the gain of an acid or the loss of $NaHCO_3$ (Flow Chart 3-2). There are three additional considerations to improve the clinical approach to determine the basis of metabolic acidosis.

### DETECT ADDITION OF ACIDS BY FINDING NEW ANIONS IN THE BLOOD AND/OR THE URINE

An increase in the $P_{Anion\ gap}$ is used to detect the addition of new acids. As was discussed in Chapter 2, because of differences in laboratory methods (e.g., measurement of $P_{Cl}$), there is a large difference in the mean value of the normal $P_{Anion\ gap}$ reported by different clinical laboratories. Furthermore, and regardless of the method used, there is a wide range of what is considered a normal value of the $P_{Anion\ gap}$ in a certain clinical laboratory. There are two additional pitfalls in using the $P_{Anion\ gap}$ to detect the appearance of new anions that the clinician should be aware of. First, the baseline value for the $P_{Anion\ gap}$ must be adjusted for the $P_{Albumin}$. A rough guide for correcting the baseline value of the $P_{Anion\ gap}$ for the $P_{Albumin}$ is that for every 1.0 g/dL (10 g/L) decrease in $P_{Albumin}$, the $P_{Anion\ gap}$ is lower by close to 2.5 mEq/L. The converse is true for a rise in the $P_{Albumin}$.

Second, there is a much smaller rise in the $P_{Anion\ gap}$ if the anions of the added acids are excreted in the urine at a rapid rate (e.g., hippurate anions in a patient with metabolic acidosis caused by glue sniffing; see the discussion of Case 3-1). To detect the presence of new anions in the urine, we calculate the urine anion gap ($U_{Anion\ gap}$) (Eqn 2).

### ABBREVIATIONS

$U_{Osmolal\ gap}$, osmolal gap in the urine

$U_{NH_4}$, concentration of $NH_4^+$ ions in the urine

$U_{Creatinine}$, concentration of creatinine in the urine

$U_{Na}$, concentration of sodium ions in the urine

$U_K$, concentration of potassium ions in the urine

$U_{Cl}$, the concentration of chloride ions in the urine

$P_{Cl}$, concentration of chloride ions in plasma

$P_{L\text{-lactate}}$, concentration of L-lactate anions in plasma

$U_{Urea}$, concentration of urea in the urine

PCT, proximal convoluted tubule

$P_{Glucose}$, concentration of glucose in plasma

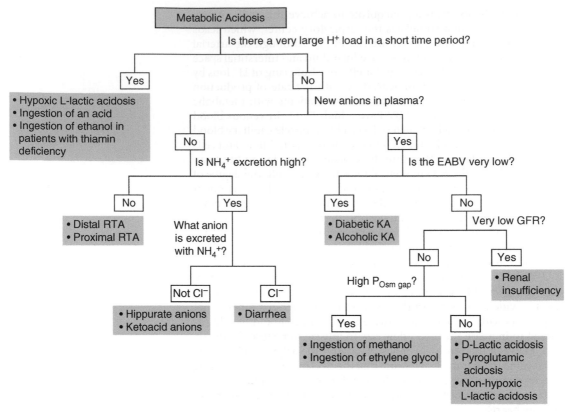

**Flow Chart 3-2 Determine the Basis of Metabolic Acidosis.** Metabolic acidosis could be caused by the gain of an acid or the loss of $NaHCO_3$. The flow chart provides an overall approach to help identify the cause of metabolic acidosis based on initial clinical evaluation and laboratory data. The specific causes will be discussed in the following chapters, with further clinical and laboratory data that are needed to confirm the diagnosis. *EABV,* Effective arterial blood volume; *GFR,* glomerular filtration rate; *KA,* ketoacidosis; *RTA,* renal tubular acidosis.

The concentration of $NH_4^+$ ions in the urine ($U_{NH4}$) is estimated from the urine osmolal gap ($U_{Osmolal\,gap}$) (see Chapter 2).

$$U_{Anion\,gap} = (U_{Na} + U_K + U_{NH4}) - U_{Cl} \qquad (2)$$

## DETECT CONDITIONS WITH FAST ADDITION OF H⁺ IONS

The first of these conditions is obvious; hypoxic L-lactic acidosis (i.e., when the supply of oxygen to tissues is too low to match their demand for ATP regeneration). Another setting where the input of $H^+$ ions can be very fast is the ingestion of a large quantity of an acid (e.g., metabolic acidosis caused by ingestion of citric acid). Fast addition of $H^+$ ions (L-lactic acid) also occurs because of the ingestion of ethanol in a patient who is thiamin deficient. These conditions are discussed in more detail in Chapter 6.

## ASSESS THE RENAL RESPONSE TO METABOLIC ACIDOSIS

The expected renal response to chronic metabolic acidosis is the excretion of 200 to 250 mmol of $NH_4^+$ ions per day in an adult. The calculation of the $U_{Osmolal\,gap}$ provides the most reliable indirect estimate of the concentration of $NH_4^+$ ions in the urine (see Chapter 2). The rate of excretion of $NH_4^+$ ions per day can be estimated by dividing the $U_{NH_4}$ by $U_{Creatinine}$ in a spot urine sample and multiplying this ratio by the expected rate of excretion of creatinine per day.

3-1 *In a patient with cholera and metabolic acidosis caused by the loss of $NaHCO_3$ in diarrheal fluid, the ECF volume is severely contracted, yet $O_2$ delivery to tissues is adequate and hence production of L-lactic acid is not increased. Might this patient have an elevated value for the $P_{Anion\ gap}$?*

3-2 *Why might pulmonary edema develop before the ECF volume is fully re-expanded in this patient?*

# PART B
# DISCUSSIONS

## DISCUSSION OF CASES

### CASE 3-1: STICK TO THE FACTS

#### What dangers were present on admission?

*Marked degree of contraction of EABV*

Based on a hematocrit of 0.50, his plasma volume (and by extrapolation his ECF volume) is reduced by one-third of its normal value (see Chapter 2 for how to use the hematocrit to estimate ECF volume). On the other hand, this patient does not have a severe degree of decreased tissue perfusion because there is no appreciable rise in the $P_{L\text{-}lactate}$. Thus, one need not re-expand the ECF volume with very great haste because there are potential dangers in doing so (see the discussion of the next question).

*Severe degree of hypokalemia*

The dangers related to hypokalemia are cardiac arrhythmias and respiratory muscle weakness. The electrocardiogram showed only prominent U waves. Analysis of his arterial blood gases shows that the patient had the appropriate fall in arterial $PCO_2$ for the fall in $P_{HCO3}$, and hence does not have a superimposed respiratory acidosis. Therefore, although the patient had a severe degree of hypokalemia that would require aggressive $K^+$ ion therapy, he does not have an emergency related to hypokalemia at present.

*Hyponatremia*

Hyponatremia was likely chronic because there were no symptoms that would strongly suggest an appreciable acute component to the hyponatremia and there was no history of a recent intake of a large amount of water.

*Binding of $H^+$ ions to proteins in cells*

Because the brachial venous $PCO_2$ (60 mm Hg) was considerably higher than the arterial $PCO_2$ (25 mm Hg), buffering of $H^+$ ions by the BBS in muscle is compromised and there is a risk of binding of more $H^+$ ions to proteins in cells of vital organs (e.g., the heart and the brain).

### What dangers should be anticipated during therapy?

*A more severe degree of hypokalemia*

Re-expansion of the EABV with the administration of saline can lead to a fall in α-adrenergics and thereby the release of insulin and a shift of $K^+$ into cells.

The administration of $NaHCO_3$ and of glucose-containing solutions should be avoided until the $P_K$ is raised to a safe level of about 3.5 mmol/L.

*Rapid rise in $P_{Na}$*

The $P_{Na}$ may rise rapidly if water diuresis occurs with re-expansion of EABV. As $K^+$ ions are administered, there will be a shift of $K^+$ ions into muscle cells in exchange for $Na^+$ ions, which will also lead to a rise in $P_{Na}$. Patients who are malnourished and/or hypokalemic are at high risk of osmotic demyelination syndrome with a rapid rise in $P_{Na}$. In our opinion, the maximum rise in $P_{Na}$ in patients who are at high risk for the development of osmotic demyelination syndrome should not exceed 4 mmol/L in the first 24 hours.

*Further fall in $P_{HCO_3}$*

Expansion of the EABV with rapid administration of saline may also lead to a further fall in $P_{HCO_3}$. First, there is a dilution effect. Second, with improved blood flow to muscles and the fall in their capillary $PCO_2$, there will be titration of $HCO_3^-$ ions by $H^+$ ions that were bound to intracellular proteins. The need to give $NaHCO_3$, however, must be balanced by the danger of creating a more severe degree of hypokalemia. We would not administer $NaHCO_3$ unless there is hemodynamic instability that is not responsive to the usual maneuvers to restore blood pressure, and with a central line in place to give a sufficient amount of KCl rapidly if a cardiac arrhythmia were to develop (see Chapter 14).

### Plan for initial therapy

On arrival to the emergency department, the patient was given 1 L of isotonic saline via the intravenous route. To correct hypokalemia and prevent a rapid rise in $P_{Na}$, the intravenous solution was changed to a saline solution with 40 mEq of KCl that was designed to have a tonicity similar to that in the plasma of the patient. To prevent water diuresis, dDAVP was administered at the onset of therapy, while water restriction was imposed. The hemodynamic status, $P_K$, $P_{Na}$, arterial pH, arterial $PCO_2$, brachial venous $PCO_2$, and $P_{HCO_3}$ were monitored closely.

### What is the basis for the metabolic acidosis?

Because the $P_{Anion\ gap}$ was not increased despite the high value for the $P_{Albumin}$, it was thought that the metabolic acidosis was not caused by a gain of acids. In fact, the initial diagnosis was distal RTA to explain the findings of the metabolic acidemia, a urine pH of 6.0 (which is thought by some to represent a renal acidification defect), and hypokalemia. Calculation of the $U_{Osmolal\ gap}$ (90 mosmol/kg $H_2O$), however, revealed a high urine concentration of $NH_4^+$ ion (45 mmol/L). Furthermore, the rate of excretion of $NH_4^+$ ions, as assessed by the $U_{NH_4}/U_{Creatinine}$, was about 15 mmol $NH_4^+$/mmol creatinine. Therefore, the diagnosis was not distal RTA because the rate of excretion of $NH_4^+$ ions was high (see margin note).

**CALCULATION OF THE RATE OF EXCRETION OF $NH_4^+$ IONS**

- Measured $U_{Osm}$ = 400 mosmol/kg $H_2O$
- Calculated $U_{Osm}$ = $2(U_{Na} + U_K)$ + $U_{Urea}$ = $2(50 + 30) + 150 = 310$ mosmol/kg $H_2O$
- $U_{Osmolal\ gap}$ = Measured $U_{Osm}$ - Calculated $U_{Osm}$ = 90 mosmol/kg $H_2O$
- $U_{NH_4}$ = $U_{Osmolal\ gap}/2 = 90/2 = 45$ mmol/L
- $U_{NH_4}/U_{Creatinine}$ = $45/3 = 15$
- Rate of excretion of creatinine in this patient was estimated to be 10 mmol/day.
- The rate of excretion of $NH_4^+$ ions = 150 mmol/day

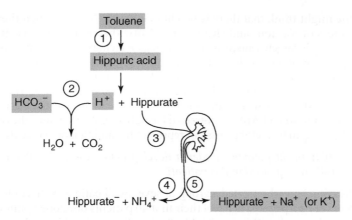

**Figure 3-2 Metabolic Acidosis Caused by the Metabolism of Toluene.** The metabolism of toluene occurs in the liver, where benzoic acid is produced via alcohol and aldehyde dehydrogenases. Conjugating benzoic acid with glycine produces hippuric acid (all represented as *site 1* for simplicity). The $H^+$ ions are titrated by $HCO_3^-$ ions for the most part (*site 2*). The hippurate anions are filtered and also secreted in the PCT (*site 3*). Therefore, instead of accumulating in blood and causing a rise in the $P_{Anion\ gap}$, they are excreted in the urine. Some of the hippurate anions are excreted in the urine with $NH_4^+$ ions (*site 4*) and others with $Na^+$ and $K^+$ ions (*site 5*), when the capacity to excrete $NH_4^+$ ions is exceeded. The excretion of hippurate anions with $Na^+$ and/or $K^+$ ions leads to worsening metabolic acidemia, EABV contraction, and hypokalemia.

Because the anion that was excreted with $NH_4^+$ ions was not $Cl^-$, diarrhea was not the cause of the metabolic acidosis. Hence, the patient had an acid gain type of metabolic acidosis with a high rate of excretion of the anion of that acid in the urine. Because his $P_{Anion\ gap}$ was not elevated, very few of the new anions could have entered the urine by glomerular filtration. Therefore, we deduced that these new anions were more likely to have entered the urine via secretion in the proximal convoluted tubule (PCT), akin to para-aminohippurate anions. The major chemical in glue is toluene. Toulene is converted to benzoic acid in the liver by cytochrome $P_{450}$. Benzoic acid is then conjugated to the amino acid glycine to form hippuric acid. After hippuric acid is formed, the PCT actively secretes these hippurate anions, which keeps their concentration in plasma very low and their concentration in urine very high. In fact, the rate of excretion of hippurate anions in the urine exceeds the rate of excretion of $NH_4^+$ ions because there is a limited amount of $NH_4^+$ ions that can be made in the PCT (Figure 3-2). The remaining hippurate anions are excreted in the urine along with $Na^+$ ions, resulting in the indirect loss of $NaHCO_3$ (see Fig. 4-1) and EABV contraction. The low EABV via activating the renin-angiotensin II-aldosterone system leads to high levels of aldosterone in plasma. Aldosterone increases the rate of electrogenic reabsorption of $Na^+$ ions in the cortical distal nephron, which results in a high rate of excretion of $K^+$ ions in the urine and therefore the development of hypokalemia (see Chapter 13).

## DISCUSSION OF QUESTIONS

3-1 *In a patient with cholera and metabolic acidosis caused by the loss of $NaHCO_3$ in diarrheal fluid, the ECF volume is severely contracted, yet $O_2$ delivery to tissues is adequate to avoid increased production of L-lactic acid. Might this patient have an elevated value for the $P_{Anion\ gap}$?*

One might think that there is no change in the $P_{Anion\ gap}$ when there is a loss of $Na^+$ ions and $HCO_3^-$ ions. Notwithstanding, because the $P_{Anion\ gap}$ is largely caused by the net negative charge on albumin, the $P_{Anion\ gap}$ would be higher if the $P_{Albumin}$ were to rise because of a contracted plasma volume. In quantitative terms, the baseline value of the $P_{Anion\ gap}$ rises by close to 2.5 mEq/L for every 1.0-g/dL (10-g/L) rise in $P_{Albumin}$. Moreover, there appears to be an increase in the negative valence on albumin when EABV is contracted (see Chapter 2). Therefore, the rise in $P_{Anion\ gap}$ in this setting does not represent the addition of new acids.

3-2 *Why might pulmonary edema develop before the ECF volume is fully re-expanded in this patient?*

The clinicians who treated a group of severely ill patients with cholera were very surprised when 5 of their first 40 patients developed pulmonary edema when they received isotonic saline at a rapid rate. In fact, the positive balance of saline was significantly less than what would be needed to fully re-expand their ECF volume. Even more surprising was the fact that pulmonary edema was ameliorated when isotonic $NaHCO_3$ was infused at a rapid rate, whereas the administration of diuretics was not successful. One speculation to help understand these observations was that the more severe degree of acidemia that developed following partial re-expansion of the ECF volume with isotonic saline led to a more intense constriction of the peripheral venous capacitance vessels and thus a larger increase in the central blood volume. Therefore, the fluid that is administered to these patients to expand their ECF volume, should contain $NaHCO_3$, or anions that can be metabolized to produce $HCO_3^-$ ions (e.g., lactated Ringer's solution). One must be extremely cautious if the patient has hypokalemia because the administration of $NaHCO_3$ may lead to worsening hypokalemia.

# Metabolic Acidosis Caused by a Deficit of NaHCO$_3$

# Introduction

Metabolic acidosis could be caused by the gain of acids or the loss of sodium bicarbonate ($NaHCO_3$). In this chapter, we focus on metabolic acidosis caused by the loss of $NaHCO_3$. In this type of metabolic acidosis, there are almost no new anions present in plasma; therefore, the anion gap in plasma ($P_{Anion\ gap}$) is not increased, hence the term "nonanion gap" metabolic acidosis. Because the fall in the concentration of bicarbonate ($HCO_3^-$) anions in plasma ($P_{HCO_3}$) is matched by a rise in the concentration of chloride ($Cl^-$) ions in plasma ($P_{Cl}$), this type of metabolic acidosis is also called hyperchloremic metabolic acidosis (HCMA).

There are two major groups of causes for this type of metabolic acidosis: direct and indirect loss of $NaHCO_3$. The direct loss of $NaHCO_3$ may be via the gastrointestinal (GI) tract (e.g., patients with diarrhea) or via the urine in patients in the initial phase of a disease process that causes proximal renal tubular acidosis (pRTA). The indirect loss of $NaHCO_3$ may be due to a low rate of excretion of ammonium ($NH_4^+$) ions that is insufficient to match the daily rate of production of sulfuric acid ($H_2SO_4$) from the metabolism of sulfur-containing amino acids (e.g., in patients with chronic renal failure or distal renal tubular acidosis [dRTA]). Indirect loss of $NaHCO_3$ may also be due to the overproduction of an acid (e.g., hippuric acid formed during the metabolism of toluene) with the excretion of its conjugate base (hippurate anions) in the urine at a rate that exceeds the rate of excretion of $NH_4^+$ ions (see Chapter 3).

Assessment of the rate of excretion of $NH_4^+$ ions in the urine reveals the cause of HCMA. The rate of excretion of $NH_4^+$ ions in adults who consume a typical Western diet is 20 to 40 mmol/day. In a patient with chronic metabolic acidosis and normal renal function, the expected rate of excretion of $NH_4^+$ ions is ~200 mmol/day (~200 mmol $NH_4^+$ ions/g creatinine or ~20 mmol $NH_4^+$ ions/mmol creatinine). If the rate of excretion of $NH_4^+$ ions is low enough that it is not sufficient to generate enough new $HCO_3^-$ ions to replace that lost while titrating the $H^+$ ion load produced from usual dietary intake of sulfur-containing amino acids, the diagnostic category is renal tubular acidosis (RTA). In contrast, if the rate of excretion of $NH_4^+$ ions is high, the cause of HCMA is a loss of $NaHCO_3$ via the GI tract or the overproduction of an acid with the excretion of its anion in the urine at a higher rate than the rate of excretion of $NH_4^+$ ions.

## ABBREVIATIONS

$P_{Anion\ gap}$, anion gap in plasma
$P_{HCO_3}$, concentration of bicarbonite ($HCO_3^-$) ions in plasma
$P_{Cl}$, concentration of chloride ($Cl^-$) ions in plasma
$U_{Osmolal\ gap}$, osmolal gap in urine
HCMA, hyperchloremic metabolic acidosis
pRTA, proximal renal tubular acidosis
dRTA, distal renal tubular acidosis
ECF, extracellular fluid
ICF, intracellular fluid
GFR, glomerular filtration rate
EABV, effective arterial blood volume
RTA, renal tubular acidosis
PCT, proximal convoluted tubule
SLGT1, sodium-linked glucose transporter 1
$CA_{IV}$, carbonic anhydrase type IV
$CA_{II}$, carbonic anhydrase type II
NBCe1, sodium bicarbonate cotransporter 1
NHE-3, sodium hydrogen exchanger 3

---

### OBJECTIVES

■ To explain the pathophysiology of the disorders that lead to metabolic acidosis caused by a deficit of $NaHCO_3$.
■ To provide an approach to the diagnosis of metabolic acidosis caused by a deficit of $NaHCO_3$.
■ To discuss issues related to therapy with $NaHCO_3$ in these patients.

---

# PART A
# OVERVIEW

## DEFINITIONS

Before proceeding, a number of terms should be clearly defined.
- *Acidemia*: Acidemia is a low pH or a high $H^+$ ion concentration in plasma. When it is due to metabolic acidosis, both the blood pH and the $P_{HCO_3}$ are low.

- Metabolic acidosis is a process that leads to the accumulation of $H^+$ ions and the decrease in the content of $HCO_3^-$ ions in the body. Nevertheless, acidemia may not be present and the plasma pH and $P_{HCO_3}$ may be close to normal if there is another condition present that raises the $P_{HCO_3}$. For example, this second condition may be one that results in the addition of new $HCO_3^-$ to the body (e.g., the loss of HCl from the stomach; see Fig. 7-2) The concentration of $HCO_3^-$ ions in the extracellular fluid (ECF) compartment is a function of its content of $HCO_3^-$ ions divided by the ECF volume. Therefore, $P_{HCO_3}$ may rise if the ECF volume is appreciably contracted (contraction alkalosis).
- *Hyperchloremic metabolic acidosis (HCMA)*: HCMA refers to the presence of metabolic acidosis that is due to a deficit of $NaHCO_3$. This is simply a descriptive term based on the observation of an associated rise in the $P_{Cl}$ with the fall in the $P_{HCO_3}$. This, however, does not imply a primary role for $Cl^-$ ions in the pathogenesis of the metabolic acidosis. There are two possible mechanisms that explain the higher value for the $P_{Cl}$ in these patients:

1. Same content of $Cl^-$ ions but a contracted ECF volume: The first step is a loss of $NaHCO_3$. As a result of the deficit of $Na^+$ ions, the ECF volume declines. If there is no intake of NaCl, the content of $Cl^-$ ions in the ECF compartment remains unchanged, but because the ECF volume is contracted, the concentration of $Cl^-$ ions rises.
2. Higher content of $Cl^-$ ions but a normal ECF volume: The first step is also a loss of $NaHCO_3$. As a result of the deficit of $Na^+$ ions, the ECF volume declines. If there is an intake of NaCl, $Na^+$ and $Cl^-$ ions will be retained by the kidney in response to the low effective arterial blood volume (EABV). The net result is a normal ECF volume and a positive balance of $Cl^-$ ions; hence, the $P_{Cl}$ rises.

## PATHOGENESIS OF METABOLIC ACIDOSIS CAUSED BY NaHCO₃ LOSS

There are two ways to create a deficit of $NaHCO_3$ while preserving electroneutrality (Figure 4-1). First, the direct loss of $NaHCO_3$ occurs when both $Na^+$ and $HCO_3^-$ ions are lost via one route (e.g., via the GI tract or in the urine). Second, the indirect loss of $NaHCO_3$. This occurs in two steps as follows:

1. Addition of an acid: The $H^+$ ions of the added acid react with $HCO_3^-$ ions, resulting in the formation of $CO_2 + H_2O$; this $CO_2$ is exhaled via the lungs. At this point, there is a deficit of $HCO_3^-$ anions together with an equivalent gain of new anions in the ECF compartment.
2. Excretion of the anions with $Na^+$ ions: The second step is the excretion of the anions in the urine with a cation other than $H^+$ or $NH_4^+$ ions (i.e., with $Na^+$ and/or $K^+$ ions). The net effect of steps 1 and 2 is the loss of $NaHCO_3$ from the body.

A list of causes for an indirect loss of $NaHCO_3$ is provided in Table 4-1. Based on the rate of excretion of $NH_4^+$ ions, there are two subgroups of disorders that cause metabolic acidosis due to the indirect loss of $NaHCO_3$:

1. Acid overproduction with a higher rate of excretion of the new anions than the rate of excretion of $NH_4^+$ ions: In this subgroup, the major lesion is an overproduction of acids with a high rate of excretion of their anions in the urine. Even though the rate of excretion of $NH_4^+$ ions is high, the rate of excretion of the new anions exceeds that of $NH_4^+$ ions; hence, some of these anions are excreted in the urine with $Na^+$ or $K^+$ ions. These new anions are excreted at a high rate either because they are secreted by the proximal convoluted

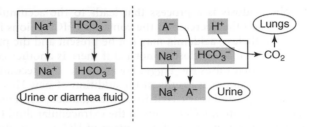

**Figure 4-1 Deficit of NaHCO₃.** The *rectangle* represents the extracellular fluid (ECF) compartment. As shown in the *left portion* of the figure, NaHCO₃ can be lost directly in gastrointestinal (GI) fluids or in the urine. As shown in the *right portion* of the figure, there is an indirect loss of NaHCO₃ when an acid (depicted as H⁺ + A⁻) is added and the rate of excretion of new anions (A⁻) exceeds the rate of excretion of $NH_4^+$ ions. There are two subgroups here, based on the rate of excretion of $NH_4^+$ ions. Individuals with a high rate of excretion of $NH_4^+$ ions have a primary high acid load, whereas those with a low rate of excretion of $NH_4^+$ ions have renal tubular acidosis (RTA) or renal insufficiency.

TABLE 4-1    **METABOLIC ACIDOSIS DUE TO AN INDIRECT LOSS OF NaHCO₃**

**Acid Overproduction with a Higher Rate of Excretion of New Anions Than the Rate of Excretion of $NH_4^+$ Ions**

- Glue-sniffing (hippuric acid overproduction)
- Diabetic ketoacidosis with rate of excretion of ketoacid anions that exceeds the rate of excretion of $NH_4^+$ ions

**Normal Acid Production but a Low Urinary Excretion of $NH_4^+$ Ions**

- Low glomerular filtration rate (GFR)
- Renal tubular acidosis
  - Low $NH_3$ type
  - Low net distal H⁺ ion secretion type
  - Low $NH_3$ and low net distal H⁺ ion secretion type

tubule (PCT) (e.g., hippurate⁻ anions produced from the metabolism of toluene in a glue sniffer) or because they are filtered and an appreciable quantity is not reabsorbed in the PCT (e.g., ketoacid anions early in the course of diabetic ketoacidosis).

2. Normal acid production but a low rate of excretion of $NH_4^+$ ions: In this subgroup of patients, the rate of production of acids is not increased. Rather, the major defect is a low rate of excretion of $NH_4^+$ ions (*low* is defined as a rate of excretion of $NH_4^+$ ions that is insufficient to generate enough new $HCO_3^-$ ions to dispose of the daily acid load produced in metabolism of sulfur-containing amino acids). Patients in this subgroup are heterogeneous with regard to the pathophysiology of their disorder; nevertheless, they are grouped together under the diagnostic category of RTA.

# PART B
# CONDITIONS THAT CAUSE A DEFICIT OF NaHCO₃

The initial steps to define why a patient has metabolic acidosis without the accumulation of new anions in plasma (i.e., HCMA) are outlined in Flow Chart 4-1. Assessing the rate of excretion of $NH_4^+$ ions in the urine is key to determine the pathophysiology of the metabolic acidosis in these patients.

## DIRECT LOSS OF NaHCO₃

In these conditions, both $Na^+$ and $HCO_3^-$ ions are lost via the same route. $NaHCO_3$ may be lost via the GI tract (e.g., in a patient with diarrhea) or via the urine (e.g., in a patient in the initial phase of a disease state causing pRTA).

### Loss of NaHCO₃ in the Gastrointestinal Tract

There are two major sites where $HCO_3^-$ ions are added to the lumen of the GI tract and thus possibly two sites for its loss.

### Secretion of HCO₃⁻ ions by the pancreas

$NaHCO_3$ is secreted by the pancreas. This process is stimulated by secretin, which is released by special enterocytes located in the duodenum in response to the $H^+$ ion load from the stomach. HCl secretion in the stomach (~100 mmol/day) adds $HCO_3^-$ ions to the body. Because somewhat in excess of 100 mmol of $NaHCO_3$ are secreted by the pancreas to ensure neutralization of this $H^+$ ion load, a modest net deficit of $NaHCO_3$ may occur if most of this pancreatic secretion is lost. Therefore, a mild degree of metabolic acidosis may develop in these patients unless the duration of these losses is prolonged and/or there is another disorder that diminishes the rate of excretion of $NH_4^+$ ions in the urine. Loss of pancreatic secretions may occur due to tube drainage, pancreatic or upper intestinal fistulae, or vomiting if the pyloric sphincter is patent as is the case in children and some adults. Fluid rich in $NaHCO_3$ may also be retained in the lumen of the intestine (e.g., due to ileus), and hence metabolic acidosis may develop.

### Secretion of HCO₃⁻ ions by the late small intestine and the colon

Two luminal transport mechanisms are involved in this process: an $Na^+/H^+$ exchanger (NHE) and a $Cl^-/HCO_3^-$ anion exchanger (AE)

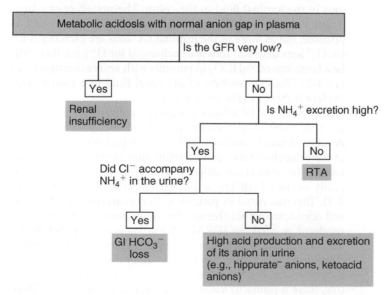

**Flow Chart 4-1 Approach to the Patient with Metabolic Acidosis and a Normal P**$_{Anion\,gap}$**.** The P$_{Anion\,gap}$ should be adjusted for the concentration of albumin in plasma (P$_{Albumin}$). Patients with proximal renal tubular acidosis (pRTA) who are in a steady state acid–base balance have a low rate of excretion of $NH_4^+$ ions; this is discussed in detail later in the chapter. *GFR*, Glomerular filtration rate; *GI*, gastrointestinal; *RTA*, renal tublar acidosis.

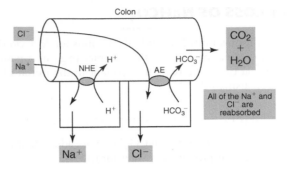

**Figure 4-2 Absorption of NaCl in the Colon.** The *cylindrical structure* represents the colon: the two *rectangles* represent colonic cells. $H^+$ ions and $HCO_3^-$ ions are formed in colonic cells from $CO_2 + H_2O$ by a reaction that is catalyzed by the enzyme carbonic anhydrase. When $Na^+$ and $Cl^-$ are delivered to the colon, both are absorbed using separate, electroneutral ion exchangers. $Na^+$ ions are absorbed in exchange for $H^+$ ions on the $Na^+/H^+$ exchanger (NHE). $Cl^-$ ions are is absorbed in exchange for $HCO_3^-$ ions on the $Cl^-/HCO_3^-$ anion exchanger (AE). In normal physiology, virtually all the $Na^+$ ions and $Cl^-$ ions are absorbed and $CO_2 + H_2O$ are produced.

(Figure 4-2). Whether the net result is a loss of $NaHCO_3$ depends on the rate of delivery of $Na^+$ and $Cl^-$ ions and the maximum transport capacity of each exchanger:

1. Low delivery of $Na^+$ and $Cl^-$ ions to the colon: In this setting, virtually all of the $Na^+$ and $Cl^-$ ions are reabsorbed while the secreted $H^+$ and $HCO_3^-$ ions are converted to $CO_2 + H_2O$. There is no loss of $NaHCO_3$ in this setting.
2. Very large delivery of $Na^+$ and $Cl^-$ ions to the colon: This may result in a loss of $NaHCO_3$ or HCl depending on the maximum transport capacity of NHE and AE.
   a. Loss of NaCl and $NaHCO_3$: Normally, the maximum transport capacity of NHE is less than that of AE because the rate of flux via NHE will be limited by the rise in the concentration of $H^+$ ions in the luminal fluid in the colon. The net effect of a large delivery of $Na^+$ and $Cl^-$ ions is to reabsorb as much NaCl as possible, but as more of the luminal $Cl^-$ ions are exchanged for $HCO_3^-$ ions than $Na^+$ ions are exchanged for $H^+$ ions, there will be a large loss of $NaHCO_3$ in patients with severe diarrhea (Figure 4-3). The composition of diarrheal fluid in a patient with cholera is shown in the margin note.
   b. Loss of NaCl and HCl: Some patients with diarrhea may not have a loss of $NaHCO_3$ in their diarrheal fluid, and therefore do not develop metabolic acidosis. In fact, these patients may lose HCl in their diarrheal fluid, and therefore may develop metabolic alkalosis. The underlying defect is a decrease in the transport capacity of the $Cl^-/HCO_3^-$ anion exchanger in the colon (Figure 4-4). This was noted in patients with certain colonic adenomas and adenocarcinomas (hence, this AE is given the name *downregulated in adenoma* [DRA]). A low transport capacity of AE may also be due to an inborn error (e.g., patients with congenital chloridorrhea) or in certain inflammatory disorders that involve the colon (e.g., some patients with ulcerative colitis). In this setting, there is primarily a loss of NaCl in the diarrheal fluid. There may be also a loss of $H^+$ and $Cl^-$ ions in diarrheal the fluid, which results in the addition of $HCO_3^-$ ions to the body and the development of metabolic alkalosis. Because the colonic NHE cannot raise the concentration of $H^+$ ions in luminal fluid to higher than 0.1 mmol/L (or lower the pH below 4), the presence of $H^+$ ion

**COMPOSITION OF DIARRHEAL FLUID IN A PATIENT WITH SEVERE DIARRHEA**

| | |
|---|---|
| $HCO_3^-$ | 40-45 mmol/L |
| $Cl^-$ | 110-115 mmol/L |
| $K^+$ | 15 mmol/L |
| $Na^+$ | 140 mmol/L |

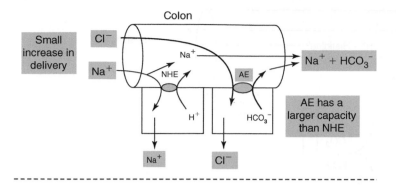

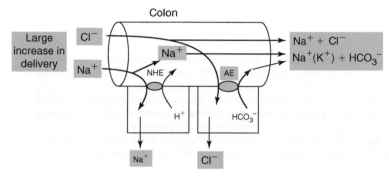

**Figure 4-3 Loss of NaHCO₃ from the colon.** The *cylindrical structure* represents the colon; the two *rectangles* represent colonic cells. The portion of
the figure above the horizontal *dashed line* reflects the effects of a modest
increase in the delivery of Na⁺ and Cl⁻ ions to the colon. The Cl⁻/HCO₃⁻
anion exchanger (AE) has a larger maximum transport capacity than Na⁺/H⁺
exchanger (NHE) because of the rise in the luminal concentration of H⁺
ions limits the secretion of H⁺ ions. Therefore, not all of the Na⁺ ions delivered are absorbed by NHE, whereas much of the Cl⁻ ions delivered are
absorbed by AE. Hence, the diarrhea fluid contains Na⁺ and HCO₃⁻ ions,
but only a small quantity of Na⁺ and Cl⁻ ions. In contrast, the portion of the
figure below the horizontal dashed line reflects the effects of a very large
increase in the delivery of Na⁺ and Cl⁻ ions to the colon. The diarrheal fluid
now contains a very large quantity of Na⁺ and Cl⁻ ions and there is also a
large loss of Na⁺, K⁺, and HCO₃⁻ ions.

acceptors in the luminal fluid in the colon are required to have an
appreciable loss of HCl. The H⁺ ion acceptors in this setting may
be histidines in the proteins of bacteria in the lumen of the colon.

## Clinical Picture

The clinical history is usually obvious, although some patients may
deny the use of laxatives. Urine electrolytes may provide a helpful clue
in this setting. The concentration of Na⁺ ions in the urine should be
low because of decreased effective arterial blood volume (EABV), but
the concentration of Cl⁻ ions in the urine may be high because of the
enhanced rate of excretion of NH₄⁺ ions in response to chronic acidemia. The ECF volume becomes contracted if the loss of Na⁺ ions
significantly exceeds their intake. Therefore, the $P_{HCO_3}$ may be close
to normal despite a significant deficit of HCO₃⁻ ions. In this setting,
the presence of metabolic acidosis and the magnitude of the deficit of
HCO₃⁻ ions are detected if the HCO₃⁻ ion content in the ECF compartment is calculated; this requires a quantitative assessment of the
ECF volume (using the hematocrit; see Chapter 2).

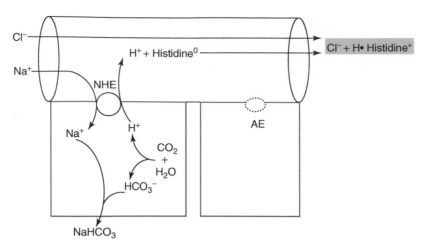

**Figure 4-4  Loss of H⁺ and Cl⁻ Ions from the Colon.** The *cylindrical structure* represents the colon: the two *rectangles* represent colonic cells. When a large quantity of Na⁺ and Cl⁻ ions are delivered to the colon, if there is downregulation of its Cl⁻/HCO₃⁻ anion exchanger (AE), there is a loss of primarily NaCl in the diarrheal fluid. There may also be a loss of H⁺ and Cl⁻ ions in diarrheal fluid, which results in addition of HCO₃⁻ ions to the body. Because the rise in the luminal concentration of H⁺ ions limits the secretion of H⁺ ions, to have an appreciable loss of HCl requires the presence of H⁺ ion acceptors in the luminal fluid in the colon; perhaps histidines in proteins of bacteria in the lumen of the colon may be the H⁺ ion acceptors. *DRA,* Downregulated in adenoma; *NHE,* Na⁺/H⁺ exchanger.

The degree of metabolic acidemia is more severe in a patient with diarrhea for two reasons. First, if there is an overproduction of organic acids in the colon (e.g., acetic acid, butyric acid, propionic acid, and D-lactic acid) caused by fermentation of carbohydrates by colonic bacteria. Second, if the rate of excretion of $NH_4^+$ ions is low because of a low GFR due to the very contracted EABV. The degree of acidemia may become more severe after the ECF volume is re-expanded for a number of reasons. First, if the ECF volume is re-expanded with the administration of a solution that does not contain enough $HCO_3^-$ ions or anions that can be metabolized to produce $HCO_3^-$ ions (e.g., lactate anions). Second, the loss of $NaHCO_3$ may also be increased with the restoration of the EABV because of the increase in blood flow and the delivery of Na⁺ and Cl⁻ ions to the small intestine. In addition, with expansion of the EABV, the blood flow rate to muscle rises and the $PCO_2$ in muscle capillaries and in muscle cells falls. This drives the bicarbonate buffer system reaction to the right, causing a fall in H⁺ ions concentration in muscle cells (see Eqn 1). As a result, many H⁺ ions that are bound to proteins in muscle cells will be released. Some of these H⁺ ions are exported out of muscle cells on the sodium-hydrogen exchanger-1 (NHE-1) because this cation exchanger is activated by a rise in the intracellular fluid (ICF) H⁺ ions concentration. These H⁺ ions titrate $HCO_3^-$ ions in the ECF compartment; hence the concentration of $HCO_3^-$ ions decreases, and a more severe degree of acidemia develops (see Figure 3-1).

$$H^+ + HCO_3^- \rightleftharpoons CO_2 + H_2O \qquad (1)$$

The $P_{Anion\ gap}$ may be increased, even in the absence of overproduction of acids, if there is a marked degree of ECF volume contraction. This is because of the rise in $P_{Albumin}$ and perhaps an increase in the anionic valence on albumin.

Patients with diarrhea may have a severe degree of K⁺ ion depletion. Nevertheless, hypokalemia may not be evident on presentation because of a shift of K⁺ ions out of cells caused by a deficiency of insulin (because of inhibition of its release by an α-adrenergic surge due

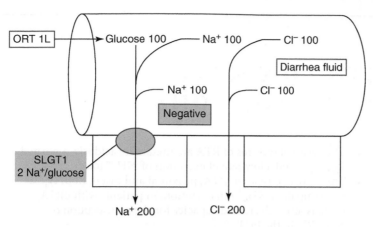

**Figure 4-5 Effects of Early Oral Replacement Therapy (ORT) on the Volume of Diarrheal Fluid.** The *cylindrical structure* represents the small intestine, the two *rectangles* represent intestinal cells. One liter of oral rehydration solution contains 100 mmol each of Na⁺ ions, Cl⁻ ions, and glucose. The stoichiometry of sodium-linked glucose transporter 1 (SLGT1) is that 2 mmol of Na⁺ ions are absorbed per mmol of glucose. The absorption of 100 mmol of glucose on SLGT1 leads to the absorption of 200 mmol of Na⁺ ions. The source of the other 100 mmol of Na⁺ ions is Na⁺ ions that are secreted in the diarrheal fluid. Although the exact mechanism of Cl⁻ ion reabsorption is not clear, it is possible that it is paracellular, driven by the negative luminal voltage created by the electrogenic absorption of Na⁺ ions via SLGT1.

to marked EABV contraction). A severe degree of hypokalemia may develop when the EABV is re-expanded.

## TREATMENT

One must first identify and treat emergencies that may be present on admission (e.g., hemodynamic instability) as well as anticipate and avoid those that might develop with therapy (e.g., hypokalemia). The volume of diarrheal fluid can be diminished by enhancing the reabsorption of NaCl that is secreted in the intestinal tract. This can be achieved by giving oral rehydration therapy, an oral solution that contain equimolar amounts of glucose and NaCl (Figure 4-5). The design of this oral rehydration fluid takes advantage of the stoichiometry of the sodium-linked glucose transporter 1 (SLGT1), which mediates the absorption of glucose from the lumen of the small intestine to decrease the volume of diarrheal fluid. The stoichiometry of SLGT1 is that 2 mmol of Na⁺ ions are absorbed per each mmol of glucose. One liter of oral rehydration solution contains 100 mmol of each Na⁺ ions, Cl⁻ ions, and glucose. The absorption of 100 mmol of glucose on SLGT1 leads to the absorption of 200 mmol of Na⁺ ions. The source of the other 100 mmol of Na⁺ ions is Na⁺ ions that are secreted in the diarrheal fluid. Although it is not exactly known, it is possible that the negative luminal voltage created by the electrogenic absorption of Na⁺ via SLGT1 provides the driving force for the paracellular reabsorption of 200 mmol of Cl⁻ ions. In more modern versions of this solution, a form of alkali is added (e.g., by replacing 25 to 50 mEq of Cl⁻ ions with citrate anions).

## RENAL LOSS OF NaHCO₃

Renal loss of NaHCO₃ may occur as a result of diminished reabsorption of filtered NaHCO₃ by the PCT. This disorder is called proximal RTA (pRTA). This topic is discussed in detail in Part C.

# PART C
# DISEASES WITH LOW RATE
# OF EXCRETION OF NH₄⁺ IONS

- The cardinal features of RTA are metabolic acidosis, a normal $P_{Anion\ gap}$, and a low rate of excretion of $NH_4^+$ ions.
- There are two types of RTA, proximal and distal. Both types have impaired $NH_4^+$ ion excretion; in patients with pRTA, there is also a decreased capacity for the reabsorption of $NaHCO_3$ in the PCT.

Patients with metabolic acidosis of renal origin have a low rate of net acid excretion. There are three groups of disorders in this diagnostic category: first, pRTA; second, dRTA; and third, disorders with a very low GFR. From a pathophysiologic perspective, the renal defect results in a low rate of excretion of $NH_4^+$ ions. pRTA is also characterized by a decreased capacity to reabsorb $NaHCO_3$.

## PROXIMAL RENAL TUBULAR ACIDOSIS

The pathophysiology of metabolic acidosis in patients with pRTA has two components:

1. Decreased reabsorption of $NaHCO_3$ in PCT:
   Although renal $HCO_3^-$ wasting and bicarbonaturia are present at the onset of disease, this is not a feature in the chronic steady state. In more detail, a decrease in the rate of $H^+$ ion secretion in the PCT diminishes the reabsorption of $HCO_3^-$ ions in the initial phase of the disease. As a result, delivery of $HCO_3^-$ ions to distal nephron segments exceeds their capacity to secrete $H^+$ ions, and $HCO_3^-$ ions are lost in the urine. As the $P_{HCO_3}$ falls, the filtered load of $HCO_3^-$ ions decreases until a point is reached where the capacity for $H^+$ ion secretion in the PCT and the distal nephron is sufficient to reclaim all the filtered load of $HCO_3^-$ ions. Thus, there is no further bicarbonaturia. In fact, the urine pH is characteristically low in patients with isolated pRTA (Table 4-2). Bicarbonaturia with a urine pH close to 7.0 may be noted, however, during times of the alkaline tide because of the secretion of HCl in the stomach, causing the addition of $HCO_3^-$ ions to the ECF compartment and a transient rise in $P_{HCO_3}$.

2. A low rate of excretion of $NH_4^+$ ions:
   The rate of excretion of $NH_4^+$ ions is low in patients with pRTA despite the presence of chronic metabolic acidemia. This low rate of excretion of $NH_4^+$ ions is due to an alkaline proximal cell pH (discussed later) in patients with the isolated form of pRTA and to a generalized PCT cell dysfunction in patients with the Fanconi syndrome type of disorder. A low rate of excretion of $NH_4^+$ ions compared to control subjects was demonstrated in a study of patients with the familial form of isolated pRTA after $NH_4Cl$ loading. In other patients with pRTA, a low rate of excretion of $NH_4^+$ ions can be deduced from the absence of bicarbonaturia in the steady state of the disease. If the kidneys were able to generate the expected close to 200 mmol/day of $HCO_3^-$ ions in these patients, the capacity for $HCO_3^-$ ion reabsorption would be exceeded, and this should have resulted in bicarbonaturia, which is not present in the chronic steady state of the disease.

TABLE 4-2   **RENAL HANDLING OF $HCO_3^-$ IONS IN PATIENTS WITH PROXIMAL RENAL TUBULAR ACIDOSIS**

In all of the examples, the GFR is 180 L/day. The normal filtered load of $HCO_3^-$ ions is 4500 mmol/day ($P_{HCO_3}$ 25 mmol/L × GFR 180 L/day). The lesion in patients with pRTA is a reduced $H^+$ ion secretion in PCT, and so the proximal reabsorption of $HCO_3^-$ ions falls. Because the distal nephron has a much lower capacity for $H^+$ ion secretion, only 900 mmol of $HCO_3^-$ per day (in this example) will be reabsorbed into the distal nephron, all the extra $HCO_3^-$ ions that are delivered to the distal nephron in excess of this amount will be excreted in the urine. As the filtered load of $HCO_3^-$ ions declines to the limits of the tubular reabsorption of $HCO_3^-$ ions, all the filtered load of $HCO_3^-$ ions is reabsorbed, there is no bicarbonaturia, and the urine pH is low in steady state.

| STATE | FILTERED $HCO_3^-$ (mmol/day) | PROXIMAL $HCO_3^-$ REABSORPTION (mmol/day) | DISTAL $HCO_3^-$ DELIVERY (mmol/day) | $HCO_3^-$ EXCRETION (mmol/day) |
|---|---|---|---|---|
| Normal | 4500 | 3600 | 900 | <5 |
| **Low $H^+$ Ion Secretion in the PCT** | | | | |
| Initial phase | 4500 | 2700 | 1800 | 900 |
| Steady state | 3600 | 2700 | 900 | <5 |

TABLE 4-3   **CONDITIONS LEADING TO PROXIMAL RENAL TUBULAR ACIDOSIS (pRTA)**

**Conditions Causing Fanconi Syndrome**
- Genetic disorders: e.g., cystinosis, galactosemia, hereditary fructose intolerance, Wilsons disease, Lowe's syndrome, tyrosinemia
- Toxin induced: e.g., Chinese herbs containing aristolochic acid, heavy metals such as lead
- Drug induced: e.g., tenofovir, ifosfamide
- Miscellaneous disorders: e.g., dysproteinemias including multiple myeloma, autoimmune diseases such as Sjögren's syndrome, chronic active hepatitis, postrenal transplantation

**Isolated Proximal RTA**
- Genetic disorders: e.g., mutations in the gene encoding the basolateral electrogenic sodium bicarbonate cotransporter 1 (NBCe1), familial isolated proximal RTA
- Drug induced: e.g., carbonic anhydrase IV inhibitors (e.g., acetazolamide, topiramate, dichlorphenamide)

**Combined Proximal and Distal RTA**
- Genetic disorders: carbonic anhydrase II deficiency

## CLINICAL SUBTYPES OF PROXIMAL RTA

### PROXIMAL RTA WITH FANCONI SYNDROME

In addition to a defect in $NaHCO_3$ reabsorption, patients with this syndrome exhibit defects in other $Na^+$-linked transport functions in the PCT. Hence, these patients may also have renal glucosuria, aminoaciduria, as well as increased excretion of urate, phosphate, and citrate. This syndrome might be due to a genetic defect or it might be acquired in a number of disorders (Table 4-3). The most common cause in the pediatric population is cystinosis, whereas common causes in the adult population are paraproteinemias and autoimmune disorders. Chinese herb ingestion is a common cause of Fanconi syndrome in Asian patients; the toxin implicated is aristolochic acid. Fanconi syndrome is also associated with the use of drugs such as tenofovir and the cyclophosphamide analog ifosfamide.

### ACQUIRED ISOLATED PROXIMAL RTA

This is caused by the use of drugs that inhibit carbonic anhydrase IV in the brush border of PCT cells, such as acetazolamide, topiramate, and dichlorphenamide. These patients may be at increased risk for formation of calcium phosphate stones. This is because the effect of these drugs to inhibit the reabsorption of $NaHCO_3$ in the PCT causes an alkaline urine pH, which increases the concentration of the divalent phosphate ions in the urine. In addition, hypocitraturia (because of the effect of metabolic acidemia to stimulate the reabsorption of citrate in the PCT) results in an increase in the concentration of the ionized calcium ions in the urine.

## HEREDITARY ISOLATED PROXIMAL RTA

**HEREDITARY ISOLATED PROXIMAL RTA**

• These findings are from studies in a single family from Costa Rica with hereditary autosomal dominant isolated pRTA.
• The molecular mechanism involved has not been identified.

Hereditary isolated pRTA has been described as an autosomal dominant disease, an autosomal recessive disease, or in some cases as a sporadic disease. Patients with isolated pRTA have both reduced capacity to reabsorb $HCO_3^-$ ions in their PCT and a low rate of excretion of $NH_4^+$ ions (see margin note). One possible explanation for this combination of defects is a more alkaline pH in PCT cells. This hypothesis could also explain the high rate of excretion of citrate observed in these patients. In more detail, the rate of excretion of citrate provides a "window" on the pH in PCT cells. An acidified PCT cell pH is associated with an enhanced reabsorption of citrate. Therefore, patients with metabolic acidemia have a very low rate of excretion of citrate. The sole exception to the previous statement is in patients with isolated pRTA who, despite metabolic acidemia, have a high rate of excretion of citrate. This may suggest that these patients have an alkaline PCT cell pH.

### Possible molecular lesions

There are three possible targets for a molecular lesion to cause isolated pRTA: the electrogenic sodium bicarbonate cotransporter 1 (NBCe1) at the basolateral membrane, the intracellular carbonic anhydrase II enzyme ($CA_{II}$), and the sodium-hydrogen exchanger-3 (NHE-3) in the luminal membrane of the PCT cells. Only two of these three possible lesions have been demonstrated to be associated with pRTA (Figure 4-6).

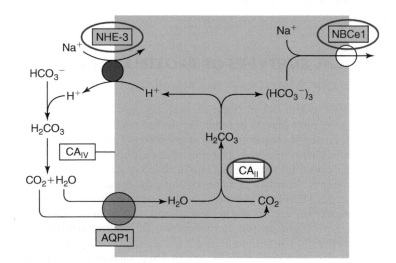

**Figure 4-6 Possible Molecular Lesions Causing Proximal Renal Tubular Acidosis (pRTA).** The structure represents the proximal convoluted tubule (PCT). The identified sites of lesions causing pRTA are inactivating mutations involving the electrogenic sodium bicarbonate cotransporter 1 (NBCe1) in the basolateral membrane or carbonic anhydrase II ($CA_{II}$) in PCT cells. Mutations in the gene encoding the sodium-hydrogen exchange-3 (NHE-3) have not been reported in patients with hereditary isolated pRTA. *AQP1*, Aquaporin 1.

## NBCe1 defect

HCO$_3^-$ ions reabsorbed in the PCT exits the cell as an ion complex (Na[HCO$_3$]$_3^{2-}$) which contains one Na$^+$ ion and three HCO$_3^-$ ions (or one HCO$_3^-$ ion and one CO$_3^{2-}$ ion), via NBCe1. Mutations in the gene encoding NBCe1 have been reported in children with the autosomal dominant hereditary isolated pRTA associated with ocular abnormalities. These mutations result in either a decreased maximum velocity ($V_{max}$) or a lower affinity for Na(HCO$_3$)$_3^{2-}$ ion complex (higher $K_m$) such that a higher concentration of HCO$_3^-$ ions (a more alkaline pH) in cells of the PCT are needed to export all HCO$_3^-$ ions that are reabsorbed.

## Carbonic anhydrase II defect

H$^+$ ions that are secreted in the PCT are derived from the dissociation of H$_2$O in PCT cells. The OH$^-$ ions formed in PCT cells are removed as HCO$_3^-$ ions in a reaction that is catalyzed by the enzyme CA$_{II}$. Mutations involving CA$_{II}$ lead to a more alkaline PCT cell pH because the OH$^-$ ion is a stronger base than the HCO$_3^-$ ion. Because CA$_{II}$ is also present in cells of the late distal nephron segments, these patients develop a clinical picture of both pRTA and dRTA. CA$_{II}$ is also involved in bone resorption. Hence, these patients may have dense bones (osteopetrosis) that are fragile, and therefore are at an and increased risk for bone fractures. They may also have cranial nerve compression due to excess bone, which can cause blindness, deafness, and/or facial paralysis.

## NHE-3 defect

Although in theory a molecular defect in the NHE-3 could cause pRTA, mutations in the gene encoding this transporter have not been reported in patients with hereditary isolated pRTA. Perhaps the reason is that NHE-3 mediates the reabsorption of an amount of HCO$_3^-$ ions (~3600 mmol/day), which is close to tenfold higher than the content of HCO$_3^-$ ions in the ECF compartment (~375 mmol). Therefore, even a relatively moderate defect in its transport activity would lead to a profound degree of acidemia. In fact, when NHE-3 was knocked out in mice, virtually all of them died at an early age.

## DIAGNOSTIC ISSUES IN THE PATIENT WITH PROXIMAL RENAL TUBULAR ACIDOSIS

Making the diagnosis of pRTA is usually not difficult. These patients have metabolic acidosis without an elevated P$_{Anion\ gap}$, and even large doses of NaHCO$_3$ fail to correct the acidemia because HCO$_3^-$ ions are lost in the urine if the filtered load exceeds the capacity for reabsorption. In patients with Fanconi syndrome, one finds other features of generalized PCT cell dysfunction (e.g., renal glucosuria). The absence of hypocitraturia despite metabolic acidemia also suggests the diagnosis of pRTA due to Fanconi syndrome.

In the chronic steady state, patients with pRTA do not have bicarbonaturia; in fact their urine pH is usually well below 6.0 (see Table 4-2). If a patient with pRTA does have bicarbonaturia, suspect one of the following:

1. A recent ingestion of alkali.
2. A disease process that is in evolution and thus a steady state has not been yet achieved (e.g., recent intake of Chinese herbs containing aristolochic acid).
3. A disease that also causes decreased distal H$^+$ secretion (e.g., a mutation involving the enzyme CA$_{II}$).

4. Intake of a drug (e.g., acetazolamide) that inhibits the enzyme $CA_{IV}$ (e.g., acetazolamide).

One may wish to confirm that there is a reduced capacity to reabsorb $HCO_3^-$ ions in the PCT by measuring the fractional excretion of $HCO_3^-$ ions ($FE_{HCO_3}$) after enough $NaHCO_3$ is given to raise the $P_{HCO_3}$ to 25 mmol/L. In patients with pRTA, the $FE_{HCO_3}$ is generally greater than 15%. In addition, the $P_{HCO_3}$ should fall promptly when the infusion of $NaHCO_3$ is stopped. In our view, it is not necessary to measure the $FE_{HCO_3}$ to confirm the diagnosis of pRTA because failure to correct the metabolic acidosis with large doses of alkali strongly suggests a PCT lesion. There is a caution here: administration of $NaHCO_3$ can be dangerous if the patient has hypokalemia because it may cause a significant fall in the $P_K$. Therefore, this test should be performed only after the $K^+$ ion deficit is replaced.

In patients with pRTA, there is usually no defect in distal $H^+$ secretion; therefore, the $PCO_2$ in alkaline urine is not low. A low $PCO_2$ in alkaline urine is observed in patients with combined pRTA and dRTA due to $CA_{II}$ deficiency. It is also possible that paraproteinemias or autoimmune disorders may involve both proximal and distal nephron sites.

### TREATMENT OF THE PATIENT WITH PROXIMAL RTA

This depends on the specific cause. Drugs that may cause pRTA (see Table 4-3) should be discontinued if feasible. In general, do not be overaggressive with treatment with $NaHCO_3$—the $P_{HCO_3}$ is rarely maintained near the normal range in patients with pRTA because bicarbonaturia ensues when the capacity for $HCO_3^-$ ion reabsorption is exceeded. Bicarbonaturia may lead to the development of hypokalemia and may increase the risk of formation of calcium phosphate kidney stones. Conversely, the administration of $NaHCO_3$ seems to be beneficial in children with pRTA and growth retardation.

## DISTAL RENAL TUBULAR ACIDOSIS

### CASE 4-1: A MAN DIAGNOSED WITH TYPE IV RENAL TUBULAR ACIDOSIS

A 51-year-old man has a long-standing history of poorly controlled type 2 diabetes mellitus and persistent HCMA. On physical examination, his blood pressure is 160/100 mm Hg, his pulse rate is 80 beats per minute, and there is no evidence of a contracted EABV. He is noted to have hyperkalemia. Further investigation revealed a low plasma renin mass and a somewhat low plasma aldosterone level. His current laboratory results are summarized in Table 4-4.

TABLE 4-4 **VALUES IN PLASMA AND A SPOT URINE SAMPLE**

|  |  | CASE 4-1 |  | CASE 4-2 |  |
|---|---|---|---|---|---|
|  |  | PLASMA | URINE | PLASMA | URINE |
| $Na^+$ | mmol/L | 140 | 140 | 140 | 75 |
| $K^+$ | mmol/L | 5.5 | 60 | 3.1 | 35 |
| $Cl^-$ | mmol/L | 112 | 130 | 113 | 95 |
| $HCO_3^-$ | mmol/L | 16 | — | 15 | — |
| pH | — | 7.30 | 5.0 | 7.30 | 6.8 |
| $PCO_2$ | mm Hg | 30 | — | 30 | — |
| Anion gap | mEq/L | 12 | — | 12 | — |
| Glucose | mg/dL (mmol/L) | 180 (10) | 20 | 90 (5.0) | 0 |
| Creatinine | mg/dL (μmol/L) | 2.3 (200) | 6 mmol/L | 0.7 (60) | 5 mmol/L |
| BUN (urea) | mg/dL (mmol/L) | 28 (10) | (250) | 14 (5.0) | (200) |
| Osmolality | mosmol/kgH₂O | 295 | 700 | 290 | 450 |

## Questions

What is the basis of the metabolic acidosis?
What is the cause of the low rate of excretion of $NH_4^+$ ions?

### CASE 4-2: WHAT IS THIS WOMAN'S "BASIC" LESION?

A 23-year-old woman suffers from Southeast Asian ovalocytosis. She is referred for assessment of HCMA and hypokalemia. Her physical examination was not remarkable, and her laboratory results are summarized in Table 4-4.

## Questions

What is the basis of the metabolic acidosis?
What is the cause of the low rate of excretion of $NH_4^+$ ions?

### NOMENCLATURE

Numeric terms are currently used to describe patients who have metabolic acidosis caused by a low rate of excretion of $NH_4^+$ ions (i.e., type I RTA, type II RTA, type IV RTA). These terms, however, do not provide insights into the pathophysiology of the disorder in each type; moreover, patients with different reasons for the low rate of excretion of $NH_4^+$ ions are grouped into a single type of RTA. In addition, terms such as distal or proximal may not reflect the site of the lesion in an individual patient. Hence, we prefer a classification of RTA based on the pathophysiology of the disorder (Table 4-5).

### CLINICAL APPROACH: INITIAL STEPS

Normal subjects who are given a large acid load for several days increase their rate of excretion of $NH_4^+$ ions to greater than 200 mmol/day. Hence, the expected renal response to chronic metabolic acidosis is a large increase in the rate of excretion of $NH_4^+$ ions. Two steps are involved. First, metabolic acidemia stimulates the production of $NH_4^+$ ions in the cells of the PCT, which results in a high concentration of $NH_4^+$ ions in the medullary interstitial compartment. Second, metabolic acidemia stimulates $H^+$ ion secretion in the distal nephron, which augments the transfer of $NH_4^+$ ions from the medullary interstitial compartment into the lumen of the medullary collecting duct. A detailed discussion of the physiology of the excretion of $NH_4^+$ ions is provided in Chapter 1.

### Assess the rate of $NH_4^+$ ion excretion

The hallmark of RTA is a low rate of $NH_4^+$ ion excretion in a patient with chronic metabolic acidosis. Hence, assessment of the rate of excretion of $NH_4^+$ ions is the first diagnostic step in these patients. The urine pH is

**HETEROGENEITY OF PATIENTS WITH RTA AND A HIGH $P_K$**

- In some patients, a high $P_K$ might cause the low rate of excretion of $NH_4^+$ ions.
- In other patients, however, separate lesions may cause the high $P_K$ and the low rate of $NH_4^+$ ion excretion.

**ABBREVIATIONS**

$P_K$, concentration of potassium ($K^+$) ions in plasma
$U_{NH_4}$, concentration of ammonium ($NH_4^+$) ions in the urine
$U_{Creatinine}$, concentration of creatinine in the urine
$U_{Osmolal\ gap}$, urine osmolal gap
AE-1, $Cl^-/HCO_3^-$ anion exchanger 1
$U_{Na}$, concentration of sodium ($Na^+$) ions in the urine
$U_K$, concentration of potassium ($K^+$) ions in the urine
$U_{Cl}$, concentration of chloride ($Cl^-$) ions in the urine
$U_{Ca}$, concentration of calcium ions in the urine
$U_{Mg}$, concentration of magnesium ions in the urine
$U_{Phosphate}$, concentration of phosphate ions in the urine
MCD, medullary collecting duct

TABLE 4-5 **NOMENCLATURE USED IN THE CLASSIFICATION OF RENAL TUBULAR ACIDOSIS**

We prefer a classification based on the pathophysiology of the disorder rather than numerical labels.

| COMMONLY USED | SUGGESTED CHANGE |
| --- | --- |
| Type I RTA or distal RTA | Low $NH_4^+$ excretion disease |
| Type II RTA or proximal RTA | Low $NH_4^+$ excretion with renal $HCO_3^-$ wasting disease |
| Type IV RTA (see margin note) | Low $NH_4^+$ excretion associated with hyperkalemia |

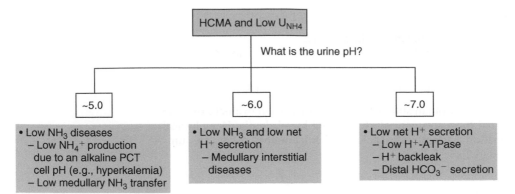

**Flow Chart 4-2 Approach to the Patient with Hyperchloremic Metabolic Acidosis (HCMA) and a Low Rate of Excretion of NH$_4^+$ Ions.** In a patient with HCMA and a low rate of excretion of NH$_4^+$ ions, the next step is to measure the urine pH to determine the basis for the low rate of excretion of NH$_4^+$ ions. *PCT*, Proximal convoluted tubule.

not a reliable indicator for the rate of excretion of NH$_4^+$ (see Chapter 1, Fig. 1-17). Therefore, it is not correct to use the urine pH to make the diagnosis of RTA. To evaluate the rate of excretion of NH$_4^+$ ions, the concentration of NH$_4^+$ in the urine should be estimated by calculating the urine osmolal gap (U$_{Osmolal\ gap}$) (see Chapter 2). If the U$_{NH_4}$/U$_{Creatinine}$ is less than 3 in a random urine sample while acidemia is present, the rate of NH$_4^+$ ion excretion is low enough to be the sole cause of the metabolic acidosis.

### Determine the basis of the low rate of excretion of NH$_4^+$ ions

Once it has been established that the rate of excretion of NH$_4^+$ ions is low in a patient with HCMA, examining the urine pH helps one to determine the basis of this low rate of NH$_4^+$ ion excretion. If H$^+$ ion secretion in the distal nephron occurs but little NH$_3$ is available to bind these H$^+$ ions, the urine pH will be close to 5.0. Conversely, if H$^+$ ion secretion in the distal nephron is low in the presence of ample NH$_3$, the urine pH will be close to 7.0. A urine pH value close to 6.0 suggests that there is a lesion causing defects in both NH$_3$ availability and distal H$^+$ ion secretion (Flow Chart 4-2).

## SUBTYPES OF DISORDERS CAUSING LOW NH$_4^+$ ION EXCRETION

### SUBTYPE WITH LOW NH$_3$

#### Pathophysiology

The pathophysiology of this subtype of low rate of excretion of NH$_4^+$ ions is a low rate of production of NH$_4^+$ ions in cells of the PCT. The usual causes of a low production of NH$_4^+$ ions are an alkaline PCT cell pH due to hyperkalemia and/or a low availability of ADP in PCT cells due to a low GFR (see Chapter 1) (Table 4-6). The rate of excretion of NH$_4^+$ ions is low in patients with pRTA despite the presence of chronic metabolic acidemia. This low rate of production of NH$_4^+$ ions may be due to an alkaline PCT cell pH. In patients with the isolated form of pRTA (e.g., due to a genetic defect), the alkaline PCT cell pH may be due to a defect involving NBCe1. In patients with the Fanconi syndrome (e.g., due to a paraproteinemia or an autoimmune disorder), the alkaline PCT cell pH may be due to a generalized PCT cell dysfunction. Less common causes of low NH$_4^+$ ion production include decreased availability of glutamine due to malnutrition and/or high levels of other

TABLE 4-6   **CAUSES OF A LOW RATE OF PRODUCTION OF NH₄⁺ IN THE PROXIMAL CONVOLUTED TUBULE**

**Alkaline Proximal Cell pH**
- Hyperkalemia
- Carbonic anhydrase II deficiency
- Some subtypes of pRTA (e.g., autosomal dominant hereditary isolated pRTA)

**A Low Rate of Oxidation of Glutamine**
- Low GFR causing low availability of ADP in PCT cells
- Low availability of glutamine (e.g., malnutrition)
- Provision of alternate fuels that compete with glutamine for oxidation (e.g., fatty acids in patients given parenteral nutrition)

fuels that PCT cells can oxidize to regenerate the body's requisite ATP (e.g., free fatty acids in patients on total parenteral nutrition).

## Clinical features

The two most common causes of a low production of $NH_4^+$ ions are hyperkalemia and a low GFR.

### Hyperkalemia

The term type IV RTA is commonly used to describe the constellation of findings of hyperkalemia and metabolic acidosis due to a low rate of excretion of $NH_4^+$ ions (see Table 4-5). Nevertheless, there are two distinct ways that hyperkalemia and a low rate of excretion of $NH_4^+$ ions may coexist:

1. Hyperkalemia is responsible for the low rate of excretion of $NH_4^+$ ions. Hyperkalemia may cause a low rate of $NH_4^+$ ion excretion by inhibiting $NH_4^+$ ion production (hyperkalemia is associated with an alkaline PCT cell pH) and/or the transfer of $NH_4^+$ ions in the loop of Henle ($K^+$ ions compete with $NH_4^+$ ions for transport on the $Na^+$, $K^+$, 2 $Cl^-$ cotransporter, NKCC-2). In these patients, the urine pH is low (~5). If this is the case, the patient should have a sufficient increase in the rate of excretion of $NH_4^+$ ions to correct the metabolic acidosis, as the $P_K$ is returned to the normal range. In some patients, however, it might be difficult to establish a "cause and effect" relationship if there is another factor that may also contribute to the low rate of excretion of $NH_4^+$ ions (e.g., a low GFR due to a contracted EABV in a patient with adrenal insufficiency) because this will also be corrected during therapy.
2. Hyperkalemia is not the major reason for the low rate of excretion of $NH_4^+$ ions. In this subgroup of patients, the low rate of excretion of $NH_4^+$ ions is not causally linked to the hyperkalemia. This is suggested by the finding that the metabolic acidemia persists and the rate of excretion of $NH_4^+$ ions remains low, after the hyperkalemia is corrected. In general, the basis of the low rate of excretion of $NH_4^+$ ions in this subgroup is a combination of low $NH_3$ availability and low distal $H^+$ ion secretion; hence, the urine pH is close to 6. For chronic hyperkalemia to be present, the disease process must also involve the late cortical distal nephron, the site of $K^+$ ion secretion.

### Consequences of a persistently low urine pH

A persistently low urine pH increases the risk of uric acid stone formation, especially if the urine volume is low. The pK of uric acid in the urine is ~5.3 and its solubility is ~0.6 mmol/L. The focus of the therapy is to raise the urine pH to ~6.5 by administration of alkali.

## Treatment

### Emergency management

The most important threat to the patient is a cardiac arrhythmia due to hyperkalemia. Hyperkalemia should be treated as an emergency if there are EKG changes that are related to hyperkalemia; treatment of emergency hyperkalemia is discussed in Chapter 15.

### Acid–base management

In a subset of patients, bringing the $P_K$ down to the normal range leads to an increase in the rate of excretion of $NH_4^+$ ions and correction of the metabolic acidemia. In other patients, treatment with $NaHCO_3$ may be necessary because chronic metabolic acidemia may lead to catabolism of lean body mass, progression of chronic kidney disease, and formation of uric acid stones (because of the persistently low urine pH). Excessive bicarbonaturia, however, should be avoided because it might predispose to the formation of calcium phosphate kidney stones should the urine pH rise excessively. Therefore, the dose of $NaHCO_3$ should be distributed throughout the day to ensure that the urine pH is not greater than 6.5 throughout the 24-hour period.

## SUBTYPE WITH LOW NET DISTAL H⁺ ION SECRETION

### Pathophysiology

These patients have a low rate of excretion of $NH_4^+$ ions because of a low net addition of $H^+$ ions into the lumen of the distal nephron. The urine pH is close to 7. The potential causes of this low net distal $H^+$ ion secretion are listed in Table 4-7. The possible etiologies can be distinguished by examining the $PCO_2$ in alkaline urine and the rate of excretion of citrate (Flow Chart 4-3).

### Low number of H⁺ ATPase pumps in the distal nephron

This group includes children with rare inborn errors affecting the $H^+$-ATPase, usually associated with sensorineuronal deafness. The common causes in adult patients are autoimmune and hypergammaglobulinemic disorders (e.g., Sjogren's syndrome). In some patients with low distal $H^+$ ion secretion, the $H^+$ ATPase was not detected in luminal membranes of $\alpha$-intercalated cells by immunohistologic staining of renal biopsy specimens. Although it is possible that circulating antibodies

---

TABLE 4-7    **CAUSES OF A LOW RATE OF EXCRETION OF NH₄⁺ IONS DUE TO DECREASED NET H⁺ ION SECRETION**

**Low H⁺ APTase Activity (PCO₂ in Alkaline Urine Is Low)**
- Mutations involving the $H^+$ APTase (±sensorineuronal deafness)
- Alkaline distal cell pH due to carbonic anhydrase II deficiency or acquired disorders causing an alkaline distal cell pH (e.g., autoimmune diseases and hypergamma-globulinemic states such as Sjögren's disease and systemic lupus erythematosus)

**High Distal Secretion of HCO₃⁻ Ions in α-Intercalated Cells (PCO₂ in Alkaline Urine Is High)**
- Some patients with Southeast Asian ovalocytosis (these patients have two mutations in the gene encoding AE-1: the usual one that leads to ovalocytosis and a second one that causes the AE-1 to be targeted abnormally to the luminal membrane of α-intercalated cells)
- Possibly in some patients with autoimmune disorders

**Back-Leak of H⁺ Ions (PCO₂ in Alkaline Urine Is High)**
- Drugs (e.g., amphotericin B)

may damage the H⁺-ATPase, it is also possible that the low amount of H⁺ ATPase is secondary to a persistently alkaline α-intercalated cell pH (see margin note). In patients with this defect, the $PCO_2$ in alkaline urine should be close to the arterial $PCO_2$ or ~40 mm Hg. Citrate excretion in these patients is low because of the effect of acidemia to enhance the reabsorption of citrate in the PCT.

### Inhibition of existing H⁺-ATPase pumps by an alkaline cell pH (Figure 4-7)

There are two subgroups of patients in this category. The first consists of patients with autoimmune disorders that lead to damage of the Cl⁻/HCO₃⁻ anion exchanger (AE-1) in the basolateral membrane of α-intercalated cells, leading to a persistently alkaline cell pH, with decreased expression of H⁺ APTase in the luminal membrane. The second subgroup consists of patients with a lesion that leads to $CA_{II}$

**DISTAL RTA DUE TO AUTOIM-MUNE DISORDERS**

• It is difficult to explain how circulating antibodies could have entered the cell and remained intact to cause damage to the H⁺-ATPase.
• Although high titers of autoantibodies against $CA_{II}$ were detected in some patients with Sjogren's syndrome, the same question as earlier arises.
• It is possible that the antibodies in these patients cause damage to the Cl⁻/HCO₃⁻ anion exchanger in the basolateral membrane of α-intercalated cells.

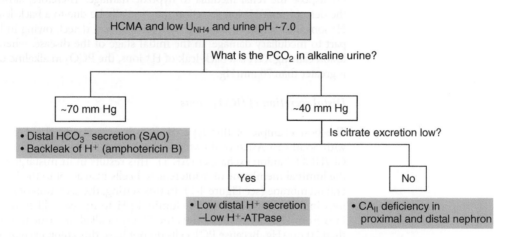

**Flow Chart 4-3 Approach to the Patient with Distal Renal Tubular Acidosis (RTA) and a Urine pH Close to 7.** RTA is present because the rate of excretion of $NH_4^+$ ions is low; its basis is a low net rate of H⁺ ion secretion in the distal nephron when the urine pH ~7.0. The steps to define the underlying disorders are summarized here. $CA_{II}$, Carbonic anhydrase II; *HCMA*, hyperchloremic metabolic acidosis; *SAO*, Southeast Asian ovalocytosis.

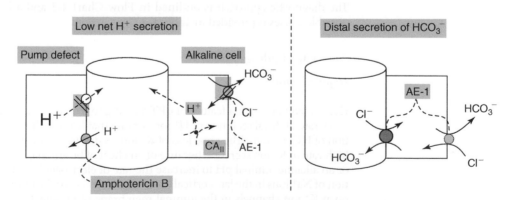

**Figure 4-7 Lesions Compromising Distal Net H⁺ Secretion.** The *cylindrical structure* represents the late distal nephron; the *rectangles* represent α-intercalated cells. Lesions causing a decrease in net H⁺ ion secretion are shown to the *left* of the dashed line, whereas those causing the secretion of HCO₃⁻ ions are shown to the *right* of the dashed line. The major causes of low net H⁺ ion secretion are an H⁺ APTase pump defect, back-leak of H⁺, or an alkaline intercalated cell (i.e., failure to remove OH⁻ ions via $CA_{II}$ deficiency or failure to export HCO₃⁻ ions out of the cell via the Cl⁻/HCO₃⁻ anion exchanger [AE-1] on their basolateral membrane). Enhanced distal secretion of HCO₃⁻ ions is shown in the *right portion* of the figure; this occurs due to mistargeting of AE-1 to the luminal membrane of α-intercalated cells.

deficiency (see pRTA section earlier in this chapter). In both subgroups, the $PCO_2$ in alkaline urine would be close to 40 mm Hg because of a low rate of distal secretion of $H^+$ ions. The rate of excretion of citrate, however, would be low in the first subset of patients but could be high in patients with $CA_{II}$ deficiency because this disorder causes an alkaline PCT cell pH, which leads to diminished reabsorption of citrate.

### Back-leak of $H^+$ ions in the distal nephron

Amphotericin B is thought to cause the insertion of nonspecific cationic channels in the luminal membrane of cells in the distal nephron. This leads to a low net $H^+$ ion secretion in the distal nephron as secreted $H^+$ ions back-leak into α-intercalated cells. With a large back-leak of $H^+$ ions, there would be a continuously high rate of distal $H^+$ ion secretion with a considerable expenditure of energy in an area of the kidney with a low blood flow rate and therefore a marginal supply of oxygen. This might predispose the renal medulla to hypoxic damage. Therefore, although the defect in net $H^+$ ion secretion may initially be due to a back-leak of $H^+$ ions, this might be followed by a longer-term defect, owing in large part to medullary damage. In the initial stage of the disease, when the lesion causing RTA is a back-leak of $H^+$ ions, the $PCO_2$ in alkaline urine is greater than 70 mm Hg.

### Distal secretion of $HCO_3^-$ ions

The best example of this type of disorder is seen in those patients with Southeast Asian ovalocytosis who have a second mutation in the $Cl^-/HCO_3^-$ anion exchanger (AE-1). This results in its mistargeting to the luminal membrane of α-intercalated cells instead of to the basolateral membrane (see Figure 4-7). In this setting, the secretion of $HCO_3^-$ ions into the lumen causes the luminal pH to increase, liberating $H^+$ ions from $H_2PO_4^-$, which raises the $PCO_2$ in alkaline urine to greater than 70 mm Hg. Because PCT cells do not have this anion exchanger as their exit step for $HCO_3^-$ ions, their ICF pH will be reduced because of the acidemia; hence, these patients have a low rate of excretion of citrate.

## Clinical features

The diagnostic approach is outlined in Flow Chart 4-3 and a list of possible causes is provided in Table 4-7.

## Associated findings

### Hypokalemia

Hypokalemia is often a feature of dRTA owing to a defect that leads to a low rate of distal secretion of $H^+$ ions or one that leads to distal secretion of $HCO_3^-$ ions. The renal loss of $K^+$ ions is due to an unexpectedly high rate of $K^+$ ion secretion because of an effect of bicarbonaturia and/or an alkaline luminal pH to increase the rate of electrogenic reabsorption of $Na^+$ ions in the late cortical distal nephron and/or the number of open $K^+$ ion channels in the luminal membrane of principal cells (see Chapter 13).

Hypokalemia may be severe and cause muscle weakness. At times, this may be the symptom that brings the patient to clinical attention.

### Nephrocalcinosis

Patients with dRTA that is associated with hypokalemia have an increased incidence of calcium deposition in the medullary interstitial

TABLE 4-8   **EFFECT OF RAISING THE URINE pH ON THE URINARY DIVALENT PHOSPHATE CONCENTRATION**

For this calculation, we used a total 24-hour excretion of inorganic phosphate of 30 mmol, a urine volume of 1 L, and a pH of 6.8. At a urine pH of 7.1, two-thirds of the total phosphate in the urine is in the divalent form ($HPO_4^{2-}$), while one third will be in the monovalent form ($H_2PO_4^-$). There is a small percentage increase in $HPO_4^{2-}$ concentration when the urine pH rises from 7.1 to 7.5.

| URINE PH | $H_2PO_4^-$ (mmol/L) | $HPO_4^{2-}$ (mmol/L) |
|---|---|---|
| 6.8 | 15 | 15 |
| 7.1 | 10 | 20 |
| 7.3 | 7.5 | 22.5 |
| 7.4 | 6 | 24 |
| 7.5 | 5 | 25 |

compartment—this is called nephrocalcinosis. The reasons that calcium salts are more likely to precipitate in this region are higher concentrations of ionized calcium in the medullary interstitial compartment and/or the anions ionized calcium might precipitate with. Medullary alkalinization is required to form a precipitate of calcium with divalent phosphate ($HPO_4^{2-}$) or carbonate anions. We provide a more detailed discussion of possible mechanisms in Part D.

## Consequences of a high urine pH

### Calcium phosphate (CaHPO₄) stones

There are two major factors that permit $CaHPO_4$ stones to form: a higher concentration (activity) of ionized calcium and a higher concentration (higher activity) of $HPO_4^{2-}$ in the urine. The major risk factor for the former is a low rate of excretion of citrate because this anion chelates ionized calcium. The low rate of excretion of citrate can be due to acidemia and/or hypokalemia, both of which are present in this group of patients with dRTA. The major reason to have a high concentration of $HPO_4^{2-}$ in the luminal fluid is a high urine pH, which converts monovalent phosphate ($H_2PO_4^-$) to divalent phosphate ($HPO_4^{2-}$) which precipitates with ionized calcium ($Ca^{2+}$). Histological examination of kidney tissue from patients with dRTA and $CaHPO_4$ stones revealed calcium phosphate deposits plugging the inner medullary collecting ducts and ducts of Bellini, with interstitial inflammation and fibrosis. This may lead to progressive renal insufficiency, and emphasizes the importance of prevention of $CaHPO_4$ precipitation. Although alkali therapy with K citrate may be beneficial in these patients if it increases the rate of excretion of citrate, it may, however, cause a further rise in the urine pH, thereby increasing the risk of precipitation of $CaHPO_4$. Notwithstanding, the effect of a rise in urine pH on increasing the concentration of $HPO_4^2$ becomes progressively smaller as the urine pH rises above 6.8 (Table 4-8).

## Treatment

### Emergency issues

The most important threat to the patient is a cardiac arrhythmia due to hypokalemia. Hypokalemia may also cause respiratory muscle weakness and thus severe acidemia due to superimposed respiratory acidosis. $NaHCO_3$ should not be given until the $P_K$ is raised to a safe level (~3.5 mmol/L) to avoid a dangerous decline in the $P_K$ because of a shift of $K^+$ ions into cells. The emergency treatment of hypokalemia is discussed in Chapter 14.

*Acid–base issues*

Alkali therapy is usually needed because these patients are unable to excrete enough $NH_4^+$ ions to regenerate the $HCO_3^-$ ions consumed by the dietary acid load. Bicarbonaturia, however, should be minimized because it might predispose to excessive renal $K^+$ ion loss and $CaHPO_4$ kidney stone formation. Therefore, the dose of $NaHCO_3$ should be as small as possible and be distributed throughout the day. After the $P_{HCO_3}$ is corrected, the dose of $NaHCO_3$ needed to maintain $P_{HCO_3}$ in the normal range is usually less than 30 to 40 mmol/day (i.e., enough to titrate the daily acid load produced from the metabolism of dietary sulfur-containing amino acids).

## SUBTYPE WITH LESIONS INVOLVING BOTH DISTAL $H^+$ ION SECRETION AND $NH_3$ AVAILABILITY

### Pathophysiology

Diseases involving the renal medulla can compromise collecting duct cells and thereby cause a low $H^+$-ATPase activity and also diminish $NH_3$ availability in the medullary interstitium. Hence, the rate of excretion of $NH_4^+$ ions is low and the urine pH is usually close to 6.0. Because of the presence of acidemia, the rate of excretion of citrate is low. The defect in distal $H^+$ ion secretion can be confirmed by finding a $PCO_2$ in alkaline urine that is close to 40 mm Hg.

### Clinical features

The list of causes of disorders that affect the renal medullary interstitial compartment is long and includes infections, drugs, infiltrations, precipitations, inflammatory disorders, and sickle cell anemia, among others. Because of the medullary interstitial disorder, these patients may also have a reduced urinary concentrating ability. Hyperkalemia may be present if the disease process also involves the late cortical distal nephron. Nevertheless, the acidemia persists even after the $P_K$ is returned to the normal range.

### Treatment

Administration of alkali is needed to correct the acidemia. The issues for alkali therapy that were discussed in the subgroup with diminished net $H^+$ ion secretion apply here.

## INCOMPLETE RENAL TUBULAR ACIDOSIS

The label "incomplete RTA" originated in an era when the linchpin in the diagnosis of dRTA was a high urine pH in patients with HCMA. Hence, when patients present with recurrent $CaHPO_4$ stones, especially at a young age, and they have a high urine pH in the absence of HCMA, the label given to this constellation of findings was incomplete RTA. This combination of findings, however, may be present in three circumstances, which are discussed in the following paragraphs. Only the third represents incomplete RTA.

### DISTAL RENAL TUBULAR ACIDOSIS CAUSED BY LOW NET DISTAL SECRETION OF $H^+$ IONS

Although these patients usually have metabolic acidosis, acidemia may not be present if they ingest a low net $H^+$ ion load (i.e., if their diet were to have more alkali, such as more fruit and vegetables [see Fig. 1-5] and/or fewer precursors of $H_2SO_4$, such as low protein intake [see Fig. 1-3]). Accordingly, the key diagnostic step in this setting is to find a low rate of excretion of $NH_4^+$ ions after chronic acidemia is induced by the administration of an acid load (e.g., $NH_4Cl$) for several days.

## LARGE INTERMITTENT INTAKE OF ALKALI IN A NORMAL SUBJECT

The diet in these subjects provides a large episodic load of alkali (e.g., large intake of fruit and vegetables). These patients have a normal plasma pH and $P_{HCO_3}$ along with a high urine pH. Additional clues to suggest that a large episodic load of alkali is the basis for the high urine pH are the following: (1) the rate of excretion of $NH_4^+$ ions is low when compared with that of $SO_4^{2-}$ anions in mEq terms (diet alkali load titrates $H^+$ ions from $H_2SO_4$) and (2) the calculated dietary net alkali intake is large (e.g., as reflected by the rate of excretion of organic anions including citrate in the urine; see margin note). The patients in this subgroup resemble the patients with dRTA due to low net $H^+$ ion secretion described previously, except that they do not develop acidemia when they consume a typical Western diet, and they are able to increase their rate of excretion of $NH_4^+$ ions appropriately when given an acid load (e.g., $NH_4Cl$) for several days.

## PATIENTS WITH TRUE "INCOMPLETE RENAL TUBULAR ACIDOSIS"

These patients usually come to medical attention because they have recurrent $CaHPO_4$ kidney stones. The initial diagnostic workup reveals a persistently high urine pH for much of the day (>6.5 for at least 12 out of 24 hours [admittedly an arbitrary definition]). The key diagnostic feature in this group of patients is a high rate of excretion of $NH_4^+$ ions relative to their dietary acid load from metabolism of sulfur-containing amino acids, as reflected by the rate of excretion of $SO_4^{2-}$ anions in mEq terms. Normal subjects have near-equal daily excretions of $NH_4^+$ and $SO_4^{2-}$ ions in mEq terms, and patients with dRTA excrete less $NH_4^+$ ions than $SO_4^{2-}$ ions in mEq terms. Hence, the term incomplete RTA is misleading because RTA is a disorder with the principal finding of a low rate of excretion of $NH_4^+$ ions, and patients with the so-called "incomplete RTA" have a high rate of excretion of $NH_4^+$ ions relative to their rate of excretion of $SO_4^{2-}$ ions. We envisage two subtypes of lesions that may lead to the high rate of $NH_4^+$ ions in these patients:

1. Acidified PCT cell pH: An acidified PCT cell pH could be due to a lesion that causes activation of the exit step for the $Na(HCO_3)_3^{2-}$ complex ion in the basolateral membrane of these cells. As a result of the low intracellular pH, there is a greater rate of production of $NH_4^+$ ions and thus a higher concentration of $NH_4^+$ ions in the renal medullary interstitial compartment. If this were to lead to a greater rate of $NH_3$ entry into the lumen of the medullary collecting duct (MCD), the urine pH would be greater than 6.5 and the rate of excretion of $NH_4^+$ ions would also be high. As a result of the low pH in the PCT cells, the rate of reabsorption of citrate should rise and the excretion of citrate would be extremely low. This contributes in a major way to the likelihood of formation of calcium stones because citrate is a chelator of ionized calcium in the urine. A high medullary $NH_4^+$ ion concentration may activate the complement system and thereby lead to secondary medullary interstitial damage. If this were to lead to a decrease in the rate of excretion of $NH_4^+$ ions, the patient may develop dRTA later in life.

**CALCULATION OF DIET ALKALI INTAKE**

- A high rate of excretion of organic anions (including citrate) is suspected when their "electrical shadow" is present in the urine, that is, $(U_{Na}+U_K+U_{NH_4}+U_{Ca}+U_{Mg})$ is greater than $(U_{Cl}+U_{HPO_4}+U_{SO_4})$, all in mEq/L terms.
- Because the major source of $Na^+$ and $Cl^-$ in the urine comes from ingestion of NaCl, the rate of excretion of these ions is virtually always equal in mEq terms and they can be removed from the preceding calculation.
- In most subjects, the rates of excretion of $NH_4^+$ and $SO_4^{2-}$ ions are virtually equal in mEq terms, so they too can be removed from the calculation.
- Because the rates of excretion of calcium and magnesium are relatively small, they can be ignored for the purpose of this calculation. Therefore, the rate of excretion of organic anions in a 24 hour period can be estimated from the difference in the rate of excretion of $K^+$ ions and the rate of excretion of monovalent phosphate during that time period (i.e., if the source of $K^+$ ions is from the ingestion of protein, they are excreted in the urine with monovalent phosphate anions. The source of $K^+$ ions excreted in the urine in excess of monovalent phosphate anions is from the ingestion of fruit and vegetables; these $K^+$ ions are excreted in the urine with organic anions).
- The usual rate of excretion of organic anions in the urine in subjects consuming a typical Western diet is about 40 mEq/day.

**2.** A primary increase in the medullary $NH_3$ transport: The current model is that $NH_3$ is transported from the medullary interstitial compartment into the lumen of the collecting duct via Rh glycoproteins, Rhbg and Rhcg, that function as gas channels (see Fig. 1-14). It is possible to have a high rate of excretion of $NH_4^+$ ions relative to the rate of excretion of $SO_4^{2-}$ anions and a high urine pH if there were a higher rate of entry of $NH_3$ into the lumen of the MCD via these channels. This speculation is based on the finding that hypocitraturia is not present in some patients with incomplete RTA, and hence the lesion in these patients is not likely to be one of an acidified PCT cell. These patients would form $CaHPO_4$ stones because of the high urine $HPO_4^{2-}$ concentration, especially if they had another lesion that leads to a high rate of excretion of calcium (e.g., idiopathic hypercalciuria) and/or if they have a low urine flow rate (which may raise the concentrations of calcium ions and $HPO_4^{2-}$ anions in the urine).

## METABOLIC ACIDOSIS IN PATIENTS WITH RENAL FAILURE

When the GFR is markedly reduced, the following changes could be expected:

### $H_2PO_4^-$ ion excretion

This still matches the input of $H_2PO_4^-$ because the urine pH is well below 6.8, the pK of $HPO_4^{2-}/H_2PO_4^-$. Hence, this form of dietary $H^+$ ion load does not contribute to the development of metabolic acidosis in these patients (see Chapter 1).

### $NH_4^+$ ion excretion

The excretion of $NH_4^+$ ions declines markedly because of low availability of ADP in PCT cells (less filtered load of $Na^+$ ions so less renal work; see Fig. 1-12). The quantity of $H^+$ ions retained depends on how much protein is ingested and thereby how much $H_2SO_4$ is produced and to what degree the excretion of $NH_4^+$ ions is reduced. The retention of $H^+$ ion load can be as high as 30 to 40 mEq/day if the dietary protein intake is not reduced and the excretion of $NH_4^+$ ions is very low.

#### Diet alkali

This is often ignored in this analysis because the traditional view of acid-base balance focuses mainly on acid balance. The alkali load is derived mainly from dietary fruit and vegetables (e.g., $K^+$ + citrate anions), and it is normally eliminated with the excretion of $K^+$ ions and organic anions in the urine (see Fig. 1-5). Notwithstanding, once metabolic acidosis develops, the excretion of organic anions (including citrate) in the urine declines, as acidemia stimulates their reabsorption in PCT. Therefore, dietary alkali is retained, and these $HCO_3^-$ ions are used to titrate the $H^+$ ions from $H_2SO_4$ produced in the metabolism of sulfur-containing amino acids and thereby diminish the net $H^+$ ion load that must be eliminated each day by the excretion of $NH_4^+$ ions. Because patients with renal insufficiency are usually placed on a low $K^+$ ion diet, they eat less alkali and, as a result, are more likely to become acidemic. On the other hand, if their intake of fruit and vegetables were not restricted, the degree of acidemia is likely to be less severe, but the large price to pay is hyperkalemia.

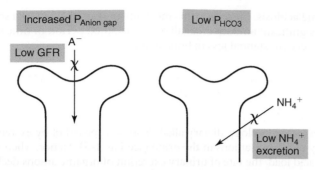

**Figure 4-8 Basis of High Plasma Anion Gap and Acidosis in Patients with Renal Failure.** The basis of the increased $P_{Anion\ gap}$ is the low glomerular filtration rate (GFR) with reduced excretion of anions, such as phosphate and sulfate (*left side*). The acidosis is due to a low rate of excretion of $NH_4^+$ ions (*right side*).

The $P_{Anion\ gap}$ usually does not rise appreciably in patients with chronic renal insufficiency until the GFR has fallen to <20 mL/min. The high $P_{Anion\ gap}$ in these patients does not represent the production of an unusually high amount of new acids; rather it is due to accumulation of $SO_4^{2-}$ and phosphate anions because of the very low GFR (Figure 4-8).

Experimental evidence from studies in rats strongly suggests that acidemia is a catabolic signal in uremia, although the evidence from human data is less robust. NaHCO₃ supplementation has also been shown to slow the progression of chronic kidney disease. It is now recommend that acidemia in patients with chronic kidney disease be corrected. After the $P_{HCO_3}$ is returned to normal, the dose of NaHCO₃ required to maintain a normal $P_{HCO_3}$ is likely to be less than 30 to 40 mmol/day. This small salt load should not represent a problem to most patients with chronic kidney disease.

# PART D

# INTEGRATIVE PHYSIOLOGY

## STEADY-STATE ACID–BASE BALANCE IN PATIENTS WITH RENAL TUBULAR ACIDOSIS

Patients with RTA are in steady state acid–base balance for a long period of time, despite having a low rate of excretion of $NH_4^+$ ions relative to their dietary H⁺ ion load from metabolism of sulfur-containing amino acids, as reflected by the rate of excretion of $SO_4^{2-}$ anions in the urine. Hence, there appears to be other mechanisms that permit them to achieve acid–base balance. The possible mechanisms are discussed subsequently.

### GENERATE NEW HCO₃⁻ IONS BY DISSOLVING THE ALKALINE SALTS IN BONE

If this were the case, there would be very close to 1 mEq of calcium ions excreted per mEq of HCO₃⁻ ions gained (see margin note). A transient, modest increase in calcium ion excretion is noted in human subjects during acute acidosis. There is no evidence, however, to suggest an appreciable increase in calcium ion excretion in patients with

**HCO₃⁻ ION GAIN FROM DISSOLVING BONE ALKALI SALTS**

- The calcium salts in bone are calcium carbonate (CaCO₃) and apatite (Ca₃[PO₄]₂). When they dissolve, there is a net addition of calcium and HCO₃⁻ ions in the body.
- For this to represent a gain of alkali, the calcium ions must be lost without forming a precipitate in the body (e.g., excreted in the urine). If calcium ions were to precipitate again as CaCO₃ and Ca₃(PO₄)₂ in bone or in other sites, the gain of HCO₃⁻ ions would be removed.

chronic acidosis. Moreover, this mechanism is unlikely to be a source for a significant amount of alkali for a sustained period of time without a very substantial loss of bone mass.

### FEWER ORGANIC ANIONS IN THE URINE ARE EXCRETED SO DIETARY ALKALI TITRATES SOME OF THE DIETARY ACID LOAD

In normal physiology, dietary alkali load is disposed of by excreting a family of organic anions in the urine (see Fig. 1-5). Hence, when there is an acid load, the rate of urinary excretion of organic anions declines, and thus dietary alkali would be used to titrate some of the dietary acid load. In quantitative terms, the decline in $NH_4^+$ ion excretion would be matched by the decline in the urinary excretion of organic anions (potential $HCO_3^-$) and as a result, acid–base balance is maintained.

## NEPHROCALCINOSIS IN PATIENTS WITH DISTAL RENAL TUBULAR ACIDOSIS

The subgroup of patients with dRTA, a urine pH close to 7.0, and a low $P_K$ are prone to deposit calcium salts in the renal medullary interstitial compartment. The factors that increase the likelihood of this deposition of calcium salts are those that raise the activity of ionized calcium and/or of $HPO_4^{2-}$, the anion that precipitates with ionized calcium. Hypokalemia likely plays an important role.

### MECHANISMS

#### Raise the medullary interstitial ionized calcium concentration

The most important risk factor for the development of nephrocalcinosis is the addition of calcium without water to the medullary interstitial compartment. Although most of the absorption of filtered calcium occurs in PCT, this does not increase the risk for interstitial calcification because the PCT has constitutively expressed aquaporin 1 water channels, and thus this nephron segment is always permeable to water. In fact, the absorption of water is the initial step to permit the absorption of calcium because it creates the driving force for this process by rising in the concentration of ionized calcium in the lumen of the PCT. In addition, a large volume of water is reabsorbed in the late cortical distal nephron. In contrast calcium is reabsorbed without water in the water-impermeable medullary thick ascending limb (mTAL) of the loop of Henle. Although calcium reabsorption in this nephron is also passive, it is driven by the lumen-positive voltage, which is created by the re-entry of $K^+$ ions into its lumen via renal outer medullary potassium (ROMK) channels. The greatest risk for a large rise in the interstitial calcium concentration is in the area immediately adjacent to the basolateral membrane of the mTAL.

Although a low rate of blood flow and a countercurrent exchange in the vasa recta should increase the risk of precipitation of calcium salts, there are five major defense mechanisms that diminish this risk. First, binding of ionized calcium to the calcium-sensing receptor (Ca-SR) at the basolateral membrane of the mTAL of the loop of Henle generates a signal to inhibit the flux of $K^+$ ions through ROMK, and this diminishes the lumen positive voltage and hence the driving force for reabsorption of ionized calcium. Second, because of the process of urea recycling in the renal inner medulla, there is delivery of water (with urea) without calcium ions or $HPO_4^{2-}$ anions to this interstitial region, which lowers the concentrations of ionized calcium ions and $HPO_4^{2-}$ anions in the medullary interstitial compartment. Third, the ascending vasa recta have fenestra, which carry the very small precipitates of $CaHPO_4$ and calcium carbonate that may form in the medullary interstitial compartment. Fourth, the high ionic strength in the renal medullary interstitial compartment leads to a diminished activity of ionized calcium ions. Fifth, because the bulk of filtered magnesium ($Mg^{2+}$) ions is also reabsorbed in the mTAL of the loop of Henle, a high interstitial concentration of $Mg^{2+}$ ions may decrease the precipitation of calcium salts because $Mg^{2+}$ ions bind more avidly than calcium ions to $HPO_4^{2-}$ and carbonate anions (see Chapter 9 for more discussion of this topic).

### Raise the medullary interstitial concentration of $HPO_4^{2-}$ and $CO_3^{2-}$

This requires alkalinization of the medullary interstitium. In a patient with hypokalemia, the $H^+/K^+$-ATPase activity in the MCD is increased. The net effect of this $H^+$ ion secretion into the lumen of the MCD is the addition of $K^+$ and $HCO_3^-$ ions to the interstitial compartment (Figure 4-9). As a result, the pH in this compartment rises, converting $H_2PO_4^-$ to $HPO_4^{2-}$ anions, which precipitates with ionized calcium. The rise in pH, however, is too small to raise the concentration of $HPO_4^{2-}$ appreciably. Notwithstanding, although the pK for carbonate is also very high (~10), there is a large pool of bicarbonate, the precursor for carbonate. Hence, precipitation of calcium carbonate may provide a nidus for the precipitation of calcium phosphate.

## STIOCHOMETRY OF SLGT1

One might ask, "Why use two mmol of $Na^+$ ions to absorb one mmol of glucose on SLGT1 when one mmol of $Na^+$ ions should suffice?" The downside in using two mmol of $Na^+$ ions for the transport of one mmol of glucose is that more ATP molecules are hydrolyzed (see margin note). Therefore, there should be an advantage for using more $Na^+$ ions because this consumes more energy. Furthermore, the absorption of 1500 mmol of glucose from dietary intake each day requires

- The Na-K-ATPase hydrolyzes one molecule of ATP for the transport of three mmol of $Na^+$ ions
- Therefore, the transport of two mmol of $Na^+$ ions requires the hydrolysis of two thirds of a molecule of ATP, whereas the transport of one mmol of $Na^+$ ions requires the hydrolysis of only one third of a molecule of ATP.

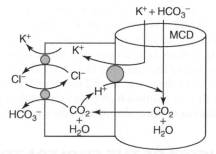

**Figure 4-9 Alkalinization of the Renal Inner Medullary Interstitial Compartment.** The structure represents the medullary collecting duct (MCD). When more $K^+$ ions are reabsorbed by the $H^+/K^+$-ATPase in the MCD, $HCO_3^-$ ions are added to the inner medullary interstitial compartment. This alkalinization raises the concentration of $CO_3^{2-}$ anions and the concentration of $HPO_4^{2-}$ anions. Precipitation of calcium carbonate may provide a nidus for the precipitation of calcium phosphate in the medullary interstitium and development of nephrocalcinosis.

the addition of about 3000 mmol of $Na^+$ ions to the lumen of the intestinal tract each day; this quantity of $Na^+$ ions is close to 150% of the entire content of $Na^+$ ions in the ECF compartment. We envision two advantages for selecting SGLT-1 in this location:

**1.** Production of L-lactic acid by enterocytes and inducing a shift of $K^+$ ions into hepatocytes.

It is well known that there is a rise in the plasma lactate ($P_{L-lactate}$) in portal venous blood after absorption of dietary glucose. We suggested that a possible function of this high portal $P_{L-lactate}$ is to prevent blood with a high $P_K$ from being delivered to the heart via hepatic venous blood following the absorption of $K^+$ ions from the diet. This mechanism to induce a shift of $K^+$ ions into hepatocytes begins by increasing the rate of glycolysis in enterocytes; as a result of performing more metabolic work, because 2 mmol of $Na^+$ ions must be absorbed for every mmol of glucose absorbed by SLGT1. Should glycolysis in enterocytes occur at a faster rate than pyruvate oxidation, L-lactate will be released into the portal vein. In the liver, the uptake of L-lactic acid on the monocarboxylic acid cotransporter (MCT) could raise the concentration of $H^+$ ions in the submembrane region of hepatocytes and hence activate the NHE-1. This electroneutral entry of $Na^+$ ions into hepatocytes and its subsequent exit via Na-K-ATPase in an electrogenic fashion will lead to a higher negative intracellular voltage and hence the retention of $K^+$ ions in hepatocytes (see Chapter 13).

**2.** Increasing osmolality at the tip of intestinal villus to prevent a water shift into the lumen of the intestinal tract.

Consumption of one liter of fruit juice provides close to 750 mmol of glucose plus fructose when its carbohydrate load is hydrolyzed by the enzyme sucrose early in the small intestine. This load of osmoles in the lumen of the small intestine creates a large osmotic force (close to 15,000 mm Hg because each mosmol exerts an osmotic pressure of ~20 mm Hg) to draw water from the body. A sudden shift of water into the intestinal lumen should cause the $P_{Na}$ to rise in the portal vein and shortly thereafter in arterial plasma. This rise in $P_{Na}$ causes thirst, and a viscious cycle is created if one were to try to quench this thirst by drinking more fruit juice.

By raising the osmolality at the tip of the villus in the small intestine, an osmotic difference that would favor the movement of water into the lumen is minimized. This is achieved because the hairpin loop of the capillaries of the villus functions as a countercurrent exchanger. The active absorption of $Na^+$ ions provides the single effect for countercurrent multiplication (Figure 4-10). With a finite permeability for $Na^+$ ions through the tight junctions between intestinal cells, a high local interstitial $Na^+$ and $Cl^-$ ion concentration (~400 mmol/L) is generated when glucose is being absorbed. This creates a local osmolality of 800 mosmol/kg $H_2O$ so there is no longer an osmotic driving force to draw water into the lumen of the intestine. Hence, another advantage of having a stoichiometry of the transport of 2 mmol of $Na^+$ ions per mmol of glucose on SGLT1 is to ensure a high osmolality at the tip of the intestinal villi when glucose is being absorbed in the small intestine.

## BIOCHEMISTRY OF THE CHOLERA TOXIN

When cholera bacteria are ingested, they do not enter the circulation; they exert their harmful effects by releasing a toxin. The first step in this toxin action is to make an irreversible linkage to the exterior of small intestinal cells in the crypt area of the villus (see Figure 4-11). This is accomplished by the five β-units of the toxin (akin to the ricin toxin and Shiga toxin, which causes the hemolytic–uremic syndrome).

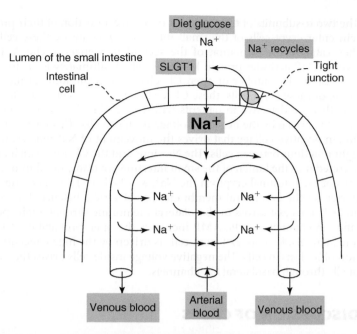

**Figure 4-10 Absorption of Glucose with Na⁺ Ions in the Villus of the Small Intestine.** The major structure is an intestinal villus, which faces into the lumen of the intestine. Two molecules of Na⁺ and one molecule of glucose are absorbed via the sodium-linked glucose transporter 1 (SLGT1). Most of the Na⁺ ions diffuse into the lumen through the tight junctions to drive the absorption of glucose. Some of the Na⁺ ions enter the subepithelial capillaries; these Na⁺ ions recycle by entering the central capillary, completing a countercurrent exchanger, which sustains the high concentration of Na⁺ ions at the tip of the villus as long as glucose is being absorbed.

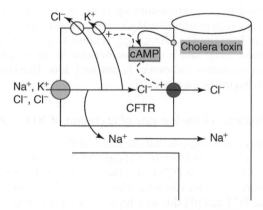

**Figure 4-11 Mechanisms of Action of the Cholera Toxin.** The *cylindrical structure* represents the small intestine and the *rectangle* to its left represents a crypt cell. The cholera toxin binds irreversibly to the luminal membrane of this cell as illustrated by the *dashed line* to the *solid dot*, and, as a result, more cyclic AMP (cAMP) is formed. This rise in cAMP leads to the insertion of a cystic fibrosis-related Cl⁻ ion channel (CFTR) in the luminal membrane, and the negative voltage in side cells drives the secretion of Cl⁻ ions. Na⁺ ions enter the lumen of the intestine between cells, driven by the luminal negative voltage. Na⁺ ions exit the cell on the Na-K-ATPase (not shown). The source of Na⁺, K⁺, and Cl⁻ ions is from portal venous blood via the Na⁺, K⁺, 2 Cl⁻ cotransporter-1 (NKCC-1) on the basolateral membrane of the cell. The rise in cAMP increases the opening probability of basolateral K⁺ ion channels, the negative voltage inside cells drives the exit of Cl⁻ ions via the basolateral Cl⁻ channel.

The two α-subunits of the toxin can now have a portion of their protein enter crypt cells of the small intestine. Once inside these cells, they catalyze the formation of the second messenger, cyclic AMP. Cyclic AMP activates protein kinase A, which ultimately leads to an increase in the number of open $Cl^-$ channels in the luminal membrane of these crypt cells; these $Cl^-$ channels are the same $Cl^-$ channels that are defective in patients with cystic fibrosis. The secretion of $Cl^-$ is driven by the negative voltage in these cells. This results in a lumen negative voltage that drives the movement of $Na^+$ ions via the tight junctions between cells. The $Na^+$ ions and the $Cl^-$ ions which are secreted into the lumen of the small intestine are transported into the cells of the intestinal crypt via the $Na^+$, $K^+$, 2 $Cl^-$ (NKCC-1) cotransporter on the basolateral membrane. For electrical balance, $K^+$ ions and $Cl^-$ ions exit across the basolateral membrane through their specific ion channels. Cyclic AMP increases the open probability of $K^+$ ion channels; $K^+$ ions' exit from cells is driven by the high concentration of $K^+$ ions in cells. The negative voltage inside cells drives the exit of $Cl^-$ through basolateral $Cl^-$ channels.

## DISCUSSION OF CASES

Both patients have metabolic acidemia, with a normal value of the $P_{Anion\ gap}$; therefore, they both have HCMA. The first step in diagnosis of the pathophysiology of HCMA is to establish whether they have a high rate of excretion of $NH_4^+$ ions (see Flow Chart 4-1).

### CASE 4-1: A MAN DIAGNOSED WITH TYPE IV RENAL TUBULAR ACIDOSIS

**What is the basis of the metabolic acidosis?**

The measured $U_{Osm}$ (700 mosmol/kg $H_2O$) is very close to the calculated $U_{Osm}$ (720 mosmol/kg·$H_2O$; see margin note); hence, his $U_{NH_4}$ is very low. The $U_{NH_4}/U_{Creatinine}$ is close to 2, and thus the rate of excretion of $NH_4^+$ ions is very low. Because his GFR (estimated by endogenous creatinine clearance) is not very low. Therefore, RTA is the correct diagnostic category.

**What is the cause of the low rate of excretion of $NH_4^+$ ions?**

The urine pH of 5.0 suggests that the basis for the low rate of $NH_4^+$ ion excretion is a low availability of $NH_3$, probably because of a low production of $NH_4^+$ ions in PCT cells. The next step is to examine Table 4-7 to identify a possible cause for a low rate of $NH_4^+$ ion production. An alkaline PCT cell pH due to a high $P_K$ is the most likely basis for his low rate of $NH_4^+$ ion excretion (the pathophysiology of hyperkalemia is discussed in detail in Chapter 15). Because his metabolic acidemia resolved when hyperkalemia was corrected, a causal role for hyperkalemia is likely.

### CASE 4-2: WHAT IS THIS WOMAN'S "BASIC" LESION?

**What is the basis of the metabolic acidosis?**

Because her measured $U_{Osm}$ (450 mosmol/kg $H_2O$) is very close to the calculated $U_{Osm}$ (420 mosmol/kg $H_2O$), her $U_{NH_4}$ is low. In fact, her $U_{NH_4}/U_{Creatinine}$ is close to 3, confirming that her $NH_4^+$ ion excretion rate is low. Because the GFR is not very low, she has a form of RTA.

**CALCULATED $U_{OSM}$**

$= 2\ (U_{Na} + U_K) + U_{Urea} + U_{Glucose}$
$= 2\ (140 + 60) + 300 + 20$
$= 720\ mosmol/kg\ H_2O$

## What is the cause of the low rate of excretion of $NH_4^+$ ions?

Because the urine pH is 6.8 (see Table 4-8), the basis for the low rate of $NH_4^+$ ion excretion is a low net secretion of $H^+$ ions in the distal nephron. The rate of excretion of citrate is low; she does not have an alkaline pH in her PCT cells.

After hypokalemia was corrected, the $PCO_2$ in alkaline urine was measured. It was 70 mm Hg; this suggests that there is no major defect in the $H^+$-ATPase. Hence, the defect is either a back-leak of $H^+$ ions or a lesion that leads to the secretion of $HCO_3^-$ ions by $\alpha$-intercalated cells in the distal nephron. Because the patient was not treated with amphotericin B, she likely suffers from Southeast Asian ovalocytosis, with another genetic abnormality affecting her with AE-1 leading to its mistargeting to the luminal membrane of $\alpha$-intercalated cells. Because the $P_{HCO_3}$ remained in the normal range after the infusion of $NaHCO_3$ (to measure $PCO_2$ in alkaline urine), pRTA was ruled out.

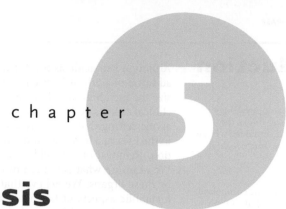
# Ketoacidosis

# Introduction

**KETOACIDS**

- A ketone is an organic compound that has a keto group (C=O) on an internal carbon atom.
- Acetone is a ketone but not an acid.
- Only acetoacetic acid is a ketoacid. β-Hydroxybutyric acid has a hydroxyl group (C–OH) on its internal carbon, so it is a hydroxy acid and not a ketoacid.

**ABBREVIATIONS**

β-HB, beta hydroxybutyrate anion
AcAc, acetoacetate anion
ADP, adenosine diphosphate
ATP, adenosine triphosphate
$NAD^+$, nicotinamide adenine dinucleotide
$NADH,H^+$, reduced form of $NAD^+$
FAD, flavin adenine dinucleotide
$FADH_2$, hydroxyquinone form of FAD
AKA, alcoholic ketoacidosis
EABV, effective arterial blood volume
$P_{Anion\ gap}$, plasma anion gap
$P_{Glucose}$, concentration of glucose in plasma
$P_{HCO_3}$, concentration of bicarbonate $(HCO_3^-)$ ions in plasma
$P_{Osmolal\ gap}$, plasma osmolal gap
TG, triglycerides

Although ketoacidosis is a form of metabolic acidosis because of the addition of acids, it is discussed separately in this chapter to emphasize the metabolic and biochemical issues required to understand the clinical aspects of this disorder (see margin note). We discuss the metabolic setting that is required to allow for the formation of ketoacids in the liver at a high rate and what sets the limit on the rate of production. Removal of ketoacids occurs mainly in the brain and kidneys. We examine what sets the limit on the rate of removal of ketoacids by these organs. We believe that understanding the biochemical and metabolic aspects of ketoacidsis provides the clinician with a better understanding of this disorder and allows for a better design of therapy in the individual patient with ketoacidosis.

## OBJECTIVES

- To discuss the pathophysiology of ketoacidosis based on an understanding of biochemistry of ketoacids formation in the liver and the principles of energy metabolism that control the rate of production and the rate of removal of ketoacids.
- To use this framework to describe the clinical aspects of the two major clinical types of ketoacidosis: diabetic ketoacidosis (DKA) and alcoholic ketoacidosis (AKA).

### CASE 5-1: THIS MAN IS ANXIOUS TO KNOW WHY HE HAS KETOACIDOSIS

This is the fourth hospital admission with a similar presentation for this 22-year-old man. As in the other episodes, his illness began with a "panic attack" that lasted for several days. During that period, he drank many liters of sweetened soft drinks on a daily basis (see margin note). He developed crampy lower abdominal pain that became severe in the 24 hours prior to coming to the hospital. He denied the intake of alcohols (including methanol or ethylene glycol). He felt well between these episodes and was taking only medications for treatment of mild depression. He had no history suggestive of diabetes mellitus. On physical examination, there was an odor of acetone on his breath, but his effective arterial blood volume (EABV) was not contracted. Arterial blood gas revealed a blood pH of 7.20, an arterial $PCO_2$ of 22 mm Hg, and a plasma bicarbonate concentration ($P_{HCO_3}$) of 8 mmol/L. Of note, his plasma osmolal gap ($P_{Osmolal\ gap}$) was not elevated. The following laboratory data were obtained from measurements in a venous blood sample on admission:

| | | |
|---|---|---|
| Glucose | mg/dL (mmol/L) | 92 (5.1) |
| Anion gap | mEq/L | 26 |
| $Na^+$ | mmol/L | 140 |
| $K^+$ | mmol/L | 4.2 |
| $Cl^-$ | mmol/L | 110 |
| Creatinine | mg/dL (μmol/L) | 1.0 (88) |
| Albumin | g/dL (g/L) | 4.1 (41) |
| β-HB | mmol/L | 4.5 |
| L-lactate | mmol/L | 1.0 |
| Osmolality | mosmol/kg $H_2O$ | 285 |

His initial therapy consisted of 1 L of isotonic saline and 1 L of 5% dextrose in water ($D_5W$). Within 24 hours, all his laboratory values returned to the normal range. Of interest, his hemoglobin $A_1C$ level was not elevated (4.4%) and his plasma insulin level was in the normal range.

## Questions

What makes diabetic ketoacidosis (DKA) an unlikely diagnosis?

What makes alcoholic ketoacidosis an unlikely diagnosis?

What makes starvation or hypoglycemic ketoacidosis an unlikely diagnosis?

How may the patient's intake of sweetened soft drinks contribute to the development of ketoacidosis?

Is ketoacidosis the only cause of metabolic acidemia in this patient?

---

# PART A
# BIOCHEMICAL BACKGROUND
## METABOLIC PROCESS ANALYSIS

- A "metabolic process" consists of a series of metabolic pathways that carry out a specific function; its control can be deduced by examining its function.
- To determine the acid–base impact of a metabolic process, count the net valence of all of its substrates and of all its final products.

Metabolic processes often consist of more than one metabolic pathway, and these pathways usually occur in more than one organ. In the metabolic process involving ketoacids, there are segments of this process that take place in adipose tissue, the liver, the brain, and the kidneys (Figure 5-1). Although each of these segments is regulated at the specific organ level, control of the whole metabolic process is in keeping with its overall function.

The function of the metabolic process involving ketoacids is to provide the brain with a water-soluble, fat-derived fuel that it can oxidize to regenerate a sufficient quantity of adenosine triphosphate (ATP) to carry out its essential functions when its major fuel in the fed state, glucose, is in short supply. Although the blood–brain barrier limits the entry of long-chain fatty acids into the brain, there is a transport system that allows ketoacids to enter brain cells at a rapid rate.

When the diet contains glucose, signals are generated to prevent the production of ketoacids in the liver. The signal system centers on the stimulation of β-cells of the pancreas by glucose to release the hormone insulin. In contrast, during prolonged starvation, insulin is not released because of a low plasma glucose ($P_{Glucose}$) level. This leads to the release of fatty acids from adipose tissue and the formation of ketoacids in the liver; therefore, the central factor in the control of the metabolic process involving ketoacids is a relative lack of insulin (see margin note).

An important element in the control of a metabolic process is to block all alternative pathways for the metabolism of its intermediates to ensure that the desired product is formed. Therefore, during ketoacid production, alternative pathways for metabolism of its substrate, acetyl-CoA formed from β-oxidation of palmitic acid in the liver, must be inhibited (i.e., oxidation and conversion to storage fat), while the pathway for production of ketoacids is stimulated (Figure 5-1).

To determine the $H^+$ ion balance in a metabolic process, examine the net valences of all of its substrates and end products. $H^+$ ions are produced if the products of a metabolic process have a greater net anionic valence than its substrates; $H^+$ ions are removed if the products of a metabolic process have a lesser net anionic valence than its substrates. In the metabolic process that involves ketoacids, there is no net

**RELATIVE LACK OF INSULIN**

This term describes the combination of low levels of insulin and high levels of hormones that oppose the actions of insulin (e.g., glucagon, cortisol, adrenaline, and the pituitary hormones: adrenocorticotropic hormone, and growth hormone).

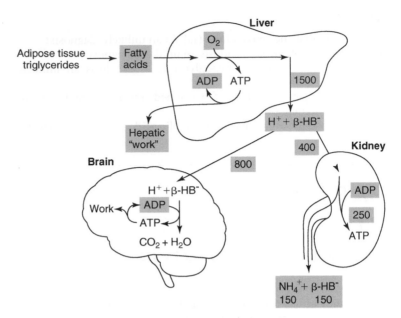

**Figure 5-1 The Metabolic Process Involving Ketoacids.** The substrate for this metabolic process is triglyceride in adipose tissue (see margin note). When the concentration of the usual brain fuel, glucose, is low in plasma, this provides a signal (low net actions of insulin) to cause the release of fatty acids from adipose tissue. The liver extracts many of these fatty acids and converts them to ketoacids when alternate metabolic pathways for their metabolism (oxidation and conversion to storage fat) are blocked. Metabolism of fatty acids in hepatic mitochondria produces acetyl-CoA and converts mitochondrial nicotinamide adenine dinucleotide ($NAD^+$) to its reduced form ($NADH, H^+$), and flavin adenine dinucleotide (FAD) to its hydroxyquinone form ($FADH_2$). $NADH, H^+$ is converted back to $NAD^+$ and $FADH_2$ is converted back to FAD when adenosine diphosphate (ADP) is converted to adenosine triphosphate (ATP) in the process of coupled oxidative phosphorylation. Therefore, the availability of ADP (which is formed from the hydrolysis of ATP to perform biological work) may set a limit on the rate of production of acetyl-CoA, the substrate for ketogenesis. The observed rate of ketoacid production during prolonged fasting (~1500 mmol/day) suggests that this limitation by rate of hepatic work is by-passed, perhaps by uncoupling of oxidative phosphorylation. Ketoacids are removed by oxidation in the brain and the kidneys. The rate of ATP utilization in these organs to perform biologic work sets an upper limit on the rate of removal of ketoacids. In this metabolic process, acid–base balance is maintained if ketoacid anions are metabolized to neutral end products ($CO_2 + H_2O$) or are excreted in the urine with $NH_4^+$ ions, as new $HCO_3^-$ ions are generated when $NH_4^+$ ions are excreted in the urine.

## TRIGLYCERIDES

- Triglycerides are the major form of storage fat in adipose tissue.
- In a triglyceride, three fatty acids are each linked by an ester bond to one of the three hydroxyl groups of glycerol. These ester bonds are formed, when a $H^+$ ion in a fatty acid and the $OH^-$ moiety in glycerol are removed.

H – C – O – C – Fatty acid
|
H – C – O – C – Fatty acid
|
H – C – O – C – Fatty acid

production or removal of $H^+$ ions if the ketoacids produced in the liver are then oxidized by the brain or the kidneys because the net valence of all substrates, triglycerides in adipose tissue, and end products ($CO_2 + H_2O$), are equal. If this metabolic process does not proceed to completion, however, the rate of production of ketoacids exceeds their rate of removal, and $H^+$ ions accumulate (see Figure 5-1).

## PRODUCTION OF KETOACIDS IN THE LIVER

### BIOCHEMISTRY OF KETOACID PRODUCTION

The metabolic process of production of ketoacids in the liver can be divided into two major steps: first, the formation of acetyl-CoA in mitochondria of hepatocytes; second, the conversion of acetyl-CoA to ketoacids.

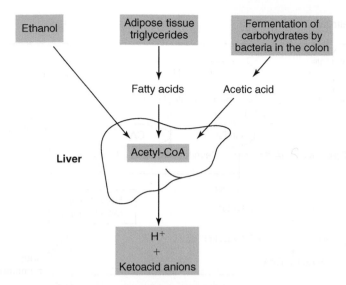

**Figure 5-2 Extrahepatic Substrates for Ketogenesis.** The three major sub-strates for the production of a large quantity of acetyl-CoA in the liver are long-chain fatty acids, ethanol, and acetic acid (produced from fermenta-tion of carbohydrates in the colon). The regulation of each of these meta-bolic pathways differs, however, as described in the text.

There are three different substrates from which acetyl-CoA can be made rapidly enough in the liver to lead to an appreciable rate of for-mation of ketoacids (see Figure 5-2): (1) long-chain free fatty acids, (2) ethanol (see Part C), and (3) acetic acid produced from fermenta-tion of carbohydrates by bacteria in the colon (see discussion of Case 5–1). Because of the tight regulation of pyruvate dehydrogenase by acetyl-CoA, fuels that can be converted to pyruvate (e.g., glucose) are not important substrates for ketoacids formation.

The only important physiologic substrate for hepatic ketogenesis is long-chain fatty acids (e.g., palmitic acid [$C_{16}H_{32}O_2$]), which are derived from storage fat (triglycerides in adipose tissue). The func-tion of this metabolic process is to provide the brain with a water-sol-uble, fat-derived brain fuel, when the $P_{Glucose}$ is low during prolonged fasting. Hence, the hormonal setting is a relative lack of insulin. In the patient with DKA, there is also a relative lack of insulin, but in this case, it is due to damage to β-cells of the pancreas. This relative lack of insulin provides the signal to activate the enzyme hormone-sensitive lipase, which catalyzes the release of palmitic acid from triglycerides in adipose tissues (Eqn 1).

$$\text{Triglycerides in adipose tissue} \rightarrow 3 \text{ Palmitic acid} \qquad (1)$$

There is a lag period before ketoacids are produced at a rapid rate when there is a relative lack of insulin actions. The underlying mechanism for this lag period is not completely understood but may be related to time needed to induce the mechanism for the trans-port of long-chain fatty acids into hepatic mitochondria. Because oxidation of fat-derived fuels inhibits the oxidation of glucose, it is advantageous to have a lag period before ketogensis occurs at a high rate to avoid hyperglycemia and its resultant osmotic diuresis and natriuresis if glucose were to become available within a relatively short period of time.

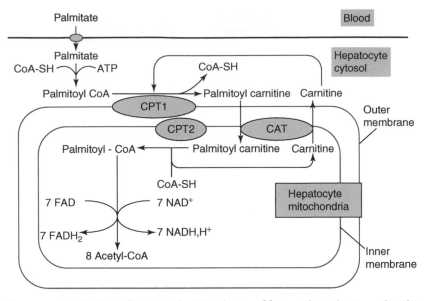

**Figure 5-3 β-Oxidation of Fatty Acids.** β-Oxidation of fatty acids (palmitic acid in this example) occurs in mitochondria. Palmitic acid must be modified so that it can enter hepatic mitochondria. The first step is to activate this long-chain fatty acid to produce palmitoyl-CoA by having it react with adenosine triphosphate (ATP) in the presence of coenzyme A with a functional sulfhydryl group (CoA-SH). Palmitoyl-CoA is then converted to palmitoyl-carnitine, a reaction that is catalyzed by the enzyme carnitine palmitoyl transferase 1 (CPT1), which is located in the outer mitochondrial membrane. Palmitoyl-carnitine crosses the inner mitochondrial membrane in exchange for intramitochondrial carnitine on a carnitine/acylcarnitine translocase (CAT). Inside the hepatic mitochondria, palmitoyl-carnitine plus CoA-SH are converted to palmitoyl-CoA plus carnitine, a reaction catalyzed by the enzyme carnitine palmitoyl transferase 2 (CPT2), which is located in the inner mitochondria membrane with its active site facing the mitochondrial matrix. Palmitoyl-CoA (16 carbon) undergoes β-oxidation, which produces eight molecules of acetyl-CoA and converts seven $NAD^+$ into seven $NADH,H^+$, and seven FAD into seven $FADH_2$.

## FORMATION OF ACETYL-CoA IN THE LIVER

- The pathways of metabolism of palmitoyl-CoA occur in two separate compartments in hepatocytes. Synthesis of fatty acids from palmitoyl-CoA occurs in the cytosol; its β-oxidation occurs inside the mitochondria.
- Carnitine plays an important role in the pathway of β-oxidation. The formation of palmitoyl-carnitine, which is catalyzed by the enzyme carnitine palmitoyl transferase 1 (CPT1), is an important site of regulation.

Once in the liver, palmitic acid must be modified so that it can enter hepatic mitochondria, the site where fatty acids are converted to acetyl-CoA in the process of β-oxidation. The first step is to activate this long-chain fatty acid to produce palmitoyl-CoA by having it react with ATP in the presence of CoA-SH (coenzyme A with functional sulfhydryl group). Adenosine monophosphate (AMP) and pyrophosphate are the other two products of this reaction (Eqn 2). Pyrophosphate is hydrolyzed nonenzymatically into two molecules of inorganic phosphate ($HPO_4^{2-}$).

$$\text{Palmitic acid} + \text{CoA-SH} + \text{ATP} \rightarrow \text{Palmitoyl-CoA} + \text{AMP} + \text{Pyrophosphate} \quad (2)$$

The next step is to convert palmitoyl-CoA to palmitoyl-carnitine, which can cross the mitochondrial membrane (Eqn 3). This reaction is catalyzed by the enzyme carnitine palmitoyl transferase 1 (CPT1).

$$\text{Palmitoyl-CoA} + \text{Carnitine} \rightarrow \text{Palmitoyl-carnitine} + \text{CoA-SH} \quad (3)$$

An important aspect of regulation is that CPT1 is inhibited by malonyl-CoA. Malonyl-CoA is formed during fatty acid synthesis in the cytosol when insulin levels are high. On the other hand, when insulin levels are low, the malonyl-CoA level falls and its inhibition of CPT1 is removed. This permits the conversion of palmitoyl-CoA to palmitoyl-carnitine, which is essential for its entry into mitochondria for β-oxidation. Hence, fatty acid synthesis and fatty acid oxidation are controlled in a reciprocal fashion and occur in different compartments in hepatocytes.

Palmitoyl-carnitine crosses the inner mitochondrial membrane in exchange for intramitochondrial carnitine on a carnitine/acylcarnitine translocase (CAT). Inside the hepatic mitochondria, palmitoyl-carnitine plus CoA-SH are converted to palmitoyl-CoA plus carnitine, a reaction catalyzed by a different enzyme with a similar name, carnitine palmitoyl transferase 2 (CPT2) (Eqn 4).

$$\text{Palmitoyl-carnitine} + \text{CoA-SH} \rightarrow \text{Palmitoyl-CoA} + \text{Carnitine} \quad (4)$$

Palmitoyl-CoA undergoes β-oxidation, a process of breaking down a long-chain acyl-CoA molecule to acetyl-CoA molecules. The number of acetyl-CoA produced depends on the carbon length of the fatty acid being oxidized. At the end of each β-oxidation cycle, an acetyl-CoA and an acyl-CoA that is two carbon atoms shorter are produced. Meanwhile, nicotinamide adenine dinucleotide ($NAD^+$) is reduced to $NADH,H^+$ and flavin adenine dinucleotide (FAD) is reduced to its hydroquinone form $FADH_2$. Hence, oxidation of palmitic acid, which has 16 carbon atoms, produces 8 acetyl-CoA, 7 $NADH,H^+$, and 7 $FADH_2$ (Eqn 5).

$$\text{Palmitoyl-CoA} + 7\,\text{CoA-SH} + 7\,NAD^+ + 7\,\text{FAD} \rightarrow$$
$$8\,\text{Acetyl-CoA} + 7\,(NADH,H^+) + 7\,FADH_2 \quad (5)$$

Acetyl-CoA is the precursor for ketoacid formation. It is important, however, to note that since $NAD^+$ and FAD are present in only tiny concentrations in mitochondria, $NADH,H^+$ must be converted to $NAD^+$ and $FADH_2$ to FAD to continue this process of β-oxidation. This occurs during coupled oxidative phosphorylation, in which ATP is regenerated from ADP plus inorganic phosphate (Pi). In turn, ADP is formed from hydrolysis of ATP when biological work is performed. Hence, the rate of performing biologic work sets a limit on the rate of coupled oxidative phosphorylation (see Chapter 1). Work can be thought of as mechanical work, electrical work (ion pumping), and biosynthesis work (e.g., protein synthesis). Unlike muscles, the liver does not perform mechanical work. Also, there is not a large leak of $Na^+$ ions into hepatocytes to drive the Na-K-ATPase. In addition, in patients with prolonged fasting and those with DKA or AKA, who are ingesting little protein, the amount of amino acids available is not sufficient to permit high rates of hepatic protein synthesis, a process that utilizes ATP. Accordingly, the liver does not perform enough work to make enough ADP and, consequently, convert enough $NADH,H^+$ to $NAD^+$ and $FADH_2$ to FAD; this sets a limit on the rate of production of ketoacids.

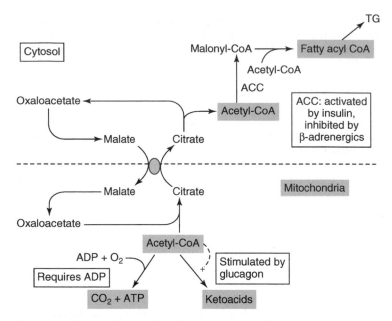

**Figure 5-4  Fates of Acetyl-CoA.** To have a metabolic process that results in the formation of ketoacids in the liver, the two major alternative pathways for removal of acetyl-CoA (i.e., its oxidation to produce adenosine triphosphate [ATP] and its conversion to long-chain fatty acids) must be inhibited. Oxidation of acetyl-CoA is limited by the availability of adenosine diphosphate (ADP) in the hepatocyte, which depends on the rate of breakdown of ATP to perform biologic work. The other major fate of acetyl-CoA is conversion into fatty acids, which occurs in the cytosol. Because acetyl-CoA cannot cross the mitochondrial membrane, it combines with oxaloacetate to form citrate, which is transported into the cytosol on the tricarboxylate carrier in exchange for malate. Acetyl-CoA carboxylase (ACC) catalyzes the first committed step in fatty acid synthesis (i.e., the conversion of acetyl-CoA to malonyl-CoA). The activity of ACC is inhibited by a relative lack of insulin and also by high levels of β-adrenergic hormones. When the oxidation of acetyl-CoA and its conversion to long-chain fatty acids are inhibited, the acetyl-CoA level in mitochondria rises and drives its conversion to ketoacids. In addition, the pathway from acetyl-CoA to ketoacids (the HMG-CoA pathway) is stimulated by glucagon. *TG*, Triglycerides.

## The Metabolic Fates of Acetyl-CoA

- To have a metabolic process that results in the formation of ketoacids in the liver, the two major alternative pathways for removal of acetyl-CoA—i.e., its oxidation to produce ATP and its conversion to long-chain fatty acids—must be inhibited (Figure 5-4).

### Inhibition of the oxidation of acetyl-CoA in the tricarboxylic acid cycle

Metabolism of one molecule of acetyl-CoA in the tricarboxylic acid cycle requires the conversion of three molecules of $NAD^+$ into $NADH,H^+$ and one molecule of FAD into $FADH_2$. Hence, as detailed previously, this oxidation pathway is limited by the availability of ADP in hepatocyte, which depends on the rate of breakdown of ATP to perform biologic work.

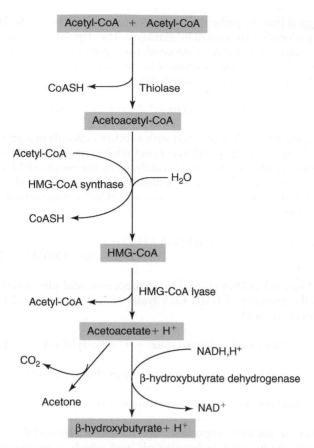

**Figure 5-5  Conversion of Acetyl-CoA to Ketoacids.** Acetyl-CoA is converted to ketoacids in the 3-hydroxy-3-methylglutaryl-CoA (HMG-CoA) pathway. The major ketoacid that is produced by the liver is β-hydroxybutyric acid. β-Hydroxybutyric acid is formed from acetoacetic acid in a reaction catalyzed by the enzyme β-hydroxybutyrate dehydrogenase and is driven by a high mitochondria ratio of NADH,H$^+$/NAD$^+$. Acetone is produced from acetoacetic acid by decarboxylation.

### Inhibition of the conversion of acetyl-CoA to long-chain fatty acids

The other metabolic fate of acetyl-CoA is its conversion to fatty acids (Figure 5-4). Fatty acid synthesis occurs in the cytosol. Because acetyl-CoA cannot cross the mitochondrial membrane, citrate (a six-carbon compound), which is made from one molecule of acetyl-CoA (a two-carbon compound) and oxaloacetate (a four-carbon compound), is shuttled out of the mitochondria on the tricarboxylate carrier in exchange for malate. In the cytosol, citrate is cleaved back into acetyl-CoA and oxaloacetate in a reaction that is catalyzed by the enzyme ATP-citrate lyase and requires the hydrolysis of one molecule of ATP, converting it to AMP and pyrophosphate. Oxaloacetate can be converted to malate, which is transported back into the mitochondria on the tricarboxylate carrier (in exchange for citrate). The enzyme acetyl-CoA carboxylase (ACC) catalyzes the first committed step in fatty acid synthesis: the conversion of acetyl-CoA to malonyl-CoA. The activity of ACC is inhibited by a relative lack of insulin and high levels of β-adrenergic hormones.

### CONVERSION OF ACETYL-COA TO KETOACIDS

When the oxidation of acetyl-CoA in the tricarboxylic acid cycle and its conversion to long-chain fatty acids are inhibited, acetyl-CoA is converted to ketoacids (see Figure 5-5). In addition, there is evidence to suggest that the pathway from acetyl-CoA to ketoacids (the HMG-CoA pathway) is stimulated by glucagon. The steps involved are:

1. Two molecules of acetyl-CoA condense together to form acetoacetyl-CoA. This reaction, a reversal of the terminal step in β-oxidation, is catalyzed by the enzyme acetoacetyl-CoA thiolase (Eqn 6).

$$2\,\text{Acetyl-CoA} \rightarrow \text{Acetoacetyl-CoA} + \text{CoA-SH} \qquad (6)$$

2. Acetoacetyl-CoA then reacts with another molecule of acetyl-CoA and water to form 3-hydroxy-3-methylglutaryl-CoA (HMG-CoA) and CoA-SH. This reaction is catalyzed by the enzyme HMG-CoA synthase, which is present exclusively in liver mitochondria. Evidence suggests that glucagon increases HMG-CoA synthase activity (Eqn 7).

$$\text{Acetoacetyl-CoA} + \text{Acetyl-CoA} + H_2O \rightarrow$$
$$\text{HMG-CoA} + \text{CoASH} \qquad (7)$$

3. HMG-CoA is then cleaved to acetoacetatic acid plus acetyl-CoA in the presence of HMG-CoA lyase; $H^+$ ions are released in this process (Eqn 8).

$$\text{HMG-CoA} \rightarrow \text{Acetoacetate}^- + H^+ + \text{Acetyl-CoA} \qquad (8)$$

4. The previous steps can be summed up as shown in Eqn 9.

$$2\,\text{Acetyl-CoA} + H_2O \rightarrow \text{Acetoacetate}^- + H^+ + 2\,\text{CoA-SH} \qquad (9)$$

There is one more important step. The major ketoacid that is produced by the liver is β-hydroxybutyric acid, which as mentioned earlier is a hydroxy acid yet is called a ketoacid. β-hydroxybutyric acid is formed from acetoacetic acid in a reaction catalyzed by the enzyme D-β-hydroxybutyrate (β-HB) dehydrogenase and is driven by a high mitochondria ratio of $NADH,H^+/NAD^+$ (Eqn 10). This provides an energy advantage because it stores an extra energy equivalent to an $NADH,H^+$ in the ketoacid that is exported to the body. Oxidation of 1 mmol of β-HB yields 27 mmol of ATP, whereas 24 mmol of ATP are regenerated from the oxidation of 1 mmol of AcAc. This more favorable ATP yield results in the need for a 10% lower rate of production of ketoacids to meet the energy demands of the brain and the kidneys, and thereby fewer $H^+$ ions may need to be transported from their site of production to their sites of oxidation and hence the degree of acidemia is less severe. In addition, the conversion of $NADH,H^+$ to $NAD^+$ regenerates the rate-limiting supply for ketogenesis in the liver, and hence it is possible to have a higher rate of production of ketoacids if needed.

$$\text{Acetoacetate} + H^+ + (NADH,H^+) \rightarrow \beta\text{-HB} + H^+ + NAD^+ \qquad (10)$$

Acetone is produced from acetoacetic acid by decarboxylation, which may occur spontaneously in a slow, nonenzymatic reaction or be catalyzed by a decarboxylase. As mentioned previously, acetone is not an acid; hence $H^+$ ions are removed in this reaction.

## BYPASSING LIMITATION BY AVAILABILITY OF ADP ON RATE OF HEPATIC KETOACID PRODUCTION

During a state of relative lack of insulin, the liver must produce enough ketoacid fuels for the brain and the kidneys to carry out their work. Hence, there must be a strategy to bypass this limitation by

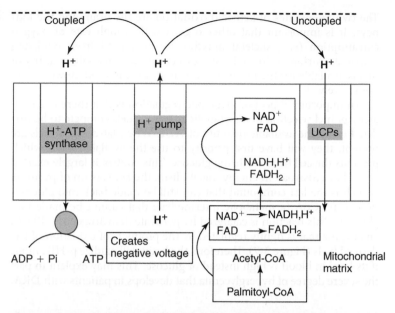

**Figure 5-6 Coupled and Uncoupled Fuel Oxidation in Mitochondria.** The structure represents the inner mitochondrial membrane with its outer layer *(outside)* and inner layer *(inside)*. The *dashed line* at top represents the outer mitochondrial membrane. Oxidation of palmitoyl-CoA in hepatic mitochondria produces acetyl-CoA and converts mitochondrial NAD$^+$ to its reduced form, NADH,H$^+$, and FAD to its hydroxyquinone form, FADH$_2$. Oxidation of NADH,H$^+$ and FADH$_2$ produces electrons. The flow of these electrons through the electron transport chain releases energy that is used to pump H$^+$ ions from the mitochondrial matrix through the inner mitochondrial membrane. This creates a large electrochemical driving force for the re-entry of H$^+$ ions. The energy is recaptured as H$^+$ ions flow through the H$^+$ ion channel portion of the H$^+$-adenosine triphosphate (ATP) synthase in the inner mitochondrial membrane, which is coupled to the conversion of adenosine diphosphate (ADP) plus inorganic phosphate (Pi) to ATP. In uncoupled oxidative phosphorylation, H$^+$ ions re-enter mitochondria through uncoupling protein channels (UPCs; usually UCP-2 and/or UCP-3); these H$^+$ ion channels are not linked to the regeneration of ATP, which permits a higher rate of conversion of NADH,H$^+$ to NAD$^+$ and FADH$_2$ to FAD when there is decreased availability of ADP.

availability of ADP on the rate of conversion of NADH,H$^+$ to NAD$^+$ and FADH$_2$ to FAD and hence the rate of formation of acetyl-CoA (if supply of long-chain fatty acids to hepatic mitochondria is not rate limiting). One such strategy is uncoupled oxidative phosphorylation, in which H$^+$ ions re-enter mitochondria via H$^+$ ion channels that are not linked to the conversion of ADP to ATP (see margin note) (Figure 5-6). Hence, it seems that in the metabolic process where ketoacids are formed from storage fat or ethanol, the maximum rate of hepatic ketogenesis is set by the rate of consumption of oxygen in hepatocytes, which limits the rates of both coupled and uncoupled oxidative phosphorylation (see Part D for further discussion of this topic).

## REMOVAL OF KETOACIDS

- The same principles of metabolic regulation will apply to ketoacid removal (i.e., the rate of ATP utilization to perform biologic work sets an upper limit on the rate of fuel oxidation in the absence of a large degree of uncoupling of oxidative phosphorylation).

**NEED FOR UNCOUPLED RESPIRATION TO AUGMENT KETOGENESIS**

- The degree of uncoupling of oxidative phosphorylation must be modest to avoid the dangers of inducing a very rapid rate of glycolysis and thereby L-lactic acidosis because of a much higher concentration of ADP in the cytosol of hepatocytes (see Chapter 6).
- Another reaction that is equivalent to uncoupling is when acetoacetate is converted to β-HB because NADH,H$^+$ is converted to NAD$^+$ in this reaction.
- As shown in Eqn 2, when palmitic acid is activated to form palmitoyl-CoA in the cytosol, ATP is hydrolyzed, which results in the formation of AMP and pyrophosphate. AMP reacts with another ATP to form two molecules of ADP. This will permit more oxidation of palmitic acid by coupled oxidative phosphorylation and thereby may diminish the need for uncoupling of oxidative phosphorylation.

The two major sites of ketoacid oxidation are the brain and the kidneys. It is important that other organs with a high rate of oxygen consumption (e.g., skeletal muscle) are prevented from oxidizing ketoacids during prolonged fasting to ensure an adequate quantity of fuel is available for the brain. The mechanisms involved, however, are not entirely clear.

An important aspect of metabolic regulation is that there is a hierarchy of fuel selection in a metabolic process. Fuels compete to be oxidized using the available quantity of ADP. When fat-derived fuels are present, they will have first priority to use the available ADP, which prevents the cell from oxidizing glucose. This control is largely exerted at the key crossroad in energy metabolism: the conversion of pyruvate (which is the last compound that can still be made back into glucose) into acetyl-CoA (a metabolic intermediate that cannot be made into glucose). This reaction is catalyzed by pyruvate dehydrogenase (PDH), an enzyme that is tightly regulated by the products of oxidation of fat-derived fuels (Figure 5-7). Therefore, the brain will oxidize β-HB anions if its level in blood is high instead of glucose. This may explain in part the severe degree of hyperglycemia that develops in patients with DKA.

## OXIDATION OF KETOACIDS IN THE BRAIN

The brain can oxidize close to 800 mmol of ketoacids per day, almost half the quantity of ketoacids that are produced when ketogenesis is most rapid (see Figure 5-1). If the rate of generation of ADP in the brain declines because of performing less biologic work (e.g., because of coma, intake of sedatives including ethanol, the effect of anesthesia), less β-HB anions can be oxidized, and the degree of acidemia becomes more severe.

## REMOVAL OF KETOACIDS BY THE KIDNEYS

The kidneys remove close to 400 mmol of ketoacids per day. If renal work (which is largely the reabsorption of filtered $Na^+$ ions) is at its usual rate, the kidneys oxidize close to 250 mmol of β-HB anions per day. Because more β-HB anions are filtered than reabsorbed, close to 150 mmol of β-HB anions are excreted daily during the ketoacidosis of prolonged fasting (see margin note). Because virtually all of these anions are excreted along with ammonium ($NH_4^+$) ions or $H^+$ ions (i.e., not with sodium [$Na^+$] ions or potassium [$K^+$] ions) during prolonged fasting, acid–base balance is maintained.

**EXCRETION OF β-HB ANIONS WITH $NH_4^+$ IONS IN THE URINE DURING PROLONGED FASTING**

- While this may be viewed as a waste of energy, it in fact may be advantageous.
- Because rates of excretion of NaCl and urea are low during prolonged fasting, excretion of β-HB with $NH_4^+$ may provide enough effective osmoles in the urine to prevent oliguria and the risk of stone formation.

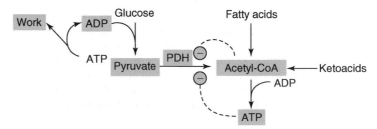

**Figure 5-7 Fuel Selection: Oxidation of Fat-Derived Fuels Prevents Oxidation of Glucose.** Fuels compete to be oxidized using the available quantity of adenosine diphosphate (ADP). When fat-derived fuels are present, they will have first priority to use the available ADP, which prevents the cell from oxidizing glucose. Control is exerted at the key crossroad in energy metabolism, the conversion of pyruvate into acetyl-CoA. This reaction is catalyzed by pyruvate dehydrogenase (PDH), an enzyme that is tightly regulated by the products of oxidation of fat-derived fuels. *ATP,* Adenosine triphosphate.

In DKA, the filtered load of $Na^+$ ions declines (because of a low glomerular filtration rate [GFR] due to decreased effective arterial blood volume (EABV) because of the loss of $Na^+$ ions in the urine because of the glucose-induced osmotic natriuresis). Accordingly, renal removal of β-HB anions decreases because the rates of excretion of $NH_4^+$ ions and of oxidation of β-HB anions are both reduced. From an energy point of view, oxidation of β-HB anions or glutamine (which produces $NH_4^+$ ions) is equivalent in terms of ADP utilization.

### KETOACID OXIDATION IN OTHER ORGANS

The intestinal tract oxidizes β-HB anions when it performs work. If digestion and absorption are proceeding at a usual rate, the intestinal tract oxidizes 200 to 300 mmol of β-HB anions per day. Notwithstanding, intestinal work is extremely low during prolonged fasting and perhaps in most patients with DKA. Skeletal muscles do not oxidize an appreciable quantity of β-HB anions when fatty acid levels are high.

### PRODUCTION OF ACETONE FROM ACETOACETIC ACID

When the level of acetoacetic acid is high, and in the absence of a high $NADH,H^+/NAD^+$ ratio, this ketoacid is converted to acetone and $CO_2$ by decarboxylation. This may occur spontaneously in a slow, nonenzymatic reaction or in a reaction catalyzed by a decarboxylase. As mentioned above, acetone is not an acid; therefore, $H^+$ ions are removed in this reaction.

### CLINICAL MESSAGES

1. Unless oxidative phosphorylation is markedly uncoupled during DKA, it is likely that the rate of ketoacid production in patients with DKA is not substantially higher than that in people with ketoacidosis due to prolonged fasting. Thus, the reason a severe degree of acidemia develops in a patient with DKA is likely to be a diminished rate of removal of ketoacids.
2. The ultimate fate of the ketoacid anions (oxidation or excretion in the urine) determines the acid–base impact of this metabolic process. If the rate of fuel oxidation declines in either of the two major organs involved in the metabolic removal of ketoacids (i.e., the brain and the kidneys), a more severe degree of acidemia may develop. $H^+$ ions also accumulate if ketoacid anions are excreted in the urine with a cation other than $NH_4^+$ ions (or $H^+$ ions).

## CLINICAL ASPECTS OF KETOACIDOSIS

The differential diagnosis of ketoacidosis is listed in Table 5-1. The causes of a relative lack of insulin are listed in Table 5-2. There are two groups of disorders that lead to a relative lack of insulin. First, those in which the β-cells of the pancreas are normal but there is absence of a stimulator or presence of an inhibitor for the release of insulin. Second, those with damage to the β-cells of the pancreas (diabetes mellitus). Diabetic ketoacidosis and alcoholic ketoacidosis are discussed in detail in the next two sections.

TABLE 5-1 **CAUSES OF KETOACIDOSIS**

| TYPES | SPECIAL FEATURES | DANGERS |
|---|---|---|
| Diabetic ketoacidosis | • Common in children with type 1 DM; uncommon in patients with type 2 DM<br>• Low EABV, very high $P_{Glucose}$<br>• $P_K$ ~5.5 mmol/L, $K^+$ ion depletion | • Cerebral edema in children<br>• Cardiac arrhythmia initially due to hyperkalemia, later to hypokalemia that may develop during therapy<br>• Neuroglycopenia ~6 hours after insulin is given |
| Alcoholic ketoacidosis | • Alcohol binge in a chronic alcoholic, prominent gastrointestinal complaints, $P_{Glucose}$ is not very high, $P_{HCO_3}$ is not very low | • $K^+$ ion depletion might be large. Thiamin deficiency |
| Hypoglycemic ketoacidosis including starvation | • $P_{Glucose}$ <3 mmol/L (54 mg/dL)<br>• Past or family history might be positive; look for drugs that inhibit glucose production or fatty acid oxidation | • Give enough glucose to raise $P_{Glucose}$ to 5 mmol/L (90 mg/dL)<br>• Seek basis of an underlying disorder |
| Other types of ketoacidosis | • Fermentation of poorly absorbed carbohydrate in gastrointestinal tract, plus inhibition of the enzyme acetyl-CoA carboxylase | • Usually there are no dangers once intake of poorly absorbed carbohydrate is discontinued |

TABLE 5-2 **CAUSES OF RELATIVE LACK OF INSULIN**

With normal β-cells of the pancreas
• Lack of stimulators for β-cells (e.g., low $P_{Glucose}$)
• Inhibitors of insulin release (e.g., high α-adrenergics)
• Hormones that oppose the actions of insulin (e.g., glucagon, α-adrenergics, cortisol, growth hormone, thyroid hormone)
With abnormal β-cells of the pancreas
• Damage to or destruction of pancreatic islets (e.g., type 1 diabetes mellitus, pancreatitis, cystic fibrosis, hemochromatosis)

# PART B
# DIABETIC KETOACIDOSIS

**DIABETES MELLITUS (DM)**

• **Type 1 DM** is the form that occurs most commonly in young patients. These patients are prone to develop DKA.
• **Type 2 DM** is the form that is most common in older, obese patients. DKA is rare in these patients.

DKA develops when there is lack of actions of insulin, together with unopposed effects of glucagon. DKA may be the initial presentation of type 1 DM in a young patient (see margin note). Failure of a patient with known type 1 DM to take insulin is a common reason for the development of DKA. The presence of elevated levels of hormones that have actions that oppose the actions of insulin (e.g., adrenaline, glucocorticoids) because of a stress state caused by underlying illness may also be a precipitating factor for development of DKA. The most common precipitating illness is an infection, usually pneumonia or urinary tract infection. Other conditions include myocardial infarction, stroke, and pancreatitis.

## CASE 5-2: HYPERGLYCEMIA AND ACIDEMIA

Andy, age 15, weighs 50 kg; he had been feeling well until he had the "flu" 2 weeks ago. During this period, his urine output increased markedly, and he felt thirsty; he drank sweetened soft drinks, but as he felt bloated and became thirstier, he changed his intake over the last 36 hours to large volumes of water. He had a 4 kg weight loss. This morning, he was confused and difficult to rouse, and he was brought to the hospital. On physical examination, respirations were rapid and deep; the odor of acetone was detected on his breath. His blood pressure was 90/60 mm Hg, his heart rate was 110 beats/min, his jugular venous pressure was flat. On laboratory examination, he had metabolic acidosis with a high value for the $P_{Anion\ gap}$, a strongly positive serum test for ketones, a hematocrit of 0.50, and the concentration of glucose in his plasma ($P_{Glucose}$) was 50 mmol/L. His plasma β-HB concentration was 12 mmol/L, and plasma L-lactate concentration was 2 mmol/L.

Other laboratory values in blood are provided in the following table. The urine osmolality was 400 mosmol/kg $H_2O$.

| PLASMA | | | | PLASMA | | | |
|---|---|---|---|---|---|---|---|
| pH | | | 7.25 | $HCO_3^-$ | mmol/L | | 10 |
| Arterial $PCO_2$ | mm Hg | | 25 | Venous $PCO_2$ | mm Hg | | 50 |
| Glucose | mg/dL | | 900 | Glucose | mmol/L | | 50 |
| Creatinine | mg/dL | | 2.1 | Creatinine | μmol/L | | 190 |
| BUN | mg/dL | | 56 | Urea | mmol/L | | 20 |
| $Na^+$ | mmol/L | | 130 | $K^+$ | mmol/L | | 3.5 |
| $Cl^-$ | mmol/L | | 90 | Anion gap | mEq/L | | 30 |
| Albumin | g/dL | | 5 | Albumin | g/L | | 50 |

## Questions

What are the major threats to Andy's life?
Should the physician administer $NaHCO_3$?

# DIAGNOSIS OF DIABETIC KETOACIDOSIS

DKA occurs most often in patients with previously diagnosed type 1 DM, often because of failure of the patient to take insulin or the presence of a precipitating illness, commonly an infection. DKA may be the initial presentation of DM in a young patient who was not previously diagnosed with this disorder.

The major complaints are polyuria (due to the glucose-induced osmotic diuresis and natriuresis), thirst, and polydipsia (because of hyperglycemia and the release of angiotensin II due to EABV contraction), fatigue, and malaise. Catabolism of lean body mass contributes to the excessive weight loss. Metabolic acidemia results in an increased rate and depth of breathing (air hunger, Kussmaul respiration [see margin note]). The conversion of acetoacetic acid to acetone imparts the characteristic fruity odor to the breath.

Decreased level of consciousness, obtundation, and even coma may be present. The state of consciousness seems to correlate with the plasma effective osmolality ($P_{Effective\ osm}$), which may reflect the degree of EABV contraction and failure of the bicarbonate buffer system (BBS) in skeletal muscle to remove the $H^+$ ion load, resulting in more $H^+$ ion binding to proteins in brain cells (see Chapter 1).

Another feature of DKA that remains unexplained is hypothermia, even in the presence of infection. This together with the fact that leukocytosis is a common finding in these patients may diminish the clinical suspicion of an underlying infection. Anorexia, nausea, vomiting, and abdominal pain are frequent gastrointestinal complaints, especially in children. These symptoms, together with the findings of abdominal tenderness, decreased bowel sounds, guarding, and leukocytosis, may mimic an acute abdominal emergency. Rebound tenderness, however, is usually absent. The cause for the abdominal pain is not entirely clear, but in some cases it may be caused by pancreatitis due to hypertriglyceridemia.

## ABBREVIATIONS

$P_{Effective\ osm}$, plasma effective osmolality

$P_{Na}$, concentration of sodium ions in plasma

$P_K$, concentration of potassium ions in plasma

$P_{Cl}$, concentration of chloride ions in plasma

$P_{Albumin}$, concentration of albumin in plasma

BBS, bicarbonate buffer system

$P_{Creatinine}$, concentration of creatinine in plasma

BUN, blood urea nitrogen

$P_{Urea}$, concentration of urea in plasma

EFW, electrolyte-free water

$P_{Osmolal\ gap}$, plasma osmolal gap

## KUSSMAUL RESPIRATIONS

- This is deep and rapid breathing caused by stimulation of the respiratory center by acidemia. The pH in the area of the respiratory center becomes low because of high brain capillary blood $PCO_2$ caused by low cerebral blood flow because autoregulation of cerebral blood flow fails in the presence of a very low EABV.

Signs and symptoms of the disorder that precipitated DKA may dominate the clinical picture. The most common precipitating factor is an underlying infection (commonly pneumonia or a urinary tract infection). In the adult patient with DKA, precipitating factors also include myocardial infarction, stroke, trauma, pancreatitis, alcohol abuse, thyrotoxicosis, and the intake of corticosteroids.

## CHANGES IN BODY COMPOSITION AND LABORATORY FINDINGS IN DKA

Typical findings in the patient with DKA include hyperglycemia, glucosuria, metabolic acidosis with an increase in the $P_{Anion\ gap}$, and a strongly positive qualitative test for acetoacetate in blood and urine. The diagnosis of DKA can be confirmed by measuring the concentration of $\beta$-HB in blood.

### Hyperglycemia

The degree of hyperglycemia varies markedly—the $P_{Glucose}$ usually exceeds 250 mg/dL (14 mmol/L). The severity of hyperglycemia is influenced mainly by the degree of contraction of the EABV and the resultant decrease in GFR, which diminishes the rate of excretion of glucose (see Chapter 16), and the quantity of glucose/sucrose ingested (usually in the form of fruit juice and sweetened soft drinks to quench thirst).

### *Sodium*

A major feature of DKA is an appreciable degree of contraction of the EABV, which may dominate the clinical picture. This is due to loss of $Na^+$ ions in the urine, caused by glucose-induced osmotic natriuresis, with a concentration of $Na^+$ ions in the urine that is often 40 to 50 mmol/L. Deficits of $Na^+$ ions are said to be 5 to 10 mmol/kg body weight (Table 5-3). The magnitude of the deficit of $Na^+$ ions, however, depends on the number of liters of osmotic diuresis, which in turn depends, for the most part, on the quantity of glucose that was ingested (see Chapter 16).

It is important to obtain a quantitative estimate of the $Na^+$ ion deficit in each individual patient with DKA (see margin note). This requires a quantitative estimate of the extracellular fluid (ECF) volume, which can be obtained using the hematocrit (see Chapter 2). If a hemodynamic emergency is not present, it is important to avoid an overzealous administration of saline early on in the course of therapy because this may be a risk factor for the development of cerebral edema in children with DKA.

### *Plasma $Na^+$ concentration ($P_{Na}$)*

**USING WEIGHT LOSS TO ESTIMATE SODIUM DEFICIT**

- Some clinicians rely on weight loss to indicate the degree of contraction of the ECF volume and the $Na^+$ ion deficit. There are, however, confounding factors that make weight loss an unreliable indictor for the degree of $Na^+$ ion deficit, such as the degree of lean mass catabolism and the unknown volume of fluid retained in the lumen of the gastrointestinal tract.

The $P_{Na}$ is the ratio of $Na^+$ ions to $H_2O$ in the ECF compartment. Although patients with DKA may have hyponatremia, their $P_{Osm}$ is usually high because of the hyperglycemia. Hyponatremia may be present in a patient with DKA for four major reasons:
1. Deficit of $Na^+$ ions: $Na^+$ ions are lost in the urine largely because of the glucose-induced osmotic natriuresis and, to a lesser degree, the excretion of $Na^+$ ions with ketoacid anions in the urine early in the course of DKA.
2. Gain of water: Because of thirst, there is a large fluid intake. In patients with DKA, a number of stimuli that cause the release of vasopressin and therefore diminished excretion of water are present (e.g., a very low EABV, pain, nausea, anxiety). Although the concentration of $Na^+$ ions in the urine during glucose-induced

TABLE 5-3    **TYPICAL DEFICITS IN A PATIENT WITH DIABETIC KETOACIDOSIS**

|  | DEFICIT | COMMENT | DANGER |
|---|---|---|---|
| $Na^+$ | 5-10 mmol/kg | Restore quickly only if a hemodynamic emergency | Rapid expansion of the ECF volume may be a risk factor for cerebral edema in children |
| $K^+$ | 5-10 mmol/kg | $K^+$ ions will shift into cells when insulin acts | Hyperkalemia on admission<br>Hypokalemia ~1-2 hours after therapy with insulin is started |
| $H_2O$ | Many liters | Do not administer hypotonic saline | A large fall in $P_{Effective\,osm}$ may be a risk factor for cerebral edema |
| $HCO_3^-$ | Variable | Most patients with DKA do not require the administration of $NaHCO_3$ | Retrospective data suggest that administration of $NaHCO_3$ is a risk factor for cerebral edema in children with DKA |

osmotic natriuresis is relatively low (~40 to 50 mmol/L), hyponatremia develops because of the large intake of hypotonic fluids.

3. Shift of water from skeletal muscle cells to the ECF compartment: Adding hypertonic glucose causes water to shift from cells that require insulin for glucose transport into the ECF compartment (see Chapter 16). It is widely held that there is a predictable fall in the $P_{Na}$ for a certain rise in $P_{Glucose}$ based on a shift of water from the intracellular fluid compartment (ICF) to the ECF compartment. This relationship is based on theoretical calculations, and different corrections are proposed based on assumptions made about the ECF volume and the volume of distribution of glucose under conditions of relative lack of insulin. This shift of water, however, would only occur when the addition of glucose to the body is as a solution that is hyperosmolar to ECF compartment. In contrast, when glucose is added, as a solution that has an osmolality similar to or lower than that of ECF compartment, there is no shift of water from cells. If glucose is added as a hypotonic solution, the $P_{Na}$ may be even lower than that which occurs with the addition of a hypertonic glucose solution for an identical rise in $P_{Glucose}$ (see Chapter 16). Because patients with hyperglycemia have variable fluid intake and also variable loss of water and $Na^+$ ions in the urine due to glucose-induced osmotic diuresis and natriuresis, one cannot assume a fixed relationship between the rise in $P_{Glucose}$ and the fall in $P_{Na}$. Therefore, calculation of the expected fall in $P_{Na}$ for a given rise in $P_{Glucose}$ or the expected rise in $P_{Na}$ with a fall in $P_{Glucose}$, based on a shift of water, should not be done because the assumptions made are not valid. More importantly, it is incorrect to assume that will be a predictable rise in the $P_{Na}$ for a fall in $P_{Glucose}$ and administer hypotonic saline to avoid the development of hypernatremia during therapy because this may increase the risk for the development of cerebral edema in children with DKA. In our view, the $P_{Effective\,osm}$ must not be permitted to fall in the first 15 hours of treatment because most cases of cerebral edema occur 3 to 13 hours after therapy is instituted.

4. Pseudohyponatremia: This is secondary to hyperlipidemia if the technique used to measure the $P_{Na}$ requires dilution of plasma (see Chapter 10).

## Potassium

Hyperkalemia with $P_K$ that is usually close to 5.5 mmol/L is observed in most patients with DKA prior to therapy, despite the fact that there is a large overall total body deficit of $K^+$ ions caused by renal $K^+$ ion loss. Hyperkalemia is largely due to a shift $K^+$ ions out of cells because of insulin deficiency. Hyperglycemia may also cause a shift of $K^+$ ions out of cells as the rise in effective osmolality in the interstitial fluid causes the movement of water out of cells via aquaporin-1 water channels in cell membranes, which raises the concentration of $K^+$ ions in the ICF and provides a chemical driving force for the movement of $K^+$ ions out of cells.

Although it is said that $K^+$ ion deficit is usually about 5 to 10 mmol/kg body weight, the magnitude of this deficit will depend on the amount of $K^+$ ions ingested because some patients, for example, consume large amounts of fruit juice, which is rich in $K^+$ (close to 50 mmol of $K^+$ ions/L), to quench thirst.

Notwithstanding, some patients with DKA may have a $P_K$ that is in the normal range, whereas others may be hypokalemic. This can occur because these patients may have had large prior losses of $K^+$ ions (vomiting or a prolonged osmotic diuresis) or if their fluid intake to quench thirst was mostly water or other fluids that are poor in $K^+$ ions. This latter group of patients may also have a very low $P_{HCO_3}$ because they have less input of alkali in the form of organic anions. These patients are at risk for developing a more severe degree of hypokalemia and perhaps cardiac arrhythmia during therapy with the administration of insulin or $NaHCO_3$.

It was observed in some patients with DKA that if insulin is administered intravenously for a prolonged period of time, hypokalemia may develop, despite the administration of $K^+$ ions. This is because of a large increase in the rate of excretion of $K^+$ ions in the urine (~30 to 40 mmol $K^+$/mmol of creatinine). This may reflect the fact that insulin activates serum and glucocorticoid kinase 1 (SGK-1) similar to the effect of aldosterone (see Chapter 13 for more discussion).

### $P_{HCO_3}$

The severity of metabolic acidemia is usually judged by the fall in the $P_{HCO_3}$. Nevertheless the $P_{HCO_3}$ may be only moderately reduced when, in fact, there is a large $HCO_3^-$ ion deficit in the setting of a severe degree of ECF volume contraction. This deficit of $HCO_3^-$ ions is detected by obtaining a quantitative estimate of the ECF volume using the hematocrit (see Chapter 2).

Accumulation of ketoacids in the ECF leads to the loss of $HCO_3^-$ ions and the gain of ketoacid anions. There is also an indirect loss of $Na^+$ ions and $HCO_3^-$ ions early in the course of DKA. This is because there is a lag period before there is a large increase in the rate of excretion of $NH_4^+$ ions in the urine and therefore, ketoacid anions are excreted in the urine with $Na^+$ and/or $K^+$ ions. When ketoacid anions are excreted with $NH_4^+$ ions, there is an addition of $HCO_3^-$ ions to the body. In contrast, if they are excreted with $Na^+$ or $K^+$ ions, there is no addition of $HCO_3^-$ ions; therefore, the degree of acidemia becomes more severe. The degree of acidemia may be less severe if the patient drank large volumes of fruit juice, which contains organic anions (e.g., citrate anions in orange juice) that can be metabolized to produce $HCO_3^-$ ions.

### $P_{Anion\ gap}$

The addition of new anions can be detected by a rise in the $P_{Anion\ gap}$ (see Chapter 2 for detailed discussion). A pitfall in using the $P_{Anion\ gap}$ is the failure to correct for the net negative valence attributable to albumin for its concentration in plasma ($P_{Albumin}$). This correction must be made not only for a fall but also for a rise in $P_{Albumin}$. The $P_{Albumin}$ is usually increased in patients with DKA because of the marked degree of ECF volume contraction. The $P_{Anion\ gap}$ is reduced (or increased) by 2.5 mEq/L for each 10 g/L decrease (or increase) in $P_{Albumin}$. Even with this

TABLE 5-4    **CHANGES IN THE $P_{HCO_3}$ AND $P_{\beta\text{-HB}}$ AND THEIR CONTENT IN DIABETIC KETOACIDOSIS**

For simplicity, in this example we ignored the ongoing loss of $\beta$-HB$^-$ in urine. Moreover, we assumed that $\beta$-HB$^-$ represents all the ketoacid anions and its concentration is equal to most of the rise in the $P_{Anion\ gap}$ (ignoring the component of the rise in $P_{Anion\ gap}$ due to a higher $P_{Albumin}$).

| CONDITION | ECF VOLUME (L) | HCO$_3^-$ (mmol/L) | HCO$_3^-$ (mmol) | $\beta$-HB$^-$ (mmol/L) | $\beta$-HB$^-$ (mmol) | HCO$_3^-$ + $\beta$-HB$^-$ (mmol) |
|---|---|---|---|---|---|---|
| Normal | 10 | 25 | 250 | 0 | 0 | 250 |
| DKA | 7 | 10 | 70 | 15 | 105 | 175 |
| Difference | −3 | −15 | −180 | +15 | +105 | −75 |

adjustment, it seems that net negative valence on albumin is increased if there is an appreciable decrease in the EABV (see Chapter 3).

The relation between the rise in the $P_{Anion\ gap}$ and the fall in $P_{HCO_3}$ (delta anion gap/delta HCO$_3^-$) is used to provide an estimate of the magnitude of the acid load and to detect the presence of coexisting metabolic acid–base disorders. Some studies indicate that in patients presenting with DKA, the ratio of the rise in $P_{Anion\ gap}$ to the fall in $P_{HCO_3}$ approximates 1. The caveat in using this relationship to gauge the magnitude of the acid load is that it is based on concentrations and not content. To illustrate this point, consider a 50-kg woman with type 1 DM whose steady-state ECF volume is 10 L, $P_{HCO_3}$ 25 mmol/L and a $P_{Anion\ gap}$ of 12 mEq/L (Table 5-4). After she developed DKA, her $P_{HCO_3}$ fell to 10 mmol/L and her $P_{Anion\ gap}$ rose to 27 mEq/L. Because of the hyperglycemia-induced osmotic diuresis and natriuresis with DKA, her current ECF volume is only 7 L. While she has the expected 1:1 ratio between the rise in $P_{Anion\ gap}$ and the fall in $P_{HCO_3}$, the HCO$_3^-$ ions deficit and the amount of ketoacid anions retained in her ECF volume are not equal. The decrease in her HCO$_3^-$ ions is 180 mmol (25 mmol/L × 10 L − 10 mmol/L × 7 L), whereas the gain of ketoacid anions is only 105 mmol (0 mmol/L × 10 L + 15 mmol/L × 7 L). Thus, there is another important aspect of the deficit of HCO$_3^-$ ions when keto-acids were added. Some of the ketoacid anions were excreted in the urine with Na$^+$ and/or K$^+$ ions (an indirect loss of NaHCO$_3$ that is not reflected by a rise in the $P_{Anion\ gap}$) (Figure 5-8). Therefore, the rise in the $P_{Anion\ gap}$ did not reveal the actual quantity of H$^+$ ions that were added during DKA, and the fall in $P_{HCO_3}$ did not reflect the actual magnitude of the deficit of HCO$_3^-$ ions. However, on re-expansion of the ECF volume with saline, the degree of deficit of HCO$_3^-$ ions will become evident. In addition, the fall in the $P_{Anion\ gap}$ will not be matched by a similar rise in the $P_{HCO_3}$.

## PCO$_2$

Acidemia in arterial blood stimulates the respiratory center and leads to a predictable degree of decrease in the arterial PCO$_2$ (a fall of approximately 1.2 mm Hg in the arterial PCO$_2$ for every 1 mmol/L fall in $P_{HCO_3}$). As discussed in Chapter 1, although the arterial PCO$_2$ sets a lower limit on the PCO$_2$ in capillaries, it does not guarantee that the PCO$_2$ in skeletal muscle capillary blood, which reflects the PCO$_2$ in their ICF and the interstitial space, will be low enough to ensure effective buffering of H$^+$ ions by the bicarbonate buffer system (BBS). Because most patients with DKA have a markedly decreased EABV, the rate of blood flow to muscles will be low and hence their capillary PCO$_2$ will be higher, which diminishes the effectiveness of the BBS in skeletal muscles to remove an H$^+$ ion load. As a result, the degree of acidemia may become more pronounced and more H$^+$ ions may be titrated by proteins in the ECF and intracellular fluids in other organs, including the brain. Because of autoregulation of cerebral blood flow, however, it is likely that the PCO$_2$ in brain capillary blood will change minimally with

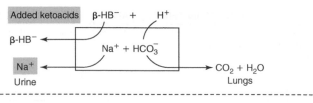

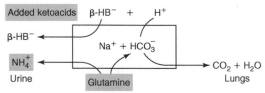

**Figure 5-8 Acid–Base Impact of Excretion of Ketoacid Anions.** The liver produces $H^+$ ions and β-$HB^-$ anions. $H^+$ ions are removed after reacting with $HCO_3^-$ anions to form $CO_2 + H_2O$; the result is a deficit of $HCO_3^-$ anions and a gain of β-$HB^-$ anions in the ECF compartment. Early in ketoacidosis, the kidneys have not yet increased their rate of excretion of $NH_4^+$ ions; hence, β-$HB^-$ anions are excreted with $Na^+$ ions (*upper portion*), and a deficit of $HCO_3^-$ ions develops. Because the loss of $HCO_3^-$ ions and the loss of $Na^+$ ions occur via two different routes, the term indirect loss of $NaHCO_3$ is used to describe this process. When the rate of production of $NH_4^+$ ions by the kidney rises, $NH_4^+$ ions and β-$HB^-$ anions are excreted in the urine while $HCO_3^-$ ions are added to the body to replace the $HCO_3^-$ ions that were lost when $H^+$ ions were added (*lower portion*). Hence, the excretion of β-HB anions with $NH_4^+$ ions results in nil balance for the sum of $H^+$ ions and $HCO_3^-$ ions.

all but a severe degree of contraction of EABV. Hence, the BBS in the brain will continue to titrate this $H^+$ ion load. Nevertheless, considering the limited quantity of BBS in the brain, and because the brain receives a relatively larger proportion of the blood flow, there is a risk that more of the $H^+$ ion load will bind to intracellular proteins in the brain. If cerebral autoregulation fails because of a severe degree of EABV contraction, the $PCO_2$ in capillary blood in the brain will rise and its BBS will fail and an even larger $H^+$ ion load will bind to proteins in brain cells.

### Ketoacids

In DKA, serum ketones are usually strongly positive in a dilution of 1 in 8 with the nitroprusside test (Acetest) used for clinical screening for ketoacids. However, only acetoacetic acid and acetone yield a positive reaction with this test. As mentioned previously, the major ketoacid that is produced by the liver is β-hydroxybutryic acid, which is not detected by Acetest. Furthermore, if there is a further increase in the $NADH,H^+/NAD^+$ ratio in the liver, as occurs with hypoxia or due to metabolism of ethanol, the vast majority of ketoacids will be in the form of β-HB. Direct assays for β-hydroxybutyric acid have largely replaced the Acetest for diagnosis of ketoacidosis.

### GFR

Because patients with DKA often have a very low EABV, their GFR will be reduced and the concentration of creatinine in plasma ($P_{Creatinine}$) will be elevated. There may be errors in the measurement of $P_{Creatinine}$, depending on the method used. Higher $P_{Creatinine}$ values are reported with the picric acid method if the level of acetoacetate in plasma is elevated, whereas lower $P_{Creatinine}$ values are reported with severe hyperglycemia, if the enzymatic assay for creatinine is performed on the Kodak analyzer. The rise in blood urea nitrogen (BUN) or in the concentration of urea in plasma ($P_{Urea}$) may be out of proportion with the rise in $P_{Creatinine}$, reflecting the increase in renal reabsorption of urea with marked decrease in EABV. Although there is tissue catabolism in patients with DKA, the rate of production of urea may not be substantially increased because the intake of protein is usually markedly decreased.

## NATURAL HISTORY

A patient with type 1 DM who stops taking insulin may not feel well for a period of days to weeks, but the symptoms lack specificity during that time period. The actual symptoms attributable to DKA develop very slowly, with a lag time of many days. When hyperglycemia and acidemia become prominent, a vicious cycle develops. As the patient starts to become confused, cerebral metabolism of ketoacids declines, and the degree of acidemia suddenly becomes more severe. Because the GFR also declines, renal work is reduced as a result of a low filtered load of $Na^+$ ions, and this also contributes to the development of a more severe degree of acidemia because both the rate of renal ketoacid ion oxidation and rate of excretion of $NH_4^+$ ions fall.

## CEREBRAL EDEMA IN CHILDREN WITH DKA

The major complication that may develop during therapy of DKA in children is cerebral edema. We discuss its possible pathophysiology before proceeding to a discussion of therapy of DKA because understanding the pathophysiology of cerebral edema has implications for the design of therapy.

Cerebral edema is the major cause of mortality and morbidity in children with DKA. Clinically evident cerebral edema occurs in close to 0.5 to 1% of cases of DKA. It commonly occurs in younger children during their first episode of DKA, which is often more severe possibly because of a long delay before the diagnosis is made. Most cases of cerebral edema occur 3 to 13 hours after therapy is instituted, and often with little warning. Cerebral edema should be suspected when there is complaint of headache, vomiting, deterioration in neurologic status, the persistence of a comatose state without an obvious cause, or an unexpected rise in blood pressure and a fall in heart rate—signs that may suggest an increased intracranial pressure. Therefore, children with DKA should be admitted to a unit where they can be observed very closely because therapy must commence without delay to minimize the risk of permanent brain damage.

Cerebral edema is primarily a clinical diagnosis. The presumptive diagnosis of cerebral edema is supported if there is a rapid improvement in neurologic status in response to intravenous administration of 3% NaCl or hypertonic mannitol solution. Making a clinical diagnosis and providing urgent therapy should take precedence over performing a diagnostic study such as a computed tomography scan or magnetic resonance imaging because provision of care may suffer if the patient is transported to an area of the hospital where continuous monitoring may be less than ideal.

## PATHOPHYSIOLOGY

Because water cannot be compressed and the skull is a rigid box, it is obvious that if the volume of one of the brain compartments (ECF or ICF) were to expand, and if this was not accompanied by an equivalent decrease in the volume of the other, there would be a rise in intracranial pressure. Hence, risk factors for the development of cerebral edema can be thought of as those that lead to an increase in the volume of brain cells and those that lead to an increase in the ECF volume of the brain.

### Intracellular fluid issues

Water moves rapidly across cell membranes through aquaporin water channels to achieve equal concentrations of effective osmoles in the ICF and ECF compartments. Effective osmoles are osmoles that are restricted to the ICF compartment or the ECF compartment. There are two major factors that could cause the ICF volume to expand: a rise in the number of effective osmoles in the ICF compartment or a fall in the the number of effective osmoles in the ECF compartment. The latter will be reflected by a fall in effective osmolality in plasma ($P_{\text{Effective osm}}$). $P_{\text{Effective osm}}$ in patients with DKA is calculated as shown in Eqn 11. $P_{\text{Urea}}$ is not included in the calculation of $P_{\text{Effective osm}}$ because urea molecules are transported across cell membranes and achieve equal concentrations in the ECF and the ICF compartments, and therefore, urea is not an effective osmole.

$$P_{\text{Effective osm}} = 2\,(P_{\text{Na}}) + (P_{\text{Glucose}}), \text{ all in mmol/L terms} \qquad (11)$$

### Extracellular fluid issues

The interstitial compartment of the ECF can expand if there is a higher capillary hydrostatic pressure, a lower plasma colloid osmotic pressure, or an increase in permeability of capillaries such that they no longer effectively restrict the movement of albumin.

Based on these considerations, we suggest that the following may be risk factors for the development of cerebral edema.

### An increase in number of effective osmoles in brain cells

The $Na^+/H^+$ exchanger 1 (NHE-1) is normally inactive in cell membranes. NHE-1 is activated by a high $H^+$ ion concentration in the ICF and a high insulin concentration in plasma. Entry of β-hydroxybutyric acid into cells on the monocarboxylic acid cotransporter (MCT), and its subsequent dissociation into β-HB⁻ anions and $H^+$ ions, may lead to a large increase in $H^+$ ion concentration in the submembrane area where NHE-1 is located. Following the administration of an intravenous bolus of insulin in the presence of a severe degree of acidemia, NHE-1 in brain cell membranes could become active. This will lead to a gain of $Na^+$ ions in, and a loss of $H^+$ ions from, the ICF compartment. This increases the number of effective osmoles in cells because the bulk of $H^+$ ions exported from the cell were bound to ICF proteins and hence were not effective osmoles. To the extent that $Na^+$ ions that entered these cells via NHE-1 are exported by the electrogenic Na-K-ATPase (which is also activated by actions of insulin), the resultant increase in the intracellular negative voltage causes the retention of $K^+$ ions in these cells. Therefore, whether this process leads to a gain of $K^+$ ions or $Na^+$ ions, the net effect is an increase in the number of effective osmoles in brain cells (Figure 5-9).

### A fall in the $P_{\text{Effective osm}}$

This could occur if there is a rapid fall in $P_{\text{Glucose}}$ and/or a gain of electrolyte-free water (EFW).

#### A rapid fall in the $P_{\text{Glucose}}$

A major factor that leads to a rapid fall in the $P_{\text{Glucose}}$ is glucosuria as a result of a rise in GFR following EABV re-expansion. The $P_{\text{Glucose}}$

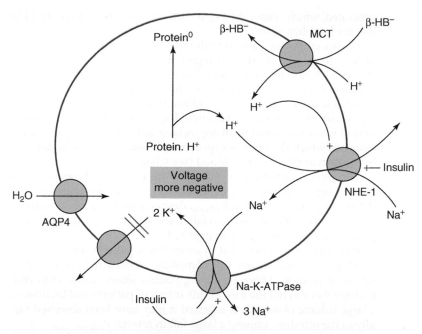

**Figure 5-9 Increased Flux Through NHE-1 Leads to an Increase in the Number of Effective Osmoles in Brain Cells.** Entry of β-hydroxybutyric acid into cells through the monocarboxylic acid cotransporter (MCT), and its subsequent dissociation into β-HB anions and $H^+$ ions, may lead to a large increase in the concentration of $H^+$ ions in the local submembrane area where the sodium-hydrogen exchanger 1 (NHE-1) is located. NHE-1 is activated by a high concentration of $H^+$ ions in the cell interior and by a high insulin concentration in interstitial fluid. Flux through NHE-1 will lead to a gain of effective osmoles because $Na^+$ ions enter cells, whereas the bulk of $H^+$ ions exported from these cells are not effective osmoles because most of these $H^+$ ions were bound to intracellular proteins. If a bolus of insulin were administered, $Na^+$ ions that entered these cells through NHE-1 may be exported by the electrogenic Na-K-ATPase, which is activated by insulin. The increased intracellular negative voltage can cause retention of $K^+$ ions in these cells. Whether this process leads to a gain of $K^+$ ions, $Na^+$ ions, or both, the net effect is an increase in the number of effective osmoles in brain cells, which promotes water flux through aquaporin water channels (AQP4) in their cell membranes.

may also fall because of increased metabolism of glucose. When the concentrations of ketoacids in plasma decline, glucose becomes the primary brain fuel. Furthermore, more glucose may be oxidized in skeletal muscle because fewer circulating free fatty acids are available because of actions of insulin to inhibit hormone-sensitive lipase in adipocytes. In addition, after a lag period of about several hours, actions of insulin will induce the enzymes required for the synthesis of glycogen in muscle and the liver.

### Gain of EFW

There are several possible sources of EFW in this setting, including the administration of hypotonic saline and administration of 5% dextrose in water solution ($D_5W$). Although administration of glucose is necessary to prevent neuroglycopenia when the $P_{Glucose}$ falls, one must recognize that after the glucose contained in 1 L of $D_5W$ is removed by oxidation or via glycogen synthesis, 1 L of solute-free water is generated, which causes the $P_{Na}$ to fall. Another two sources of EFW that are less obvious are:

Gastric emptying: Patients with DKA often consume large volumes of fluid to quench thirst. This ingested fluid may be retained in the stomach because hyperglycemia slows stomach emptying. This, however, will result in a gain of water when absorbed, if water has been ingested or after glucose is metabolized if fruit juice or sugar-containing soft drinks have been consumed. Rapid absorption of a large volume of water may result in an appreciable fall in $P_{Effective\ osm}$ in arterial blood, to which the brain is exposed and which may not be detected by measurements in venous blood (see Chapter 11).

The clinician should take a detailed history of fluid ingestion and look for signs that indicate recent gastric emptying. Such signs include the absence of a large fall in $P_{Glucose}$ despite a high rate of excretion of glucose in the urine or a sudden fall in the $P_{Effective\ osm}$, which will happen if water without sugar was ingested.

It is interesting to note that in about 5% of patients with DKA who developed cerebral edema, this complication occurred prior to institution of therapy. Although hyperglycemia slows gastric emptying, perhaps this was not the case in this subset of patients and therefore if a large volume of water was ingested it may have been absorbed rapidly in the intestine, causing a large fall in arterial $P_{Effective\ osm}$.

Desalination of administered saline: The usual clinical practice is to administer large volumes of saline to patients with DKA. If vasopressin is released (due to a number of nonosmotic stimuli that may be present in this setting), water reabsorption in the cortical and medullary collecting ducts will increase. As glucose excretion diminishes and its concentration in the urine falls, the concentration of $Na^+$ ions in the urine will rise. The excess saline that was administered may be excreted in the urine as a hypertonic (to the patient) solution, and therefore, EFW is generated in the body (see Chapter 10).

### Increase ECFV in the brain

A large bolus of saline distributes initially in the plasma that reaches the blood–brain barrier before mixing with the entire ECF compartment. This may increase the interstitial volume of the brain ECF compartment and lead to cerebral edema because it causes an increase in the capillary hydrostatic pressure and a decrease in colloid osmotic pressure. There is some evidence to suggest that the blood–brain barrier is somewhat leaky in some patients with DKA. This is based on the fact that the brain appeared to be swollen on computed tomography scan in some patients with DKA at the time of presentation to hospital. At that time, the volumes of both the ECF and the ICF compartments of the brain should have been decreased.

### *Clinical implications*

Based on the previous analysis, we suggest the following modifications to the current management of children with DKA:
1. Do not administer an intravenous bolus of insulin.
2. Prevent a fall in $P_{Effective\ osm}$. The $P_{Effective\ osm}$ must not be permitted to fall in the first 15 hours of treatment. The goal of fluid therapy should be to raise the $P_{Na}$ by one-half of the fall in $P_{Glucose}$ in mmol/l.
3. Use 10% dextrose in water ($D_{10}W$) in 0.9% NaCl instead of $D_5W$ to minimize the amount of EFW generated after glucose is metabolized.
4. Monitor for signs of gastric emptying.
5. Avoid overzealous saline administration.

# TREATMENT OF THE PATIENT WITH DIABETIC KETOACIDOSIS

The approach to the design of therapy in the patient with DKA involves nine major issues:

1. Re-expand the EABV to maintain hemodynamic stability.
2. Minimize the risk for development of cerebral edema: do not administer a bolus of insulin, prevent an appreciable fall in the $P_{Effective\ osm}$, and avoid excessive infusion of saline.
3. Stop ketoacids production.
4. Replace the deficit of $K^+$ ions.
5. Replace the deficit of $Na^+$ ions.
6. Consideration of $NaHCO_3$ therapy.
7. Consideration of phosphate therapy.
8. Identify and deal with underlying events that may have precipitated DKA.
9. Anticipate and prevent complications that may arise during therapy.

## TREAT A HEMODYNAMIC EMERGENCY IF PRESENT

A large bolus of saline should be given only if there is a hemodynamic emergency. This is because a large bolus of intravenous saline can be a risk factor for the development of cerebral edema. In general, we limit the amount of $Na^+$ ions to infuse in the first 120 minutes of therapy to about 3 mmol/kg body weight (see margin note).

In the absence of a hemodynamic emergency, we use the brachial venous $PCO_2$ as a guide to the rate of infusion of saline. Enough saline should be administered to lower the brachial venous $PCO_2$ to a value that is no more than 6 mm Hg above the arterial $PCO_2$. We think this is important to ensure effective buffering of $H^+$ ions by the BBS in muscle and thus decrease binding of $H^+$ ions to intracellular proteins in vital organs (e.g., the brain and the heart; see Chapter 1 and Fig. 1–7).

## AVOID A LARGE FALL IN THE $P_{Effective\ osm}$

A large fall in the $P_{Effective\ osm}$ may occur early during therapy due to the fall in $P_{Glucose}$ caused by the glucosuria that occurs with the re-expansion of the EABV and the resultant rise in the GFR. Therefore, design of therapy needs to achieve a rise in the $P_{Na}$ by an amount that is one-half of the fall in the $P_{Glucose}$ (both $Na^+$ ions and their accompanying anions contribute to the $P_{Effective\ osm}$) (Figure 5-10). As discussed previously, the clinician should not correct the $P_{Na}$ for the degree of hyperglycemia.

To prevent a fall in the $P_{Effective\ osm}$, the effective osmolality of the infusate should be equal to or greater than that of the urine in this polyuric state. When $K^+$ ion infusion is needed, this goal can be achieved if KCl is added to 0.9% saline at a concentration of 30 to 40 mmol per liter. This solution has an effective osmolality that is reasonably close to that of the urine (which is about 400 mosmol/kg $H_2O$) in children with DKA at that time. Because children with DKA often present with near-normal $P_{Na}$, a degree of hypernatremia would develop with such an infusion, but that would be an important tradeoff to prevent a fall in the $P_{Effective\ osm}$.

When administration of glucose is needed to prevent neuroglycopenia as the $P_{Glucose}$ falls, use $D_{10}W$ in 0.9% NaCl instead of $D_5W$ to minimize the amount of EFW generated after glucose is metabolized.

The clinician should take a detailed history of fluid ingestion and look for signs that indicate recent gastric emptying. The $P_{Effective\ osm}$ in arterial blood must be monitored if the history reveals an intake of a large volume of water. Infusion of hypertonic saline may be needed if

**EXPRESSING VOLUME OF SALINE TO INFUSE PER KILOGRAM OF BODY WEIGHT**

- Because patients with DKA differ in size, it is better to express the volume to infuse per kilogram of body weight rather than to infuse an absolute volume.
- An infusion of 3 mmol $Na^+$ ions/kg body weight as an isotonic solution provides a volume that is equivalent to 10% of the normal ECF volume in a given subject.
- For example, in a 50-kg patient, normal ECF volume is 10 L, 3 mmol $Na^+$/kg body weight = 150 mmol $Na^+$ ions = 1 L of isotonic saline.

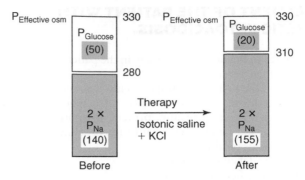

**Figure 5-10 Defense of the Effective Osmolality of Plasma.** A rise in the $P_{Na}$ is needed to prevent a fall in the $P_{Effective\ osm}$ when there is a fall in the $P_{Glucose}$. If the $P_{Na}$ on admission is close to 140 mmol/L, the $P_{Na}$ should be raised to 155 mmol/L when the $P_{Glucose}$ falls from 50 mmol/L to 20 mmol/L to maintain a constant $P_{Effective\ osm}$.

## USE OF HEMATOCRIT TO ESTIMATE ECF VOLUME

- Blood volume is ~70 mL/kg body weight. Therefore, in a 70 kg adult subject, blood volume is close to 5 L. With a hematocrit of 0.40, red blood cells (RBC) volume is 2 L and plasma volume is 3 L.
- If the hematocrit is 0.50, assuming that the RBC volume remains 2 L, the new blood volume (X), can be calculated as follows:

**Hematocrit = RBC volume/ blood volume**

**0.50 = 2 L/X L blood volume**

**X = 4 L**

- Because the RBC volume is 2 L, the plasma volume is 2 L (i.e., decreased by 33%).
- The following table relates the value hematocrit to the ECF volume. Of note, the percent decline in the ECF volume is larger than the percent decline in the plasma volume in the patient with DKA because of changes in Starling forces (the plasma hydrostatic pressure is lower and the plasma oncotic pressure is higher when the $P_{Albumin}$ is increased), which increases the plasma volume at the expense of the interstitial fluid volume.

| HEMATOCRIT | % ↓ IN ECF VOLUME |
|---|---|
| 40 | 0 |
| 50 | 33 |
| 60 | 57 |

there is a large fall in $P_{Effective\ osm}$ in arterial blood. EFW may be also generated by desalination of body fluids as described above. Hence the urine osmolality and composition should be followed. If a large volume of hypertonic urine is being excreted, the tonicity of the fluid infused should match the tonicity of the urine to prevent a fall in the $P_{Effective\ osm}$.

### Replace the Na⁺ ion deficit

Having defined the safe rate and the tonicity of the fluid to infuse, the issue now is to define what is a reasonable total volume of saline to infuse. Enough saline should be given initially to restore hemodynamic stability.

The deficit of Na⁺ ions on presentation can be estimated from the $P_{Na}$, and a quantitative estimate of the ECF volume using the hematocrit can be made (see margin note). This avoids the overzealous administration of saline and the excessive expansion of the ECF volume, which occurs commonly during therapy in patients with DKA. In general, in patients who are hemodynamically stable, we aim to replace ~30% of the deficit of Na⁺ ions over the first 4-6 hours. We monitor the brachial venous $PCO_2$ and the arterial $PCO_2$ and adjust the rate of infusion to achieve a value of brachial venous $PCO_2$ that is no more than 6 mm Hg higher than the arterial $PCO_2$. We replace the remaining deficit of Na⁺ ions over the rest of the 24 hour period.

In addition to the calculated Na⁺ ion deficit on presentation, ongoing losses of Na⁺ ions in the urine must be replaced. Because glucose is an effective osmole in the ECF compartment when there is a relative lack of insulin, glucose molecules that accumulated in the ECF compartment helped to maintain EABV by causing a shift of water from the ICF compartment to the ECF compartment. Therefore, this amount of glucose should be replaced during therapy with an equimolar amount of NaCl (see margin note).

### STOP KETOACIDS PRODUCTION

Insulin plays a central role in arresting ketogenesis; there may be, however, a lag period of a few hours before there is an appreciable decline in the rate of production of ketoacids. This is usually not an urgent aspect of therapy because, based on data from adult subjects with starvation ketosis, the maximum rate of hepatic production of ketoacids is about 1 mmol/min. Hence, the administration of insulin can be delayed if required, as in the case of a patient with DKA and an initial $P_K$ of less than 4 mmol/L (see the following discussion). In our view, the only circumstance in which insulin must be administered urgently in a patient with DKA is the presence of ECG changes related to hyperkalemia because of its effect to induce a shift of $K^+$ ions into cells. The effects of insulin to treat hyperglycemia are minimal early in therapy. Rather, the $P_{Glucose}$ will fall initially as a result of re-expansion of the ECF volume (dilution) and glucosuria caused by the rise in GFR. Six to eight hours after therapy begins, insulin will lower $P_{Glucose}$ by increasing the rate of oxidation of glucose because competing fat fuels are no longer available, and by promoting the synthesis of glycogen.

A bolus of insulin should *not* be used in children because it may lead to brain cell swelling (see Figure 5-9). Insulin therapy has potentially detrimental side effects that should be anticipated and avoided. The major ones are hypokalemia and hypoglycemia. The risk of hypoglycemia is minimized by infusing glucose when the $P_{Glucose}$ falls to ~250 mg/dL (~14 mmol/L).

## DEFICIT OF $K^+$ IONS

The $P_K$ is usually close to 5.5 mmol/L in most patients with DKA prior to therapy. This is despite the fact that there is a large overall total body deficit of $K^+$ ions due to the loss of $K^+$ ions in the urine. Hyperkalemia is usually due to insulin deficiency, which causes $K^+$ ions to shift out of cells. Although it is said that deficit of $K^+$ ions in patients with DKA is usually ~5 to 10 mmol/kg body weight, the magnitude of this deficit may vary among patients depending on the intake of $K^+$ ions. For instance, some patients consume large amounts of fruit juice, which is rich in $K^+$ ions (close to 50 mmol of $K^+$ ions/L), to quench thirst.

If the $P_K$ is less than 5 mmol/L, KCl should be added to each liter of intravenous fluids once insulin is given. The $P_K$ should be monitored closely because the actual $K^+$ ion deficit may vary among patients.

Both the American Diabetes Association guidelines and the Canadian Diabetes Association guidelines for the treatment of DKA suggest that the administration of insulin be delayed if the initial $P_K$ is <3.3 mmol/L. These patients are likely to be severely depleted in $K^+$ ions and are likely to be at risk for cardiac arrhythmias because the administration of insulin may induce a shift of $K^+$ ions into cells, which will result in a more severe degree of hypokalemia. We think that avoiding insulin only if $P_K$ is <3.3 mmol/L is in fact too low a threshold. The administration of insulin may cause a fall in $P_K$ of ~1 mmol/L. Furthermore, the effect of insulin to cause a shift of $K^+$ ions into cells may be more pronounced in the presence of acidemia because a rise in $H^+$ ion concentration inside cells also activates NHE-1 and increases the electroneutral entry of $Na^+$ ions into cells (see Chapter 13). We suggest that the administration of insulin be delayed in patients with $P_K$ of <4 mmol/L. Aggressive therapy with the administration of KCl via the intravenous route should be instituted promptly to bring $P_K$ close to 4 mmol/L before starting insulin.

## $NaHCO_3$ THERAPY

Most patients with DKA do not require administration of $NaHCO_3$ because administered insulin will slow the rate of production of ketoacids, and $HCO_3^-$ ions will be produced when ketoacid anions are oxidized.

Only three randomized controlled trials (n = 73 patients) examined the effect of $NaHCO_3$ in adult patients with DKA. Patients with serious concomitant illnesses (e.g., acute myocardial infarction, gastrointestinal hemorrhage, chronic renal failure, or intraabdominal sepsis) were excluded. The administration of $NaHCO_3$ was found to not be beneficial, based on outcome measurements such as the change in arterial pH, $P_{HCO_3}$ and of the metabolites measured. There was only one study

---

**CALCULATION OF QUANTITY OF GLUCOSE IN THE ECF COMPARTMENT**

• In a patient with a $P_{Glucose}$ of 50 mmol/L and an ECF volume that has fallen from 10 L to 7 L, the current content of glucose in the ECF compartment is 350 mmol (50 mmol/L × 7 L). Prior to developing DKA, the content of glucose in the ECF compartment was 50 mmol (5 mmol/L × 10 L). Therefore, 300 mmol of glucose were added to the ECF compartment and should be replaced with 150 mmol of NaCl to prevent a fall in the quantity of effective osmoles in the ECF compartment and thereby maintain its volume.

that reported the impact of $NaHCO_3$ on mean arterial blood pressure. Although the consensus of opinion is not to administer $NaHCO_3$ in patients with DKA unless the plasma pH is close to 6.90, we suggest that this decision should be individualized and not based solely on an arbitrary blood pH value. We suggest that therapy with $NaHCO_3$ be considered in the initial treatment of a subset of patients who have moderately severe acidemia (plasma pH <7.20, $P_{HCO_3}$ <12 mmoL/L), who are hemodynamically unstable, and those are at risk for developing a more severe degree of acidemia before a dangerous fall in plasma pH develops. One must remember that in patients with a very low $P_{HCO_3}$, a quantitatively small additional $H^+$ ion load will produce a proportionately larger fall in the $P_{HCO_3}$ and plasma pH. It may take a number of hours after insulin is administered for an appreciable decrease in the rate of production of ketoacids to occur. Meanwhile, the rate of ketoacid oxidation and production of $HCO_3^-$ ions will be diminished if there is a lower rate of work in the brain (e.g., coma, intake of sedatives, including ethanol) and the kidneys (e.g., patients with advanced renal dysfunction and estimated GFR <30 mL/min). The target of $NaHCO_3$ therapy in these patients would be at least to avoid a significant fall in the $P_{HCO_3}$. To achieve this goal, the rate of infusion of $NaHCO_3$ should match the expected rate of production of ketoacids by the liver. This, based on data from subjects with starvation ketosis, is ~60 mmol/hr. We think that this is a reasonable start, which can be re-evaluated based on serial measurements of the $P_{HCO_3}$. We would give $NaHCO_3$ as an infusion in a solution with a similar tonicity to the calculated $P_{Effective\ osm}$. Clinical trials designed to evaluate the potential benefits of this approach on outcome measures such as restoration of hemodynamic stability and the incidence of complications such as acute kidney injury, myocardial infarction, and stroke have not been performed.

A multicenter, case-controlled, retrospective study in pediatric patients with DKA found that patients who were treated with $NaHCO_3$ had a significantly greater risk of developing cerebral edema. This association does not prove causation or rule out other confounding factors (see margin note). Nevertheless, because of the potential of causing harm, in our opinion, $NaHCO_3$ should not be administered to children with DKA unless acidemia is very severe and hemodynamic instability is unresponsive to the usual maneuvers to restore blood pressure.

## PHOSPHATE THERAPY

Patients with DKA are catabolic and therefore have large deficits of phosphate ions. In addition, because the plasma phosphate levels decline markedly once insulin acts, there seems to be a rationale to administer phosphate to patients with DKA. On the other hand, there are no compelling data to suggest that administration of phosphate alters the course of recovery. We would recommend treating hypophosphatemia if severe (serum phosphate concentration <1 mg/dL [0.32 mmol/L]), particularly in the presence of cardiac dysfunction, respiratory muscle weakness, or hemolytic anemia. Notwithstanding, if a decision is made to give phosphate, the maximum dose is about 6 mmol/hour to avoid the danger of development of hypocalcemia due to precipitation of calcium ions with phosphate ions.

### Identify and deal with underlying events that may have precipitated DKA

Always look for an underlying illness (e.g., an infection, commonly pneumonia or urinary tract infection) that may have initiated this metabolic emergency.

**$NaHCO_3$ AND RISK OF CEREBRAL EDEMA**

- Confounding factors may include the administration of a large volume of saline in response to hemodynamic instability because of a severe degree of acidemia and/or the administration of a bolus of insulin.

**Anticipate and prevent complications that may arise during therapy**

One should also be on the lookout for complications that may arise during therapy, such as deep venous thrombosis or aspiration pneumonia.

# PART C
# ALCOHOLIC KETOACIDOSIS

## CASE 5-3: SAM HAD A DRINKING BINGE YESTERDAY

Sam is a patient with chronic alcoholism; he does not have a history of diabetes mellitus. After a large intake of a liquor that he bought from the store, he had several bouts of vomiting. He was taken to the emergency room by a friend. On physical examination, he responded only to painful stimuli. He had a low blood pressure and tachycardia. Acetone was not detected on his breath. His arterial plasma pH was 7.30, and arterial $PCO_2$ was 30 mm Hg. His hematocrit was 0.50. The following laboratory values were obtained from a venous blood sample:

| | | |
|---|---|---|
| Glucose | mg/dL (mmol/L) | 45 (2.5) |
| Na$^+$ | mmol/L | 116 |
| K$^+$ | mmol/L | 3.5 |
| Cl$^-$ | mmol/L | 76 |
| HCO$_3^-$ | mmol/L | 18 |
| Anion gap | mEq/L | 24 |
| Creatinine | mg/dL (μmol/L) | 2.0 (175) |
| Osmolality | mosmol/kg H$_2$O | 290 |
| Albumin | g/dL (g/L) | 4.5 (45) |
| β-HB | mmol/L | 6 |
| L-lactate | mmol/L | 2 |

## Questions

What is Sam's acid–base disorder?
What are the issues for therapy?

## BIOCHEMISTRY OF ALCOHOLIC KETOACIDOSIS

The biochemical features of ketoacids formation from ethanol are very similar to those of the process of ketoacid formation during prolonged fasting, even though the substrate for the formation of acetyl-CoA is different. Metabolism of ethanol in the liver occurs in the cytoplasm and results in formation of acetic acid. Acetic acid enters the mitochondria, where it is metabolized to acetyl-CoA, the precursor for ketoacids synthesis. There are, however, important differences between the process of ketoacid formation when fatty acids are its major substrate and when ethanol is its major substrate. The most notable of these differences is how each pathway is regulated. To gain insights into the control of each of these metabolic processes, one must focus on its function. In prolonged fasting, the substrate for ketogenesis is long-chain fatty acids, and the function of the process is to produce a water-soluble, fat-derived fuel

## THE CONVERSION OF CYTOSOLIC NADH,H⁺ TO NAD⁺

- The inner mitochondrial membrane lacks an NADH,H⁺ transport protein.
- The electrons from cytosolic NADH,H⁺ are transported into mitochondria by the malate–aspartate shuttle.

## ETHANOL AND THE UNCOUPLING OF OXIDATIVE PHOSPHORYLATION

- When rats were given a very large load of ethanol, a swift initial accelerated metabolism of ethanol was observed; this was accompanied by an increased rate of consumption of oxygen that persisted for a period of time after ethanol disappeared. This is consistent with uncoupled oxidative phosphorylation in the liver (see Part D for more discussion). It is not certain what triggers this accelerated metabolic rate.
- Another reaction that is equivalent to uncoupling of oxidative phosphorylation is the conversion of acetoacetic acid to β-hydroxybutyric acid because NADH,H⁺ is converted to NAD⁺ in this reaction.

(ketoacids) for the brain at a rate that is sufficient to match the rate of removal of ketoacids by the brain and the kidneys. Conversely, when ethanol is the substrate, the function of the metabolic process of ketoacids formation is to remove as much ethanol as possible via alcohol dehydrogenase in the liver to avoid a depressant effect on the central nervous system. Therefore, while there is a lag period before ketoacids are produced at a rapid rate when long-chain fatty acids are the substrate, there is no lag period when ethanol is the substrate. Simply put, the rate of formation of acetyl-CoA is regulated when fatty acids are the substrate but not when ethanol is the substrate. In alcoholic ketoacidosis, there is no regulation to speak of once the ethanol level in blood rises other than if the rate of ethanol oxidation is limited by the rate of removal of NADH,H⁺ via its oxidation in mitochondria to convert it back to NAD⁺ (see margin note). Oxidation of NADH,H⁺ to NAD⁺ requires the consumption of oxygen and either the availability of ADP (produced from the hydrolysis of ATP when biologic work is performed) in coupled oxidative phosphorylation, or the uncoupling of oxidative phosphorylation to bypass this limitation of availability of ADP. To allow for a larger amount of ethanol to be removed, the final product of ketogenesis must be β-hydroxybutyric acid.

### STEPS IN KETOACIDS FORMATION FROM ETHANOL

1. The first step in the metabolic process is to remove a large quantity of ethanol in the liver is catalyzed by an NAD⁺-linked enzyme: alcohol dehydrogenase. The products of this reaction are acetaldehyde + NADH,H⁺ (Eqn 12).

$$\text{Ethanol} + \text{NAD}^+ \rightarrow \text{Acetaldehyde} + \text{NADH,H}^+ \qquad (12)$$

2. Because aldehydes bind avidly to proteins and hence are toxic in the body, acetaldehyde must be converted into a safe product. This conversion is catalyzed by another NAD⁺-linked enzyme: acetaldehyde dehydrogenase. The product of this reaction is acetic acid, which dissociates completely at body pH into acetate anions and H⁺ ions (Eqn 13).

$$\text{Acetaldehyde} + \text{NAD}^+ \rightarrow \text{Acetic acid} + \text{NADH,H}^+ \qquad (13)$$

3. Acetic acid enters the mitochondria on a monocarboxylic acid transporter, where it is converted to acetyl-CoA. This step is catalyzed by the enzyme acetic acid thiokinase and requires the presence of CoA-SH and ATP; ATP is hydrolyzed to form AMP and pyrophosphate (Eqn 14).

$$\text{Acetic acid} + \text{CoA-SH} + \text{ATP} \rightarrow \text{Acetyl-CoA} + \\ \text{AMP} + \text{Pyrophosphate} \qquad (14)$$

4. If a large amount of ethanol is consumed, and a large amount of acetyl-CoA is produced at a rapid rate, oxidation of acetyl-CoA will be limited by the rate of regeneration of ADP during performance of hepatic work. As acetyl-CoA accumulates, two molecules of acetyl-CoA condense to form acetoacetyl-CoA. Acetoacetyl-CoA is metabolized to acetoacetic acid in the HMG-CoA pathway. Because of the high mitochondria ratio of NADH,H⁺/NAD⁺ due to metabolism of ethanol, the majority of acetoacetic acid is converted to β-hydroxybutyric acid.

## REMOVAL OF KETOACIDS IN THE PATIENT WITH ALCOHOLIC KETOACIDOSIS

Decreased rate of removal of ketoacids is a critical factor in determining the severity of acidemia in patients with alcoholic ketoacidosis. Ketoacids are oxidized primarily in the brain and the kidneys. To have high rates of oxidation in these organs, there must be a high rate of consumption of oxygen.

- *Brain*: The consumption of oxygen in the brain can be diminished by the sedative effect of ethanol. In addition, removal of ketoacids by the brain may be decreased because, although there is no lag period before ketoacids are produced at a rapid rate from the metabolism of ethanol in the liver, there appears to be a lag period before the transporter for ketoacids in the blood–brain barrier is induced.
- *Kidneys*: The kidneys oxidize fewer ketoacids if the filtered load of $Na^+$ ions is decreased due to the fall of GFR because of decreased EABV.
- *Acetone*: A minor pathway for $H^+$ ions removal during ketoacidosis is the conversion of acetoacetic acid to acetone. Because of the high $NADH,H^+/NAD^+$ ratio in the liver secondary to the oxidation of ethanol, more of the acetoacetic acid produced is converted to β-hydroxybutyric acid and thus a smaller proportion is converted to acetone.

## DIAGNOSIS OF ALCOHOLIC KETOACIDOSIS

Patients with alcoholic ketoacidosis usually have a history of chronic alcohol abuse and present after a large, recent intake of ethanol. Presence of ethanol in blood is suggested by the finding of an elevated osmolal gap in plasma $P_{Osmolal\ gap}$ and confirmed by direct measurement of ethanol in blood. In addition to the large intake of ethanol, a key factor to the development of ketoacidosis is a large release of catecholamines, caused by a decreased EABV and/or repetitive bouts of vomiting and the pain secondary to alcohol-induced gastritis. Other factors that cause an adrenergic surge may be also present (e.g., a large intake of caffeine). This adrenergic surge has important metabolic effects with regard to the development of ketoacidosis, including inhibition of the release of insulin, enhanced lipolysis, and inhibition of acetyl-CoA carboxylase, the enzyme that catalyzes the first committed step in fatty acid synthesis (see Figure 5-4).

### Low EABV

Patients with alcoholic ketoacidosis often present with an appreciable degree of EABV contraction. This may be due to prior NaCl depletion. Although there is little $Na^+$ ions in the gastric secretions, the contents of the stomach that are lost during vomiting may contain some $Na^+$ ions from swallowed saliva or from entry of intestinal secretions that are rich in $NaHCO_3$ through a patent pyloric sphincter. There could also be some loss of $Na^+$ ions in the urine because alkalemia (caused by vomiting) may increase the renal excretion of $NaHCO_3$ and/or the $Na^+$ salts of organic acids. In addition, redistribution of the ECF volume because of alcohol-induced acute pancreatitis and/or paralytic ileus, or pooling of blood in the venous capacitance vessels, could also contribute to the low EABV. A decreased EABV may also be due to the presence of alcoholic cardiomyopathy.

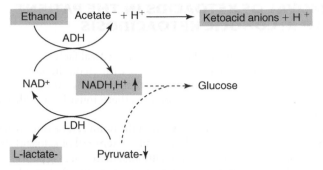

**Figure 5-11 Biochemical Consequences of Ethanol Metabolism in the Liver.** The metabolism of ethanol leads to inhibition of the production of glucose and a low $P_{Glucose}$ in those patients who have poor glycogen stores in the liver. Key to this metabolic pattern is the high level of reduced nicotinamide adenine dinucleotide (NADH,H+) in the cytosol of hepatocytes, which "drives" the conversion of pyruvate to L-lactate instead of its metabolism to produce glucose. *ADH*, Alcohol and aldehyde dehydrogenases; *LDH*, L-lactate dehydrogenase; *NAD+*, nicotinamide adenine dinucleotide.

## $P_{Glucose}$

During metabolism of ethanol, there is diminished hepatic production of glucose because the high NADH,H+/NAD+ ratio drives the conversion of pyruvate to L-lactate because these two metabolic intermediates can be interconverted by lactate dehydrogenase, an enzyme with a very large catalytic capacity (Figure 5-11). This reduces the rate of formation of glucose from pyruvate. The $P_{Glucose}$ is within the normal limits in most patients with alcoholic ketoacidosis. Hypoglycemia, however, is present in some patients who are particularly malnourished and therefore have limited glycogen storage in their liver. Hyperglycemia is present in some other patients, but the $P_{Glucose}$ is usually only modestly elevated with levels that are usually less than 270 mg/dL (15 mmol/L).

### β-Hydroxybutyric Acidosis

Because of the high NADH,H+/NAD+ ratio in the liver caused by the metabolism of ethanol, the majority of acetoacetic acid is converted to β-hydroxybutyric acid. This provides a pathway to regenerate NAD+ that does not require the availability of ADP (performance of biologic work) or the consumption of $O_2$, and thus a larger amount of ethanol can be removed. The price to pay is a more severe degree of acidemia, especially if the rate of removal of ketoacids is compromised (discussed previously).

## $P_K$

There are two opposing forces on the $P_K$, caused by the high levels of adrenergic hormones that affect the distribution of K+ ions between the ICF and ECF compartments. On the one hand, a $\beta_2$-adrenergic effect leads to a shift of K+ ions into cells because it activates the Na-K-ATPase, which makes the cells' interior voltage more negative. On the other hand, a high α-adrenergic action leads to inhibition of the release of insulin. As a result, there is a shift of K+ ions out of cells because the cell interior voltage becomes less negative (see Chapter 13 for more discussion). Hence, the $P_K$ in these patients may be low, normal, or high depending on which of these effects predominates.

If the patient had vomiting for a long period of time, K+ ion depletion may be present because of a large kaliuresis (see Chapter 7 for more discussion). Hypomagnesemia is common in patients with chronic alcoholism, and it may be a contributing factor to $K^+$ ion depletion. On the other hand, hyperkalemia may be present if the patient had rhabdomyolysis.

## NUTRITIONAL DEFICIENCIES

Patients with chronic alcoholism may have a number of nutritional deficiencies, including components of vitamin B. These patients should be given thiamin (vitamin $B_1$) at the onset of therapy to avoid the development of Wernicke's encephalopathy (see Chapter 6).

## ACID–BASE DISORDERS

### Mixed metabolic acidosis and metabolic alkalosis

Even though ketoacidosis (which tends to lower $P_{HCO_3}$) is present, the patient might not be acidemic because of the presence of coexisting metabolic alkalosis (which tends to raise the $P_{HCO_3}$). The metabolic alkalosis may be caused by vomiting, which results in a gain of $HCO_3^-$ ions. A higher $P_{HCO_3}$ may also be caused by contraction alkalosis because of the loss of ECF volume. The key to the diagnosis of this mixed acid–base disturbance is that the increase in the $P_{Anion\ gap}$ is larger than the fall in the $P_{HCO_3}$. A note of caution is important. A low $P_{Albumin}$ might mask the rise in the $P_{Anion\ gap}$; therefore, the baseline value for the $P_{Anion\ gap}$ must be adjusted for $P_{Albumin}$ (for every 1.0-g/dL [10-g/L] decline in the $P_{Albumin}$, the $P_{Anion\ gap}$ falls by 2.5 mEq/L). In addition, the content of $HCO_3^-$ ions in the ECF compartment could be calculated using the $P_{HCO_3}$ and a quantitative estimate of the ECF volume from the hematocrit value; many of these patients, however, may have prior anemia. Some patients, however, might have reduced gastric HCl secretion (e.g., because of intake of drugs such as proton pump inhibitors for relief of heartburn or dyspepsia caused by gastritis), hence there is a low net addition of $HCO_3^-$ ions to the body during vomiting. In some patients there may be loss of $NaHCO_3$ during vomiting if the pyloric sphincter is patent, and hence there is loss of pancreatic secretions rich in $HCO_3^-$ ions (see Chapter 7).

### L-Lactic acidosis

A mild degree of L-lactic acidosis may be present in patients with AKA because metabolism of ethanol raises the $NADH,H^+/NAD^+$ in the cytosol of hepatocytes, and this results in the conversion of pyruvate to L-lactate. If a more severe degree of L-lactic acidosis is present (plasma lactate concentration >10 mmol/L), reasons in addition to ethanol metabolism should be suspected. Two of the most common causes of L-lactic acidosis are obvious: first, tissue hypoxia due to a very low EABV; second, muscular contractions (e.g., the tremors in delirium tremens, or a recent seizure). The most important cause of a severe degree of L-lactic acidosis, however, is thiamin deficiency (see Chapter 6), which may also cause permanent cerebral damage (Wernicke's encephalopathy) if it is not recognized and treated promptly. Other B vitamin deficiencies (e.g., vitamin $B_2$ [riboflavin]) can also cause L-lactic acidosis (see Chapter 6).

### Respiratory alkalosis

There are a number of reasons why patients with alcoholic ketoacidosis may have a superimposed respiratory alkalosis. These include aspiration pneumonia, hyperventilation because of a high adrenergic state caused by alcohol withdrawal, and/or chronic liver disease.

## TREATMENT OF ALCOHOLIC KETOACIDOSIS

### HYPOGLYCEMIA

**DOSE OF GLUCOSE NEEDED TO RAISE $P_{Glucose}$ BY 5 mmol/L**

- Because the volume of distribution of glucose under conditions of lack of insulin in a 70 kg subject is close to 20 L (ECF volume [15 L] +5 L of ICF), give a total of 100 mmol of glucose (18 g) (=0.4 L of $D_5W$ or 30 mL of $D_{50}W$). A larger amount of glucose will be needed later to permit the usual rate of glucose oxidation in the brain once the level of ketoacids in blood declines appreciably.

A small amount of glucose is usually sufficient to correct hypoglycemia and maintain a normal $P_{Glucose}$ because the rate of metabolism of glucose is low in this setting (see margin note). Avoid hyperglycemia because high levels of insulin may lead to a shift of $K^+$ ions into cells and a sudden fall in $P_K$. In addition, inhibition of insulin release by α-adrenergic actions may no longer be present once the EABV is re-expanded.

### LOW EABV

In patients with a contracted EABV, isotonic saline can be infused rapidly to restore hemodynamic stability. One must be cautious, however, because some of these patients may have alcoholic cardiomyopathy and may not tolerate a rapid, large infusion of saline. In the absence of hemodynamic instability, we infuse enough saline to lower brachial venous $PCO_2$ to a value that is not more than 6 mm Hg higher than arterial $PCO_2$ as a guideline that enough saline has been infused. This also allows for buffering of $H^+$ ions by BBS in the interstitial space and ICF of muscles and prevents their binding to intracellular proteins in cells of vital organs (e.g., brain cells). One may not be able to use the hematocrit or total plasma proteins concentration to provide a quantitative assessment of the ECF volume to estimate the total $Na^+$ ion deficit because some patients may not have had normal hematocrit or albumin values to begin with. Nevertheless, changes in hematocrit or plasma total proteins concentration with therapy may provide rough guides to the degree of re-expansion of the ECF volume.

Of great importance, if the patient has chronic hyponatremia and is malnourished, a rapid rise in the $P_{Na}$ must be avoided because of the risk of developing osmotic demyelination. Administration of 1-desamino-8-D-arginine vasopressin (dDAVP) to prevent a large water diuresis that may occur once the EABV is re-expanded should be considered (see Chapter 10 for more discussion). Water intake must be restricted if dDAVP is given.

### K$^+$ ION DEFICIT

As the EABV is re-expanded, the α-adrenergic surge disappears, and insulin will be released (if the $P_{Glucose}$ is not low). This may cause a shift of $K^+$ ions into cells, resulting in hypokalemia. One should not wait for hypokalemia to develop before administering KCl. The actual amount of KCl to give depends on the $P_K$ during therapy; the deficit could be several hundreds of mmols in a patient with chronic alcoholism.

There are a number of reasons why the administration of KCl may cause a rapid or excessive rise in $P_{Na}$ and hence the risk of osmotic demyelination in a patient with chronic hyponatremia (see Case 5-3 for discussion of management of hypokalemia in this setting).

### THIAMIN

It is critical that thiamin (and probably riboflavin) be added early in therapy of a patient with chronic alcoholism. This will permit aerobic oxidation of glucose in the brain once ketoacids disappear and prevent the development of Wernicke's encephalopathy (for more discussion, see Chapter 6).

## PHOSPHATE

Although phosphate depletion is quite marked, it takes time before anabolic reactions occur subsequent to the actions of insulin. Hence, as in DKA, replacing the majority of the phosphate ion deficit (with $K^+$ ions) should be delayed. If phosphate is to be infused, the rate should not exceed 6 mmol per hour and it should never be given as a bolus infusion because of the risk of hypocalcemia.

## KETOACIDOSIS

There is usually no specific therapy needed to deal with the ketoacidosis because excessive production of ketoacids falls once ethanol disappears and the EABV is re-expanded (insulin is released from β-cells of the pancreas). Moreover, the utilization of ketoacids improves when the GFR rises because of re-expansion of the EABV and when ethanol levels fall sufficiently to permit normal cerebral function. Therapy with $NaHCO_3$ is not needed in most patients.

---

# PART D
# INTEGRATIVE PHYSIOLOGY

## CONTROL OF KETOGENESIS: A MORE DETAILED ANALYSIS

Control of the maximum rate of production of ketoacids in the liver when there is hormonal permission for ketogenesis to occur (low net actions of insulin) can be due to a limited supply of its extrahepatic and/or intrahepatic substrates. In this section, we provide a quantitative analysis to define whether the availability of any of the substrates for ketogenesis may limit the rate of ketoacid production during prolonged fasting and in patients with DKA.

### CONTROL BY SUPPLY OF FATTY ACIDS TO THE LIVER

A conservative estimate of the content of fatty acids in 1 L of blood is close to 1 mmol. Because blood flow to the liver is close to 1 L/minute, and 4 mmol of ketoacids are formed per 1 mmol of palmitic acid (16 carbons; see Eqn 15), the liver could make 4 mmol of ketoacids per minute. Some of these fatty acids, however, are tightly bound to albumin. Nevertheless, even if only 0.5 mmol of palmitic acid is taken up by the liver per minute, it should be sufficient to support the observed rate of ketogenesis during prolonged fasting (close to 1 mmol/min).

Palmitic acid $(C_{16}H_{32}O_2) + 6\,O_2 \rightarrow 4\,\text{ketoacids}\,(C_4H_7O_3) + 2\,H_2O$   (15)

In the patient with DKA, there is a lower rate of blood flow to the liver because of the markedly contracted EABV, which may reduce the delivery of fatty acids to the liver sufficiently to lower the rate of ketogenesis in these patients. On the other hand, there could be a higher content of fatty acids in each liter of plasma in these patients because of a higher $P_{Albumin}$. Nevertheless, it is possible that the rate of production of ketoacids may be limited by the supply of fatty acids in patients with DKA.

## CONTROL BY SUPPLY OF INTRAHEPATIC SUBSTRATES

Oxidation of long-chain fatty acids (e.g., palmitic acid) in hepatic mitochondria produces acetyl-CoA and converts $NAD^+$ to $NADH,H^+$ and FAD to $FADH_2$. Because these substrates are present in tiny amounts in cells, one limiting factor for the rate of hepatic ketoacid formation could be the availability of mitochondial $NAD^+$ and FAD. $NADH,H^+$ is converted back to $NAD^+$ and $FADH_2$ to FAD during coupled oxidative phosphorylation, which converts ADP and Pi to ATP. The availability of ADP depends on the rate of utilization of ATP to perform biologic work.

Hepatic work consists primarily of biosynthesis and flux through the Na-K-ATPase. Notwithstanding, the liver does very little biosynthetic work or ion pumping when there are low net actions of insulin. In patients with DKA who have little protein ingestion, there are insufficient amino acids available to permit high rates of protein synthesis, a process that utilizes ATP. Accordingly, the liver does not perform enough work to hydrolyze ATP and make enough ADP and Pi to permit mitochondria to have a high rate of coupled oxidative phosphorylation to convert $NADH,H^+$ to $NAD^+$ and $FADH_2$ to FAD.

Hence, this problem must be overcome when an augmented rate of ketogenesis is needed for the brain to have an alternate fuel when glucose is not available, and for the kidneys to excrete enough effective osmoles to avoid oliguria and the formation of precipitates in the urine. The observed ketoacid production rate during prolonged fasting is ~1500 mmol/day, which suggests that there are other ways for the liver to bypass this limitation from insufficient ADP. The process that is most likely to achieve this task is uncoupling of oxidative phosphorylation.

## UNCOUPLED OXIDATIVE PHOSPHORYLATION

In coupled oxidative phosphorylation, $H^+$ ions are pumped out of mitochondria using the energy derived from the oxidation of fuels. These $H^+$ ions re-enter mitochondria via special $H^+$ ion channels that are linked to the conversion of ADP + Pi to ATP (Figure 5-6). In contrast, if $H^+$ ions re-enter mitochondria through another $H^+$ ion channel that is not linked to the conversion of ADP + Pi to ATP, this results in an uncoupled oxidative phosphorylation. The net effect of this uncoupling is to increase the rate of oxidation of fuels in the presence of $O_2$ because this process removes the absolute need for ADP availability to convert $NADH,H^+$ back to $NAD^+$ and $FADH_2$ to FAD to permit fuel oxidation. These $H^+$ channels are called uncoupler proteins (UCP), mainly UCP2 and/or UCP3.

There is a second mitochondrial mechanism to increase the rate of $H^+$ ion entry into the mitochondria without converting ADP + Pi to ATP. This occurs when weak acids enter mitochondria ($H^+$ entry) and have their anions exit the mitochondria without an $H^+$ ion. So, in effect, this weak acid recycles. Two examples of this type of uncoupler of oxidative phosphorylation are metformin (discussed in more detail in Chapter 6) and salicylic acid (discussed in more detail in Chapter 8). Therefore, the ingestion of acetyl-salicyclic acid may augment the rate of hepatic ketogenesis in a patient with DKA.

CONTROL BY SUPPLY OF OXYGEN TO THE LIVER

Each liter of arterial blood has close to 8 mmol of $O_2$ (see margin note). Although the liver receives 1 L of blood per min, most of this blood arrives via the portal vein, where one-fourth to one-third of its oxygen was extracted by the intestinal tract. As a result, the liver receives close to 6 mmol of oxygen per liter of blood. If the liver extracted all 6 mmol of $O_2$, it could convert 1 mmol of palmitic acid to ketoacids in coupled or uncoupled oxidative phosphorylation (see Eqn 15). Because the liver receives close to 1 mmol of palmitic acid in 1 L of blood, it seems that the supply of oxygen may be a limiting factor for the rate of ketoacids production by the liver.

**OXYGEN CONTENT PER LITER OF BLOOD**

- The concentration of hemoglobin in blood is 140 g/L. Because the molecular weight of hemoglobin is ~70,000, the concentration of hemoglobin in blood is 2 mmol/L.
- 4 mmol $O_2$ bind to 1 mmol hemoglobin.
- Therefore, the content of $O_2$ in 1 L of arterial blood is 8 mmol.

## REGULATION OF KETOACIDS FORMATION DURING PROLONGED FASTING

There is little variation in the concentrations of AcAc and β-HB in plasma during prolonged fasting. In addition, there is a fairly robust turnover of these metabolic intermediates. When quantities are examined, the need for regulatory mechanisms that exert control on the rate of ketoacid production becomes obvious. First, close to 1500 mmol of ketoacids are produced each day during prolonged fasting (~1 mmol/min). Second, the content of ketoacid anions in the ECF compartment of a 50-kg person is only 50 mmol (ECF volume 10 L, and a total concentration of AcAc and β-HB in plasma of ~5 mmol/L). If the ketoacid anions were distributed in total body water, the overall content would be 150 mmol (5 mmol/L × total body water 30 L). Because the production rate is ~1500 mmol/24 hours, in one-tenth of this time (i.e., 2.4 hours), the patient would have produced 150 mmol, which would double the content of ketoacid anions if there were no removal. Based on these quantitative considerations, feedback regulation of ketogenesis is very likely to be present.

There are data to suggest that the rate of ketogenesis in the liver might be regulated by changes in the plasma pH and $P_{HCO_3}$. The administration of an acid load ($NH_4Cl$) to obese subjects who fasted for a prolonged period led to a marked decline in the concentration of ketoacid anions in plasma and in the rate of ketoacid anion excretion. Conversely, both the concentration of ketoacid anions in plasma and the rate of ketoacid anion excretion rose appreciably when $NaHCO_3$ was administered to these subjects. Taken together, it is possible that changes in the plasma pH and $P_{HCO_3}$ might play an important role in the control of hepatic ketogenesis in this setting. We are not certain about the mechanism(s) involved, but a change in the rate of uncoupled oxidative phosphorylation via a change, for example, in the gating of uncoupler $H^+$ ion channels is a reasonable hypothesis.

## DISCUSSION OF CASES

### CASE 5-1: A MAN IS ANXIOUS TO KNOW WHY HE HAS KETOACIDOSIS

**What makes DKA an unlikely diagnosis?**

DKA is unlikely because his $P_{Glucose}$ is in the normal range despite a large intake of sugar, he does not have a history of diabetes mellitus, his EABV is not contracted, and his previous two episodes of ketoacidosis resolved without the administration of insulin. Moreover, his plasma insulin level, which was measured during this admission, was in the expected range for his $P_{Glucose}$.

### What makes alcoholic ketoacidosis an unlikely diagnosis?

Alcoholic ketoacidosis is unlikely because the patient denies the intake of alcohol and his $P_{Osmolal\ gap}$ is not elevated (although he could have metabolized the alcohol by the time he presented).

### What makes starvation or hypoglycemic ketoacidosis an unlikely diagnosis?

Starvation and hypoglycemic ketoacidosis are ruled out because he does not have a low $P_{Glucose}$ and he has had a large intake of sugar.

### How may the patient's intake of sweetened soft drinks contribute to the development of his ketoacidosis?

To develop ketoacidosis, one requires a source of carbon for the synthesis of acetyl-CoA in hepatic mitochondria at a rate that exceeds its removal via oxidation to $CO_2 + ATP$ and mechanisms to inhibit the synthesis of long-chain fatty acids from acetyl-CoA.

The source for acetyl-CoA formation in the liver in this patient is not fatty acids (there is no lack of insulin). The source of acetyl-CoA does not seem to be ethanol. We suggest that the source of acetyl-CoA is the fructose in the large amount of sweetened soft drinks he consumed. In more detail, there is no specific transporter for fructose in the intestinal tract. Although some absorption of fructose occurs via one of the glucose transporters, it is largely delivered to the colon, where it is a major fuel for bacteria in the lumen of the colon. The major product of fermentation of fructose by bacteria is acetic acid. In fact, fermentation of poorly absorbed carbohydrates by bacteria in the colon normally leads to the absorption of close to 200 mmol/day of acetic acid.

The major metabolic fate of this acetic acid is its conversion to acetyl-CoA in the mitochondria of liver cells. The usual site of regulation of formation of acetyl-CoA from long-chain fatty acids in mitochondria of the liver is the entry of palmitoyl-CoA into mitochondria via a carnitine-dependent transport step. Because this is not required for the entry of acetic acid into the mitochondria (which is probably via a monocarboxylic acid cotransporter), acetyl-CoA is produced at a rapid rate. If the rate of acetyl-CoA production exceeds its possible rate of removal via oxidation (as determined by the rate of ATP utilization to perform biologic work in the liver), ketogenesis may occur, providing that the other pathway for metabolism of acetyl-CoA, fatty acid synthesis, is inhibited. The rate-limiting enzyme for fatty acid synthesis (which occurs in the cytosol), is acetyl-CoA carboxylase, which is inhibited by $\beta_2$ adrenergics (see Figure 5-5). Recall that this patient is suffering from an anxiety attack; furthermore, he drank large amounts of soft drinks that contained a large quantity of caffeine, which causes an adrenergic surge (see margin note).

### Is ketoacidosis the only cause of metabolic acidosis in this patient?

His metabolic acidosis is not simply due to ketoacidosis because his plasma $\beta$-HB is only 4.5 mmol/L, yet his $P_{Anion\ gap}$ is elevated by close to 18 mEq/L. Perhaps there is an unusually high concentration of AcAc. Alternatively, other short-chain fatty acids produced by

**CAFFEINE AND RELEASE OF CATECHOLAMINES**

Each liter of soda contains close to 100 mg of caffeine, and he drank many liters per day. One of the effects of caffeine is to block adenosine receptors and thereby create an adrenergic surge (see Chapter 14).

bacterial fermentation in the colon could account for the remaining unmeasured anions in plasma.

## CASE 5-2: HYPERGLYCEMIA AND ACIDEMIA

The diagnosis of DKA was quite obvious and was confirmed with the measurement of plasma β-HB. Andy has no previous history of DM, so this was his first presentation with type 1 DM.

**What are the major threats to Andy's life?**

The major immediate threat to Andy's life is hypokalemia causing a cardiac arrhythmia. Although most patients with DKA are severely $K^+$ ion depleted, with $K^+$ ion deficit of about 5 to 10 mmol/kg body weight, the $P_K$ at presentation is usually about 5.5 mmol/L, reflecting a shift of $K^+$ ions out of cells, largely caused by the lack of actions of insulin. The fact that Andy's $P_K$ was only 3.5 mmol/L indicates that he may be severely $K^+$ ion depleted. He is at risk of a more severe degree of hypokalemia with the risk for cardiac arrhythmia if insulin were administered and caused a shift of $K^+$ ions into cells. Therefore, insulin should be withheld initially and aggressive intravenous therapy with KCl should be started to raise his $P_K$ to close to 4 mmol/L. We would add 30 to 40 mmol of KCl to 1 L of 0.9% saline and infuse it over 2 hours. While some suggest using 0.45% saline, we think this is dangerous because this solution has an osmolality that is substantially lower than the $P_{Effective\ osm}$ and hence may increase the risk of cerebral edema. Because there is a risk of phlebitis with the rapid infusion of a solution with a high concentration of $K^+$ ions, it is preferable to use a large caliber peripheral vein. We cannot overemphasize that the $P_K$ must be followed very closely because one does not know how much of the administered $K^+$ ions will shift into his cells.

Andy has an appreciable decrease in his EABV. As Andy weighed 50 kg before he fell ill, his total body water was 60% of his body weight, or 30 L, with ECF volume of 10 L and ICF volume of 20 L. His blood volume was 3500 mL (50 kg body weight × 70 mL blood/kg body weight). With an initial hematocrit of 0.40, his initial RBC volume was 1400 mL and his plasma volume was 2100 mL. As his hematocrit on presentation was 0.50, his plasma volume has decreased to 1400 mL, a fall of 33%. Ignoring changes in Starling forces, his ECF volume has declined by 33% (i.e., from 10 L to 6.6 L). The volume of saline administered initially should be just enough to ensure hemodynamic stability and lower his brachial venous $PCO_2$ to a value that is no more than 6 mm Hg greater than his arterial $PCO_2$ to ensure effective buffering of the $H^+$ ion load primarily by his BBS in skeletal muscles.

The other major threat to Andy's life is the development of cerebral edema. This dreaded complication usually develops 3 to 13 hours after initiation of therapy in children during their first episode of DKA. We were particularly concerned about Andy because he had been drinking large volumes of water to quench his thirst. Because hyperglycemia slows gastric emptying, he may have a large volume of water sitting in his stomach. If gastric emptying were to occur, rapid absorption of water from his intestine may lead to an appreciable fall in $P_{Effective\ osm}$ in arterial blood (to which his brain is exposed), which may not be detected in measurements performed in venous blood. We had an arterial line inserted and monitored the $P_{Effective\ osm}$ in both the arterial and venous blood. To minimize the risk for cerebral edema, the following measures were taken:

- No bolus of insulin was given.
- Overzealous administration of saline was avoided.

- To prevent a fall in $P_{Effective\ osm}$, the effective osmolality of the fluid infused was equal to that of the urine in a polyuric patient. A solution of 0.9% saline plus KCl 40 mmol/L has an osmolality of 380 mosmol/kg $H_2O$, which is reasonably close to Andy's urine osmolality of 400 mosmol/kg $H_2O$.

- Eight hours after initiation of therapy, there was an appreciable fall in the $P_{Effective\ osm}$ in arterial blood to a value that was 15 mosmol/kg $H_2O$ lower than the $P_{Effective\ osm}$ in brachial venous blood. To restore the $P_{Effective\ osm}$, if his ECF volume now (estimated from current hematocrit value of 0.45) is ~8 L, then we need to administer about 120 mmol of effective osmoles (15 mosmol/L × 8 L of ECF). Because hypertonic 3% saline has an osmolality of close to 1000 mosmol/kg $H_2O$, our decision was to administer 100 mL of 3% saline slowly and to monitor $P_{Effective\ osm}$ in arterial and brachial venous blood.

The $Na^+$ ion deficit was replaced over several hours. One needs a quantitative approximation of his $Na^+$ ion deficit to avoid overexpansion of his ECF volume, which commonly occurs in therapy of patients with DKA. If Andy had an initial ECF volume of 10 L and initial $P_{Na}$ of 140 mmol/L, the content of $Na^+$ ions in his ECFV was 1400 mmol. His ECF volume on presentation was calculated, based on hematocrit of 0.50, to be 6.6 L, and his $P_{Na}$ was 130 mmol/L; therefore, the content of $Na^+$ ions in ECF volume was about 860 mmol. Therefore, he has a deficit of $Na^+$ ions of about 540 mmol. There is also ongoing loss of $Na^+$ ions in the urine, which can be calculated from measurements of urine volume and the concentration of $Na^+$ in the urine. In addition, because his $P_{Glucose}$ was 50 mmol/L and his ECF volume on presentation was estimated to be about 6.6 L, the content of glucose in his ECF volume was 330 mmol. This is about 280 mmol more than the content of glucose in his ECF volume before he fell ill (ECF volume of 10 L × $P_{Glucose}$ of 5 mmol/L). Because these 280 mmol of glucose represented effective osmoles that maintained ECF volume, their loss in the urine should be replaced with 150 mmol of NaCl.

When the $P_{Glucose}$ fell to ~250 mg/dL (~14 mmol/L), to prevent neuroglycopenia, intravenous glucose was given with a small volume of water by adding 50 g of glucose (100 mL $D_{50}W$) to 1 L of 0.9% NaCl instead of infusing $D_5W$.

### Should the physician administer $NaHCO_3$?

Because of the association with increased risk of cerebral edema, $NaHCO_3$ should not be administered to children with DKA unless acidemia is very severe and hemodynamic instability is unresponsive to the usual maneuvers to restore blood pressure).

### CASE 5-3: SAM HAD A DRINKING BINGE YESTERDAY

### What is Sam's acid–base disorder?

Metabolic acidosis with a high $P_{Anion\ gap}$ was present. We do not know Sam's normal value for his $P_{Anion\ gap}$. Normal value for $P_{Anion\ gap}$ in our hospital laboratory is 8 to 16 mEq/L. If we assume that Sam's baseline $P_{Anion\ gap}$ was 12 mEq/L, then the rise in his $P_{Anion\ gap}$ is higher than what can be accounted for by the measured values of β-HB and L-lactate anions in his plasma. This may be due to the presence of other unmeasured anions in his plasma (e.g., acetate) or it may in fact reflect a rise in the $P_{Anion\ gap}$ because of a rise in the $P_{Albumin}$ and also in its negative valence, secondary to the contracted ECF volume. The rise in the $P_{Anion\ gap}$ is larger than the fall in $P_{HCO_3}$ if we assume that his normal $P_{HCO_3}$ was 25 mmol/L (normal value for $P_{HCO_3}$ in our hospital laboratory is 22 to 30 mmol/L). This may be due to coexisting metabolic alkalosis caused by the loss of HCl in vomiting. The markedly contracted EABV also raises the $P_{HCO_3}$ because the same amount of $HCO_3^-$ ions in the ECF compartment is now in a smaller ECF volume.

### What are the issues for therapy?

- *Thiamin deficiency*: Thiamin must be added at the outset in therapy so that energy metabolism in the brain is not compromised once ketoacids disappear (see Chapter 6 for more discussion).
- *Hypovolemia*: The EABV should be re-expanded to avoid a circulatory problem; this should be done rapidly only if there are signs of hemodynamic instability. The dangers of this therapy are raising the $P_{Na}$ too rapidly if water diuresis were to occur with restoration of EABV. Patients with chronic alcoholism who are $K^+$ depleted and malnourished are at high risk for development of osmotic demyelination syndrome with rapid correction of chronic hyponatremia. In these patients, we limit the rate of rise of $P_{Na}$ to 4 mmol/L/day. Administration of dDAVP should be considered at the outset to avoid the development of water diuresis and thereby a rapid rise in the $P_{Na}$. Be vigilant about restricting the intake of water while dDAVP acts.
- *Potassium*: Sam might have a large deficit of $K^+$ ions if there is a source for their loss together with a poor prior intake of $K^+$ ions. Despite this deficit, a shift of $K^+$ ions out of cells caused by the low levels of insulin could have caused a higher $P_K$. Anticipate a significant shift of $K^+$ ions into cells during therapy; because when EABV is restored, the $\alpha$-adrenergic response, which inhibits the release of insulin from $\beta$-cells of the pancreas, will be removed. In addition, insulin will be released when hypoglycemia is corrected with the administration of glucose. Hence, sufficient amounts of $K^+$ ions must be administered to keep the $P_K$ in the normal range. There are a number of reasons why the administration of KCl may cause a rapid or excessive rise in $P_{Na}$ and hence the risk of osmotic demyelination in a patient with chronic hyponatremia. In terms of body tonicity, $Na^+$ ions (the main ECF cation) and $K^+$ ions (the main intracellular cation) are equivalent in osmolal terms. As the administered $K^+$ ions enter cells, $Na^+$ ions that entered these cells to replace the $K^+$ ions that were lost from cells will exit from these cells. Hence, the administration of $K^+$ ions will cause a rise in body tonicity, which will be reflected by a rise in $P_{Na}$ similar to that with the administration of an equivalent amount of $Na^+$ ions if there is no change in total body water. Therefore, $K^+$ ions should be administered in a solution that is isotonic to the patient. Furthermore, because $Na^+$ ions are retained in the ECF compartment, the EABV may become expanded and water diuresis may ensue.

# Metabolic Acidosis: Acid Gain Types

# Introduction

The focus in this chapter is on metabolic acidosis due to the accumulation of acids. Two disorders that can cause this type of metabolic acidosis are not discussed in this chapter. Ketoacidosis was discussed in Chapter 5. Metabolic acidosis caused by hippuric acid production from the metabolism of toluene in patients who sniff glue was discussed in Chapter 4, because the hippurate anion is uniquely secreted into the urine, resulting in a hyperchloremic form of metabolic acidosis due to an indirect loss of $NaHCO_3$.

It is important to recognize that the term *metabolic acidosis* is not a specific diagnosis—rather, it is a disorder that can be the result of a number of disease processes. Therefore, the clinician must determine the basis for metabolic acidosis in each patient because this has major implications for the management of the patient. Even in a single category such as L-lactic acidosis, there are different pathophysiologic mechanisms that may lead to the accumulation of L-lactic acid; hence, a definitive diagnosis is needed to address the specific underlying pathophysiology in the an individual patient.

## OBJECTIVE

- To provide an understanding of the pathophysiology of the different disease processes that may cause metabolic acidosis due to the accumulation of acids.
- To provide an approach to the clinical diagnosis and management of patients with the different disease processes that may cause metabolic acidosis due to the gain of acids, emphasizing that the presence of metabolic acidosis is a red flag to alert the physician about an ominous danger to the patient.

## CASE 6-1: PATRICK IS IN FOR A SHOCK

Patrick, a large, muscular man, has a long history of alcohol abuse. He was perfectly well until he drank a solution containing an unknown substance about 6 hours ago. In the past hour, he began to feel very unwell. He denied blood loss, vomiting, or diarrhea. His clinical condition deteriorated very quickly. On presentation to the emergency room, his respirations were rapid and deep, his blood pressure was 80/50 mm Hg, his pulse rate was 150 beats per minute, and his jugular venous pressure was flat. His electrocardiogram revealed changes due to hyperkalemia with tall, peaked T waves. His arterial blood gas revealed a pH of 7.20 and a $PCO_2$ of 25 mm Hg. The concentration of bicarbonate ($HCO_3^-$) ions in plasma ($P_{HCO_3}$) in a venous blood sample was 11 mmol/L. Other laboratory data are provided in the following table. Shortly after he was given intravenous calcium gluconate for the emergency treatment of hyperkalemia, his blood pressure rose and he felt much better.

| $P_{Na}$ | mmol/L | 143 | $P_K$ | mmol/L | 6.3 |
| $P_{Cl}$ | mmol/L | 99 | $P_{HCO_3}$ | mmol/L | 11 |
| $P_{Glucose}$ | mg/dL (mmol/L) | 180 (10) | $P_{Albumin}$ | g/dL (g/L) | 4.5 (45) |
| $P_{Creatinine}$ | mg/dL (µmol/L) | 1.8 (160) | BUN | mg/dL | 8.4 |
| | | | $P_{Urea}$ | mmol/L | 3.0 |
| $P_{Ca}$(total) | mg/dL (mmol/L) | 10 (2.5) | $P_{L\text{-lactate}}$ | mmol/L | 2.0 |

## Questions

Judging from the time frame for his illness, what is (are) the likely cause(s) of metabolic acidosis?

Why did his blood pressure fall so precipitously?

Why did he have hyperkalemia?

Why did the administration of intravenous calcium cause a rapid recovery?

### CASE 6-2: METABOLIC ACIDOSIS ASSOCIATED WITH DIARRHEA

One week ago, this 40-year-old man began to have several bouts of diarrhea during a trip abroad. He was treated with an antimotility drug and an antibiotic. In the past 24 hours, however, his diarrhea has increased. His only intake has been popsicles to satisfy his desire for cold liquids. On physical examination, he appeared very ill and was confused. He had poor balance and an ataxic gait. He did not have signs of an appreciable decrease in his effective arterial blood volume (EABV).

His abdomen was distended and bowel sounds were scanty. There were no masses or enlarged organs. Acetone was not detected on his breath, and the urine test for ketones was negative. His arterial blood gas revealed a pH of 7.22 and a $PCO_2$ of 27 mm Hg. His $P_{HCO_3}$ in a venous blood sample was 11 mmol/L. Other laboratory data from measurements in a venous blood sample are provided in the following table.

| | | | | | | |
|---|---|---|---|---|---|---|
| $P_{Na}$ | mmol/L | 138 | $P_K$ | mmol/L | | 3.8 |
| $P_{Cl}$ | mmol/L | 101 | $P_{Glucose}$ | mg/dL (mmol/L) | | 108 (6) |
| $P_{Albumin}$ | g/dL (g/L) | 3.8 (38) | $P_{Osm}$ | mosmol/kg $H_2O$ | | 289 |
| BUN | mg/dL | 14 | $P_{Creatinine}$ | mg/dL | | 1.2 |
| $P_{Urea}$ | mmol/L | 5.0 | $P_{Creatinine}$ | μmol/L | | 106 |

### Question

What is the cause for the metabolic acidosis in this patient?

### CASE 6-3: SEVERE ACIDEMIA IN A PATIENT WITH CHRONIC ALCOHOLISM

A 52-year-old man presented to the emergency room with abdominal pain, visual disturbances, and shortness of breath. He had a history of drinking excessive amounts of alcohol on a regular basis. He admitted to drinking approximately 1 L of vodka the day before but denied ingesting any other substances. During the 24 hours before admission, he had not eaten at all. In the 5 hours before his admission, he had several bouts of vomiting and did not drink any alcohol. His dietary intake has been generally very poor over the last several months because he had no appetite.

On physical examination, he was conscious and oriented. His respiratory rate was rapid (40 breaths per minute). His pulse rate was also rapid (150 beats per minute), and his blood pressure was 120/58 mm Hg. Neurological examination was unremarkable. His urine tested strongly positive for ketones. His initial laboratory results on admission to the emergency department are shown in the following table. The plasma pH and $PCO_2$ are from an arterial blood sample; the other measurements are from a venous blood sample.

| | | | | | |
|---|---|---|---|---|---|
| $P_{Na}$ | mmol/L | 132 | pH | | 6.78 |
| $P_K$ | mmol/L | 5.4 | $PCO_2$ | mm Hg | 23 |
| $P_{Cl}$ | mmol/L | 85 | $P_{Glucose}$ | mmol/L | 3.0 |
| $P_{HCO_3}$ | mmol/L | 3.3 | | | |
| $P_{Anion\ gap}$ | mEq/L | 44 | $P_{Albumin}$ | g/L | 36 |
| $P_{Osm}$ | mOsm/L | 325 | $P_{Osm\ gap}$ | mosmol/kg $H_2O$ | 42 |
| Hematocrit | | 0.46 | | | |

### Question

What dangers may be present on admission or arise during therapy?

# PART A
# GENERAL CONSIDERATIONS

## MAJOR THREATS IN THE PATIENT WITH METABOLIC ACIDOSIS

There are a number of threats for the patient with metabolic acidosis caused by added acids, depending on the underlying cause of the metabolic acidosis (Table 6-1). The emphasis in therapy should be to deal with the underlying cause of the metabolic acidosis rather than just focusing on how to deal with the $H^+$ ion load. For example, although L-lactic acid may be produced at an extremely rapid rate during hypoxia, an energy crisis because of failure to regenerate adenosine triphosphate (ATP) in vital organs, rather than the acidemia per se, is the most important danger for the patient. In a patient with methanol or ethylene glycol intoxication, toxic aldehydes formed during metabolism of these alcohols pose the major danger to the patient. In patients with pyroglutamic acidosis, the major danger is accumulation of reactive oxygen species (ROS) due to depletion of glutathione. In patients with D-lactic acidosis, a number of compounds produced by intestinal bacteria can cause cerebral dysfunction. In patients with metabolic acidosis due to end stage kidney disease, the danger may be a cardiac arrhythmia because of associated hyperkalemia.

## BUFFERING OF $H^+$ IONS IN A PATIENT WITH METABOLIC ACIDOSIS

Binding of $H^+$ ions to proteins in cells alters their charge, shape, and perhaps their functions. This may be particularly detrimental if it occurs in cells of vital organs (e.g., the brain and heart). To prevent this "bad" form of buffering of $H^+$ ions, $H^+$ ions must be "forced" to bind to $HCO_3^-$ ions in the extracellular fluid (ECF) and intracellular fluid (ICF) compartments of skeletal muscle because this is where the bulk of the bicarbonate buffer system (BBS) exists. For this to occur, the $PCO_2$ in capillary blood of skeletal muscle must be low. There are two requirements to achieve a low $PCO_2$ in capillary blood of skeletal muscle. First, an appropriate fall in arterial $PCO_2$ in response to the effect of acidemia to stimulate the respiratory center. Second, a high enough blood flow rate to skeletal

TABLE 6-1   **THREATS TO LIFE ASSOCIATED WITH THE CAUSE OF THE ADDITION OF ACIDS**

Although other emergencies may be present, only those that are specific to the cause of the metabolic acidosis are included in this table.

| CONDITION | MAJOR THREAT |
|---|---|
| • L-Lactic acidosis due to hypoxia | • Inadequate delivery of $O_2$ to vital organs, causing depletion of ATP |
| • Diabetic ketoacidosis in children | • Cerebral edema |
| • Alcoholic ketoacidosis with thiamin deficiency | • Wernicke's encephalopathy |
| • Toxin-induced metabolic acidosis (e.g., methanol) | • Toxic aldehyde metabolites (e.g., formaldehyde) |
| • Metabolic acidosis with a high $P_K$ (e.g., renal failure) | • Cardiac arrhythmia |
| • Metabolic acidosis with a low $P_K$ (e.g., glue sniffing) | • Cardiac arrhythmia, respiratory failure |
| • Pyroglutamic acidosis | • Accumulation of reactive oxygen species due to depletion of glutathione |

muscle relative to their rate of production of $CO_2$. If this fails to titrate the $H^+$ ion load, the degree of acidemia may become more pronounced and more $H^+$ ions may bind to proteins in the ECF and ICF in other organs, including the brain (see Figure 1-7). Because of autoregulation of cerebral blood flow, however, it is likely that the $PCO_2$ in brain capillary blood will not change appreciably unless there is a severe degree of contraction of the EABV. Hence, the BBS in the brain will continue to titrate much of this large $H^+$ ion load. Considering the limited content of $HCO_3^-$ ions in the brain, and that the brain receives a relatively larger proportion of blood flow, there is a risk that more $H^+$ ions will bind to proteins in the brain cells, further compromising their functions.

Therefore, an important aim in therapy in patients with metabolic acidosis is to improve ventilation and to restore blood flow to skeletal muscles to lower their capillary $PCO_2$ (which is reflected by the $PCO_2$ in their venous blood). At the usual rates of blood flow and metabolic work at rest, the $PCO_2$ in venous blood of skeletal muscle is about 46 mm Hg—that is, ~6 mm Hg greater than the arterial $PCO_2$. If the blood flow rate to the skeletal muscles declines because of a low EABV, the brachial venous $PCO_2$ will be increased to >6 mm Hg higher than the arterial $PCO_2$. It is our opinion that in patients with metabolic acidemia and a low EABV, enough saline should be administered to increase the blood flow rate to muscle to restore the differences between the brachial venous $PCO_2$ and the arterial $PCO_2$ to its usual value of ~6 mm Hg.

## ISSUES IN DIAGNOSIS

Accumulation of acids ($H^+ + A^-$) in the ECF compartment will result in the loss of $HCO_3^-$ ions and the gain of new anions. This addition of new anions can be detected by their electrical presence. Because electroneutrality must be maintained, the sum of all the valences of cations and the sum of all the valences of anions in plasma must be equal. For convenience, however, one need not measure the concentrations of all the cations and all the anions in plasma, but rather that of the major cation in plasma, sodium ($Na^+$) ions, and the major anions in plasma, chloride ($Cl^-$) and $HCO_3^-$ ions. The term *plasma anion gap* ($P_{Anion\ gap}$) is used for the difference between the concentration of $Na^+$ ions and the sum of the concentrations of $Cl^-$ ions and $HCO_3^-$ ions in plasma. This difference reflects the usual excess of the other anions in plasma over that of the other cations in plasma, which is largely due to the net anionic valence on plasma proteins, principally plasma albumin ($P_{Albumin}$). If the difference is larger than the "normal" value of the $P_{Anion\ gap}$, then other anions are present in plasma. Note, however, that because of differences in laboratory methods (e.g., measurement of $P_{Cl}$), there is a large difference in the mean value for the $P_{Anion\ gap}$ reported by different clinical laboratories. Furthermore, regardless of the laboratory method used, there is a wide range for the normal values of the $P_{Anion\ gap}$. Although it is imperative that the clinician knows the normal values of the $P_{Anion\ gap}$ for his or her clinical laboratory, it would be difficult to know what the individual patient's baseline $P_{Anion\ gap}$ was within the wide range of normal values. Another pitfall in the use of the $P_{Anion\ gap}$ is the failure to correct for the net negative valence attributable to the most abundant unmeasured anion in plasma, albumin. This adjustment should be made for a fall (or an increase) in the $P_{Albumin}$. The $P_{Anion\ gap}$ is reduced (or increased) by 2.5 mEq/L for each 1g/dL (10 g/L) decrease (or increase) in the $P_{Albumin}$. One must also be aware of other causes for a spurious reduction in the $P_{Anion\ gap}$ (e.g., cationic proteins in a patient with multiple myeloma, lithium intoxication).

If metabolic acidosis develops over a short period of time, the likely causes are overproduction of L-lactic acid (e.g., shock, ingestion of alcohol in a patient with thiamin deficiency) or ingestion of acids (e.g., metabolic acidosis due to ingestion of a large quantity of citric acid).

Disorders causing metabolic acidosis due to added acids are often associated with a marked decrease in the EABV. If not, suspect a toxin-induced form of metabolic acidosis (methanol or ethylene glycol), renal failure, or L-lactic acidosis due to causes other than tissue hypoxia (discussed in the following).

# PART B
# SPECIFIC DISORDERS

## L-LACTIC ACIDOSIS

To understand the pathophysiology that leads to the development of L-lactic acidosis, we begin the discussion with a synopsis of the biochemistry of glucose oxidation. This is followed by a description of the biochemistry of the process that leads to the accumulation of L-lactic acid.

### SYNOPSIS OF BIOCHEMISTRY OF GLUCOSE OXIDATION IN SKELETAL MUSCLES

**ABBREVIATIONS**

NAD+, nicotinamide adenine dinucleotide
NADH,H+, reduced form of NAD+
FAD, flavin adenine dinucleotide
FADH$_2$, hydroxyquinone form of FAD
ADP, adenosine diphosphate
AMP, adenosine monophosphate
CoA-SH, coenzyme A with functional sulfhydryl group
GDP, guanosine diphoshate
GTP, guanosine triphoshate
Pi, inorganic phosphate

The process of oxidation of glucose can be divided into three phases: the first is glycolysis, the second is the citric acid cycle, and the third is the electron transport chain (Figure 6-1):

1. **Glycolysis:** In glycolysis, one molecule of glucose is split into two molecules of pyruvate. Oxygen is not required in the process. Two molecules of ATP are utilized in the initial reactions in glycolysis, which are catalyzed by kinases hexokinase and phosphofructokinase-1 (PFK-1). Four molecules of ATP are ultimately generated; hence, there is net generation of two molecules of ATP. Also 2 molecules of nicotinamide adenine dinucleotide (NAD+) are converted to its reduced form, NADH,H+ (Eqn 1).

$$Glucose + 2\,ATP + 2\,NAD^+ \rightarrow 2\,Pyruvate + 4\,ATP + 2\,NADH,H^+ \quad (1)$$

PFK-1 is a key regulatory enzyme in glycolysis in skeletal muscle. PFK-1 catalyzes an important committed step in the process of glycolysis: the conversion of fructose 6-phosphate and ATP to fructose 1,6-bisphosphate and adenosine diphosphate (ADP). The activity of this enzyme is under direct allosteric regulation by ATP (i.e., when concentration of ATP in the cytosol is high as a result of low metabolic demand, PFK-1 is inhibited, causing flux through glycolysis to be low. In contrast, when the concentration of ATP in cytosol is low, PFK-1 is activated and flux through glycolysis is high to replenish the pool of ATP). Notwithstanding, there is little variation (<10%) in the concentration of ATP in the cytosol of skeletal muscle between resting condition and vigorous exercise, yet flux in glycolysis can increase by more than 100-fold. Therefore, the signal related to a change in the ATP concentration must be amplified. In more detail, hydrolysis of ATP to perform biological work results in formation of ADP. ADP is converted back to ATP in a near-equilibrium reaction catalyzed by the enzyme adenylate kinase (also known as myokinase), and adenosine monophosphate (AMP) is generated (Eqn 2).

$$2\,ADP \rightarrow ATP + AMP \quad (2)$$

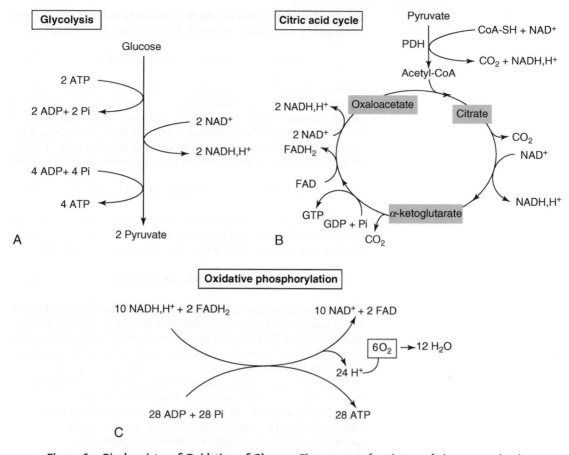

**Figure 6-1 Biochemistry of Oxidation of Glucose.** The process of oxidation of glucose can be divided into three phases as illustrated in the three panels. Glycolysis (Panel A): One molecule of glucose is split into two molecules of pyruvate. There is net generation of two molecules of adenosine triphosphate (ATP) and two nicotinamide adenine dinucleotide (NAD$^+$) are reduced to two NADH,H$^+$. Citric acid cycle (Panel B): Pyruvate is transported into the mitochondria where it is converted into acetyl-CoA by the enzyme pyruvate dehydrogenase (PDH). In this process, one molecule of CO$_2$ is produced and one NAD$^+$ is reduced to NADH,H$^+$. Acetyl-CoA combines with oxaloacetate to form citric acid. Citric acid then undergoes a series of reactions in the citric acid cycle, which lead to the oxidation of the acetyl group into two CO$_2$ molecules and the regeneration of oxaloacetate. In this process, three molecules of NAD$^+$ are reduced to three molecules of NADH,H$^+$, one molecule of flavin adenine dinucleotide (FAD) is made into its hydroxyquinone form FADH$_2$, and one molecule of guanosine diphosphate (GDP) is made into guanosine triphosphate (GTP). Electron transport chain (Panel C): Oxidation of the electrons from NADH,H$^+$ and those from FADH$_2$ by O$_2$ to form H$_2$O, which takes place inside the mitochondrial matrix, is the major process used by cells to regenerate ATP in coupled oxidative phosphorylation. *ADP*, Adenosine diphosphate ; *Pi*, inorganic phosphate.

Because the concentration of ATP in muscle is about 50 times higher than the concentration of AMP and about 10 times higher than the concentration of ADP, a small decrease in the concentration of ATP results in a large increase in the concentration of AMP. Therefore, the signal of a decrease in the concentration of ATP is markedly amplified via an increase in AMP concentration to produce a large increase in PFK-1 activity.

To maintain a high flux in glycolysis, NADH,H$^+$ that is produced must be converted back to NAD$^+$. Under aerobic conditions, NADH,H$^+$ is oxidized in mitochondria to NAD$^+$. Because the inner mitochondrial membrane lacks an NADH,H$^+$ transport protein, the electrons from cytosolic NADH,H$^+$ are transported into the mitochondria using the malate/aspartate shuttle. Under anaerobic conditions, NADH,H$^+$ can be converted to NAD$^+$ in the cytosol, in an equilibrium reaction in which pyruvate is reduced to L-lactate, catalyzed by the enzyme lactate dehydrogenase (LDH) (Eqn 3).

$$Pyruvate + NADH,H^+ \rightarrow Lactate^- + NAD^+ \qquad (3)$$

2. **Citric acid cycle:** Pyruvic acid is transported into the mitochondria by a monocarboxylic acid cotransporter. Once in the mitochondrial matrix, pyruvate is converted into acetyl-CoA by the multienzyme complex pyruvate dehydrogenase (PDH). In this process, one molecule of $CO_2$ is produced and one $NAD^+$ is reduced to $NADH,H^+$ (Eqn 4). A derivative of thiamin is an important cofactor for PDH.

$$Pyruvate + CoA\text{-}SH + NAD^+ \rightarrow Acetyl\text{-}CoA + CO_2 + NADH,H^+ \quad (4)$$

Acetyl-CoA (a two-carbon compound) combines with oxaloacetate (a four-carbon compound), to form citrate (a six-carbon compound), in a reaction catalyzed by the enzyme citrate synthase (Eqn 5).

$$Acetyl\text{-}CoA + Oxaloacetate \rightarrow Citrate \qquad (5)$$

Citrate then enters the citric acid cycle (also called the tricarboxylic acid cycle or the Krebs cycle), where it undergoes a series of reactions, catalyzed by a number of enzymes, which leads to the oxidation of the acetyl group into two $CO_2$ molecules and the regeneration of the four-carbon molecule oxaloacetate. In this process, three molecules of $NAD^+$ are reduced to three molecules of $NADH,H^+$, one molecule of flavine adenine dinucleotide (FAD) is made into its hydroxyquinone form $FADH_2$, and one molecule of guanosine diphosphate (GDP) and one molecule of inorganic phosphate (Pi) are made into one molecule of guanosine triphosphate (GTP) (the latter is equivalent to the conversion of one molecule of ADP and one molecule of Pi into one molecule of ATP) (Eqn 6). Because two molecules of pyruvate are produced from one molecule of glucose in glycolysis, two molecules of ATP are regenerated per one molecule of glucose in the citric acid cycle.

$$Acetyl\text{-}CoA + Oxaloacetate + 3\,NAD^+ + 1\,FAD + 1\,GDP + Pi$$
$$\rightarrow 2\,CO_2 + 3\,NADH,H^+ + 1\,FADH_2 + 1\,GTP\,(ATP) + Oxaloacetate \quad (6)$$

Although the citric acid cycle does not require $O_2$, it can only take place in the presence of $O_2$, because it requires the regeneration of $NAD^+$ and FAD, which takes place in the process of oxidative phosphorylation.

3. **Electron transport chain:** Oxidation of the electrons from $NADH,H^+$ and those from $FADH_2$ by $O_2$ is the major process used by cells to regenerate ATP (see Chapter 5). Flow of electrons through the electron transport chain (coenzyme Q, flavin mononucleotide [FMN] and flavin adenine dinucleotide [FAD], and ultimately to cytochrome C) from electron donors ($NADH,H^+$ and $FADH_2$) to electron acceptors ($O_2$) releases energy. This energy is used to pump $H^+$ ions from the mitochondrial matrix through the inner mitochondrial membrane. This creates a very large electrical (~150 mV) and a smaller chemical (equivalent to ~30 mV) driving force for $H^+$ ion re-entry. This energy is recaptured as $H^+$ ions flow through the $H^+$ channel portion of the $H^+$-ATP synthase in the inner mitochondrial membrane, which is coupled (linked) to ATP regeneration, providing that ADP and inorganic phosphate (Pi) molecules are available inside these mitochondria. Oxidation of one molecule of $NADH,H^+$ leads to regeneration of 2.5 molecules

## ATP REGENERATION FROM OXIDATION OF NADH,H⁺ AND FADH₂

- This approximation of the rate of ATP regeneration from oxidation of NADH,H⁺ and FADH₂ takes into account the possible leak of electrons from the electron transport chain.
- Ten molecules of NADH,H⁺ and two molecules of FADH₂ are produced per molecule of glucose that undergoes metabolism in glycolysis and the citric acid cycle.
- Oxidation of the electrons from 10 molecules of NADH,H⁺ and 2 molecules of FADH₂ in the electron transport chain leads to regeneration of 28 molecules of ATP.
- Oxidation of 1 molecule of glucose can lead to the regeneration of 32 molecules of ATP (2 molecules in glycolysis, 2 molecules in the citric acid cycle, 28 molecules in the electron transport chain). This is summarized in Figure 6-1.

of ATP, while only 1.5 molecules of ATP are regenerated from oxidation of one molecule of $FADH_2$ (see margin note). Hence, there is net regeneration of approximately 32 mmol of ATP from the oxidation of one molecule of glucose.

The process of oxidation of glucose can be summarized as shown in Eqn (7).

$$\text{Glucose } (C_6 H_{12} O_6) + 6 O_2 + 32 \text{ (ADP + Pi)} \rightarrow 6 CO_2 + 6 H_2O + 32 \text{ ATP} \tag{7}$$

In the cytosol, energy needed to perform biological work (e.g., ion pumping by Na-K-ATPase) is provided by hydrolysis of the terminal high-energy bond of ATP. This results in formation of ADP. ADP enters the mitochondria on the adenine nucleotide translocator in exchange for ATP, which is produced in the mitochondria in coupled oxidative phosphorylation in the electron transport chain.

## SYNOPSIS OF THE BIOCHEMISTRY OF L-LACTIC ACIDOSIS

A rise in the concentration of L-lactate$^-$ anions and H$^+$ ions can be caused by an increased rate of production and/or a decreased rate of removal of L-lactic acid. Although both of these mechanisms are involved in most cases, usually one mechanism predominates.

## INCREASED PRODUCTION OF L-LACTIC ACID

Increased production of L-lactic acid occurs under conditions in which the rate of regeneration of ATP in mitochondria is largely insufficient to meet the requirement for ATP to perform its biological work (Figure 6-2). Under these conditions of diminished rate of regeneration of ATP, the concentration of ADP in the cytosol in cells rises. As stated previously, when ADP is converted back to ATP in the near-equilibrium reaction catalyzed by the enzyme adenylate kinase, AMP is generated (Eqn 2). The increase in AMP concentration produces a robust signal that leads to a large increase in PFK-1 activity and hence the flux in glycolysis in muscle is augmented. The accumulation of pyruvate in the cytosol, coupled with an increase in NADH,H$^+$/NAD$^+$ ratio, drives the equilibrium reaction catalyzed by the enzyme LDH, in which pyruvate is reduced to L-lactate and NADH,H$^+$ is converted to NAD$^+$. Contrary to common belief, glycolysis is not a metabolic pathway that causes net production of H$^+$ ions (count the valences in the following equations individually and then together to see where H$^+$ ions are produced). One can see that the hydrolysis of ATP$^{4-}$ to perform biological work is what produces the H$^+$ ions, rather than the conversion of one molecule of glucose to two L-lactate anions (Eqns 8 and 9).

$$\text{Work} + 2 \text{ ATP}^{4-} \rightarrow 2 \text{ ADP}^{3-} + 2 H^+ + 2 HPO_4^{2-} \tag{8}$$

$$\text{Glucose} + 2 \text{ ADP}^{3-} + 2 HPO_4^{2-} \rightarrow 2 \text{ ATP}^{4-} + 2 \text{ L} - \text{lactate}^- \tag{9}$$

Although only 2 mmol of ATP are regenerated per mmol of glucose in glycolysis (versus approximately 32 mmol of ATP when 1 mmol of glucose is oxidized), the rate of ATP production by glycolysis can be 100 times faster than that in oxidative phosphorylation. The price to pay, however, is the production of 1 mmol of L-lactic acid per 1 mmol of ATP regenerated. An increase in H$^+$ ion concentration inhibits PFK-1. Although this minimizes the drop in intracellular pH, there is a huge price to pay because this may lead to a critical shortage of energy, especially in cells of vital organs (e.g., the brain).

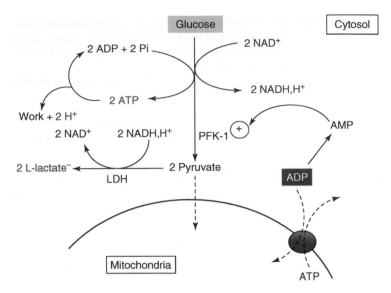

**Figure 6-2 Biochemistry of L-Lactic Acid Production.** In the cytosol, energy needed to perform biological work is provided by hydrolysis of the terminal high-energy bond of adenosine triphosphate (ATP); this results in formation of adenosine diphosphate (ADP). ADP enters mitochondria in exchange for ATP, produced in coupled oxidative phosphorylation. Under conditions of diminished rate of regeneration of ATP, the concentration of ADP in the cytosol rises. ADP is converted back to ATP in a near equilibrium reaction catalyzed by the enzyme adenylate kinase, in which adenosine monophosphate (AMP) is generated. The increase in the AMP concentration produces a robust signal that leads to a large increase in phosphofructokinase-1 (PFK-1) activity and the flux in glycolysis in muscle. Accumulation of pyruvate in the cytosol, coupled with an increase in NADH,H$^+$/NAD$^+$ ratio, drives the equilibrium reaction catalyzed by the enzyme lactate dehydrogenase (LDH), in which pyruvate is reduced to L-lactate and NADH,H$^+$ is converted to NAD$^+$.

## DECREASED REMOVAL OF L-LACTIC ACID

In normal physiology, glycolysis is an obligatory pathway for the regeneration of ATP in red blood cells because they lack mitochondria; therefore, red blood cells always produce L-lactic acid. L-Lactic acid may be also produced by fast-twitch muscle fibers during muscle contraction and by enterocytes when glucose and amino acids are absorbed. This load of L-lactic acid produced under normal circumstances is removed via gluconeogenesis in the liver. Hence, under conditions of severe loss of liver tissue (e.g., due to hepatitis, shock liver, infiltration by tumor cells), L-lactic acidosis may develop. In this setting, L-lactic acid accumulates and the level of L-lactate anions in plasma rises until the level of pyruvate in hepatocytes in the remaining liver tissue is sufficient to saturate the critical enzymes in gluconeogenesis (pyruvate carboxylase [PC] and phosphoenolpyruvate carboxykinase [PEPCK]) with their substrates to drive the reactions catalyzed to their maximum velocity. When this level of L-lactate anions in plasma is reached, all the L-lactic acid produced is removed, and therefore a chronic steady state develops.

There are two major ways to remove L-lactic acid: oxidation and conversion to glucose in the liver and the kidney (Figure 6-3). In both processes, the first step is the conversion of L-lactate into pyruvate in the equilibrium reaction catalyzed by LDH (Eqn 10). An important point to emphasize here is that one cannot overcome a rapid rate of production of lactic acid by enhancing its rate of removal.

$$\text{L-lactate}^- + \text{NAD}^+ \rightarrow \text{Pyruvate} + \text{NADH,H}^+ \qquad (10)$$

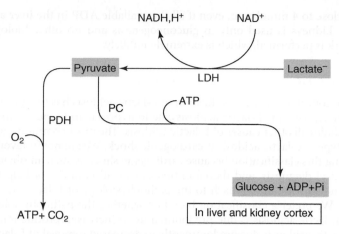

**Figure 6-3 Biochemistry of L-Lactic Acid Removal.** L-Lactate and pyruvate are linked by an enzyme-catalyzed step, L-lactate dehydrogenase (LDH), which is present in such a large amount that pyruvate and L-lactate can be interconverted very quickly; thus, their concentrations are determined by the ratio of $NADH,H^+$ to $NAD^+$ in the cytosol of cells. There are two major fates of pyruvate: first, it can be fully oxidized in the citric acid cycle if pyruvate dehydrogenase (PDH) is active; second, it can be converted to glucose, where the initial step is catalyzed by pyruvate carboxylase (PC). The latter process occurs in the liver and in the kidney cortex. *ATP,* Adenosine triphosphate; *ADP,* adenosine diphosphate.

### Oxidation of L-lactic acid

Pyruvic acid is transported into the mitochondria via a mono-carboxylic acid cotransporter and is then metabolized by PDH into acetyl-CoA. Metabolism of acetyl-CoA follows the pathway described previously. To oxidize 1 mmol of L-lactic acid, 3 mmol of oxygen must be consumed, and 16 mmol of ATP are formed in coupled oxidative phosphorylation. Therefore, if (theoretically) all organs could be persuaded to oxidize L-lactic acid to yield 100% of their requirement to regenerate ATP, only 4 mmol of L-lactic acid could be oxidized per minute at rest ($O_2$ consumption is 12 mmol/min at rest).

It is important to note the large imbalance of the rate of ATP regeneration when $H^+$ ions are produced in glycolysis and when they are removed via the oxidation of L-lactic acid. While 18 mmol of $H^+$ ions are produced per 18 mmol of ATP regenerated in glycolysis, only 1 mmol of $H^+$ ions is removed when 16 mmol of ATP are regenerated via oxidation of 1 mmol of L-lactic acid.

### Gluconeogenesis

L-lactic acid can be made into glucose in the liver and in the kidney cortex. L-Lactate is converted to pyruvate as shown in Eqn 10. Pyruvic acid is transported into the mitochondria, where it is metabolized into oxaloacetate by the enzyme pyruvate carboxylase. Oxaloacetate is then reduced to malate, which is transported into the cytosol by the malate transporter. In the cytosol, malate is made back into oxaloacetate. Oxaloacetate then feeds into the gluconeogenic pathway via its conversion to phosphoenolpyruvate by the biotin (vitamin $B_2$)-requiring enzyme PEPCK. The conversion of 2 mmol of pyruvate to 1 mmol of glucose uses 6 mmol of ATP.

Because the liver and the kidneys each consume 2 mmol of $O_2$ per minute, they both regenerate a total of 24 mmol of ATP per minute. Thus, the maximum rate of L-lactic acid removal via gluconeogenesis is close to 4 mmol/min, even if all the available ADP in the liver and the kidneys is used only in gluconeogenesis and no other biologic work is performed, which is extremely unlikely.

## CLASSIFICATION OF L-LACTIC ACIDOSIS

The commonly used classification of L-lactic acidosis has two groups: type A, which is L-lactic acidosis due to hypoxia, and type B, which includes all other causes of L-lactic acidosis. The most common cause of type A L-lactic acidosis is cardiogenic shock. We are not in favor of using this classification because cardiogenic shock is such an obvious clinical diagnosis, and therefore this classification does not help the clinician with an approach to the pathophysiology of L-lactic acidosis. We prefer a classification based on whether the pathophysiology of L-lactic acidosis is due predominantly to increased production of L-lactic acid or is due predominantly to decreased removal of L-lactic acid.

## CLINICAL SETTINGS WITH PREDOMINANTLY OVERPRODUCTION OF L-LACTIC ACID

### Inadequate delivery of oxygen

The commonest clinical setting for rapid overproduction of L-lactic acid is cardiogenic shock. Other examples of conditions that lead to an inadequate delivery of $O_2$ to tissues include acute airway obstruction, hypovolemic shock, and carbon monoxide poisoning. In patients with sepsis, tissue hypoxia may be present due to decreased delivery of $O_2$ because of both decreased EABV and impaired tissue extraction of $O_2$.

The crucial issue in therapy is to improve the rate of regeneration of ATP in vital organs rather than correction of the metabolic acidemia per se. Measures to improve hemodynamics and restore adequate cardiac output and tissue perfusion (e.g., use of inotropic agents) are absolutely critical, as are measures to ensure that the blood has an adequate content of $O_2$. The use of $NaHCO_3$ during severe hypoxia may be of little value because of the large and rapid rate of production of $H^+$ ions. Nevertheless, $NaHCO_3$ may buy a little time while therapeutic interventions to correct the underlying disorder are administered in cases in which hypoxia is marginal and potentially reversible, but this issue remains controversial (see margin note). The load of $Na^+$ ions poses a major limit on the amount of $NaHCO_3$ that can be administered in patients with cardiogenic shock and pulmonary edema.

## EXCESSIVE DEMAND FOR OXYGEN

L-Lactic acidosis due to excessive demand for $O_2$ occurs during seizures or extreme exercise. Another example of this pathophysiology may be seen in some patients taking the drug isoniazid (isonicotinylhydrazide [INH]), which is commonly used to treat tuberculosis (Figure 6-4). This may be due to the rapid development of vitamin $B_6$ (pyridoxine) deficiency because of the formation of an isoniazid/vitamin $B_6$ complex. Pyridoxine is a cofactor for the reaction catalyzed by the enzyme glutamic acid decarboxylase, in which glutamate is converted to the inhibitory neurotransmitter γ-amino butyric acid (GABA). A deficiency of GABA could result in increased muscle excitability, leading to muscle twitching and at times mini-seizures. Patients on chronic hemodialysis who are given isoniazid are at increased risk of this complication because they tend to be deficient in vitamin $B_6$ due to the efficient removal of this water-soluble vitamin by hemodialysis.

**ALKALI ADMINISTRATION AND REMOVAL OF INHIBITION OF PFK-1**

- An increase in $H^+$ ion concentration in cells inhibits the key glycolytic enzyme PFK-1 and therefore the flux in glycolysis. Removal of $H^+$ ions may result in deinhibition of PFK-1 and therefore may increase the flux in glycolysis and the rate of regeneration of ATP.
- The price to pay, however, is the production of 1 mmol of $H^+$ ions per 1 mmol of ATP regenerated.
- This can be of benefit only if it were to occur in vital organs (e.g., the brain and the heart) and if the $H^+$ ions produced are titrated by the BBS and thus do not bind to intracellular proteins.

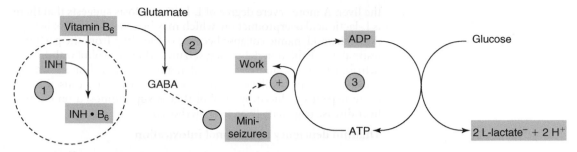

**Figure 6-4  L-Lactic Acidosis due to Isoniazid.** (1) Patients taking the drug isoniazid (isonicotinyl-hydrazide [INH]) may develop vitamin B$_6$ (pyridoxine) deficiency because of the formation of a complex of INH and vitamin B$_6$. (2) Pyridoxine is a cofactor for the reaction catalyzed by the enzyme, glutamic acid decarboxylase, in which glutamate is converted to the inhibitory neurotransmitter, γ-amino butyric acid (GABA). (3) A deficiency of GABA could result in increased muscle excitability and at times mini-seizures and the development of L-lactic acidosis due to increased demand for O$_2$. *ADP,* Adenosine diphosphate; *ATP,* adenosine triphosphate.

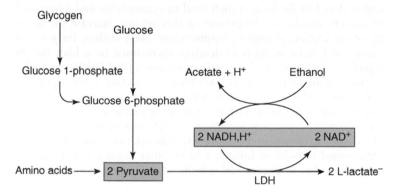

**Figure 6-5  Production of L-Lactic Acid During Ethanol Metabolism.** Ethanol is metabolized in cytosol of hepatocytes to acetaldehyde in a reaction catalyzed by the enzyme alcohol dehydrogenase. Acetaldehyde is metabolized into acetic acid, a reaction catalyzed by the enzyme acetaldehyde dehydrogenase. In both reactions, nicotinamide adenine dinucleotide (NAD$^+$) is reduced to NADH,H$^+$. The rise in cytosolic NADH,H$^+$/NAD$^+$ ratio drives the equilibrium reaction catalyzed by the enzyme lactate dehydrogenase (LDH), in which pyruvate is reduced to L-lactate$^-$ and NADH,H$^+$ is converted to NAD$^+$. The source of pyruvate is gluconeogenesis from amino acids, and perhaps also from the breakdown of glycogen.

## CLINICAL SETTINGS WITH INCREASED PRODUCTION OF L-LACTIC ACID IN THE ABSENCE OF HYPOXIA

### Ethanol intoxication

The development of L-lactic acidosis in patients with ethanol intoxication reflects the higher NADH,H$^+$/NAD$^+$ ratio in hepatocytes due to the ongoing production of NADH,H$^+$ caused by ethanol metabolism. This high NADH,H$^+$/NAD$^+$ ratio drives the equilibrium reaction catalyzed by the enzyme LDH, in which pyruvate is reduced to L-lactate and NADH,H$^+$ is converted to NAD$^+$. The source of pyruvate is gluconeogenesis from amino acids and perhaps the breakdown of glycogen, if there is glycogen stored in the liver (Fig. 6-5). A high level of epinephrine and a low level of insulin, which may be present in this setting, increase the activity of the enzyme glycogen phosphorylase. The degree of L-lactic acidosis in patients with ethanol intoxication is usually mild, with a plasma L-lactate concentration of ~5 mmol/L, because other organs are capable of removing L-lactic acid made by the liver. A more severe degree of L-lactic acidosis suggests that there is L-lactic acid overproduction, which may be caused by hypoxia (e.g., due to hemodynamic collapse because of bleeding from the gastrointestinal tract), thiamin deficiency, seizures (due to alcohol withdrawal, delirium tremens, and/or a central nervous system lesion), and/or L-lactic acid underutilization from severe liver disease caused by an acute hepatitis induced by alcohol that is superimposed on chronic liver disease (e.g., fatty liver, liver cirrhosis).

### Thiamin deficiency and ethanol intoxication

A severe degree of L-lactic acidosis may develop rapidly in these patients. A derivation of thiamin (vitamin $B_1$) is a key cofactor for the enzyme PDH. The site of L-lactic acid production in this setting is likely to be the liver because it is the site where there is accumulation of pyruvate (caused by the diminished activity of PDH) and also a high $NADH,H^+/NAD^+$ ratio (caused by metabolism of ethanol) (Figure 6-6). The source of pyruvate is gluconeogenesis from amino acids and perhaps also from the breakdown of glycogen if there is remaining glycogen stored in the liver. A high level of epinephrine and a low level of insulin, which may be present in this setting, increase the activity of the enzyme glycogen phosphorylase. Nevertheless, for a severe degree of L-lactic acidosis to develop, there must be a high flux in glycolysis. Perhaps a high rate of conversion of $NADH,H^+$ to $NAD^+$ in the cytosol, as pyruvate is converted to L-lactate, limits the availability of $NADH,H^+$ for mitochondrial oxidative phosphorylation and the regeneration of ATP at a rate sufficient to match the rate of its hydrolysis to perform biologic work. There may be also an effect of ethanol to uncouple oxidative phosphorylation (see Chapter 5). Diminished removal of L-lactic acid by other organs is also likely to be present due to diminished activity of PDH and the presence of

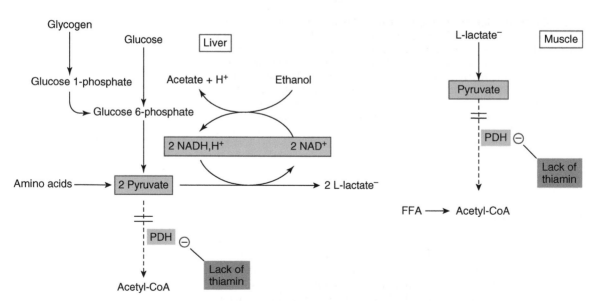

**Figure 6-6  L-Lactic Acidosis in Patients With Thiamin Deficiency and Ethanol Intoxication.** A derivative of thiamin (vitamin $B_1$) is a key cofactor for the enzyme pyruvate dehydrogenase (PDH). A severe degree of L-lactic acidosis may develop rapidly in patients with ethanol intoxication, who are thiamin deficient. The *left part* of the figure shows that the site of L-lactic acid production is likely to be the liver because it is the site where there is accumulation of pyruvate (caused by diminished activity of PDH) and also a high $NADH,H^+/NAD^+$ ratio (due to metabolism of ethanol). The source of pyruvate is gluconeogenesis from amino acids, and perhaps also from the breakdown of glycogen. The *right part* of the figure shows that diminished removal of L-lactic acid by other organs is also likely to be present due to diminished activity of PDH and also due to the presence of alternative fuels that are used preferentially to regenerate adenosine triphosphate (ATP) (e.g., free fatty acids [FFA] for muscles).

alternative fuels that are used preferentially to regenerate ATP (e.g., free fatty acids for muscles, ketoacids for the brain) (see Figure 6-6).

Although the degree of acidemia may be severe, damage to the brain is the major concern in these patients. In more detail, the brain must regenerate ATP as fast as it is being used to perform biologic work. Keto-acids are the preferred fuel for the brain if they are present. This is because ketoacids are derived from storage fat; therefore, there is an advantage in using ketoacids as the preferred fuel for the brain during prolonged starvation because this avoids the need for glucose, which would be derived from catabolism of endogenous proteins. After successful treatment of alcoholic ketoacidosis, the concentration of ketoacids in blood will decline; the brain must regenerate its ATP from the oxidation of glucose. This, however, will be limited by the diminished activity of PDH because of the lack of thiamin. Probably of greater significance is the likelihood of an increased demand for ATP regeneration in this setting (e.g., due to delirium tremens or the use of salicylates, which may uncouple oxidative phosphorylation). Therefore, there will be a sudden rise in the production of L-lactic acid in areas of the brain in which the metabolic rate is the most rapid and/or the reserve of thiamin is the lowest.

The clinical manifestations include Wernicke–Korsakoff syndrome, in which the patient disguises the cerebral deficit by confabulating; hence, a high degree of suspicion is needed to make this diagnosis.

The obvious treatment is to administer thiamin intravenously *before* the concentration of ketoacids in plasma falls to low levels (i.e., before the patient receives glucose, which stimulates the release of insulin, or the administration of sufficient saline to re-expand the contracted EABV, which removes the $\alpha$-adrenergic inhibition of the release of insulin). The background of malnutrition that leads to thiamin deficiency might also lead to deficiency of other B vitamins (e.g., riboflavin), which should also be corrected.

### Riboflavin deficiency and the use of tricyclic antidepressants

The active metabolites formed from vitamin $B_2$ (riboflavin), FMN and FAD, are components of the mitochondrial electron transport system (Figure 6-7). Riboflavin must be activated via an ATP-dependent kinase

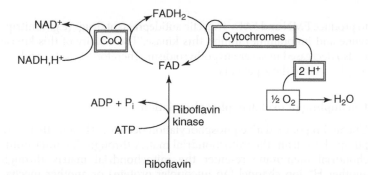

**Figure 6-7 L-Lactic Acidosis due to Riboflavin Deficiency.** Flow of electrons through the electron transport chain (coenzyme Q [CoQ], flavin mononucleotide [FMN] and flavin adenine dinucleotide [FAD], and ultimately to cytochrome C) from electron donors (reduced nicotinamide adenine dinucleotide [NADH,H+]) to electron acceptors ($O_2$) is the principal pathway for the cell to regenerate adenosine triphosphate (ATP) in coupled oxidative phosphorylation. Riboflavin (vitamin $B_2$) must be activated by riboflavin kinase to FMN or FAD to become a component in the electron transport system. A deficiency of riboflavin or inhibition of riboflavin kinase by tricyclic antidepressant drugs can lead to low levels of FMN and/or FAD. *ADP,* Adenosine diphosphate; *Pi,* inorganic phosphate; *NAD+,* nicotinamide adenine dinucleotide; *FADH₂,* hydroxyquinone form of FAD.

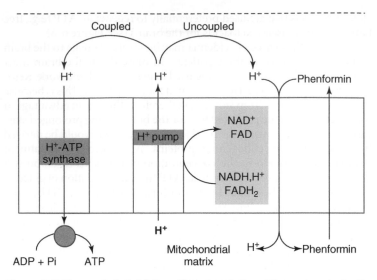

**Figure 6-8 Uncoupled Oxidative Phosphorylation.** The rectangle in the middle of the figure represents the inner mitochondrial membrane with its inner and outer bilayers. The dotted line at the top of the figure represents the outer mitochondrial membrane. Uncoupling of oxidative phosphorylation occurs if $H^+$ ions that were pumped from the mitochondrial matrix through the inner mitochondrial membrane re-enter through another pathway that is *not* linked to the conversion of adenosine diphosphate (ADP) and inorganic phosphate (Pi) to adenosine triphosphate (ATP). The biguanide phenformin has a large hydrophobic end, which enables it to cross the lipid-rich mitochondrial membrane rapidly, bringing $H^+$ ions with it into the mitochondial matrix. This re-entry of $H^+$ ions into the mitochondial matrix is not linked to the conversion of ADP to ATP. Metformin is another biguanide that does not, however, have a large hydrophobic end. Therefore, it cannot cross the mitochondrial membrane as easily as phenformin and so is a very weak uncoupler of oxidative phosphorylation. *FAD*, Flavin adenine dinucleotide; *FADH₂*, hydroxyquinone form of FAD; *NAD⁺*, nicotinamide adenine dinucleotide; *NADH,H⁺*, reduced form of NAD⁺.

to produce FMN and FAD. Tricyclic antidepressant drugs (e.g., amitriptyline and imipramine) inhibit this kinase. The activity of this kinase is also decreased in severe hypothyroidism. Therefore, L-lactic acidosis may be seen in these patients.

### Uncoupling of oxidative phosphorylation

Uncoupling of oxidative phosphorylation occurs if $H^+$ ions that were pumped out from the mitochondrial matrix through the inner mitochondrial membrane re-enter the mitochondrial matrix through another $H^+$ ion channel (an uncoupler protein) or another mechanism that is *not* linked to the conversion of ADP to ATP.

Phenformin is a biguanide that is no longer in clinical use because it was associated with a high incidence of L-lactic acidosis in patients with type 2 diabetes mellitus. This drug has a large hydrophobic end, which enabled it to cross the lipid-rich mitochondrial membrane rapidly bringing $H^+$ ions with it into the mitochondrial matrix. This re-entry of $H^+$ ions into the mitochondrial matrix uncouples oxidative phosphorylation because it is not linked to the conversion of ADP to ATP (Figure 6-8). Metformin is another biguanide, but because it does not have a large hydrophobic end, it is a very weak uncoupler of oxidative phosphorylation and hence rarely (in the absence of acute renal failure, in which case the drug may accumulate sufficiently) is the sole cause of L-lactic acidosis. Acetyl salicylic acid is another drug that uncouples oxidative phosphorylation (see Chapter 8).

## CLINICAL SETTINGS WITH PREDOMINANTLY DECREASED REMOVAL OF L-LACTIC ACID

This type of L-lactic acidosis does not have the same urgency as the type with primary overproduction of L-lactic acid because it is not associated with a problem in regenerating ATP. In addition, the rate of $H^+$ ion accumulation is usually much slower. A chronic steady state of L-lactic acidosis is often present. The causes of a low rate of removal of L-lactic acid are usually related to problems with the liver, either hepatitis, replacement of normal liver cells (e.g., by tumor cells or large fat deposits), or destruction of the liver due to prior hypoxia (e.g., shock liver).

In patients with a malignancy and hepatic metastases, a number of mechanisms may contribute to the development of L-lactic acidosis. First, the replacement of a substantial number of liver cells with tumor cells sufficient to impair L-lactic acid removal. Second, the production of metabolites by tumor cells, such as the amino acid tryptophan, which may inhibit the conversion of pyruvate to glucose in the liver. Third, the overproduction of L-lactic acid by ischemic tumor cells. Administration of $NaHCO_3$ to these patients may have detrimental long-term effects. This is because the load of alkali might deinhibit PFK-1 and hence enhance the flux in glycolysis in tumor cells; a considerable amount of lean body mass may be lost if the source of pyruvate is glucose that is made from amino acids in gluconeogenesis.

## ANTIRETROVIRAL DRUGS

L-Lactic acidosis has been reported with the use of a number of antiretroviral drugs in patients with human immunodeficiency virus (HIV) infection. The agent that is most frequently associated with L-lactic acidosis is zidovudine, but didanosine, stavudine, lamivudine, and indinavir have also been implicated. There are two possible mechanisms whereby antiretroviral agents may cause L-lactic acidosis. First, these drugs may block the electron transport system and may lead to mitochondrial myopathy, as manifested by ragged-red fibers and mitochondrial DNA depletion. These effects may lead to increased production of L-lactic acid. Second, these drugs may lead to a severe degree of hepatic steatosis with replacement of liver tissue with storage fat, which decreases the removal of L-lactic acid.

## QUESTIONS

6-1 Consider the following example. An anoxic limb needs to regenerate 18 mmol/min of ATP (25% of the ATP needed in the body) via glycolysis. If the rest of the body could be persuaded to oxidize L-lactic acid as its only fuel to regenerate all its needed ATP (54 mmol/min), would L-lactic acid still accumulate?

6-2 $NaHCO_3$ was given to a patient for the treatment for L-lactic acidosis, but there was no rise in the $P_{HCO_3}$. Is it correct to conclude that the administration of $NaHCO_3$ had no beneficial effect?

# D-LACTIC ACIDOSIS

## PATHOPHYSIOLOGY

Under normal circumstances, gut flora, which is largely located in the colon, does not have access to glucose because virtually all of the ingested glucose is absorbed in the upper small intestine (Figure 6-9). Disruption of this geographic separation of bacteria and glucose is a major factor in the development of D-lactic acidosis. Three factors that make this possible are slow intestinal transit (drugs that decrease intestinal motility, blind loops, intestinal obstruction), a change of the normal gut flora (usually due to prior antibiotic therapy), and the supply of carbohydrate substrate to these bacteria (foods containing cellulose or fructose). In addition, the intake of antacids or other drugs that inhibit gastric $H^+$ ion secretion may lead to a higher pH in the lumen of the intestinal tract that is more favorable for bacterial growth and metabolism.

A number of organic acids may be produced in this fermentation process (e.g., butyric acid, propionic acid, acetic acid), but D-lactic acid is the most prevalent at times. Although humans lack the enzyme D-lactate dehydrogenase, metabolism of D-lactate occurs via the enzyme D-2-hydroxyacid dehydrogenase, but at a slow rate. Because the rate of production of these organic acids, however, is not rapid, the degree of acidemia is usually not severe unless the patient also has a defect in the renal excretion of ammonium ($NH_4^+$) ions. Noxious alcohols, aldehydes, amines, and mercaptans are produced during fermentation of carbohydrates and may lead to many of the CNS symptoms that are observed in this disorder.

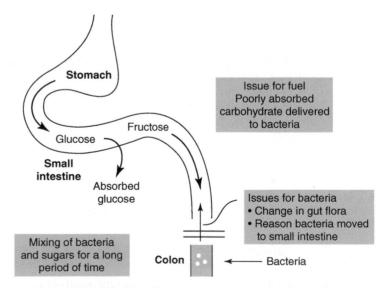

**Figure 6-9 Organic Acid Production in the Gastrointestinal Tract.** Bacteria are normally separated from dietary sugar by gastrointestinal (GI) geography. For overproduction of D-lactic acid, a change in gut flora needs to be present (e.g., because of the intake of antibiotics). These bacteria from the lower GI tract must mix with nonabsorbed sugars. Either bacteria migrate up to and proliferate in the small intestine, or sugars are delivered to the colon. More D-lactic acid (and other organic acids) can be produced if bacteria and sugars are mixed together for long time periods (e.g., because of low GI motility, blind loops).

### DIAGNOSIS AND TREATMENT

The usual clinical laboratory test for lactate anions is specific for the L-lactate isomer; therefore, specific assay for D-lactate anions is needed if one wants to confirm the diagnosis.

The metabolic acidosis in patients with D-lactic acidosis is associated with increased $P_{Anion\,gap}$. There may also be a component of hyperchloremic metabolic acidosis if the fall in $P_{HCO_3}$ is larger than the rise in $P_{Anion\,gap}$. This may occur for two reasons. First, if there is an appreciable loss of $NaHCO_3$ in diarrheal fluid. Second, if the $H^+$ ions of D-lactic acid produced are retained in the body while the D-lactate anions are lost in the stool or in the urine with $Na^+$ ions or $K^+$ ions (indirect loss of $NaHCO_3$) (see Chapter 4).

Treatment should be directed at the GI problem. The oral intake of fructose and complex carbohydrates should be stopped. Antacids and oral $NaHCO_3$ should be avoided because they could lead to a higher intestinal luminal fluid pH and thereby an increased production of toxic products of fermentation. Drugs that diminish GI motility should be discontinued. Intravenous $NaHCO_3$ can be given if the acidemia is severe, but this is usually not needed. Poorly absorbed antibiotics (e.g., vancomycin) could be used to change the bacterial flora. Insulin may be helpful because it decreases the rate of oxidation of fatty acids and thus permits a higher rate of oxidation of absorbed organic acids (Figure 6-10).

## METABOLIC ACIDOSIS DUE TO TOXIC ALCOHOLS

### METHANOL INTOXICATION

Methanol ($CH_3OH$), also known as methyl alcohol, wood spirit, and wood alcohol, has a molecular weight of 32. It is used as antifreeze, an additive to gasoline, and a solvent in the manufacture of various drugs.

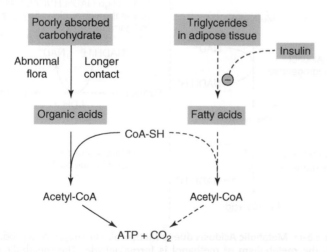

**Figure 6-10 Possible Role of Insulin for Therapy in D-Lactic Acidosis.** Organic acids, including D-lactic acid, are produced during fermentation of poorly absorbed carbohydrate in the gastrointestinal tract. The metabolic removal of these organic acids by the liver and skeletal muscle is slower if fatty acids are being oxidized to produce acetyl-CoA. Hence, administering insulin, which inhibits the release of fatty acids from adipose tissues, may permit more organic acids to be oxidized. *ATP,* Adenosine triphosphate; *CoA-SH,* coenzyme A with active sulfhydryl group.

Methanol itself is not toxic, but its metabolic product, formaldehyde, is the major cause of toxicity because it rapidly binds to tissue proteins.

Methanol is converted to formaldehyde by the enzyme alcohol dehydrogenase in the liver. A high concentration of methanol, however, is required for rapid rates of oxidation. Formaldehyde is rapidly converted to formic acid by the enzyme aldehyde dehydrogenase (Figure 6-11). The latter step is much faster; therefore, the blood level of formaldehyde is only slightly increased, yet it may still be in the toxic range. In each step, $NAD^+$ is converted to $NADH,H^+$.

The metabolic acidosis of methanol poisoning is associated with an increased $P_{Anion\ gap}$ due to the accumulation of formate anions and L-lactate anions. The concentration of L-lactate anions often exceeds that of formate anions. L-Lactic acidosis results from inhibition of cytochrome oxidase by formate anions and the conversion of pyruvate to L-lactate anions in the liver because of an increased $NADH,H^+/NAD^+$ ratio caused by the metabolism of methanol. $HCO_3^-$ anions are produced when formate anions are metabolized to neutral end products; folic acid is a cofactor in this metabolism. Filtered formate anions are reabsorbed in the proximal convoluted tubule via the formate/chloride exchanger, and thus the rate of excretion of formate anions in the urine is low.

Early on, symptoms of intoxication (e.g., inebriation, ataxia, and slurred speech) dominate the clinical picture. Later, blurred vision, blindness, abdominal pain, malaise, headache, and vomiting develop. Fundoscopic examination may reveal the presence of papilledema. Visual impairment is related to metabolism of methanol to formaldehyde via an alcohol dehydrogenase in the retina (retinol dehydrogenase). Fixed and dilated pupils may result from reduced light perception caused by optic neuropathy. Abdominal pain and tenderness often result from acute pancreatitis.

Methanol intoxication should always be considered in the differential diagnosis of metabolic acidosis with an increased $P_{Anion\ gap}$,

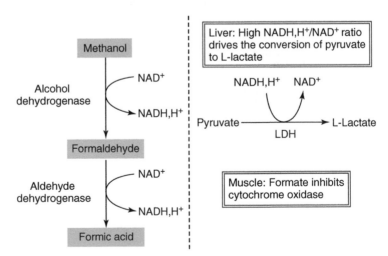

**Figure 6-11 Metabolic Acidosis due to Methanol.** The major toxin produced from the metabolism of methanol is formaldehyde. The metabolic conversion of methanol to formaldehyde is catalyzed by the enzyme alcohol dehydrogenase. Formaldehyde is metabolized rapidly into formic acid in a reaction catalyzed by the enzyme aldehyde dehydrogenase. The *right part* of the figure shows the mechanisms for L-lactic acidosis in this setting. L-Lactic acidosis results from inhibition of cytochrome oxidase in muscle by formate anions, and also from the conversion of pyruvate to lactate in the liver because of an increased $NADH,H^+/NAD^+$ ratio caused by the metabolism of methanol. *NAD+*, Nicotinamide adenine dinucleotide; *NADH,H+*, reduced form of NAD+; *LDH*, lactate dehydrogenase.

particularly if the EABV volume is not appreciably contracted and renal failure is not present. This diagnosis should be suspected by finding of an elevated $P_{Osmolal\ gap}$ and confirmed by a direct assay for methanol in the blood.

## ETHYLENE GLYCOL (ANTIFREEZE) INTOXICATION

Ethylene glycol ($OH–CH_2–CH_2–OH$), a colorless liquid with a sweet taste, has a molecular weight of 62. Ethylene glycol is widely used as antifreeze, in hydraulic brake fluids, as a solvent in the paint and plastics industries, and in the formulation of inks for printers, stamp pads, and ballpoint pens. The lethal dose is approximately 1.4 mL/kg body weight (about 100 mL in an average-sized adult). Ethylene glycol is converted to glycoaldehyde by the enzyme alcohol dehydrogenase in the liver (Figure 6-12); the affinity of this enzyme to ethylene glycol is close to 100 times lower than for ethanol; thus, the rate of metabolism of ethylene glycol is rapid only when its concentration is high. Glycoaldehyde is further metabolized to glycolic acid by hepatic aldehyde dehydrogenase. Glycolic acid is the major acid that accumulates in ethylene glycol poisoning. Only 1% or less of glycolic acid is converted to oxalic acid, mainly by the action of the enzyme lactate dehydrogenase. Virtually all the oxalate produced is precipitated as calcium oxalate, causing hypocalcemia and contributing to acute renal failure. The major end product of glycolic acid metabolism is glycine, which occurs in a transamination reaction with alanine and is catalyzed by the enzyme alanine glyoxylate aminotransferase; vitamin $B_6$ (pyridoxine) is a cofactor in this reaction.

CNS symptoms, such as inebriation, ataxia, and slurred speech, are the effects of ethylene glycol itself. At this stage, the $P_{Osmolal\ gap}$ is high. After a period of about 4 to 12 hours, patients may develop nausea, vomiting, hyperventilation, elevated blood pressure, tachycardia, tetany, and convulsions. At this stage, an increased $P_{Anion\ gap}$ type of metabolic acidosis is present. Tetany is most likely caused by

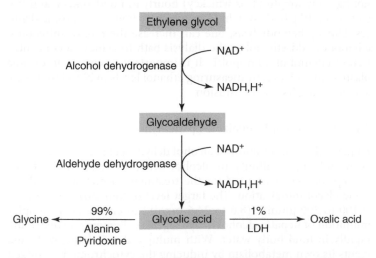

**Figure 6-12 Pathway for the Metabolism of Ethylene Glycol.** Ethylene glycol is converted to glycoaldehyde by alcohol dehydrogenase in the liver. Glycoaldehyde is further metabolized to glycolic acid by hepatic aldehyde dehydrogenase. Only 1% or less of glycolic acid is converted to oxalic acid, mainly by the action of lactate dehydrogenase. The major end product of glycolic acid metabolism is glycine in a transamination reaction with alanine that is catalyzed by the enzyme alanine glyoxylate aminotransferase; vitamin $B_6$ (pyridoxine) is a cofactor. *LDH*, Lactate dehydrogenase.

hypocalcemia, which may be the result of deposition of calcium oxalate crystals. Cranial nerve palsies may be present; calcium oxalate deposition in the vessels and in the meninges of the brain has been noted at autopsy. Leukocytosis is frequently observed; the mechanism is unknown.

Renal failure is common and usually develops 36 to 48 hours after the ingestion of ethylene glycol; glycoaldehyde appears to be the main toxin. It is not clear whether the deposition of calcium oxalate monohydrate crystals plays an important role in pathogenesis of renal failure in these patients (see margin note). In patients who survive, calcium oxalate crystals can persist in the kidneys for months.

### Therapy of methanol or ethylene glycol intoxication

The most important goal of therapy is to stop the metabolism of these alcohols into toxic aldehydes by the enzyme alcohol dehydrogenase in the liver. This is followed by the removal of these alcohols and their toxic metabolites by hemodialysis.

The major difference in treating ethylene glycol poisoning is that when acute oliguric renal failure is present, the amount of $NaHCO_3$ that can be administered when a severe degree of acidemia is present; therefore, early institution of dialysis may be required.

### Administration of ethanol

Maintenance of a plasma ethanol level of about 20 mmol/L (100 mg/dL) almost completely inhibits methanol and ethylene glycol metabolism by alcohol dehydrogenase. Because ethanol distributes throughout total body water, administer a bolus of 0.6 g of ethanol/kg of body weight intravenously to increase its plasma level to 100 mg/dL; this amount of alcohol is contained in 4 ounces of whiskey (40% by volume). The maintenance dose should be equal to the expected rate of metabolic removal of ethanol; about 0.16 g of ethanol/kg body weight (1 oz whiskey) hourly in nondrinkers, and 0.32 g of ethanol/kg body weight (2 oz whiskey) hourly in chronic drinkers. During hemodialysis, one can increase the rate of infusion of ethanol or add ethanol to the dialysis bath to achieve a concentration of ethanol of 20 mmol/L. It is important to ensure an optimal plasma ethanol level by measuring ethanol levels in blood frequently and adjusting its rate of infusion.

### Administration of fomepizole (4-methylpyrazole)

Fomepizole is an inhibitor of alcohol dehydrogenase that has almost 8000-fold higher affinity to alcohol dehydrogenase than ethanol. Fomepizole has been used for the treatment of methanol and ethylene glycol intoxication. The target level of fomepizole in humans is 100 to 300 μmol/L (8.6 to 24.6 mg/dL) to ensure near-complete inhibition of hepatic alcohol dehydrogenase. Fomepizole distributes rapidly in total body water. With multiple doses, fomepizole augments its own metabolism by inducing the cytochrome $P_{450}$ mixed-function oxidase system; this increases its elimination rate by about 50% after about 30 to 40 hours. Therefore, the rate of infusion will need to be increased.

The side effects of fomepizole include headache, nausea, dizziness, and allergic reactions (rash and eosinophilia). Venous irritation and phlebitis may occur if the drug is not diluted prior to infusion. The main disadvantage of using fomepizole is its high cost.

---

**CALCIUM OXALATE CRYSTALS IN THE URINE IN PATIENTS WITH ETHYLENE GLYCOL INTOXICATION**

- The crystals are usually monohydrates, which are needle shaped on microscopic examination of the urine. Less often, there may be the envelope-shaped dihydrate crystals.

## PROPANE 1,2-diol (PROPYLENE GLYCOL)

This compound is commonly used as a diluent for many drug preparations (e.g., intravenous lorazepam, which is commonly used in large doses as a sedative in the intensive care unit and to treat delirium tremens, see margin note).

### Biochemistry

Propane 1,2-diol (molecular weight 76) is a 50:50 mixture of D- and L-isoforms (see margin note). Of the administered dose, 40% is excreted unchanged in the urine, and 60% is metabolized in the liver by alcohol dehydrogenase to lactaldehyde. L-lactaldehyde is metabolized by the enzyme aldehyde dehydrogenase to L-lactic acid (Figure 6-13). D-Lactaldehyde, however, is not a good substrate for aldehyde dehydrogenase; it accumulates and leads to many of the toxic effects observed in this setting. D-Lactaldehyde can be metabolized to D-lactic acid by an alternate pathway in the liver, which uses reduced glutathione as a cofactor. Because L-lactic acid is metabolized much faster than D-lactic acid, the acid that accumulates is largely D-lactic acid.

### Clinical manifestations

The major findings are seizures, cardiac dysfunction, and progressive renal failure. It is likely that D-lactaldehyde is responsible for much of this toxicity. When given in large quantities, this alcohol can be detected by finding a large increase in $P_{Osmolal\ gap}$. The metabolic acidosis is a sign of the metabolic abnormality rather than posing a major threat to the patient.

### Treatment

One must stop the drug. The most important step in treatment is to stop the formation of D-lactaldehyde by giving ethanol or fomepizole. This must be followed up by removal of propane 1,2-diol by hemodialysis.

**PROPANE 1,2-diol**

- A vial of lorazepam contains 2 mg/mL, of which 0.8 mL is propylene glycol. Because its molecular weight is 76, a vial of lorazepam contains 0.83 g of propylene glycol. If a patient were to receive 10 mg/hr of lorazepam, this will result in the administration of 96 g (1300 mmol)/day of propylene glycol. Hence, its presence can be detected by the finding of a large increase in $P_{Osmolal\ gap}$.

**ASYMMETRICAL CARBON IN PROPANE 1,2-diol**

- The middle carbon of this three-carbon compound has four different chemical groups attached to it. Hence, it is an asymmetrical carbon. Because propane 1,2-diol can be metabolized to lactic acid, both the D- and the L-isomers are produced.

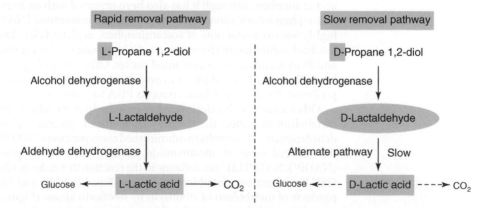

**Figure 6-13 Metabolism of Propane 1,2-diol to L- and D-Lactic Acid.** When a large quantity of propane 1,2-diol is ingested, the body is presented with a racemic mixture; the middle carbon of this three-carbon chain has four different groups attached. Both the L-form (shown to the *left*) and the D-form (shown to the *right*) are substrates for alcohol dehydrogenase; hence, their metabolism occurs in the liver. The products are L-lactaldehyde and D-lactaldehyde. L-Lactaldehyde is a good substrate for aldehyde dehydrogenase. D-lactaldehyde accumulates and is responsible for most of the toxicity. The acid that accumulates is D-lactic acid because it is metabolized much more slowly than L-lactic acid. To simplify the figure, the cofactors, NAD⁺ and NADH,H⁺, are not shown.

# PYROGLUMATIC ACIDOSIS

Pyroglutamic acidosis is a unique form of metabolic acidosis. It was thought to represent only rare inborn errors of metabolism in the γ-glutamyl cycle (defects in 5-oxoprolinase or in glutathione synthetase). It has been recently increasingly recognized as the cause of metabolic acidosis with an increased $P_{Anion\ gap}$, which occurs most often in critically ill, malnourished patients who have a history of chronic acetaminophen ingestion. It is interesting to note that the vast majority of reported cases are in women; the reason for this is not clear. The importance of this disorder is not the acidemia but that it signals that there is a serious metabolic stress present caused by a high level of reactive oxygen spices (ROS) due to depletion of glutathione.

Glutathione is made up of three amino acids: glutamate, cysteine, and glycine. It is the sulfhydryl moiety of cysteine that endows this compound with an ability to detoxify ROS. In this process, the reduced form of glutathione (GSH) is converted to the oxidized form of glutathione (GS-SG; see Eqn 11).

$$2\,GSH + ROS \rightarrow GS\text{-}SG + Inactive\ ROS \qquad (11)$$

**ABBREVIATIONS**

GSH, reduced from of glutathione
GS-SG, oxidized form of glutathione
PGA, pyroglutamic acid
$NADP^+$, nicotinamide adenine dinucleotide phosphate
$NADPH, H^+$, reduced form of $NADP^+$

Key to understanding the basis for the accumulation of pyroglutamic acid (PGA) is that GSH inhibits the enzyme γ-glutamyl cysteine (γ-GC) synthase, which catalyzes the first step in the reaction that converts glutamate to γ-GC. This reaction, however, has two steps. First, glutamate is phosphorylated to form γ-glutamyl phosphate, a step which requires the hydrolysis of ATP. γ-Glutamyl phosphate remains within the active site of the enzyme γ-GC synthase, and cysteine is added in the second step of the reaction; γ-GC is formed and released. Hence, when ROS accumulate, as in a patient with sepsis, the concentration of GSH declines and its inhibitory effect on γ-GC synthase is removed. This results in accelerated formation of γ-glutamyl phosphate. If the patient is cysteine deficient, γ-GC will not be formed; instead, γ-glutamyl phosphate will be transformed to PGA by the enzyme cyclotransferase (see Figure 6-14).

A number of drugs have been identified as causes of PGA accumulation. Pyroglutamic acidosis has been associated with chronic use of acetaminophen, although it has also been reported with an acute acetaminophen intoxication. N-acetyl-p-benzoquinoneimine (NAPQI), a highly reactive metabolite of acetaminophen, depletes GSH. Thus, the feedback inhibition of the enzyme γ-GC synthase by GSH is removed, and PGA accumulates as explained earlier. Other drugs (e.g., the antibiotic flucloxacillin and the anticonvulsant vigabatrin) inhibit 5-oxoprolinase, the enzyme which converts PGA to glutamate.

Other causes of this disorder may include drugs or inborn errors of metabolism that affect the activity of the enzyme glucose 6-phosphate dehydrogenase. This results in a diminished concentration of $NADPH, H^+$, the reduced form of nicotinamide adenine dinucleotide phosphate ($NADP^+$). $NADPH, H^+$ is a cofactor in the reaction that reduces GS-SG to GSH by the enzyme glutathione reductase (Eqn 12). FMN and FAD, the products of metabolism of riboflavin by riboflavin kinase (Figure 6-15), are cofactors for the enzyme glutathione reductase because they are transformed to their reduced form in the first step of the reaction in which GS-SG is reduced to GSH. This may explain, at least in part, why malnutrition seems to be a risk factor for the development of pyroglutamic acidosis. Severe hypothyroidism decreases the activity of riboflavin kinase and may contribute to the development of pyroglutamic acidosis.

$$GS\text{-}SG + NADPH, H^+ \rightarrow 2\,GSH + NADP^+ \qquad (12)$$

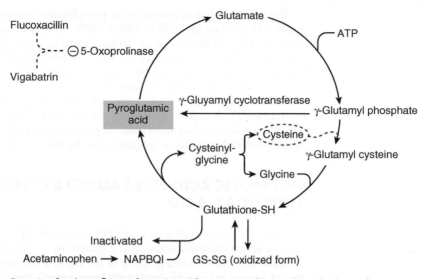

**Figure 6-14 Production of Pyroglutamic Acid.** Key to understanding the basis for the accumulation of pyroglutamic acid (PGA) is that the reduced form of glutathione (GSH) inhibits the enzyme γ-glutamyl cysteine (γ-GC) synthase, which catalyzes the conversion of glutamate to γ-GC. This reaction has two steps. First, glutamate is phosphorylated to form γ-glutamyl phosphate via hydrolysis of adenosine triphosphate (ATP). Second, cysteine is added to γ-glutamyl phosphate, and γ-GC is formed and released. When reactive oxygen species (ROS) accumulate, as in a patient with sepsis, the concentration of GSH declines and its inhibitory effect on γ-GC synthase is removed. This results in accelerated formation of γ-glutamyl phosphate. If the patient is cysteine deficient, γ-GC will not be formed; instead, γ-glutamyl phosphate will be transformed to PGA by the enzyme cyclotransferase. N-acetyl-p-benzoquinonimide (NAPBQ I), a highly reactive metabolite of acetaminophen, depletes GSH. Thus, the feedback inhibition of the enzyme γ-GC synthase is removed, and PGA develops as explained earlier. The antibiotic flucloxacillin and the anticonvulsant vigabatrin inhibit 5-oxoprolinase, the enzyme that converts PGA to glutamate. GS-SG, oxidized form of glutathione.

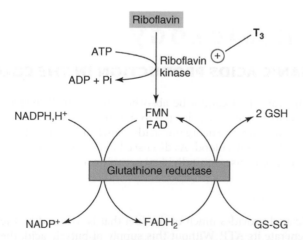

**Figure 6-15 Role of Riboflavin Deficiency and Hypothyroidism in the Pathophysiology of Pyroglutamic Acidosis.** Flavin mononucleotide (FMN) and flavin dinucleotide (FAD), the products of metabolism of riboflavin by riboflavin kinase, are cofactors for the enzyme glutathione reductase because they are transformed to their reduced form in the first step of the reaction in which GS-SG (oxidized form of glutathione) is reduced to glutathione (GSH). Severe hypothyroidism decreases the activity of riboflavin kinase and may contribute to the development of pyroglutamic acidosis. *ATP,* Adenosine triphosphate; *ADP,* adenosine diphosphate; *NADP+,* nicotinamide adenine dinucleotide phosphate; *NADPH,H+,* reduced form of NADP+.

The major danger in patients with pyroglutamic acidosis related to sepsis is tissue damage by ROS. While $NaHCO_3$ may be needed, treatment of sepsis is the key issue. Drugs that may cause pyroglutamic acidosis should be discontinued. *N*-acetyl cysteine should be given in patients with acetaminophen overdose and is also likely beneficial in patients with pryoglutamic acidosis related to sepsis, since deficiency of cysteine seems to play a role in the pathophysiology of this disorder. Malnutrition is thought to be a risk factor for the development of pyroglutamic acidosis and so nutritional support must be provided. As suggested previously, riboflavin deficiency may be important in this regard.

## METABOLIC ACIDOSIS CAUSED BY THE INGESTION OF AN ACID

Patients may occasionally ingest a sufficient quantity of an organic acid to cause severe metabolic acidosis. The symptoms may be due to the acidemia or may result from a property of the anion of the acid (e.g., chelation of ionized calcium by citrate with ingestion of citric acid; see Case 6-1). The clue for this diagnosis is that the patient presents with hyperacute metabolic acidosis with an increased $P_{Anion\ gap}$. L-Lactic acid is the only acid of endogenous origin that may be produced at an extremely rapid rate during hypoxia or in patients with ethanol intoxication who also have deficiency of thiamin. Therefore, suspect the ingestion of an acid in patients with hyperacute metabolic acidosis with an increased $P_{Anion\ gap}$ if the plasma L-lactate level is not very high and the $P_{Osmolal\ gap}$ is not markedly increased (unless ethanol, methanol, or ethylene glycol was also ingested).

Treatment consists of administration of $NaHCO_3$ if the acidemia is severe, and dealing with any adverse effect of the anion of the ingested acid (e.g., hypotension due to hypocalcemia caused by chelation of ionized calcium by citrate with ingestion of citric acid).

# PART C
# INTEGRATIVE PHYSIOLOGY

## ORGANIC ACIDS PRODUCTION IN THE COLON

Carbohydrates that cannot be absorbed in the small intestine (e.g., some fructose, fiber) are delivered to the colon. Colonic bacteria convert them to a mixture of organic acids, which are absorbed and added to the portal venous blood. As discussed in the following paragraphs, there are specific uses for individual organic acids.

### BUTYRIC ACID

Butyric acid provides much of the fuel that is oxidized by the colon to regenerate its ATP. Without this supply of butyric acid, the colon may not function properly (starvation colitis), possibly due in part to a deficiency of ATP.

### PROPIONIC ACID

Although propionic acid represents just 20% of the total amount of organic acids produced each day in the colon, it may have an important metabolic function. Propionic acid is converted in the liver to propionyl-CoA. There are two major fates for this compound. In the fed state, it can be converted to pyruvate, which can then be oxidized or be made into glucose. Between meals there may be a need to synthesize four-carbon catalysts for the citric acid cycle in organs other than the liver (e.g., in the heart). This may be also the case in a catabolic state, during which some of these four-carbon catalysts may have been depleted. To ensure that propionic acid is not fully metabolized in the liver, propionyl-CoA combines with a molecule of acetyl-CoA to produce a five-carbon keto-acid, which then exits the liver. When the heart extracts this five-carbon ketoacid, propionyl-CoA is formed. Propionyl-CoA is then converted to succinyl-CoA, an intermediate in the citric acid cycle.

## DISCUSSION OF CASES

### CASE 6-1: PATRICK IS IN FOR A SHOCK

**Judging from the time frame for his illness, what is (are) the likely cause(s) of metabolic acidosis?**

The only acid that is made endogenously at a very rapid rate is L-lactic acid during hypoxia or in patients with ethanol intoxication and deficiency of thiamin. The concentration of L-lactate anions in blood was only 2 mmol/L. Therefore, the most likely cause of the development of acute metabolic acidosis in this patient is that he ingested an acid. The properties of its anion can help deduce which acid he ingested.

**Why did his blood pressure fall so precipitously?**

Blood pressure is a function of the cardiac output and the peripheral vascular resistance. Cardiac output is directly related to the heart rate and the stroke volume. Because his heart rate was rapid, one should look for a process that could compromise his stroke volume and/or his peripheral vascular resistance. Because he had no evidence of blood loss, sepsis, or a disorder that can cause salt depletion (e.g., a history of diarrhea), one should suspect that there is a problem with the contractility of his heart and/or the vaso-constrictor tone of his blood vessels. The factor essential for cardiac contractility is ionized calcium. Therefore, it is possible that the anion of the acid that he ingested might have removed ionized calcium. Because citrate is a chelator of ionized calcium, it was thought that he may have ingested citric acid. This was confirmed later when the composition of the solution he ingested became known.

**Why did he have hyperkalemia?**

To shift $K^+$ ions out of cells, the voltage in cells must become less negative. Inorganic acids (e.g., HCl) or non-monocarboxylic organic acids (e.g., citric acid) cannot enter cells by the monocarboxylic acid cotransporter. Therefore, a different mechanism is needed to permit some of these $H^+$ ions to be titrated using $HCO_3^-$ ions in the ICF compartment. This may involve activation of the $Cl^-/HCO_3^-$ anion exchanger (AE) (perhaps because of a low $P_{HCO_3}$, but the exact mechanism is not known), which leads to the transport of $HCO_3^-$ ions out of cells and $Cl^-$ ions into cells. Because this exchange of anions has a 1:1 stoichiometry, it is electroneutral, and it does not change the magnitude of the negative voltage in these cells. Nevertheless, as a result of the combination of the higher concentration of $Cl^-$ ions in cells and the negative intracellular voltage,

Cl⁻ ions are forced out of cells in an electrogenic fashion via open Cl⁻ ion channels in the cell membrane. As a result, the voltage in these cells becomes less negative, and K⁺ ions exit from the cells if K⁺ ion channels in the cell membrane are open (see Figure 13-7).

### Why did the administration of intravenous calcium cause a rapid recovery?

As part of the emergency treatment of hyperkalemia, his physician infused calcium gluconate. This caused a rise in the concentration of ionized calcium in plasma, which increased myocardial contractility as well as caused vasoconstriction; both effects raised his blood pressure. This was another piece of the puzzle that alerted his physicians to the possibility that this patient may have ingested citric acid.

### CASE 6-2: METABOLIC ACIDOSIS ASSOCIATED WITH DIARRHEA

### What is the cause of the metabolic acidosis in this patient?

Metabolic acidosis in this patient was not simply the result of loss of $NaHCO_3$ in diarrheal fluid because the $P_{Anion\ gap}$ was 26 mEq/L. L-Lactic acidosis is unlikely because there was no hemodynamic problem, liver function tests were normal, and the time period was too short for a nutritional deficiency (e.g., thiamin and/or riboflavin deficiency) that may have caused L-lactic acidosis. Moreover, he did not ingest drugs that may be associated with L-lactic acidosis. There was no history of diabetes mellitus or the intake of ethanol, and his blood sugar was normal. Later, L-lactic acidosis and ketoacidosis were ruled out because the concentrations of L-lactate anions and β-hydroxybutyrate anions were not elevated in his blood. Toxic alcohol ingestion was not likely from the history or the laboratory data (no increase in the $P_{Osmolal\ gap}$). Renal failure was not present ($P_{Creatinine}$ is near the normal range). There was no known history of intake of an organic acid. Therefore, the most likely diagnosis is D-lactic acidosis.

The factors that might lead to overproduction of D-lactic acid and other organic acids in his GI tract include a change in his GI bacterial flora caused by the use of antibiotics, provision of substrates to these bacteria (popsicles contain sucrose and fructose; fructose is poorly absorbed in the intestinal tract), and a slower transit time because of the drug used to decrease intestinal motility to treat his diarrhea.

### CASE 6-3: SEVERE ACIDEMIA IN A PATIENT WITH CHRONIC ALCOHOLISM

### What dangers may be present on admission or arise during therapy?

The dangers that may present on admission or may arise during therapy include:
1. Severe acidemia: The patient had a severe degree of metabolic acidemia with a large increase in the $P_{Anion\ gap}$ suggesting overproduction of acids. Binding of H⁺ ions to proteins in cells alters their charge, shape, and perhaps functions. This may be particularly detrimental if it occurs in cells of vital organs (e.g., the brain and heart). Although he was hemodynamically stable, a quantitatively small additional H⁺ ion load will produce a proportionately larger fall in the $P_{HCO_3}$ and plasma pH. For instance, reducing the

$P_{HCO_3}$ by half will cause the arterial pH to drop by 0.30 units if the arterial $PCO_2$ does not change.

2. Toxic alcohol ingestion: Because the patient had a severe degree of metabolic acidemia with a large $P_{Osmolal\ gap}$, ingestion of methanol or ethylene glycol was suspected. Aldehydes produced from the metabolism of these alcohols by the enzyme alcohol dehydrogenase in the liver are the major cause of toxicity because they rapidly bind to tissue proteins. Although he ingested a large amount of ethanol, which could have caused the large $P_{Osmolal\ gap}$, and his urine was strongly positive for ketones, such a severe degree of acidemia is not usual in patients with alcoholic ketoacidosis. Because of the strong clinical suspicion of toxic alcohol ingestion, the patient was started on fomepizole while awaiting the results of the measurements of the level of these alcohols in his blood.

3. Thiamin deficiency: Malnourished patients who present with alcoholic ketoacidosis are at risk of developing encephalopathy due to thiamin deficiency.

### More information

Plasma L-lactate was 23 mmol/L; blood assays for methanol and ethylene glycol were negative.

### What is the cause of the severe L-lactic acidosis in this patient?

A rise in the concentration of L-lactate$^-$ anions and $H^+$ ions can be caused by an increased rate of production and/or a decreased rate of removal. The rapid development and the severity of L-lactic acidosis suggest that it is largely due to overproduction of L-lactic acid.

The degree of L-lactic acidosis in patients presenting with alcohol intoxication is usually mild (concentration of L-lactate anions in plasma ~5 mmol/L) because it reflects the increased $NADH,H^+/NAD^+$ ratio due to the ongoing production of $NADH,H^+$ caused by ethanol metabolism, which is largely restricted to the liver. Other organs in the body are capable of oxidizing the L-lactic acid produced by the liver because they lack the enzyme alcohol dehydrogenase and hence do not have a high $NADH,H^+/NAD^+$ ratio in this setting.

A severe degree of L-lactic acidosis may develop rapidly if there is a large intake of alcohol in a patient who is thiamin deficient. The site of L-lactic acid production is likely to be the liver because there is accumulation of pyruvate (caused by diminished activity of PDH) and also a high $NADH,H^+/NAD^+$ ratio (due to metabolism of ethanol). Diminished removal of L-lactic acid by other organs is also likely to be present due to diminished activity of PDH and the presence of alternative fuels that are used preferentially to regenerate ATP. Vitamin $B_2$ (riboflavin) deficiency may be also present in this malnourished patient with chronic alcoholism, another cause for increased production of L-lactic acid.

### DISCUSSION OF QUESTIONS

6-1 *Consider the following example. An anoxic limb needs to regenerate 18 mmol/min of ATP (25% of the ATP needed in the body) via glycolysis. If the rest of the body could be persuaded to oxidize L-lactic acid to regenerate all its needed ATP (54 mmol/min), would L-lactic acid still accumulate?*

The answer to this question focuses on the stoichiometry of $H^+$ ion production and removal relative to the rate of ATP regeneration during the production and the removal of L-lactic acid. For this anoxic limb to regenerate 18 mmol of ATP via glycolysis, 18 mmol of L-lactic acid are produced. Oxidation of 1 mmol of L-lactic acid causes the regeneration of about 18 mmol of ATP. Therefore, if the rest of the body could be persuaded to oxidize L-lactic acid to regenerate all its needed ATP (54 mmol/min), only 3 mmol of L-lactic acid per minute are removed (compared to 18 mmol/min of L-lactic acid that were produced). Clearly L-lactic acid will accumulate. The obvious message from this quantitative analysis is that one cannot overcome a rapid rate of production of L-lactic acid by accelerating its rate of removal. Therefore, drugs such as dichloroacetate, which activate PDH, are not beneficial in patients with hypoxic L-lactic acidosis.

6-2 *NaHCO₃ was given to a patient for the treatment for L-lactic acidosis, but there was no rise in the $P_{HCO_3}$. Is it correct to conclude that the administration of NaHCO₃ was not beneficial?*

In patients with hypoxic L-lactic acidosis, it is the depletion of ATP in vital organs (e.g., the brain and the heart) and the binding of $H^+$ ions to proteins in cells of these organs that are detrimental, rather than the concentration of $H^+$ ions in the ECF compartment. Therefore, there are two possible ways the administration of $NaHCO_3$ may have had a beneficial effect, even if it did not cause a rise in $P_{HCO_3}$. First, if the administered $HCO_3^-$ ions titrated $H^+$ ions that were bound to intracellular proteins, this would be beneficial. Second, if the administration of $NaHCO_3$ caused a rise in intracellular pH to remove the inhibition of the enzyme PFK-1, and therefore resulted in an increase in flux in glycolysis, this would be beneficial because it increases the rate of regeneration of ATP. The $P_{HCO_3}$ may not rise because the administered $HCO_3^-$ ions are titrated by the L-lactic acid produced.

# Metabolic Alkalosis

# Introduction

## ABBREVIATIONS

$P_{HCO_3}$, concentration of bicarbonate ions ($HCO_3^-$) in plasma

$U_{Cl}$, concentration of chloride ions ($Cl^-$) in urine

$P_{Glucose}$, concentration of glucose in plasma

$P_K$, concentration of potassium ions ($K^+$) in plasma

$P_{Na}$, concentration of sodium ions ($Na^+$) in plasma

$P_{Albumin}$, concentration of albumin in plasma

$P_{Anion\ gap}$, anion gap in plasma

GFR, glomerular filtration rate

ECF, extracellular fluid

ICF, intracellular fluid

EABV, effective arterial blood volume

PCT, proximal convoluted tubule

Metabolic alkalosis is principally an electrolyte disorder that is accompanied by changes in acid–base parameters in plasma, namely an elevated concentration of bicarbonate ($HCO_3^-$) ions ($P_{HCO_3}$) and elevated pH. Most patients with metabolic alkalosis have a deficit of chloride ($Cl^-$)-containing compounds: sodium chloride (NaCl), potassium chloride (KCl) and/or hydrochloric acid (HCl). A deficit of NaCl raises the $P_{HCO_3}$ primarily by lowering the extracellular fluid (ECF) volume, whereas a deficit of HCl or KCl raises the $P_{HCO_3}$ by adding new $HCO_3^-$ ions to the body. In some patients, however, metabolic alkalosis may be due to the retention of $NaHCO_3$. For example, patients with disorders causing primary high mineralocorticoid activity may develop metabolic alkalosis due to the retention of $NaHCO_3$ when they become hypokalemic, although they do not have a deficit of $Cl^-$ ions. The most common causes of metabolic alkalosis are chronic vomiting and the use of diuretics. Measuring the concentration of $Cl^-$ ions in the urine ($U_{Cl}$) is often very helpful for diagnosis of the cause of metabolic alkalosis. The goal for therapy in patients with metabolic alkalosis is to replace the specific electrolyte deficits.

---

### OBJECTIVES

- ■ To illustrate that metabolic alkalosis is an electrolyte disorder that is commonly due to deficits of compounds that contain $Cl^-$ ions: NaCl, KCl, and/or HCl. Patients with primary high mineralocorticoid activity may develop metabolic alkalosis because of retention of $NaHCO_3$ when they become hypokalemic, although they do not have a deficit of $Cl^-$ ions.
- ■ To describe how deficits of NaCl, KCl, and/or HCl may increase the ratio of $HCO_3^-$ ion content/ECF volume by influencing its numerator and/or its denominator. To describe the pathophysiology of the metabolic alkalosis in patients with primary high mineralocorticoid activity.
- ■ To describe the clinical approach to the diagnosis of the cause of metabolic alkalosis.
- ■ To emphasize that the goal for therapy should be to replace the specific electrolyte deficits.

---

## CASE 7-1: THIS MAN SHOULD NOT HAVE METABOLIC ALKALOSIS

After a forced 6-hour intense training exercise in the desert, in the heat of the day, an elite corps soldier was the only one in his squad who collapsed. He perspired profusely during the training exercise and drank a large volume of water and glucose-containing fluids. He did not vomit and denied the intake of any medications. Physical examination revealed a markedly contracted effective arterial blood volume (EABV). Initial laboratory data are provided in following table. The pH and $PCO_2$ data are from an arterial blood sample, whereas all other data are from a venous blood sample.

| | | | | | |
|---|---|---|---|---|---|
| $P_{Na}$ | mmol/L | 125 | pH | | 7.50 |
| $P_K$ | mmol/L | 2.7 | $P_{HCO_3}$ | mmol/L | 38 |
| $P_{Cl}$ | mmol/L | 70 | Arterial $PCO_2$ | mm Hg | 47 |
| Hematocrit | | 0.50 | | | |

## Questions

What are the major threats to the patient and how should these dictate the initial therapy?

What is the basis for the metabolic alkalosis in this patient?
What is the therapy for the metabolic alkalosis in this patient?

## CASE 7-2: WHY DID THIS PATIENT DEVELOP METABOLIC ALKALOSIS SO QUICKLY?

A 52-year-old Asian man has chronic lung disease. Prior to this admission, his arterial pH was 7.40, $PCO_2$ was 40 mm Hg, and $P_{HCO_3}$ was 24 mmol/L. In the past 24 hours, he developed an acute attack of asthma with marked exertional dyspnea and very prominent wheezing that was resistant to his usual medications (inhaled $\beta_2$-adrenergics and theophylline). In the emergency department, he received a large dose of intravenous steroids. He was admitted to hospital and continued on intravenous steroids for the following 4 days. On day 3, his breathing had improved markedly, and he was able to eat without difficulty. He did not vomit and was not given diuretics. Surprisingly, on day 4, he was found to have a severe degree of hypokalemia ($P_K$ 1.7 mmol/L) and metabolic alkalosis (arterial pH 7.47, arterial $PCO_2$ 50 mm Hg, $P_{HCO_3}$ in venous blood 37 mmol/L). At this time, the concentration of $Na^+$ ions in his urine ($U_{Na}$) was 54 mmol/L, the concentration of $K^+$ ions in his urine ($U_K$) was 23 mmol/L, and the concentration of $Cl^-$ ions ($U_{Cl}$) in his urine was 53 mmol/L. The concentration of glucose in his plasma ($P_{Glucose}$) was 102 mg/dL (6 mmol/L) and his calculated creatinine clearance by his Cockcroft-Gault equation was 80 mL/min.

| DAY | | 0 | 3 | 4 |
|---|---|---|---|---|
| $P_K$ | mmol/L | 4.0 | 3.2 | 1.7 |
| $P_{HCO_3}$ | mmol/L | 24 | 29 | 37 |

**Question**

Why did this patient develop metabolic alkalosis on days 3 and 4?

## CASE 7-3: MILK-ALKALI SYNDROME, BUT WITHOUT MILK

A 60-year-old man had complaints of malaise, anorexia, and constipation over the past several weeks. He denied vomiting or the intake of diuretics. He had been chewing close to 40 betel nuts on a daily basis for many years. To avoid the bitter taste of the betel nut, he had been adding to it a paste that contains calcium hydroxide ($Ca[OH]_2$). On physical examination, his EABV was contracted and his tongue, oral mucosa, and the angles of his mouth were stained brick red by the betel nut juice. The laboratory data are provided in the following table. Of note, he had hypercalcemia, and the levels of both his parathyroid hormone and 1,25-dihydroxyvitamin $D_3$ in plasma were low (data not shown).

| | | PLASMA | URINE |
|---|---|---|---|
| pH | | 7.47 | — |
| $HCO_3^-$ | mmol/L | 36 | — |
| $Na^+$ | mmol/L | 137 | 21 |
| $K^+$ | mmol/L | 3.2 | 21 |
| $Cl^-$ | mmol/L | 91 | 42 |
| Creatinine | mg/dL (μmol/L) | 9.7 (844) | 108 (9400) |
| Calcium | mg/dL (mmol/L) | 12.8 (3.2) | 23.4 (5.9) |
| Phosphate | mg/dL (mmol/L) | 5.7 (1.8) | 5.9 (2.1) |
| Albumin | g/dl (g/L) | 3.9 (39) | |

**Questions**

What is the basis for the metabolic alkalosis?
What should the initial therapy be?

# PART A
# PATHOPHYSIOLOGY

## OVERVIEW

Metabolic alkalosis is a process that leads to a rise in the $P_{HCO_3}$ and the arterial blood pH.

The following principles are fundamental to understanding why metabolic alkalosis develops and how it is maintained:

1. *The concentration of $HCO_3^-$ ions in the ECF compartment is the ratio of its content of $HCO_3^-$ ions (numerator) and the ECF volume (denominator).*

    A rise in the concentration of $HCO_3^-$ ions might be due to an increase in its numerator (addition of $HCO_3^-$ ions) and/or a decrease in its denominator (loss of ECF volume). A quantitative estimate of the ECF volume is required to assess the quantity of $HCO_3^-$ ions in the ECF compartment and thereby to determine the basis of the metabolic alkalosis.

2. *Electroneutrality must be present. Hence, the term $Cl^-$ depletion alkalosis does not provide an adequate description of the pathophysiology of metabolic alkalosis.*

    The deficit of $Cl^-$ ions must be defined as being due to a deficit of HCl, KCl, and/or NaCl to determine why the $P_{HCO_3}$ has risen and what changes have occurred in the composition of the ECF and intracellular fluid (ICF) compartments and therefore what is the appropriate therapy.

    Even though balance data are not available in most patients, available laboratory measurements such as the hematocrit can help the clinician to obtain a quantitative assessment of ECF volume and reach a reasonable conclusion about the contribution of deficits of the different $Cl^-$-containing compounds to the development of the metabolic alkalosis (see Case 7-1).

3. *Critical to the understanding of the pathophysiology of metabolic alkalosis is that there is no tubular maximum for $HCO_3^-$ ion reabsorption in the kidney.*

    It is widely thought that there is a tubular maximum for renal reabsorption of $HCO_3^-$ ions, and therefore a derangement in renal handling of $HCO_3^-$ ions are needed to prevent the excretion of the excess $HCO_3^-$ ions and maintain the metabolic alkalosis. Because of its importance for the understanding of the pathophysiology of metabolic alkalosis and implications for its therapy, this issue will be discussed in more detail in the following paragraphs.

### RENAL REABSORPTION OF NaHCO₃: A MORE DETAILED ANALYSIS

The traditional view of the renal handling of $HCO_3^-$ ions is that there is a tubular maximum for the reabsorption of $HCO_3^-$ ions in the proximal convoluted tubule (PCT). This view is based largely on experimental studies performed by Pitts many decades ago. Before examining the results of these experiments, it is important to consider first some pertinent aspects of regulation of $HCO_3^-$ ion reabsorption by PCT cells.

### Stimuli for the reabsorption of filtered $NaHCO_3$

The vast majority of filtered $HCO_3^-$ ions are reabsorbed in the PCT via $H^+$ ion secretion, which is largely mediated by the electroneutral $Na^+/H^+$ exchanger-3 (NHE-3) (see Chapter 1 for more details). The usual circulating levels of angiotensin II and the usual concentration of $H^+$ ions in PCT cells provide sufficient stimuli for NHE-3 to permit the reabsorption of most of the filtered $NaHCO_3$.

### Experiments carried out by Pitts

These experiments were designed to define the physiologic renal response to an administered load of $HCO_3^-$ ions in dogs. In fact, these experiments examined the renal response to the administration of a load of $NaHCO_3$. This, however, would diminish the stimuli for the reabsorption of $NaHCO_3$ that are normally present in the PCT. This is because the $Na^+$ ion load would expand the EABV, which would lead to suppression of the release of angiotensin II, and the load of $HCO_3^-$ ions would increase the peritubular concentration of $HCO_3^-$ ions, which would lead to diminished reabsorption of $HCO_3^-$ ions in the PCT.

Therefore, the results of these experiments are predictable: all the extra $NaHCO_3$ that is filtered will be excreted in the urine. These results, however, were interpreted to indicate that there is a tubular maximum for the rate of reabsorption of $NaHCO_3$ by the kidney.

### Renal response to a physiologic load of $HCO_3^-$ ions

Evidence to support the physiology of an absence of a tubular maximum for the reabsorption of $HCO_3^-$ ions is that while the $P_{HCO_3}$ rises to ~30 mmol/L during the daily alkaline tide caused by the secretion of HCl in the stomach, there is no appreciable bicarbonaturia. As shown in Figure 7-1, the gain of $HCO_3^-$ ions in the ECF compartment that occurs when the stomach secretes HCl is accompanied by an equivalent deficit of $Cl^-$ ions in the ECF compartment. Accordingly, there is no increase in the ECF volume with this rise in $P_{HCO_3}$. Hence, there is no suppression of the release of angiotensin II and no inhibition of the reabsorption of $HCO_3^-$ ions by the PCT. Therefore, virtually all the surplus of $HCO_3^-$ ions is retained in this setting.

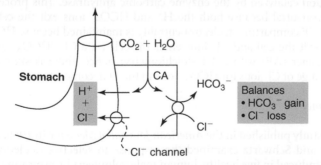

**Figure 7-1 Secretion of HCl in the Stomach.** The *stylized structure* is the stomach with a parietal cell on its right border. In the cell, $CO_2 + H_2O$ are converted to $H^+$ ions and $HCO_3^-$ ions, a reaction that is catalyzed by the enzyme carbonic anhydrase (CA). $H^+$ ions are secreted into the lumen of the stomach by an $H^+/K^+$-ATPase, while $K^+$ ions recycle back into the parietal cell *(not shown, for simplicity)*. $Cl^-$ ions from the extracellular fluid compartment enter parietal cells on their basolateral $HCO_3^-/Cl^-$ anion exchanger. $HCO_3^-$ ions are added to the extracellular fluid compartment, while $Cl^-$ enter the lumen of the stomach via $Cl^-$ ion channels. Overall, there is a loss of $Cl^-$ ions and a gain of $HCO_3^-$ ions in the body during vomiting.

We have carried out experimental studies in rats in which a loss of NaCl, induced with the administration of a loop diruetic, was replaced with an equivalent amount of $NaHCO_3$. Although $P_{HCO_3}$ rose to ~50 mmol/L, there was no appreciable bicarbonaturia. This suggests that there is no tubular maximum for the reabsorption of $NaHCO_3$ (see Figure 1-9).

QUESTION

7-1  *What might be the advantages of not having a tubular maximum for the renal reabsorption of* $NaHCO_3$?

## DEVELOPMENT OF METABOLIC ALKALOSIS

Patients with metabolic alkalosis can be divided into two groups based on the pathophysiology of their disorder. In most patients, metabolic alkalosis is due to deficits of $Cl^-$ salts (HCl, KCl, and/or NaCl). In some patients, metabolic alkalosis is the result of retention of $NaHCO_3$.

### METABOLIC ALKALOSIS CAUSED BY DEFICITS OF $Cl^-$ SALTS

A deficit of HCl, KCl, and/or NaCl causes the $P_{HCO_3}$ to rise (Flow Chart 7-1). Understanding how electroneutrality and balance are achieved has implications for understanding the pathophysiology of metabolic alkalosis in a given patient and what changes have occurred in the composition of the ECF and ICF compartments and hence for designing appropriate therapy.

### Deficit of HCl

#### *Gain of $HCO_3^-$ ions*

The steps involved in the gain of $HCO_3^-$ ions in the ECF compartment from the loss of HCl in vomiting are illustrated in Figure 7-1. The process that adds $H^+$ ions to the lumen of the stomach is electroneutral because there is an equivalent secretion of $H^+$ and $Cl^-$ ions. Within the gastric parietal cells that secrete HCl, the source of $H^+$ ions (and $HCO_3^-$ ions) is carbonic acid ($H_2CO_3$), which is made from $CO_2 + H_2O$, in a reaction catalyzed by the enzyme carbonic anhydrase. This process is electroneutral because both the $H^+$ and $HCO_3^-$ ions exit the cell. In the ECF compartment, electroneutrality is maintained because $HCO_3^-$ ions exit the cell and $Cl^-$ ions enter the cell via a $Cl^-/HCO_3^-$ anion exchanger (AE) with a 1:1 stoichiometry; hence, there is simply an exchange of $Cl^-$ ions for $HCO_3^-$ ions in the ECF compartment.

#### *Balance*

In a study published in the *American Journal of Medicine* in 1966, Kassirer and Schwartz examined the response to selective depletion of HCl induced in five healthy human male volunteers by aspirating gastric contents for several days. Balance data were obtained during the drainage period and for 4 to 8 days after drainage was discontinued (postdrainage period). The study's quantitative results are somewhat complex, but they do provide a very useful insight into the likely actual electrolyte deficits that occur in patients with repetitive vomiting or nasogastric suction. Two points become evident from the analysis of the results of the study:
1.  At the end of the postdrainage period, there was a cumulative negative balance for both $Cl^-$ and $K^+$ ions, which were of similar magnitude.

2. At the end of the postdrainage period, there was a gain of $HCO_3^-$ ions in the ECF compartment, with an equal gain of $H^+$ ions in the ICF. Therefore, despite the presence of metabolic alkalemia, there was no appreciable net total body gain of $HCO_3^-$ ions.

Subjects consumed a constant diet that contained 4 to 6 mmol of $Na^+$ ions, 4 to 7 mmol of $Cl^-$ ions, and 59 to 76 mmol of $K^+$ ions per day. One subject received an oral supplement of 40 mmol of $Na^+$ ions per day as a neutral phosphate salt. The amount of $Na^+$ and $K^+$ ions that were removed in gastric drainage was also given back to each subject as chloride salts that were added to the fluid ingested in the day following drainage. The average initial weight of these subjects was 65 kg. The initial $P_{HCO_3}$ was 28.6 mmol/L; it rose to 37.5 mmol/L at the end of the drainage period and was 35.7 mmol/L at the end of the postdrainage period. Average balance data for $Na^+$, $Cl^-$ and $K^+$ ions are provided in Table 7-1 (see margin note).

### Drainage period

The amount of acid removed by gastric drainage averaged 262 mmol. An equivalent amount of $HCO_3^-$ ions should have been added to the ECF compartment. Based on the observed rise in $P_{HCO_3}$ and an estimation of ECF volume, the authors calculated that on average 104 mmol of $HCO_3^-$ ions were retained in the ECF. Therefore, there was a loss of 158 mmol of $HCO_3^-$ ions, out of the 262 mmol that were generated in the process of the loss of HCl. During this gastric drainage period, there was a deficit of 128 mmol of $K^+$ ions and 26 mmol of $Na^+$ ions

**$Na^+$ ION DEFICIT**

The cumulative negative $Na^+$ ion balance for the four subjects who were not receiving Na phosphate supplementation was 85 mmol (46 mmol during the drainage period, and 39 mmol during the postdrainage period).

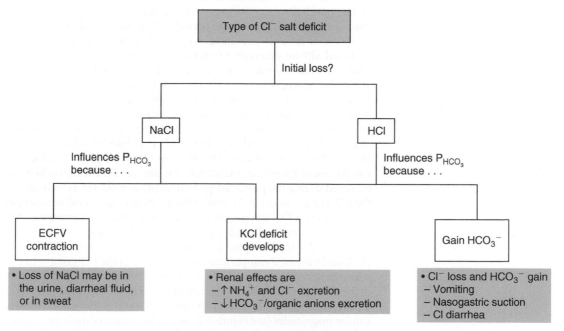

**Flow Chart 7-1  Pathophysiology of Metabolic Alkalosis due to a Deficit of $Cl^-$ Salts.** This algorithm is useful for understanding how a deficit of HCl, KCl, and/or NaCl contributes to the development of metabolic alkalosis. *ECFV*, Extracellular fluid volume.

TABLE 7-1   **BALANCE DATA FOR ELECTROLYTES IN A STUDY OF SELECTIVE HCl DEPLETION ALKALOSIS**

|  | $Na^+$ | $K^+$ | $Cl^-$ |
|---|---|---|---|
| Drainage period | −26 | −128 | −232 |
| Postdrainage period | +4 | −85 | +33 |
| Cumulative | −22 | −213 | −199 |

**BALANCE DATA**

One needs to keep in mind that with balance data obtained over several days, small errors may result in large cumulative differences.

### LOSS OF $HCO_3^-$ IONS IN THE URINE AS ORGANIC ANIONS

The following data were provided in one patient:

- Acid removed = 444 mmol.
- $HCO_3^-$ ions retained in the ECF compartment = 138 mmol, difference = 306 mmol.
- $HCO_3^-$ loss in the urine = 71 mmol.
- Therefore, bicarbonaturia was modest and the bulk of alkali loss in the urine (235 mmol) was as organic anions.

### $Na^+$ ION GAIN IN THE ICF

If $Na^+$ ions were retained in the ICF compartment, there would need to be a lower activity of the Na-K-ATPase, but the mechanism for this is not clear.

due to the loss of these cations in the urine. Therefore, it is likely these $HCO_3^-$ ions were lost in the urine largely with $K^+$ ions. More detailed data were provided for one patient and suggest that there was no appreciable bicarbonaturia, hence it is likely that most of the alkali loss in the urine was as organic anions (see margin note and Chapter 1).

The source for the $K^+$ ion deficit was $K^+$ ions from the ICF compartment. To maintain electroneutrality in cells when $K^+$ ions exit, there must be either a loss of anions from the ICF compartment (predominantly from organic phosphates such as RNA, DNA, phospholipids, phosphocreatine, and adenosine triphosphate [ATP]) or a gain of cations ($Na^+$ and/or $H^+$ ions) in the ICF. Loss of anions from the ICF is not likely because there was little negative balance for phosphate ions. Oxidation of dietary sulfur-containing amino acids yields sulfuric acid $H_2SO_4$. It is possible that $K^+$ ions were excreted in the urine with sulfate ($SO_4^{2-}$) anions, and the $H^+$ ions were retained in the ICF. Nevertheless, because $K^+$ ions were largely excreted in the urine with organic anions/$HCO_3^-$ and not with $SO_4^{2-}$ anions, it is likely that $K^+$ ion loss from the ICF compartment was in exchange for $Na^+$ ions from the ECF compartment (Figure 7-2, *A*) (see margin note).

### Postdrainage period

Based on calculation of chloride space, the author estimated that the ECF volume declined on average by 0.5 L. It was calculated (based on their estimate of the ECF volume and the measured $P_{HCO_3}$) that the amount of $HCO_3^-$ ions retained in the ECF compartment at the end of the postdrainage period was on average 82 mmol (24 mmol less than at the end of the drainage period). There was an additional loss of 85 mmol of $K^+$ ions (see Table 7-1). The loss of $K^+$ ions in the urine occurred with an anion other than $Cl^-$ (no further deficit of $Cl^-$ ions than what occurred in the drainage period) and other than $HCO_3^-$ or organic anions (no appreciable loss of $HCO_3^-$ ions). One possible scenario is that $K^+$ ions ions were excreted in the urine with $SO_4^{2-}$ anions that were produced from oxidation of dietary sulfur-containing amino acids to $H_2SO_4$. For electroneutrality in the ICF compartment, the shift of $K^+$ ions out of cells was accompanied by a shift of $H^+$ ions into cells (Figure 7-2, *B*). Because the amount of extra $HCO_3^-$ ions that were present in the ECF compartment at this stage (82 mmol) was similar to the $K^+$ ion deficit that occurred during the postdrainage period (85 mmol), the $H^+$ ion gain in the ICF compartment at the end of the postdrainage period was roughly equal to the $HCO_3^-$ ion gain in the ECF compartment. Therefore, in this model of metabolic alkalosis due to selective depletion of HCl, there is no appreciable total body net gain of $HCO_3^-$ ions. In essence, there is an alkalosis in the ECF compartment and acidosis in the ICF compartment, with a deficit of $Cl^-$ ions in the ECF compartment and a deficit of $K^+$ ions in the ICF compartment. It is interesting to note that, on mass balance, the deficit of $Cl^-$ ions (–232 mmol) and that of $K^+$ ions (–199 mmol) were of similar magnitudes (see Figure 7-2 for an illustration of these processes).

Hence, KCl must be given to replace the deficit of KCl. Although it is possible to lower the concentration of $HCO_3^-$ ions in the ECF compartment with a large infusion of saline, this does not correct the gain of $HCO_3^-$ ions in the ECF compartment or the gain of $H^+$ ions in the ICF compartment.

With the administration of KCl, $K^+$ ions enter the ICF compartment in conjunction with the net transfer of $H^+$ ions to the ECF compartment. These exported $H^+$ ions react with $HCO_3^-$ ions to form $H_2O$ and $CO_2$. After the $CO_2$ is exhaled, both the $H^+$ ion gain in the ICF compartment and the $HCO_3^-$ ion gain in the ECF compartment are corrected. In addition, $Cl^-$ ions remain in the ECF compartment, replacing their

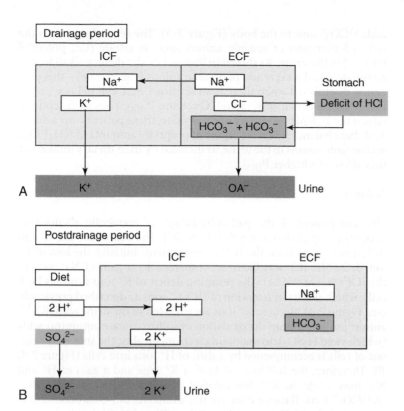

**Figure 7-2 Balances of Cations and Anions in the Extracellular Fluid (ECF) and Intracellular Fluid (ICF) Compartments in the Model of Selective Depletion of HCl. A,** The *top* part of the figure depicts events during the drainage period. **B,** The *bottom* part of the figure depicts events in the postdrainage period. *Drainage period:* There is loss of $Cl^-$ ions from the ECF compartment with a gain of $HCO_3^-$ ions in that compartment. There is loss of $K^+$ ions from the ICF compartment with some of these $HCO_3^-$ ions (in the form of organic anions) in the urine. To maintain electroneutrality in cells, $K^+$ ions exit from cells in exchange for $Na^+$ ions from the ECF compartment. *Postdrainage period:* There was an additional loss of $K^+$ ions from the ICF compartment. $K^+$ ions were excreted in the urine with sulfate $SO_4^{2-}$ anions that were produced from oxidation of dietary sulfur-containing amino acids to sulfuric acid ($H_2SO_4$). For electroneutrality in the ICF compartment, the shift of $K^+$ ions out of cells was accompanied by a shift of $H^+$ ions into cells. Because the amount of $HCO_3^-$ ions that was present in the ECF compartment was similar to the loss of $K^+$ ions that occurred during the postdrainage period, the $H^+$ ion gain in the ICF compartment at the end of the postdrainage period is roughly equal to the $HCO_3^-$ ion gain in the ECF compartment.

deficit, which preserves electroneutrality. If the loss of $K^+$ ions from the ICF compartment was accompanied by a shift of $Na^+$ ions from the ECF compartment, this process is also reversed with the administration of KCl. The retention of NaCl in the ECF compartment expands its volume and further lowers the concentration of $HCO_3^-$ ions by dilution.

## Deficit of KCl

### Gain of $HCO_3^-$ ions

The gain of $HCO_3^-$ ions in the ECF compartment is the result of two renal processes that are driven by a deficit of $K^+$ ions. $K^+$ ion depletion is associated with an acidified PCT cell pH. The first process is an enhanced excretion of $NH_4^+$ ions in the urine with $Cl^-$ ions, which adds $HCO_3^-$ ions to the body (Figure 7-3). The second process is the reduced excretion of organic anions such as citrate (i.e., potential $HCO_3^-$) in the urine. As shown in Figure 1-5, the dietary alkali load is eliminated by the excretion of organic anions (e.g., citrate)—this process is diminished when there is an acidified PCT cell pH (e.g., associated with a deficit of $K^+$ ions). Once the $P_{HCO_3}$ rises sufficiently to return the ICF pH toward its normal value, these patients can achieve acid–base balance by excreting the appropriate amounts of $NH_4^+$ ions and organic anions in the urine, as dictated by their dietary intake, but they do so at a higher $P_{HCO_3}$.

### Balance

One component of the pathophysiology of metabolic alkalosis in patients using diuretics is a deficit of KCl. The source for the $K^+$ ion deficit is $K^+$ ions from the ICF compartment. Initially, the loss of $K^+$ ions from the ICF was likely accompanied by a gain of $Na^+$ ions in the ICF (Figure 7-4, A). The resulting deficit of $K^+$ ions acidifies PCT cells, which results in retention of $HCO_3^-$ ions as described previously (see Figure 7-3). Because $K^+$ ions are excreted in the urine with $SO_4^{2-}$ anions produced from the oxidation of sulfur-containing amino acids (which yield $H_2SO_4$), to maintain electroneutrality, the shift of $K^+$ ions out of cells is accompanied by a shift of $H^+$ ions into cells (Figure 7-4, B). Therefore, the ICF has a deficit of $K^+$ ions and a gain of $H^+$ and $Na^+$ ions, while the ECF has a deficit of $Na^+$ and $Cl^-$ ions and a gain of $HCO_3^-$ ions. Balance data are not available, but bicarbonaturia is not expected with the correction of the KCl and NaCl deficits because there is not likely a large net gain of $HCO_3^-$ ions in the body.

### Deficit of NaCl

A deficit of NaCl results in an increase in the $HCO_3^-$ ion concentration in the ECF compartment primarily because of contraction of the

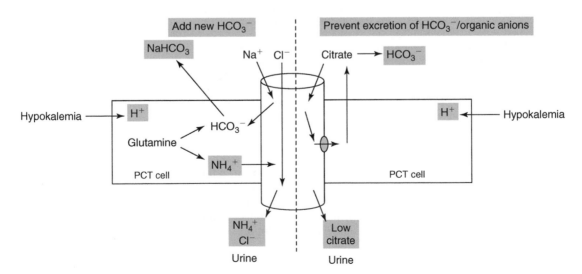

**Figure 7-3  Retention of $HCO_3^-$ ions in the Body During a Deficit of KCl.** The *central cylindrical structure* represents the lumen of the proximal convoluted tubule (PCT) with two rectangular structures representing two PCT cells. A deficit of $K^+$ ions is associated with intracellular acidosis in PCT cells. As shown *to the left of the dashed vertical line*, the production of $NH_4^+ + HCO_3^-$ ions is augmented. $NH_4^+$ ions are excreted in the urine with $Cl^-$ ions while the new $HCO_3^-$ ions are added to the body. As shown *to the right of the dashed vertical line*, intracellular acidosis augments the reabsorption of filtered organic anions (e.g., citrate), which diminishes the elimination of dietary alkali load.

ECF volume; the content of $HCO_3^-$ ions in the ECF compartment is largely unchanged. Angiotensin II, released in response to decreased EABV, is a potent stimulator of the reabsorption of $NaHCO_3$ in the PCT (see Chapter 1 for more discussion). Because there is no appreciable gain of $HCO_3^-$ ions in the body, bicarbonaturia is not likely to occur with correction of the NaCl deficit.

## Metabolic Alkalosis Caused by Retention of NaHCO₃

### Primary high mineralocorticoid activity

Patients with primary high mineralocorticoid activity may develop metabolic alkalosis when they become hypokalemic. These patients, however, do not have a deficit of $Cl^-$ ions. In this setting, there is an initial surplus of NaCl in the ECF compartment caused by the actions of mineralocorticoids to enhance the renal reabsorption of NaCl. The second primary event is the excretion of $K^+$ ions in the urine along with some of the $Cl^-$ ions that were retained. The source of these $K^+$ ions is from the ICF compartment, with electroneutrality maintained by the shift of $Na^+$ ions from the ECF compartment to the ICF compartment (Figure 7-5, $A$). Metabolic alkalosis develops because $K^+$ ion depletion is associated with an acidified PCT cell pH. This in turn results in an enhanced excretion of $NH_4^+$ ions in the urine with $Cl^-$ ions, which adds $HCO_3^-$ ions to the body. Also,

**ABBREVIATIONS**

ENaC, epithelial sodium channel
CDN, cortical distal nephron (includes the late distal convoluted tubule, the connecting segment, and the cortical collecting duct)
11 β-HSD2, the enzyme 11 β-hydroxy steroid dehydrogenase II
ROMK, renal outer medullary potassium channel

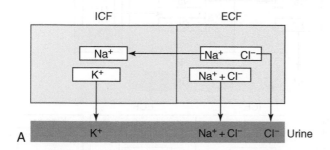

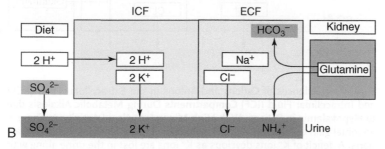

**Figure 7-4 Balances of Cations and Anions in the Extracellular Fluid (ECF) and Intracellular Fluid (ICF) Compartments During Metabolic Alkalosis due to a Deficit of KCl. A,** the initial loss of $K^+$ ions from the ICF compartment is accompanied by a gain of $Na^+$ ions. **B,** $K^+$ ion depletion is associated with acidified proximal convoluted tubule cells, which results in enhanced excretion of $NH_4^+$ ions in the urine with $Cl^-$ ions, and reduced excretion of organic anions such as citrate (i.e., potential $HCO_3^-$) in the urine; both processes add $HCO_3^-$ ions to the body (see Figure 7-3). $K^+$ ions are excreted in the urine with $SO_4^{2-}$ anions produced from the oxidation of sulfur-containing amino acids (which yields $H_2SO_4$). The shift of $K^+$ ions out of cells is accompanied by a shift of $H^+$ ions into cells. Therefore, there is a deficit of $K^+$ ions and a gain of $H^+$ and $Na^+$ ions in the ICF compartment, while in the ECF compartment there is a deficit of $Na^+$ and $Cl^-$ ions and a gain of $HCO_3^-$ ions.

because of the acidified PCT cell pH, the excretion of organic anions such as citrate (i.e., potential $HCO_3^-$) in the urine is reduced; therefore, some of the dietary alkali are retained with $Na^+$ ions. Again, because $K^+$ ions are excreted in the urine with $SO_4^{2-}$ anions produced from the oxidation of sulfur-containing amino acids (which yield $H_2SO_4$), the shift of $K^+$ ions out of cells is accompanied by a shift of $H^+$ ions into cells (Figure 7-5, *B*). Therefore, there is a net gain of NaCl and $NaHCO_3$ in ECF compartment, there is loss of $K^+$ ions from the ICF compartment, accompanied by a gain of $Na^+$ and $H^+$ ions in that compartment. Although balance data are not available in these patients, it is likely that with the correction of hypokalemia with the administration of KCl, which will lead to restoration of the usual pH in PCT cells, there will be an appreciable loss of $NaHCO_3$ in the urine because these patients have a surplus of $NaHCO_3$ in the body. The use of a blocker of the epithelial sodium channel (ENaC) in the cortical distal nephron (e.g., amiloride) or an aldosterone receptor blocker (e.g., spironolactone) will be required to induce a loss of NaCl and to prevent development of hypokalemia.

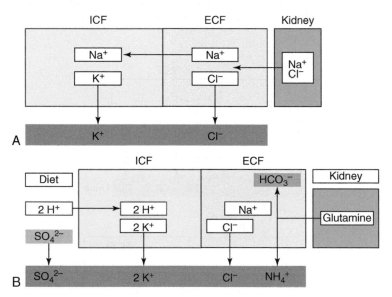

**Figure 7-5 Balances of Cations and Anions in the Extracellular Fluid (ECF) and Intracellular Fluid (ICF) Compartments During Metabolic Alkalosis due to Hypokalemia in Patients With High Mineralocorticoid Activity. A,** There is an initial gain of NaCl in the ECF compartment due to mineralocorticoid actions. A deficit of $K^+$ ions develops as $K^+$ ions are lost in the urine along with some of the $Cl^-$ ions that were retained. The source of $K^+$ ions is from the ICF; electroneutrality is maintained by the shift of $Na^+$ ions from the ECF compartment to the ICF compartment. **B,** Metabolic alkalosis develops because $K^+$ ion depletion is associated with acidified proximal convoluted tubule cells, which results in an enhanced excretion of $NH_4^+$ ions in the urine with $Cl^-$ ions, and also reduced excretion of organic anions such as citrate (i.e., potential $HCO_3^-$) in the urine and thereby the retention of some of the dietary alkali with $Na^+$ ions (see Figure 7-3). Because $K^+$ ions are excreted in the urine with $SO_4^{2-}$ anions produced from the oxidation of sulfur-containing amino acids, the shift of $K^+$ ions out of cells is accompanied by a shift of $H^+$ ions into cells. Therefore, there is a net gain of NaCl and $NaHCO_3$ in the ECF compartment and a loss of $K^+$ ions from the ICF compartment accompanied by a gain of $H^+$ and $Na^+$ ions.

### Input and retention of NaHCO₃

To understand the basis of this type of metabolic alkalosis, look for a source of $NaHCO_3$ input and also for a reason for a markedly reduced rate of renal excretion of $NaHCO_3$.

#### Source of alkali

A diet that contains fruit and vegetables provides an alkali load in the form of $K^+$ salts of organic anions (potential $HCO_3^-$; see Figure 1-5). In subjects who consume a typical Western diet, the daily intake of alkali is about 30 to 40 mEq. At times, the source of alkali is the intake of certain medications; examples include $NaHCO_3$ tablets, citrate anions (e.g., in $K^+$ supplements), and carbonate or hydroxyl anions (e.g., in some antacid preparations).

#### Renal reasons for a markedly reduced rate of excretion of NaHCO₃

The first reason for a markedly reduced rate of excretion of $NaHCO_3$ is a relatively large decrease in its filtered load because of a large reduction in the GFR. The second reason is the presence of the stimuli for $NaHCO_3$ reabsorption by PCT cells. The latter is due to an acidified PCT cell pH (usually because of hypokalemia) or a condition in which the level of angiotensin II is high despite an expanded EABV (e.g., renal artery stenosis or a renin-producing tumor).

## QUESTIONS

**7-2** *Why might a deficit of NaCl occur in patients with protracted vomiting or nasogastric suction?*

**7-3** *When HCl is secreted into the stomach during the cephalic phase of gastric secretion (before food is ingested), the $P_{HCO_3}$ rises. What is the renal response to this high $P_{HCO_3}$?*

**7-4** *Why do some infants who vomit have metabolic alkalosis, whereas others develop metabolic acidosis?*

# PART B
# CLINICAL SECTION

## CLINICAL APPROACH

A list of causes of metabolic alkalosis is provided in Table 7-1. Four aspects of the clinical picture in a patient with metabolic alkalosis merit careful attention. These include the medical history (e.g., vomiting, diuretic use), the presence of hypertension, assessment of EABV status, and the $P_K$.

Our clinical approach to a patient with metabolic alkalosis is outlined in Flow Chart 7-2. The first step is to rule out the common causes of metabolic alkalosis: vomiting and use of diuretics. Although this may be evident from the history, some patients may deny inducing vomiting or the use of diuretics; examining the urine electrolytes is particularly helpful if you suspect these diagnoses (Table 7-2). A very useful initial test to detect the cause of metabolic alkalosis is to examine the concentration of $Cl^-$ ions in the urine

TABLE 7-1 **CAUSES OF METABOLIC ALKALOSIS**

**Causes Usually Associated With a Contracted EABV**

- Low $U_{Cl}$
  - Loss of gastric secretions (e.g., vomiting, nasogastric suction)
  - Remote use of diuretics
  - Delivery of $Na^+$ ions to CDN with nonreabsorbable anions with increased reabsorption of $Na^+$ ions in CDN
  - Posthypercapnic states
  - Loss of HCl via lower gastrointestinal tract (e.g., congenital disorder with $Cl^-$ ion loss in diarrhea, acquired forms of DRA)
- High $U_{Cl}$
  - Recent use of diuretics
  - Inborn errors affecting transporters of $Na^+$ and/or $Cl^-$ ions in the thick ascending limb of the loop of Henle (e.g., Bartter syndrome) or in the distal convoluted tubule (e.g., Gitelman syndrome)
  - Pseudo-Bartter syndrome caused by ligand binding to the Ca-SR in the thick ascending limb of the loop of Henle (e.g., calcium in patients with hypercalcemia, gentamicin, cisplatin, cationic proteins)

**Causes Associated With an Expanded EABV and Possibly Hypertension**

- Disorders with primary enhanced mineralocorticoid activity causing hypokalemia
  - Primary hyperreninemic hyperaldosteronism (e.g., renal artery stenosis, malignant hypertension, renin-producing tumor)
  - Primary hyperaldosteronism (e.g., adrenal adenoma, bilateral adrenal hyperplesia, glucocorticoid, remediable aldosteronism)
  - Disorders with cortisol acting as a mineralocorticoid (e.g., apparent mineralocorticoid excess syndrome, inhibition of the enzyme 11 β-HSD2 by compounds containing glycyrrhetinic acid [e.g., licorice], ACTH-producing tumor)
  - Disorders with constitutively active ENaC in the CDN (e.g., Liddle syndrome)
- Large reduction in GFR plus a source of $NaHCO_3$

*ACTH*, Adrenocorticotropic hormone; *CDN*, cortical distal nephron; *Ca-SR*, calcium-sensing receptor; *DRA*, downregulated $Cl/HCO_3$ exchanger in adenoma/adenocarcinoma; *EABV*, effective arterial blood volume; *ENaC*, epithelial sodium channel; *GFR*, glomerular filtration rate; *11 β-HSD2*, 11 β-hydroxysteroid dehydrogenase 2.

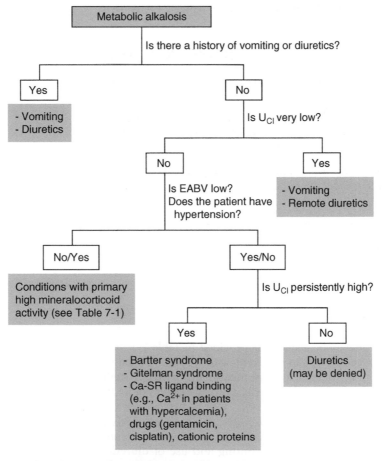

**Flow Chart 7-2 Clinical Approach to the Patient With Metabolic Alkalosis.** The $U_{Cl}$ should be very low if the cause of metabolic alkalosis is vomiting or the remote use of diuretics. If the $U_{Cl}$ is not low, an assessment of effective arterial blood volume (EABV) and blood pressure helps differentiate patients with disorders of high primary mineralocorticoid from those with diuretic abuse or Bartter or Gitelman syndromes. Serial measurements of $U_{Cl}$ in spot urine samples are helpful to separate patients with Bartter or Gitelman syndromes (persistently high $U_{Cl}$) from those with diuretic abuse (intermittently high $U_{Cl}$). *Ca-SR,* Calcium-sensing receptor in thick ascending limb of loop of Henle.

TABLE 7-2  **USE OF URINE ELECTROLYTES IN THE DIFFERENTIAL DIAGNOSIS OF EABV CONTRACTION**

In this table, "high" indicates a concentration of the electrolyte in the urine >15 mmol/L and "low" indicates a concentration <15 mmol/L. These values are based on a urine volume of 1 L/day and therefore must be adjusted for the urine volume if polyuria is present. Note that chronic diarrhea and the abuse of laxatives are usually associated with hyperchloremic metabolic acidosis. *EABV*, Effective arterial blood volume.

| | Urine Electrolyte | |
|---|---|---|
| CONDITION | Na⁺ | Cl⁻ |
| **Vomiting** | | |
| Recent | High | Low |
| Remote | Low | Low |
| **Diuretics** | | |
| Recent | High | High |
| Remote | Low | Low |
| **Diarrhea or laxative abuse** | Low | High |
| **Bartter or Gitelman syndrome** | High | High |

($U_{Cl}$). A very low $U_{Cl}$ is expected when there is a deficit of HCl and/or NaCl. Nevertheless, the $U_{Cl}$ may not be low if there is a recent intake of diuretics (see margin note). If the $U_{Cl}$ is not low, assessment of the EABV and blood pressure helps separate patients with disorders of high ENaC activity (see Table 7-1; EABV is not low, presence of hypertension) from those with diuretic abuse or Bartter or Gitelman syndromes (EABV is low, absence of hypertension). Serial measurements of $U_{Cl}$ in spot urine samples are helpful to separate patients with Bartter or Gitelman syndromes (persistently high $U_{Cl}$) from those with diuretic abuse (intermittently high $U_{Cl}$). Diuretic abuse may be confirmed by a urine assay for diuretics. This assay needs to be done, however, on a urine sample that has high concentrations of Na⁺ and Cl⁻ ions and hence may reflect the presence of a diuretic.

## EFFECT OF ALKALEMIA ON VENTILATION

Because the concentration of H⁺ ions in plasma is a major determinant of ventilation, alkalemia in patients with metabolic alkalosis depresses ventilation. In fact, there is a linear relationship between the increase in the $P_{HCO_3}$ and the increase in the arterial $PCO_2$; the slope is approximately 0.7. Thus, when patients present with $CO_2$ retention and alkalemia, the alkalemia should be corrected before attributing the $CO_2$ retention to a respiratory disease.

Hypoventilation may cause a lower arterial $PO_2$. The reduced delivery of $O_2$ to tissues is further aggravated by the effect of alkalemia to shift the $O_2$-hemoglobin dissociation curve to the left, which increases the affinity of hemoglobin for $O_2$. Hypoxemia may offset the degree of respiratory suppression by alkalemia, and thus a rise in the arterial $PCO_2$ may be observed in patients receiving $O_2$ supplementation when the hypoxemia is corrected.

Patients with chronic lung disease and chronic respiratory acidosis commonly develop edema secondary to NaCl retention and are often given diuretics. Therefore, they may develop a metabolic alkalosis superimposed on their chronic respiratory acidosis. This may return the plasma H⁺ ion concentration toward the normal range, but their clinical condition may deteriorate when they no longer have the effects of acidemia to drive ventilation (Table 7-3).

**CAVEATS IN THE USE OF URINE ELECTROLYTES TO DETECT CAUSE OF EABV CONTRACTION**

- Both Na⁺ and Cl⁻ ion concentrations may be high (e.g., recent intake of diuretics, acute tubular necrosis).
- Na⁺ ion concentration may be high in a patient with recent vomiting because the excretion of the anion $HCO_3^-$ obligates the loss of the cation Na⁺.
- Cl⁻ ion concentration in the urine may be high during diarrhea or laxative abuse because excretion of the cation $NH_4^+$ obligates the excretion of the anion Cl⁻.

# COMMON CAUSES OF CHRONIC METABOLIC ALKALOSIS

## VOMITING

The diagnosis is obvious if the patient has a history of prolonged vomiting or nasogastric suction (see margin note). The difficulty arises if the patient denies vomiting. Nevertheless, there are some helpful clues to suggest the diagnosis: the patient is particularly concerned with body image, has a profession where weight control is important (e.g., ballet dancer, fashion model), has an eating disorder, and/or has a psychiatric disorder that might lead to self-induced vomiting. The physical examination may also provide some helpful clues including a calloused lesion on the back of the finger or knuckles, which are often inserted into the mouth to induce vomiting, and erosion of dental enamel from repeated exposure to HCl.

The EABV is often mildly contracted (see the discussion of Question 7-1). If the EABV is markedly contracted, one should consider other reasons for excessive loss of $Na^+$ ions. Hypokalemia is usually present, and a deficit of KCl is a major factor in the pathophysiology of the metabolic alkalosis in these patients. Alkalemia suppresses the respiratory center, and this leads to hypoventilation. A primary respiratory acidosis may be present if respiratory muscle weakness occurs because of hypokalemia. On the other hand, a primary respiratory alkalosis may be present if the patient develops aspiration pneumonia, for example. In patients with chronic vomiting, $U_{Cl}$ is very low. If there has been recent vomiting, the $U_{Na}$ may be high due to bicarbonaturia (the urine pH will be >7.0).

## DIURETICS

The key findings in patients with metabolic alkalosis due to the use of diuretics are low EABV, hypokalemia, and intermittently high concentrations of $Na^+$ and $Cl^-$ ions in the urine (when the diuretic is acting). A large deficit of NaCl is most commonly seen in patients who have a low intake of NaCl (e.g., in the elderly). Hypokalemia is more likely to occur in patients who have a low intake of $K^+$ ions.

The use of diuretics might be denied at times, especially in patients who are particularly concerned with their body image. To help sort out these patients from those with Bartter or Gitelman syndromes, measure the urine electrolytes using multiple random urine samples (see Table 7-3). An assay for diuretics in the urine may be helpful; make sure, however, that the assay is performed in a urine sample that contains high concentrations of $Na^+$ and $Cl^-$ ions.

Some cationic agents (e.g., drugs such as gentamicin or cisplatin or cationic proteins in some patients with multiple myeloma) may bind to the calcium-sensing receptor in the thick ascending limb of the loop of

**ZOLLINGER–ELLISON SYNDROME**

- Metabolic alkalosis might be particularly severe when there is a gastrin-producing tumor because this hormone stimulates the secretion of HCl in the stomach.
- The most common symptoms are abdominal pain and diarrhea caused by intestinal irritation and destruction of digestive enzymes by HCl.

TABLE 7-3   **EFFECT OF ALKALEMIA IN PATIENTS WITH $CO_2$ RETENTION**

Data are derived from eight patients with chronic respiratory acidosis prior to and following therapy for metabolic alkalosis. All values reported are from measurements in arterial blood. There is a little difference in the [$H^+$] in plasma before and after therapy of the coexisting metabolic alkalosis in patients with chronic respiratory acidosis. After correction of the metabolic alkalosis, however, the arterial $PCO_2$ is lower and the arterial $PO_2$ is higher. The increase in the $O_2$ content of blood can be large if the changes in $PO_2$ are occurring on the steeper portion of the sigmoid shape of the $O_2$ saturation curve: the arterial $PO_2$ curve.

| | $H^+$ (nmol/L) | $P_{HCO_3}$ (mmol/L) | $PCO_2$ (mm Hg) | $PO_2$ (mm Hg) |
|---|---|---|---|---|
| Before therapy | 40 | 37 | 61 | 52 |
| After therapy | 42 | 28 | 48 | 69 |

Henle (Ca-SR) and lead to a picture that mimics Bartter syndrome (see Chapter 14 for more discussion of Bartter and Gitelman syndromes).

## LESS COMMON CAUSES OF CHRONIC METABOLIC ALKALOSIS

### CONDITIONS WITH HIGH MINERALOCORTICOID ACTIVITY

The specific disorders are listed in Table 7-1 and are discussed in detail in Chapter 14.

Hypokalemia is of major importance in the pathophysiology of the metabolic alkalosis in these patients. Because of the high mineralocorticoid activity or a constitutively active ENaC, principal cells of the cortical distal nephron (CDN) have an increased number of open ENaC in their luminal membrane. Electrogenic reabsorption of $Na^+$ ions (i.e., without $Cl^-$ ions) in CDN via ENaC generates a lumen-negative transepithelial voltage that drives the secretion of $K^+$ ions into the luminal fluid, if principal cells have open renal outer medullary potassium (ROMK) channels in their luminal membrane. Hypokalemia is associated with an acidified PCT cell pH. This results in an enhanced excretion of $NH_4^+$ ions in the urine with $Cl^-$ ions, which adds $HCO_3^-$ ions to the body. It also results in decreased excretion of organic anions such as citrate (i.e., potential $HCO_3^-$) in the urine.

### METABOLIC ALKALOSIS ASSOCIATED WITH MILK-ALKALI SYNDROME

Although milk and absorbable alkali are not used nowadays to treat duodenal ulcers, this form of metabolic alkalosis still continues to be present, but the setting has changed. Its cardinal features are still a source of dietary alkali and absence of suppression of the stimuli for the PCT to retain alkali. Hypercalcemia is the key player in this clinical scenario. The intake of calcium supplements, commonly in the form of calcium carbonate tablets, is now a common cause of hypercalcemia, particularly in elderly women. Hypercalcemia develops primarily because more calcium is absorbed in the intestinal tract (especially if the intake of calcium exceeds that of dietary phosphate; see Part C for more details). When more calcium binds to Ca-SR on the basolateral membrane of cells in the medullary thick ascending limb of the loop of Henle, it generates a signal that inhibits the flux of $K^+$ ions through the luminal ROMK. This inhibits $Na^+$ and $Cl^-$ ion reabsorption akin to the effect of a loop diuretic (see Chapter 9 for more details). Therefore, hypercalcemia leads to an excessive excretion of NaCl and KCl in the urine. The combination of a contracted EABV and direct effects of hypercalcemia can cause a marked reduction in the GFR, which itself further reduces the filtration and excretion of $HCO_3^-$ ions in the urine. Angiotensin II released in response to a contracted EABV stimulates the reabsorption of $HCO_3^-$ ions in PCT. A deficit of $K^+$ ions is associated with intracellular acidosis in PCT cells, which leads to the retention of ingested alkali. Therapy consists of stopping the intake of calcium and alkali and replacing the deficits of NaCl and KCl.

### METABOLIC ALKALOSIS ASSOCIATED WITH A POSTHYPERCAPNIC STATE

In the course of chronic hypercapnia, there is a rise in $P_{HCO_3}$. This is because of the effect of the high $PCO_2$ to cause a fall in pH cells of the PCT, which stimulates ammoniagenesis and results in the excretion of $NH_4^+$ ions with $Cl^-$ ions in the urine with the additions of $HCO_3^-$ ions to the body. If the patient has a contracted EABV after the hypercapnia resolves, $NaHCO_3$ will continue to be retained because the high angiotensin II levels stimulate the reabsorption of $NaHCO_3$ by PCT cells. Expansion of the EABV lowers angiotensin II levels and causes the excretion of the excess $NaHCO_3$.

### METABOLIC ALKALOSIS ASSOCIATED WITH THE INTAKE OF NONREABSORBABLE ANIONS

Hypokalemia may develop because of intake of a $Na^+$ salt with an anion that cannot be reabsorbed by the kidney (e.g., $Na^+$ carbenicillinate) in a patient who has a contracted EABV. Hypokalemia is due to actions of aldosterone, which increases electrogenic $Na^+$ ion reabsorption via ENaC in CDN and hence $K^+$ ion secretion, providing that the delivery of $Cl^-$ ions is low. The rise in $P_{HCO_3}$ in these patients is the result of the deficits of NaCl and KCl.

### METABOLIC ALKALOSIS ASSOCIATED WITH HYPOMAGNESEMIA

Patients with hypomagnesemia may develop hypokalemia and metabolic alkalosis. The usual clinical settings for $Mg^{2+}$ deficiency include malabsorption, chronic alcoholism, chronic use of proton pump inhibitors, use of loop diuretics, or the administration of drugs that may bind the Ca-SR in the loop of Henle (e.g., cisplatin or aminoglycosides). These patients must be distinguished from those with primary hyperaldosteronism and those with Bartter or Gitelman syndrome who may also have hypomagnesemia.

## THERAPY OF METABOLIC ALKALOSIS

There are two major groups of disorders that can cause metabolic alkalosis: those that are due to deficits of HCl, KCl, or NaCl, and those that are due to the retention of $NaHCO_3$. For the former, one must replace the appropriate deficit, whereas for the latter, one must induce a loss of $NaHCO_3$ by treating the underlying disorder.

### PATIENTS WITH METABOLIC ALKALOSIS CAUSED BY DEFICITS OF $Cl^-$ SALTS

A deficit of more than one $Cl^-$-containing compound—HCl, NaCl, or KCl—may be present in the same patient. While it is suggested to use NaCl as the main therapy for what is called "saline-responsive metabolic alkalosis," clearly NaCl will not replace a deficit of KCl. Although one can lower the $P_{HCO_3}$ by overexpanding the ECF volume, this does not return the composition of the ECF and ICF compartments to normal when there is a deficit of KCl. If the deficit of $K^+$ ions in cells was accompanied by a gain of $H^+$ ions, giving KCl will cause $K^+$ ions to enter cells and $H^+$ ions to exit; these $H^+$ ions will remove the extra $HCO_3^-$ ions in the ECF compartment, while the retained $Cl^-$ ions replace its deficit in the ECF compartment. If the deficit of $K^+$ ions in cells was accompanied by a gain of $Na^+$ ion, giving KCl will cause the exit of $Na^+$ ions from cells, and this extra NaCl will be excreted if there is no deficit of NaCl in the ECF compartment.

In a patient with hypokalemia, the emergencies to consider are cardiac arrhythmia and hypoventilation because of respiratory muscle weakness. Emergency treatment of hypokalemia is discussed in Chapter 14. It is also important to note that the administration of KCl may cause a rise in $P_{Na}$ and hence the risk of osmotic demyelination in a patient with chronic hyponatremia and hypo-kalemia. Furthermore, patients with hypokalemia are at increased risk for osmotic demyelination with rapid correction of chronic hyponatremia.

In patients with a deficit of NaCl and hemodynamic instability, one must administer an isotonic $Na^+$-containing solution quickly until hemodynamic stability is restored. One can use the hematocrit and/or the $P_{Albumin}$ to obtain a quantitative estimate of the deficit of NaCl. Caution must be exerted in patients with chronic hyponatremia to avoid a water diuresis because distal delivery of filtrate is increased and/or vasopressin release is suppressed with EABV expansion. A water diuresis may lead to a rapid rise in $P_{Na}$ and risk of osmotic demyelination (see Chapter 10).

## PATIENTS WITH METABOLIC ALKALOSIS CAUSED BY RETENTION OF NaHCO₃

In patients with disorders that cause a high mineralocorticoid effect, specific therapy depends on the underlying disease (see Chapter 14). Notwithstanding, there might be a large excretion of $NaHCO_3$ in the urine when enough KCl is given to correct this deficit of $K^+$ ions. The use of an ENaC blocker (e.g., amiloride) or an aldosterone receptor blocker (e.g., spironolactone) will be required to induce a loss of NaCl and to prevent the development of hypokalemia.

The carbonic anhydrase inhibitor acetazolamide is sometimes used (e.g., when weaning a patient who has metabolic alkalosis from mechanical ventilation) to inhibit the reabsorption of $NaHCO_3$ in PCT and hence diminish the degree of alkalemia and hypoventilation. $K^+$ ion loss can be very high when a large load of $NaHCO_3^-$-rich fluid is delivered to the CDN.

If the alkalemia is very severe, one can give $H^+$ ions in the form of HCl or $NH_4Cl$. If the patient has fixed alveolar ventilation, however, the arterial $PCO_2$ may rise with $H^+$ ion administration as production of $CO_2$ increases. This is not likely, however, to pose a significant risk if the rate of infusion is slow.

Therapy is more difficult in the group of patients in whom there is retention of alkali because of a very low GFR. It is obvious that the input of alkali must be diminished (e.g., using a dialysate fluid with a lower concentration of $HCO_3^-$ ions in patients on hemodialysis). As a preventive measure to minimize the risk of developing metabolic alkalosis in a patient with a markedly reduced GFR who requires nasogastric suction, a blocker of the gastric $H^+/K^+$-ATPase can be administered.

# PART C
# INTEGRATIVE PHYSIOLOGY

## INTEGRATIVE PHYSIOLOGY OF CALCIUM HOMEOSTASIS

We use data from Case 7-3 to provide an understanding of some aspects of the integrative physiology of calcium homeostasis and illustrate how hypercalcemia might develop. Hypercalcemia develops when the input of calcium exceeds its output; a steady state with hypercalcemia may be reached at which the excretion of calcium matches the increased input. The focus here is on the input of calcium from the gastrointestinal tract.

## INPUT OF CALCIUM FROM THE GASTROINTESTINAL TRACT

The patient discussed in Case 7-3 ingested calcium hydroxide ($Ca[OH]_2$), a sparingly soluble compound that was used to remove the bitter taste of the betel nut preparation (a form of local anesthetic to the taste buds). Calcium carbonate ($CaCO_3$) tablets are commonly used to prevent or treat osteoporosis. The use of $CaCO_3$ tablets is currently the third leading cause of hypercalcemia in adults. These poorly soluble alkaline forms of calcium are converted to ionized calcium in the stomach because of HCl secretion (Figure 7-6).

There are two possible fates of ionized $Ca^{2+}$ in the duodenum. First, it may be absorbed; the active form of vitamin D stimulates this process. Second, if sufficient $NaHCO_3$ is secreted into the duodenum, ionized $Ca^{2+}$ is precipitated as $CaCO_3$. Formation of $CaCO_3$ has two major effects. First, it stops the absorption of more calcium because it is no longer in its ionized form. Second, because of the low level of ionized $Ca^{2+}$, phosphate ions produced by digestion of dietary organic phosphates remain as ionized inorganic phosphate, which permits their absorption.

The next issue to consider is the fate of $CaCO_3$ in the lower intestinal tract (Figure 7-7). Ionized calcium is formed if the $CaCO_3$ can be redissolved; a source of $H^+$ ions is needed for this to occur. There is a large source of $H^+$ ions in the later segment of the small intestine and the colon: organic acids produced by the fermentation of carbohydrates (fiber and fructose from the diet) by bacteria. In fact, more than twice as many $H^+$ ions are produced in these segments as secreted by the stomach each day. If, because of a low phosphate intake (diet poor in meat and fish), the delivery of divalent phosphate ($HPO_4^{2-}$) ions is less than is required to precipitate all the ionized $Ca^{2+}$ as calcium phosphate, some ionized $Ca^{2+}$ could remain in the lumen and be absorbed passively and at a site where its absorption is not regulated. Hence, hypercalcemia may develop because of the intake of calcium tablets, especially when there is a low intake of phosphate (e.g., elderly individuals, patients with anorexia).

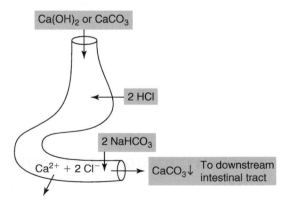

**Figure 7-6 Generation and Absorption of Ionized Calcium in the Upper Intestinal Tract.** Alkaline calcium salts, $Ca(OH)_2$ or $CaCO_3$, are poorly soluble in water but are converted by gastric HCl to ionized calcium ($Ca^{2+}$), which can be absorbed. When $NaHCO_3$ is added in the duodenum, insoluble $CaCO_3$ is formed.

# OUTPUT OF CALCIUM

Ionized $Ca^{2+}$ is reabsorbed in the thick ascending limb of the loop of Henle via the paracellular pathway, driven by the lumen-positive voltage. This lumen-positive voltage is generated via the electroneutral reabsorption of 1 $Na^+$, 1 $K^+$, and 2 $Cl^-$ ions by the Na/K/2 Cl cotransporter 2 (NKCC2), with the subsequent electrogenic exit of $K^+$ ions via the luminal ROMK channel. A rise in activity of ionized $Ca^{2+}$ in the medullary interstitial compartment because of hypercalcemia increases binding of ionized $Ca^{2+}$ to the Ca-SR on the basolateral membrane of cells in the thick ascending limb of the loop of Henle. This generates a signal to inhibit the flux of $K^+$ ions through luminal ROMK, and hence the lumen-positive voltage is decreased (Figure 7-8). As a result, less ionized $Ca^{2+}$ is reabsorbed in this nephron segment (see margin note). This results in a large increase in the delivery of calcium to the last sites where its reabsorption is regulated, the late distal convoluted tubule and the connecting segment. Reabsorption of ionized $Ca^{2+}$ in these segments will be decreased because parathyroid hormone secretion is suppressed by hypercalcemia (if hypercalcemia is not due to primary hyperparathyroidism). The net effect is an increase in the rate of excretion of calcium.

# DISCUSSION OF CASES

## CASE 7-1: THIS MAN SHOULD NOT HAVE METABOLIC ALKALOSIS

**What are the major threats to the patient and how should these dictate the therapy?**

1. *Acute hyponatremia*: The danger is brain herniation due to increased intracranial pressure caused by swelling of brain cells.

### ROLE OF CLAUDINS

- Claudins are tight junction proteins that can function as channels or barriers for movement of ions through the paracellular pathway in epithelial cells.
- In the thick ascending limb of the loop of Henle, claudin-16 and claudin-19 form cationic channels that mediate the paracellular reabsorption of ionized $Ca^{2+}$ and ionized $Mg^{2+}$. Claudin-14 inhibits claudin-16 and claudin-19 through physical interaction.
- Activation of the Ca-SR leads to decreased paracellular permeability for ionized $Ca^{2+}$ and $Mg^{2+}$. Calcineurin activates nuclear factor of activated T cells (NFAT), leading to increased transcription of two microRNAs that downregulate claudin-14 expression. Signaling though the Ca-SR inhibits calcineurin, and therefore leads to increased expression of claudin-14.

**Figure 7-7 Prevention of Absorption of Ionized Calcium Downstream in the Intestinal Tract.** The *large rectangle* represents the lower intestinal tract and the colon, where calcium can be absorbed if it exists in an ionized form. Calcium is delivered as a precipitate of $CaCO_3$. Ionized calcium ($Ca^{2+}$) is formed when $CaCO_3$ is dissolved by the $H^+$ ions of the organic acids produced by bacterial fermentation of dietary fiber and/or fructose. If the delivery of divalent inorganic phosphate ($HPO_4^{2-}$) is less than required to precipitate all the ionized $Ca^{2+}$ as calcium phosphate, some ionized $Ca^{2+}$ could remain in the lumen and be absorbed passively. Absorption and subsequent metabolism of the organic anions ($OA^-$) produced in this fermentation process to neutral end products represents the conversion of some of the alkali in $CaCO_3$ to $HCO_3^-$ ions in the body.

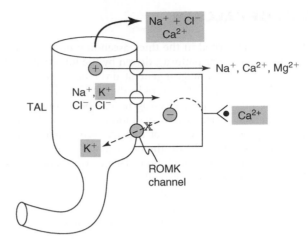

**Figure 7-8 Physiology of the Calcium-Sensing Receptor in the Loop of Henle.** The structure in the figure represents the thick ascending limb (TAL) of the loop of Henle with one of its epithelial cells. A rise in activity of ionized calcium in the medullary interstitial compartment because of hypercalcemia increases binding of calcium to the calcium-sensing receptor (Ca-SR) on the basolateral surface of cells in the TAL of the loop of Henle. This generates a signal to inhibit the flux of $K^+$ ions through luminal renal outer medullary potassium channel (ROMK) and diminishes the lumen-positive voltage, which is required to drive the paracellular reabsorption of $Na^+$, $Ca^{2+}$, and $Mg^{2+}$ ions. Hence, more $Na^+$, $Cl^-$, $Ca^{2+}$, and $Mg^{2+}$ ions are delivered to downstream nephron sites.

*What is the basis of hyponatremia?*: Because he weighed 80 kg and has a muscular build, his initial total body water was ~50 L (ECF volume was 15 L, ICF volume was 35 L). Because he has hyponatremia, his ICF volume is expanded due to water gain. The percent expansion of his ICF volume is close to the percent fall in his $P_{Na}$, i.e., ~11%. Hence, he has a water gain in his ICF of ~4 L. Because his hematocrit is 0.50, his ECF volume had decreased by close to one-third from its normal value of ~15 to ~10 L; accordingly, he lost 5 L of ECF volume. This is a loss of 5 L of water and 700 mmol of $Na^+$ ions (5 L × 140 mmol $Na^+$/L). In addition, because his $P_{Na}$ decreased from 140 to 125 mmol/L, each of the remaining 10 L of ECF volume has a loss of 15 mmol of $Na^+$ ions. Hence, his total $Na^+$ ion loss is 850 mmol. Therefore, in total body balance terms, he has a loss of 850 mmol of $Na^+$ ion and 1 L of water (a loss of 5 L of water from his ECF compartment and a gain of 4 L of water in his ICF compartment). Hence, the primary basis of his hyponatremia is a deficit of $Na^+$ ions.

2. *Hemodynamic instability*: An infusion of isotonic saline was started in the field, and he was hemodynamically stable on arrival at the emergency department.

After it was recognized that his $P_{Na}$ was 125 mmol/L, his intravenous therapy was changed from isotonic saline to 3% hypertonic saline. The goal of therapy was to raise his $P_{Na}$ by 5 mmol/L rapidly. Because his hyponatremia was acute, there was little risk (if any) of causing osmotic demyelination by rapidly correcting his hyponatremia. Furthermore, there may be a large volume of water retained in his stomach that may be absorbed (especially as intestinal motility is improved with the correction of his hypokalemia), which may cause a sudden fall in his arterial $P_{Na}$. We would continue with the infusion of 3% hypertonic saline to replace his $Na^+$ ion deficit and bring his $P_{Na}$ back to the normal range (see Chapter 10).

3. *Hypokalemia*: This did not represent an emergency because he did not have cardiac arrhythmia or respiratory muscle weakness. As discussed in the following paragraphs, the basis of the hypokalemia seemed to be largely due to an acute shift of $K^+$ ions into his ICF compartment. An intravenous infusion of isotonic saline supplemented with 40 mmol/L of KCl was started. His $P_K$ was followed closely.

### What is the basis for metabolic alkalosis?

To determine if the basis of metabolic alkalosis in this patient is a deficit of HCl, KCl, and/or NaCl, a quantitative analysis of the degree of contraction of the ECF volume is needed. As mentioned previously, based on a hematocrit of 0.50 (assuming a baseline hematocrit of 0.40), his ECF volume was decreased by close to one-third, from its normal value of ~15 to ~10 L; accordingly, he lost 5 L of ECF volume.

#### *Balance data for $Na^+$, $K^+$, and $Cl^-$ ions*

#### *Deficit of HCl*

There was no history of vomiting, so a deficit of HCl is a very unlikely basis for metabolic alkalosis.

#### *Deficit of NaCl*

The decrease in his ECF volume was ~5 L. One can now calculate how much this degree of ECF volume contraction would raise his $P_{HCO_3}$ (divide the normal content of $HCO_3^-$ ions in his ECF compartment [15 L × 25 mmol/L or 375 mmol] by his new ECF volume of 10 L). His $P_{HCO_3}$ would be 37.5 mmol/L, a value that is remarkably close to the measured $P_{HCO_3}$ of 38 mmol/L, suggesting that a major reason for the rise in his $P_{HCO_3}$ is the fall in his ECF volume.

#### *Balance for $Na^+$ ions*

As calculated previously, the deficit of $Na^+$ ions in his ECF compartment was ~850 mmol.

#### *Balance for $Cl^-$ ions*

Multiplying his $P_{Cl}$ before the training exercise (103 mmol/L) by his normal ECF volume (15 L) yields content of $Cl^-$ ions in his ECF compartment of ~1545 mmol. After the training exercise, his $P_{Cl}$ was 70 mmol/L and his ECF volume was 10 L; hence, the content of $Cl^-$ ions in his ECF compartment was now 700 mmol. Accordingly, the deficit of $Cl^-$ ions in his ECF compartment is ~840 mmol, a value that is similar to his deficit of $Na^+$ ions.

#### *Balance for $K^+$*

There was little difference between the deficits of $Na^+$ and $Cl^-$ ions; hence, there was no appreciable deficit of KCl to account for a drop in $P_K$ to 2.7 mmol/L. Accordingly, the major mechanism for his hypokalemia is likely to be a shift of $K^+$ ions into cells (due to a $\beta_2$-adrenergic surge, the release of insulin due to a large intake of sugar, and possibly the effect of alkalemia).

The next issue to examine is the possible routes for such a large loss of NaCl in such a short time period. Because diarrhea and polyuria were not present, the only route for a large NaCl loss is via sweat.

## LOSS OF ELECTROLYTES IN SWEAT IN PATIENTS WITH CYSTIC FIBROSIS

- Cystic fibrosis is caused by mutations in the cystic fibrosis transmembrane regulator (CFTR) protein, a complex chloride channel and regulatory protein found in all exocrine organs including the sweat glands.
- The concentrations of $Na^+$ and $Cl^-$ ions in sweat in patients with cystic fibrosis can be as high as 100 mmol/L as compared to <30 mmol/L in normal subjects.
- The mechanism for the loss of $K^+$ and $Cl^-$ ions is described in the legend for the figure in the margin below.

**Ion balance in sweat**

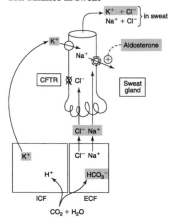

The structure with a coil represents the sweat gland with its channels for $Na^+$ ions (ENaC) and for $Cl^-$ ions (CFTR). Aldosterone causes ENaC to be open, and more $Na^+$ ions are reabsorbed than $Cl^-$ ions when CFTR is defective. To the extent that there are open $K^+$ ion channels in the luminal membrane of sweat ducts, some $K^+$ ions are lost with $Cl^-$ ions. The lower rectangles represent the body with its ECF and its ICF compartments. Electroneutrality is achieved in each compartment when $K^+$ and $Cl^-$ ions are lost— $H^+$ ions replace $K^+$ ions in the ICF compartment, and $HCO_3^-$ ions replace $Cl^-$ ions in the ECF compartment. *CFTR*, Cystic fibrosis transmembrane regulator; *ECF*, extracellular fluid; *ICF*, intracellular fluid.

To have a high electrolyte concentration in sweat and a large sweat volume, the likely underlying lesion would be cystic fibrosis (see margin note). The diagnosis of cystic fibrosis was confirmed later by molecular studies.

### What is the therapy for metabolic alkalosis in this patient?

Knowing that the basis for the metabolic alkalosis is largely an acute deficit of NaCl, he requires a positive balance of ~850 mmol of NaCl to replace his deficit. He was initially given hypertonic saline to deal with the danger of acute hyponatremia. After the administration of only 40 mmol of KCl, his $P_K$ rose to 3.8 mmol/L, adding support to our speculation that the major cause for his hypokalemia was an acute shift of $K^+$ ions into cells.

### CASE 7-2: WHY DID THIS PATIENT DEVELOP METABOLIC ALKALOSIS SO QUICKLY?

### Why did this patient develop metabolic alkalosis on days 3 and 4?

The first step is to look for the common causes of metabolic alkalosis. Because there is no history of vomiting, there is no evidence for a loss of HCl. Similarly, there is no evidence of a large loss of NaCl by any of the usual routes; the absence of a rise in hematocrit also provides evidence to support the impression that there is not a large deficit of NaCl. Therefore, only a KCl deficit is a possible explanation for the metabolic alkalosis in this patient.

He appears to have renal $K^+$ ion wasting on day 3 because he is modestly hypokalemic ($P_K$ 3.2 mmol/L) and his urine on the morning of day 4 contained more $K^+$ ions than expected (~4 mmol $K^+$ ions/mmol creatinine, expected less than 1 to 1.5 mmol $K^+$ ions/mmol creatinine). A possible reason for the excessive excretion of $K^+$ ions is the administration of high doses of cortisol. When very large amounts of cortisol are given, some of this hormone escapes destruction by the enzymes, 11 β-HSD2 in principal cells of the CDN. As a result, some cortisol binds to the mineralocorticoid receptor, resulting in aldosterone-like actions that promote kaliuresis (see Chapter 14 for more discussion).

The sudden fall in $P_K$ from 3.2 to 1.7 mmol/L in just 24 hours while the $K^+$ excretion rate was modest suggests that there had been an acute shift of $K^+$ ions into cells. Perhaps this is related to high insulin levels (dietary intake of carbohydrate), prolonged $\beta_2$-adrenergic actions of his medications for treatment of asthma, and the acute rise in his $P_{HCO_3}$.

For a rise in $P_{HCO_3}$, he needs an input of alkali and the preservation of the stimuli for the reabsorption of $NaHCO_3$ in the PCT. The input of alkali was due to his dietary intake of fruit and vegetables (but the amount needed is larger than that in the usual dietary intake). The presence of the mild degree of hypokalemia leads to an acidified PCT cell pH, which promotes the reabsorption of $HCO_3^-$ ions and diminishes the elimination of dietary alkali via the excretion of citrate and other organic anions (see Figure 7-2). Of note, he did have a high urine pH and a large excretion of $NaHCO_3$ during therapy, suggesting that the basis for the metabolic alkalosis was a net gain of alkali.

Although it is difficult to determine how large a deficit of KCl was present and to what degree an acute shift of $K^+$ ions into cells was contributing to this profound degree of hypokalemia, this will become evident from the amount of KCl that is needed to correct the hypokalemia.

## CASE 7-3: MILK-ALKALI SYNDROME, BUT WITHOUT MILK

### What is the basis for the metabolic alkalosis?

The major possibilities considered are discussed in the following.

#### Deficit of HCl

There was no history of vomiting, which means that there was likely no deficit of HCl.

#### Deficit of NaCl

He did not take a diuretic drug, but hypercalcemia can cause inhibition of the reabsorption of $Na^+$ and $Cl^-$ ions in the thick ascending limb of the loop of Henle. The fact that he had a contracted EABV and that the concentrations $Na^+$ and $Cl^-$ ions in his urine were not low is consistent with this impression. The presence of a high plasma renin activity would add support to this interpretation. A contracted ECF volume because of the deficit of NaCl is an important reason for the high $P_{HCO_3}$.

#### Deficit of KCl

There was a modest degree of hypokalemia and a high rate of $K^+$ excretion in this setting. Thus, a deficit of KCl has also contributed to the development of his metabolic alkalosis.

#### Ingestion of alkali

The patient ingested calcium salts of alkali; this, however, is not sufficient on its own to cause chronic metabolic alkalosis. Alkali were retained because of the presence of angiotensin II (caused by a contracted EABV) and an acidified PCT cell (caused by hypokalemia).

### What should the initial therapy be?

The most important component of the initial therapy in this patient is the administration of intravenous isotonic saline to re-expand his EABV. This should cause a fall in $P_{HCO_3}$. His calcium concentration in plasma fell to normal levels by the end of day 1, and this was due to both a decrease in calcium input and an enhanced excretion of calcium caused by the expanded EABV. In more detail, about 70% of filtered calcium is reabsorbed in the PCT; this process is passive and parallels the reabsorption of $Na^+$ ions. This is because the reabsorption of $Na^+$ ions and water raises the luminal concentration of ionized $Ca^{2+}$, which drives its passive reabsorption via the paracellular pathway. Expansion of the EABV diminishes the reabsorption of $Na^+$ ions and thereby of ionized $Ca^{2+}$ in the PCT.

The metabolic alkalosis resolved completely due in large part to reexpansion of his ECF volume and the correction of the KCl deficit.

## DISCUSSION OF QUESTIONS

7-1 *What might be the advantages of not having a tubular maximum for the renal reabsorption of* $NaHCO_3$?

There a number of advantages not to have a tubular maximum for the renal reabsorption of $NaHCO_3$. If there were a tubular maximum of its reabsorption, $NaHCO_3$ would be lost in the urine during the daily alkaline tide. If this were to occur, the ECF volume would decrease. This would be an important problem for subjects who have little NaCl in their diet (e.g., our Paleolithic ancestors). There are other problems as well. For example, by excreting $HCO_3^-$ ions in the urine, its pH could be high enough to cause precipitation of calcium phosphate ($CaHPO_4$) kidney stones. A high rate of excretion of $HCO_3^-$ ions in the urine would lead to high rates of $K^+$ ion excretion and $K^+$ ion depletion. In addition, there would be a deficit of $HCO_3^-$ ions when $NaHCO_3$ is secreted by the pancreas into the duodenum. The resultant metabolic acidosis would require high rates of excretion of $NH_4^+$ ions to regenerate new $HCO_3^-$ ions by the kidney. This could have caused medullary damage and perhaps chronic renal insufficiency because of tubulointerstitial inflammation caused by activation of the complement system by amidation.

*7-2  Why might a deficit of NaCl occur in patients with protracted vomiting or nasogastric suction?*

To create a negative balance for NaCl, its loss must exceed its intake. Because losses are small in this setting, a prerequisite to develop a deficit of NaCl is a low intake of this salt. There are, however, two sites of loss of NaCl in patients with vomiting or nasogastric suction.

**Loss in the gastric fluid**

Although there are no $Na^+$ ions to speak of in gastric secretions per se, nevertheless fluid lost during vomiting or nasogastric suction may contain some NaCl for two reasons. First, there is NaCl in saliva, therefore swallowed saliva adds some NaCl to gastric fluid. Second, in most subjects who vomit, the gastric fluid contains some $NaHCO_3^-$-rich fluid from the small intestine that enters the stomach via retrograde flux (notice the color of bile in vomited fluid). The combination of HCl and $NaHCO_3$ results in the loss of NaCl and the formation of some $CO_2 + H_2O$ (see Eqn 1).

$$H^+ + Cl^- + Na^+ + HCO_3^- \rightarrow Na^+ + Cl^- + CO_2 + H_2O \quad (1)$$

**Loss in the Urine**

An increase in the delivery of $HCO_3^-$ ions to the CDN may inhibit the electroneutral mechanism for the reabsorption of NaCl mediated by the parallel activity of the $Na^+$-dependent $Cl^-/HCO_3^-$ exchanger, and the $Na^+$-independent $Cl^-/HCO_3^-$ exchanger (pendrin). Although this may lead to increased electrogenic reabsorption of $Na^+$ ions in the CDN and the loss of KCl, there is also some loss of NaCl in the urine (see Chapter 13 for more discussion).

*7-3  When HCl is secreted into the stomach during the cephalic phase of gastric secretion (before food is ingested), the $P_{HCO_3}$ rises. What is the renal response to this high $P_{HCO_3}$?*

When gastric cells secrete HCl, there is a gain of $HCO_3^-$ ions and a deficit of $Cl^-$ ions in the ECF compartment in a 1:1 stoichiometry. Notice that the ECF volume should not be altered appreciably by this simple exchange of anions in the ECF compartment. Hence, without an expanded EABV, there is sufficient angiotensin II present to activate NHE-3 in PCT cells to reabsorb most of the filtered load of $HCO_3^-$ ions. Nevertheless, if alkalemia were to occur, there might be a decrease in $H^+$ ion secretion in the distal nephron and, as a result, there could be a small degree of bicarbonaturia. This contributes to the alkaline tide of urine pH. Hence, the renal response is to retain the extra $HCO_3^-$ ions until the HCl reaches the duodenum, where $NaHCO_3$ secreted by the pancreas is added. The products of the reaction of HCl and $NaHCO_3$ are $Na^+$ ions, $Cl^-$ ions, $CO_2$, and $H_2O$. $Na^+$ and $Cl^-$ ions are subsequently absorbed in the small intestine.

7-4 *Why do some infants who vomit have metabolic alkalosis, whereas others develop metabolic acidosis?*

The key to answering this question is whether fluid from the small intestine can enter the stomach through the pyloric sphincter. When the pylorus of the stomach is blocked (e.g., in patients with congenital hypertrophic pyloric stenosis), vomiting results in the loss of HCl and therefore metabolic alkalosis may develop. In contrast, with a patent pylorus, the net loss is a mixture of fluid containing HCl and fluid containing $NaHCO_3$. If the amount of $NaHCO_3$ exceeds that of HCl in the stomach, metabolic acidosis may develop when vomiting occurs. There are two settings for this scenario. First, normal young infants often have a less tight pyloric sphincter and hence may lose more $NaHCO_3$ than HCl during vomiting. Second, adults with reduced secretion of HCl as part of a disease or with aging, or following the intake of drugs that inhibit the secretion of HCl (e.g., proton pump inhibitors), may also have more $NaHCO_3$ than HCl in their stomach, so metabolic acidosis may develop when vomiting occurs.

chapter 8

# Respiratory Acid–Base Disturbances

# Introduction

Respiratory acidosis is characterized by an increased arterial blood $PCO_2$ and $H^+$ ion concentration. The major cause of respiratory acidosis is alveolar hypoventilation. The expected physiologic response is an increased $P_{HCO_3}$. The increase in concentration of bicarbonate ions ($HCO_3$) in plasma ($P_{HCO_3}$) is tiny in patients with acute respiratory acidosis, but is much larger in patients with chronic respiratory acidosis.

Respiratory alkalosis is caused by hyperventilation and is characterized by a low arterial blood $PCO_2$ and $H^+$ ion concentration. The expected physiologic response is a decrease in $P_{HCO_3}$. As in respiratory acidosis, this response is modest in patients with acute respiratory alkalosis and much larger in patients with chronic respiratory alkalosis.

Although respiratory acid-base disorders are detected by measurement of $PCO_2$ and pH in arterial blood and may reveal the presence of a serious underlying disease process that affected ventilation, it is important to recognize the effect of changes in capillary blood $PCO_2$ in the different organs on the binding of $H^+$ ions to intracellular proteins, which may change their charge, shape, and possibly their functions.

## OBJECTIVE

■ To discuss the pathophysiology and the clinical approach to the patient with a respiratory acid–base disorder.

# PART A
# REVIEW OF THE PERTINENT PHYSIOLOGY

## THE BICARBONATE/CARBONIC ACID BUFFER SYSTEM

Major changes in the $H^+$ ion concentration in the body are prevented by buffering. Buffers are primarily weak acids with their conjugate bases, which are able to take up or release $H^+$ ions so that changes in free $H^+$ ion concentration are minimized. The major buffer system in the body is the bicarbonate ($HCO_3^-$; $H^+$ ion acceptor)/carbonic acid ($H_2CO_3$; $H^+$ ion donor) buffer system (Eqn 1).

$$H^+ + HCO_3^- \rightleftharpoons H_2CO_3 \qquad (1)$$

$H^+$ ion concentration in the extracellular fluid (ECF) compartment is determined by the ratio of the concentrations of $H_2CO_3$ to $HCO_3^-$ ions as described by the Henderson equation (Eqn 2).

$$[H^+] = Ka \, \frac{[H_2CO_3]}{[HCO_3^-]} \qquad (2)$$

where $K_a$ includes the dissociation constant for $H_2CO_3$ and the solubility coefficient of the gas $CO_2$.

The content of $HCO_3^-$ ions in the body is large, and hence the bicarbonate buffer system (BBS) is able to titrate a large $H^+$ ion load. Furthermore, in response to a chronic acid load, the kidneys can generate an excess of 200 mmol of new $HCO_3^-$ ions per day via excretion of ammonium ($NH_4^+$) ions in the urine.

Because $CO_2$ partially dissolves in water, $H_2CO_3$ acid is formed from the hydration of $CO_2$ (Eqn 3).

$$CO_2 \rightleftharpoons [CO_2] \text{ dissolved} + H_2O \rightleftharpoons H_2CO_3 \qquad (3)$$

$H_2CO_3$ is a weak acid; it will only partially dissociate into $H^+ + HCO_3^-$ ions. Because the concentration of $H^+$ ions in plasma is in nanomol/L terms, while the concentration of $HCO_3^-$ ions in plasma is in mmol/L terms, and $H^+$ and $HCO_3^-$ ions are produced from dissociation of $H_2CO_3$ in a 1:1 ratio, the relative increase in $H^+$ ion concentration will be substantially higher than the relative increase in $HCO_3^-$ ion concentration (Eqn 4).

$$CO_2 \rightleftharpoons [CO_2] \text{ dissolved} + H_2O \rightleftharpoons H_2CO_3 \rightleftharpoons H^+ + HCO_3^- \qquad (4)$$

$CO_2$ is the major carbon end product of oxidative metabolism. In an adult human subject, about 15,000 mmol of $CO_2$ are produced each day. This $CO_2$ is transported to the lungs (see the following section on transport of $CO_2$), where the rate of its elimination via alveolar ventilation matches the rate of its production. The amount of $CO_2$ that dissolves in a solution is proportional to the partial pressure of $CO_2$ ($PCO_2$) in mm Hg in that solution. Hence, the amount of $H_2CO_3$ in a solution is proportional to the $PCO_2$. In humans, the $PCO_2$ in arterial blood is in equilibrium with the $PCO_2$ in alveolar air, which is normally 40 mm Hg. In arterial blood, when the $PCO_2$ is 40 mm Hg and the solubility coefficient of $CO_2$ in plasma is 0.03, the concentration of $H_2CO_3$ is 1.2 mmol/L. If alveolar ventilation is decreased, the $PCO_2$ in alveolar air will be higher and the $PCO_2$ in arterial blood will rise, as will the concentration of $H_2CO_3$, a process called *respiratory acidosis*. If alveolar ventilation is increased, the $PCO_2$ in alveolar air will be lower and the $PCO_2$ in arterial blood will decrease, as will the concentration of $H_2CO_3$, a process called *respiratory alkalosis*.

Although respiratory acid-base disorders are detected by measurement of $PCO_2$ and pH in arterial blood and reveal the presence of disease processes that lead to altered alveolar ventilation, it is important to recognize the effect of changes of $PCO_2$ in capillary blood in the individual organs on binding of $H^+$ ions to intracellular proteins, which may change their charge, shape, and possibly affect their functions (as enzymes, contractile proteins, ion transporters). In more detail, in a patient with respiratory acidosis, because the arterial $PCO_2$ sets the lower limit on the capillary blood $PCO_2$, the capillary blood $PCO_2$ will be higher. This may limit the ability of the BBS in that organ to titrate an $H^+$ ion load. Thererfore, in the steady state, intracellular $H^+$ ion concentration will be higher and intracellular proteins will be in a more protonated form. In a patient with respiratory alkalosis, the capillary blood $PCO_2$ may be lower. More of an $H^+$ ion load will be removed by the BBS. Therefore, in the steady state, intracellular $H^+$ ion concentration may be lower, and as a result, intracellular proteins will be in a less protonated form (Figure 8-1).

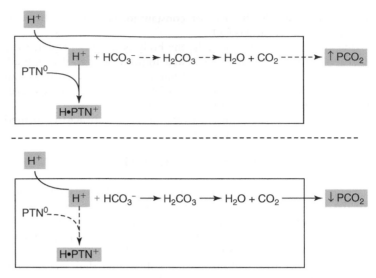

**Figure 8-1 Bicarbonate Buffer System and Respiratory Acid–Base Disorders.** In a patient with respiratory acidosis (*upper panel*), the capillary blood $PCO_2$ will be higher. This may limit the ability of the bicarbonate buffer system (BBS) in that organ to titrate an $H^+$ ion load. Hence, in the steady state, intracellular $H^+$ ion concentration will be higher and intracellular proteins will be in a more protonated form. In a patient with respiratory alkalosis (*bottom panel*), the capillary blood $PCO_2$ may be lower. More of an $H^+$ ion load will be removed by the BBS in that organ. Hence, in steady state, the intracellular $H^+$ ion concentration may be lower, and as a result intracellular proteins will be in a less protonated form. A change in $H^+$ ion binding to intracellular proteins will change their charge and shape, and may affect their functions. *PTN$^o$*, proteins with less bound $H^+$ ions; *H·PTN$^+$*, proteins with more bound $H^+$ ions.

# OVERVIEW OF CO₂ HOMEOSTASIS

The arterial $PCO_2$ reflects the balance between the rate of $CO_2$ production (metabolic $CO_2$ + acid–base $CO_2$) and the rate of $CO_2$ removal (alveolar ventilation).

## PRODUCTION OF CO₂

$CO_2$ is the major carbon end product of oxidative metabolism. When carbohydrates are oxidized, 1 mmol of $CO_2$ is produced for every mmol of $O_2$ that is consumed (the respiratory quotient [RQ] is 1.0; see margin note). In contrast, less $CO_2$ is formed per unit of $O_2$ consumed when fatty acids are oxidized (RQ ~ 0.7). In a typical Western diet, the usual RQ is close to 0.8, which reflects the oxidation of the mixture of fat and carbohydrate in the diet. The type of fuel that is being oxidized influences the rate of production of $CO_2$; this can be illustrated by considering the ratio of the rate of production of $CO_2$ and the rate of regeneration of adenosine triphosphate (ATP) from the oxidation of the different fuels (Table 8-1).

When more work is being performed, the rate of consumption of $O_2$ rises and more $CO_2$ is produced. For example, during vigorous aerobic exercise, the rate of consumption of $O_2$ can increase close to 20-fold and there is a large increase in the rate of $CO_2$ production in skeletal muscles. The rate of production of $CO_2$ decreases during hypothermia and in patients with severe hypothyroidism, conditions that result in a correspondingly lower rate of oxidative metabolism because of a lower rate of turnover of ATP. A list of clinical settings

**RESPIRATORY QUOTIENT (RQ)**

- The RQ is the quantity of $CO_2$ produced divided by the quantity of $O_2$ consumed.
- The RQ helps one deduce which type of fuel is being oxidized (e.g., when 1 mmol of palmitic acid [$C_{16}H_{32}O_2$, the most abundant fatty acid] is completely oxidized, the RQ is ~0.7 because 16 mmol of $CO_2$ are produced and 23 mmol of $O_2$ are consumed).
- Overall, on a per-minute basis at rest, 12 mmol of $O_2$ are consumed and 10 mmol of $CO_2$ are produced. This reflects the oxidation of a mixture of fatty acids and carbohydrates because the brain uses glucose as its fuel, and on a per kg basis, consumes more O2 than any other organ in the body. Thus, the average RQ for all organs in the body is ~0.8

TABLE 8-1   **PRODUCTION OF CO$_2$ PER 100 mmol OF ADENOSINE TRIPHOSPHATE (ATP) DURING OXIDATION OF MAJOR FUELS**

The oxidation of carbohydrates produces more CO$_2$ than does the oxidation of fat-derived fuels when viewed in terms of the yield of ATP. No CO$_2$ is produced when O$_2$ is consumed in the liver if fatty acids or ethanol are converted to ketoacids.

| FUEL | PRODUCTS | mmol CO$_2$/100 mmol ATP |
|------|----------|--------------------------|
| Carbohydrate | CO$_2$ + H$_2$O | 17 |
| Fatty acids | CO$_2$ + H$_2$O | 12 |
| Fatty acids | Ketoacids | 0 |
| Ethanol | CO$_2$ + H$_2$O | 11 |
| Ethanol | Ketoacids | 0 |

TABLE 8-2   **CLINICAL SETTINGS WITH ALTERED RATES OF PRODUCTION OF CO$_2$**

The numbers in the table are for an adult subject and are approximations for illustrative purposes.

| ORGAN | STATE | EFFECT ON RATE OF CO$_2$ PRODUCTION |
|-------|-------|-------------------------------------|
| Brain | Coma/anesthesia | • Decrease CO$_2$ production from 3 mmol/min to 1.5 mmol/min |
| Kidney | Low GFR | • Decrease CO$_2$ production from 2 mmol/min to <1 mmol/min |
| Muscle | Cachexia/paralysis | • Decrease CO$_2$ production from 2.4 mmol/min to <1 mmol/min |
| Muscle | Vigorous exercise | • Increase CO$_2$ production from 2.4 mmol/min to 180 mmol/min |
| Liver | Ketogenesis | • Decrease CO$_2$ production from 2.4 mmol/min to close to nil |

in which there is an altered rate of CO$_2$ production in individual organs is provided in Table 8-2.

Arterial blood contains approximately 8 mmol/L of O$_2$. Therefore, if all the content of O$_2$ in 1 L of blood is extracted, 8 mmol of CO$_2$ will be added to the venous blood, and the venous PCO$_2$ will be considerably higher than the arterial PCO$_2$. There are two conditions during which most of the O$_2$ that is delivered in a liter of blood may be consumed. First, when there is a large rise in the rate of work in an organ without a change in the rate of its O$_2$ delivery. Second, when there is delivery of a fewer liters of blood per minute with no change in the rate of work. Of clinical relevance, when the effective arterial blood volume (EABV) is contracted and the blood flow rate falls, more O$_2$ is extracted from each liter of blood delivered, and hence each liter of capillary blood must carry more CO$_2$ to the lungs. This requires a high PCO$_2$ in cells and capillary blood.

CO$_2$ is also produced during buffering of an H$^+$ load by the BBS; this is called "acid–base" CO$_2$ (e.g., buffering of L-lactic acid produced in glycolysis during a sprint). CO$_2$ is produced in the liver when acetoacetic acid is converted to acetone.

## REMOVAL OF CO$_2$

All of the CO$_2$ produced (~10 mmol/min) enters the venous blood so that it can be transported to the lungs for elimination. Because the cardiac output in adult subjects is ~ 5 L/min at rest, each liter of venous blood must carry 2 mmol of CO$_2$ (10 mmol/min ÷ 5 L/min) more than the arterial blood. These extra 10 mmol of CO$_2$ are exhaled in 5 L of alveolar ventilation per minute (the same numeric value as the cardiac output per minute). The PCO$_2$ in arterial blood is in equilibrium with the PCO$_2$ in alveolar air, which is normally 40 mm Hg. If the rate of alveolar ventilation is doubled to 10 L/min, and if there is no change in

TABLE 8-3    **QUANTITATIVE IMPACT OF DECREASED ALVEOLAR VENTILATION ON ALVEOLAR $PCO_2$**

When alveolar ventilation is 5 L/min, and 10 mmol of $CO_2$ are removed per min, the concentration of $CO_2$ in alveolar air is 2 mmol/L and its $PCO_2$ is 40 mm Hg. If alveolar ventilation were to decrease to 4 L/min and if the same amount of $CO_2$ is to be removed, the concentration of $CO_2$ in alveolar air will rise to 2.5 mmol/L and its $PCO_2$ will be 50 mm Hg.

| | $CO_2$ EXCRETION | ALVEOLAR VENTILATION | [$CO_2$] ALVEOLAR AIR | $PCO_2$ ALVEOLAR AIR |
|---|---|---|---|---|
| Normal | 10 mmol/min | 5 L/min | 2 mmol/L | 40 mm Hg |
| Chronic respiratory acidosis | 10 mmol/min | 4 L/min | 2.5 mmol/L | 50 mm Hg |

the rate of production of $CO_2$, the $PCO_2$ in alveolar air and therefore, the $PCO_2$ in arterial blood will fall by 50%. Conversely, if the rate of alveolar ventilation falls, the concentration of $CO_2$ in alveolar air must rise in the steady state to remove all the $CO_2$ that is produced (Table 8-3). Therefore, the $PCO_2$ in arterial blood will rise.

**Control of ventilation**

The quantity of $O_2$ in 1 L of arterial blood (8 mmol) is much higher than the quantity of $CO_2$ (2 mmol) (see margin note). The consumption of $O_2$ and the production of $CO_2$ occur in a ratio of close to 1:1. Because the cardiac output in an adult subject at rest is 5 L/min, and the rate of $O_2$ consumption at rest is 12 mmol/min, the supply of $O_2$ to tissues markedly exceeds their demand at rest. Accordingly, it is not surprising that the control of the rate of ventilation is to adjust the arterial $PCO_2$ rather than the arterial $PO_2$ unless the arterial $PO_2$ is quite low.

# PHYSIOLOGY OF $CO_2$ TRANSPORT

About 10 mmol of $CO_2$ are produced per minute, and they diffuse into red blood cells in capillary blood. The enzyme carbonic anhydrase in red blood cells converts $CO_2$ and $H_2O$ into $H^+$ and $HCO_3^-$ ions (Figure 8-2). This maintains a low $PCO_2$ in the red blood cells, which aids further diffusion of $CO_2$. The $HCO_3^-$ ions formed are transported into the plasma in exchange for $Cl^-$ ions ("chloride-shift") on the $Cl^-/HCO_3^-$ anion exchanger (AE) and $H^+$ ions bind to deoxyhemoglobin ($H^+\cdot Hgb$), which facilitates the release of $O_2$. In the lung, the process is reversed (see Figure 8-2). The high $PO_2$ in alveolar air drives the diffusion of $O_2$ into blood, which raises the $PO_2$ in red blood cells and thereby promotes the binding of $O_2$ to hemoglobin. As a result, the $H^+$ ions that were bound to deoxyhemoglobin are released and combine with the $HCO_3^-$ ions in red blood cells and form $CO_2$; this new $CO_2$ diffuses into the alveolar air. The lower concentration of $HCO_3^-$ ions in red blood cells leads to the entry of $HCO_3^-$ ions on AE in their cell membranes with the exit of $Cl^-$ ions. The net result is the addition of $O_2$ to, and the removal of $CO_2$ from, capillary blood in the lungs.

# RENAL RESPONSE TO A CHRONIC CHANGE IN $PCO_2$

The expected physiologic response in patients with respiratory acidosis is an increase in $P_{HCO_3}$. The increase in $P_{HCO_3}$ is tiny in patients with acute respiratory acidosis because it reflects a shift to the left in the

**$O_2$ CONTENT AND CONCENTRATION OF HEMOGLOBIN**

- The concentration of hemoglobin in blood is close to 140 g/L and the molecular weight of hemoglobin is close to 70,000. Therefore, each liter of blood contains 2 mmol of hemoglobin. When fully saturated, each mmol of hemoglobin carries 4 mmol of $O_2$. Therefore, the $O_2$ content in 1 L of blood is 8 mmol.
- With a cardiac output of 5 L/min, 40 mmol of $O_2$ are delivered to body tissues per minute. The rate of consumption of $O_2$ at rest is 12 mmol/min. Therefore, the rate of delivery of $O_2$ is three-fold higher than its rate of consumption at rest.

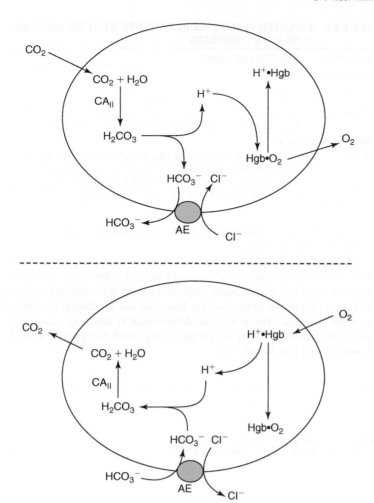

**Figure 8-2  Physiology of Transport of CO$_2$.** The *upper panel* shows the transport of CO$_2$ that is produced in cells. The two circles represent two red blood cells. CO$_2$ diffuses into red blood cells in capillary blood. The carbonic anhydrase (CA$_{II}$) in these cells converts CO$_2$ and H$_2$O into H$^+$ ions and HCO$_3^-$ ions. The HCO$_3^-$ ions formed are transported into the plasma in exchange for Cl$^-$ ions on the Cl$^-$/HCO$_3^-$ anion exchanger (AE), and H$^+$ ions bind to deoxyhemoglobin (H$^+$•Hgb), which facilitates the release of O$_2$. The *bottom panel* shows the transport of CO$_2$ at the lungs. The high PO$_2$ of alveolar air drives the diffusion of O$_2$ into blood, which raises the PO$_2$ in red blood cells and promotes the binding of O$_2$ to hemoglobin (Hgb•O$_2$). The H$^+$ ions that are bound to hemoglobin (H$^+$•Hgb) are released and combine with the HCO$_3^-$ ions in red blood cells to form CO$_2$. CO$_2$ diffuses into the alveolar air. The lower concentration of HCO$_3^-$ ions in red blood cells leads to the entry of HCO$_3^-$ ions on the AE in their cell membranes with the exit of Cl$^-$ ions. The net result is the removal of CO$_2$ from capillary blood in the lungs.

bicarbonate buffer reaction (see Eqn 1). In patients with chronic respiratory acidosis, there is much larger increase in P$_{HCO_3}$ caused by the effect of the associated intracellular acidosis in cells of the PCT to stimulate the production and excretion of NH$_4^+$ ions, and the effect of high peritubular PCO$_2$ to enhance the reabsorption of HCO$_3^-$ ions by the PCT.

The expected physiologic response in patients with respiratory alkalosis is a reduction in the P$_{HCO_3}$. As in respiratory acidosis, this response is modest in patients with acute respiratory alkalosis; it reflects the effect of the low PCO$_2$ to shift the bicarbonate buffer reaction to the right (see Eqn 1). In patients with chronic respiratory alkalosis, there is a more appreciable decrease in P$_{HCO_3}$ because of the

TABLE 8-4 **EXPECTED RESPONSES IN PATIENTS WITH RESPIRATORY ACID–BASE DISORDERS**

| DISORDER | EXPECTED RESPONSE |
|---|---|
| **Respiratory Acidosis** | |
| Acute | For every 1 mm Hg rise in the arterial $PCO_2$ from 40 mm Hg, the plasma $[H^+]$ rises by close to 0.8 nmol/L from 40 nmol/L |
| Chronic | For every 1 mm Hg rise in the arterial $PCO_2$ from 40 mm Hg, the $P_{HCO_3}$ should rise by close to 0.3 mmol/L from 25 mmol/L |
| **Respiratory Alkalosis** | |
| Acute | For every 1 mm Hg fall in the arterial $PCO_2$ from 40 mm Hg, the plasma $[H^+]$ falls by close to 0.8 nmol/L from 40 nmol/L |
| Chronic | For every 1 mm Hg fall in arterial $PCO_2$ from 40 mm Hg, the $P_{HCO_3}$ should fall by close to 0.5 mmol/L from 25 mmol/L |

effect of the low peritubular $PCO_2$ to decrease the reabsorption of $HCO_3^-$ ions by the PCT.

Thus, individuals with chronic respiratory acid–base disturbances have a different steady-state $P_{HCO_3}$, and hence $H^+$ ion concentration in plasma, than those with acute respiratory acid–base disorders (Table 8-4). It is therefore important for the clinician to clarify, on clinical grounds, whether the acid–base disturbance is acute or chronic, to avoid the misdiagnosis of the presence of a coexisting metabolic acid–base disorder (see Chapter 2).

# PART B
# RESPIRATORY ACID–BASE DISORDERS

## RESPIRATORY ACIDOSIS

Respiratory acidosis is characterized by an increased *arterial* blood $PCO_2$ and $H^+$ ion concentration. If alveolar ventilation fails to remove all the $CO_2$ produced by normal metabolism, the $PCO_2$ in alveolar air rises, and this increases the arterial $PCO_2$. In the chronic steady state, all the $CO_2$ that is produced can be removed despite the reduced ventilation, but at the expense of a higher level of $PCO_2$ in alveolar air and arterial blood and a rise in arterial blood $H^+$ ion concentration.

The diagnostic approach to the patient with respiratory acidosis is first to determine from the history, physical examination, and available past records whether the patient has an acute decrease in alveolar ventilation causing an acute respiratory acidosis, a chronic respiratory acidosis, or an acute-on-chronic respiratory acidosis. In patients with chronic respiratory acidosis, examine the $P_{HCO_3}$ to detect the presence of a coexisting metabolic acid–base disorder (i.e., metabolic acidosis is likely present if the rise in the $P_{HCO_3}$ is appreciably less than 0.3 times the rise in arterial $PCO_2$, metabolic alkalosis is likely present if the rise in the $P_{HCO_3}$ is appreciably higher than 0.3 times the rise in the arterial $PCO_2$).

The clinician should establish the cause of the decreased alveolar ventilation. Patients who have hypoventilation can be divided into two groups—those who will not breathe (e.g., because of drugs that suppress the respiratory center) and those who cannot breathe (e.g., because of respiratory muscle weakness, pulmonary parenchymal disease, or obstructive airway disease). A list of causes of chronic respiratory acidosis is provided in Table 8-5.

TABLE 8-5   **CAUSES OF CHRONIC RESPIRATORY ACIDOSIS**

| CONDITION | CAUSES |
|---|---|
| Suppression of medullary respiratory center | Drugs (e.g., opiates, sedatives), brain tumor, central sleep apnea |
| Disorders affecting respiratory muscles and/or chest wall | Muscle weakness (e.g., spinal cord injury, amytrophic lateral sclerosis, multiple sclerosis, polymyositis, diaphragmatic paralysis), kyphoscoliosis, extreme obesity |
| Increased ratio of dead space to tidal volume | Chronic obstructive lung disease, pulmonary fibrosis, chronic interstitial lung disease |

### PERMISSIVE HYPERCAPNIA

This form of hypercapnia is not "permissive" but rather "permitted" to minimize lung trauma resulting from high pressure/volume ventilation. With the traditional means of mechanical ventilation, although one could achieve better arterial blood gas values, the price to pay, especially in patients with high airway pressures, is the danger of causing barotrauma and/or a pneumothorax. Hence, the strategy is to deliberately ventilate these patients with a lower tidal volume and pressure. The lungs may be "saved"; however, the ability to exhale $CO_2$ at a low alveolar $PCO_2$ is compromised, and the result is a higher $PCO_2$ in the alveolar air and in arterial blood. In other words, hypercapnia is not the goal but rather the consequence of this therapy.

Because a high $PCO_2$ causes dilation of cerebral arterioles, permissive hypercapnia is potentially dangerous in the patient with traumatic brain injury or cerebrovascular disease. Hypercapnia may also be harmful in patients with coronary artery disease, heart failure, cardiac arrhythmias, or pulmonary hypertension with right ventricular dysfunction because hypercapnia is associated with high levels of circulating catecholamines. Another concern with this mode of ventilation is in the patient with metabolic acidemia because the high venous $PCO_2$ compromises the effectiveness of the BBS to remove an $H^+$ load. Therefore, more $H^+$ ions bind to intracellular proteins. This results in a change in their charge, shape, and perhaps function(s), and may have detrimental effects on cell function, especially in vital organs (e.g., the brain and the heart). Although observational studies suggest that permissive hypercapnia may be beneficial, no prospective, randomized controlled studies have demonstrated appreciable improvements in clinical outcome when permissive hypercapnic ventilation is compared with conventional mechanical ventilation.

## RESPIRATORY ALKALOSIS

Respiratory alkalosis is characterized by a low *arterial* blood $PCO_2$ and $H^+$ ion concentration. Respiratory alkalosis is a common acid–base disorder that is often ignored. In fact, the mortality rate in hospitalized patients with respiratory alkalosis is higher than in patients with respiratory acidosis, which likely reflects the severity of the underlying disease process.

Respiratory alkalosis occurs when the rate of removal of $CO_2$ via ventilation exceeds its rate of production. Therefore, the $PCO_2$ in alveolar air, and hence in arterial blood, falls. If this persists, a new steady state is achieved in which the daily production of $CO_2$ is removed, but a lower arterial $PCO_2$ and therefore a lower arterial plasma $H^+$ ion concentration, are maintained.

Respiratory alkalosis may result from increased alveolar ventilation caused by stimulation of the peripheral chemoreceptors (because of hypoxemia), the afferent pulmonary reflexes (because of intrinsic pulmonary disease), or the respiratory center in the brain (Table 8-6).

TABLE 8-6    **CAUSES OF RESPIRATORY ALKALOSIS**

| CONDITION | CAUSES |
| --- | --- |
| Hypoxia | Intrinsic pulmonary disease, high altitude, congestive heart failure, congenital heart disease (cyanotic) |
| Pulmonary receptor stimulation | Pneumonia, pulmonary embolism, asthma, interstitial lung disease, pulmonary edema |
| Drugs | Salicylates, catecholamines, theophylline, progesterone |
| Central nervous system disorders | Subarachnoid hemorrhage, cerebrovascular accident, encephalitis, tumor, trauma, primary hyperventilation syndrome |
| Miscellaneous | Psychosis, hepatic failure, fever, Gram-negative sepsis, pregnancy |

Salicylate intoxication, an important cause of respiratory alkalosis, is discussed in the following section.

An increase in ventilation may be difficult to recognize clinically, and the diagnosis of respiratory alkalosis is often made by determination of the arterial blood gases. The diagnostic approach to the patient with respiratory alkalosis begins by deciding on clinical grounds whether there is a disease process present that is associated with acute respiratory alkalosis; if not, the patient is presumed to have chronic respiratory alkalosis. Chronic respiratory alkalosis is the only acid–base disorder in which the concentration of $H^+$ ions and pH in plasma may be in the normal range (see Table 8-5 for the expected $P_{HCO_3}$ in a patient with chronic respiratory alkalosis). If the fall in $P_{HCO_3}$ is appreciably more than expected for the fall in arterial $PCO_2$, there is coexisting metabolic acidosis. On the other hand, if the fall in $P_{HCO_3}$ is appreciably less than expected for the fall in arterial $PCO_2$, there is a coexisting metabolic alkalosis.

**ABBREVIATIONS**

ASA, acetylsalicylic acid

SA$^-$, salicylate anions

H•SA, undissociated salicylic acid

### SALICYLATE INTOXICATION

Respiratory alkalosis is the most common acid–base disorder in adult patients with salicylate intoxication.

Toxicity of salicylate is caused by accumulation of salicylate anions (SA) in cells. Toxicity may result from direct effects of salicylate on cell functions. It is also possible that this organic anion could uncouple oxidative phosphorylation (see Chapter 6 for more discussion). This may lead to some of the central nervous system manifestations of salicylate intoxication. If the uncoupling effect is pronounced in the brain, it may lead to an increase in brain glucose consumption, and cerebral glycopenia may cause mental dysfunction. Furthermore, if an increased consumption of $O_2$ and production of $CO_2$ occurs near the respiratory center, this could stimulate alveolar ventilation and perhaps explain the respiratory alkalosis that is commonly seen in these patients. In severe intoxications, the degree of uncoupling of oxidative phosphorylation may be excessive. If this compromises the rate of conversion of adenosine diphosphate (ADP) to ATP, glycolysis is stimulated and a severe degree of L-lactic acidosis may develop.

### Effect of acidemia on the concentration of salicylates in cells

The effect of acidemia on the concentration of salicylates in blood and their concentration in cells is illustrated in Table 8-7. The following points are central to understanding this effect. First, only the undissociated salicylic acid (H•SA) can cross the cell membrane, and at equilibrium, it achieves equal concentrations in the ICF compartment and the ECF compartment (Figure 8-3). Second, the concentration of the H•SA in the compartment rises as the pH falls, and hence more H•SA enters cells. Third, inside cells, $H^+$ ions released from H•SA are immediately titrated by intracellular proteins. The concentration of intracellular salicylate

TABLE 8-7    **EFFECT OF ACIDEMIA ON THE CONCENTRATION OF SALICYLATES IN CELLS**

In the example shown below, the total salicylate concentration in the extracellular fluid (ECF) is 7 mmol/L. Because of its low pK (~3.5), only a very tiny fraction is in the undissociated form at normal blood pH values (i.e., H•SA=0.3 μmol/L). H•SA diffuses across cell membranes and at equilibrium; its concentration is equal inside and outside cells. The concentration of salicylate anion inside cells depends on the intracellular fluid (ICF) pH. Because ICF pH is normally close to 7.10, the pK of salicylic acid/salicylate is ~3.5; at H•SA concentration of 0.3 μmol/L, the concentration of salicylate anion in cells would be close to 3.5 mmol/L (i.e., half its concentration in the ECF compartment). If the pH in ECF compartment drops to 7.10, the concentration of H•SA will rise to 0.6 μmol/L. Because H•SA diffuses across cell membranes to achieve equilibrium, the concentration of H•SA in cells will be 0.6 μmol/L. At an ICF pH of close to 7.10, the concentration of salicylate anion in cells would be close to 6.0 mmol/L (i.e., 86% of its concentration in the ECF compartment).

|  | ECF | ICF | ECF | ICF |
|---|---|---|---|---|
| pH | 7.40 | 7.10 | 7.10 | 7.10 |
| H•SA (μmol/L) | 0.3 | 0.3 | 0.6 | 0.6 |
| Salicylate (mmol/L) | 7.0 | 3.5 | 7.0 | 6.0 |

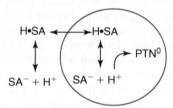

**Figure 8-3 Nonionic Diffusion of Salicylic Acid Versus Salicylate Anions.** The *circle* represents a cell. Only the undissociated salicylic acid (H•SA) can cross the cell membrane and at equilibrium achieves equal concentrations in the intracellular fluid compartment and the extracellular fluid compartment. The concentration of the H•SA in the ECF compartment rises as the pH falls, and hence more H•SA enter cells. H+ ions released inside the cell are titrated by intracellular proteins with no bound H+ ions (PTV°). Because intracellular pH is close to 7.10, the pK of salicylic acid/salicylate is ~3.50, the concentration of salicylate anion (SA−) inside cells will be almost 10,000-fold higher than that of H•SA.

anion in cells depends on intracellular pH. Because the pK of salicylic acid/salicylate is ~3.5 and intracellular pH is 7.10, the concentration of salicylate in cells will be almost 10,000-fold higher than that of H•SA.

## Signs and symptoms

The central nervous system manifestations of aspirin overdose include tinnitus, vertigo, nausea, and fever. The gastrointestinal manifestations include upper abdominal pain, vomiting, and diarrhea. Lung toxicity is manifested by noncardiogenic pulmonary edema. Cerebral edema may occur; however, the mechanism is not clear. With more severe intoxication, the degree of altered mental status is more profound (e.g., coma). Death because of salicylate poisoning is caused most often by asystole or ventricular fibrillation. Uncoupling of oxidative phosphorylation in the cardiac cells responsible for impulse conduction is a possible mechanism.

## Acid–base changes

### Respiratory alkalosis

The most common acid–base disturbance associated with salicylate intoxication in adults is respiratory alkalosis. This is thought to be caused by a direct effect of salicylate to stimulate the central respiratory center. As suggested previously, it may also be caused by the effect of salicylate to cause uncoupling of oxidative phosphorylation, which may lead to an increased $CO_2$ production near the respiratory center.

### Metabolic acidosis

Metabolic acidosis is more common in children with salicylate intoxication than in adults. In adults with salicylate intoxication, respiratory alkalosis is the most prominent acid–base disorder with only a modest degree of metabolic acidosis. Because toxicity is caused by the monovalent salicylate anion and occurs when the concentration is 3 to 5 mmol/L, the contribution of salicylic acid itself to the metabolic acidosis is small. Metabolic acidosis in these patients is usually caused by the accumulation of ketoacids and L-lactic acid. Increased glucose consumption in the brain may lead to cerebral glycopenia with increased release of catecholamines. Hypoglycemia is common in patients with salicylate intoxication, which likely reflects increased utilization of glucose by the brain (uncoupling of oxidative phosphorylation) and/or impaired hepatic gluconeogenesis (perhaps by a direct effect of salicylate anion). The relative lack of insulin action (low insulin blood level caused by hypoglycemia, and high blood level of catecholamines) may lead to increased release of fatty acids from adipose tissues. In this setting, a modest degree of uncoupling of oxidative phosphorylation can increase the production of ketoacids in the liver (see Chapter 5). In severe intoxications, the degree of uncoupling of oxidative phosphorylation may be excessive. If this compromises the rate of conversion of ADP to ATP, glycolysis is stimulated and a severe degree of L-lactic acidosis develops.

### Diagnosis

The diagnosis of salicylate intoxication should be suspected on the basis of a history of ingestion or symptoms of tinnitus and lightheadedness and a severe degree of respiratory alkalosis. An unexplained ketoacidosis, hypouricemia (high dose salicylate has a uricosuric effect), and/or noncardiogenic pulmonary edema should raise suspicion of salicylate intoxication. As a result of the excretion of salicylate anions in the urine, the sum of the concentrations of $Na^+$ and $K^+$ ions in the urine will be much higher than the concentration of $Cl^-$ ions, in the absence of a high concentration of $HCO_3^-$ ions in the urine (urine pH is not alkaline). The diagnosis is confirmed by measuring the concentration of salicylate anion in blood.

### Treatment

The focus of treatment is to reduce the intracellular concentration of salicylate anions.

Gastric lavage along with instillation of activated charcoal should be instituted even 6 to 12 hours after ingestion because of the effect of acetyl salicylic acid (ASA) to delay gastric emptying and also the delayed absorption if an enteric coated preparation was ingested.

Dialysis should be instituted if salicylate levels exceed 90 mg/dL (6 mmol/L). If levels of salicylate exceed 60 mg/dL (4 mmol/L), dialysis should be considered, particularly if further absorption is anticipated. In patients with an unexplained decreased level of consciousness, dialysis should be started at even lower levels of salicylate in blood because of the poor prognosis. Hemodialysis is more efficient for the removal of salicylate than peritoneal dialysis, but peritoneal dialysis may be considered if available and there will be a long delay before hemodialysis can be initiated.

In the absence of severe toxicity, the goals of therapy are to decrease the concentration of H•SA in blood and to promote the urinary excretion of salicylate via the following two maneuvers:

1. *Administration of NaHCO$_3^-$:* NaHCO$_3$ should be administered in a patient with salicylate intoxication who has metabolic acidosis to decrease the concentration of H•SA in the blood and thus diminish its movement into brain cells. Administration of NaHCO$_3$ may also increase the pH in the lumen of the PCT, and hence lower the concentration of H•SA and promote the excretion of salicylate anions. Notwithstanding, one should be very cautious because the patient may become very alkalemic from the coexistent respiratory alkalosis; blood pH should be monitored and kept under 7.50.

2. *Administration of acetazolamide:* This carbonic anhydrase inhibitor has been shown to increase the excretion of salicylate anions in the urine. The traditional explanation is that acetazolamide increases the excretion of the salicylate anions by raising the pH in the lumen of the PCT, thereby decreasing the concentration of H•SA. However, the effect of acetazolamide to inhibit luminal carbonic anhydrase leads to an *increase* (not a *decrease*) in the concentration of H$^+$ ions of luminal fluid in PCT. Therefore, the mechanism for acetazolamide to increase the excretion of salicylate anions cannot be a result of lowering the H•SA concentration in luminal fluid. It is possible that there is a direct effect of HCO$_3^-$ ions to inhibit the reabsorption of salicylate anions in the PCT; therefore, an increase in luminal HCO$_3^-$ ion concentration resulting from the effect of acetazolamide to decrease the reabsorption of NaHCO$_3$ in PCT may explain its effect to increase salicylate anion excretion. Caution is needed, however, because acetazolamide may increase the toxicity of salicylate because it competes with salicylate anions for binding to albumin in plasma, which may increase the free salicylate anion concentration and H•SA in blood. In addition, acetazolamide may induce acidemia by increasing the excretion of HCO$_3^-$ ions in the urine, which may increase the concentration of H•SA in blood, and hence increase the toxicity.

There is some experimental evidence in humans to suggest that 250 mg of acetazolamide has a tubular effect that lasts for about 16 hours. Therefore, little drug is needed to achieve beneficial effects, and one could use a low dose of acetazolamide instead of alkali therapy in the patient with a high blood pH and avoid the use of alkali.

# section two
# Salt and Water

# Sodium and Water Physiology

# Introduction

**ABBREVIATIONS**

ECF, extracellular fluid

ICF, intracellular fluid

$P_{Na}$, concentration of sodium ions ($Na^+$) in plasma

$P_K$, concentration of potassium ions ($K^+$) in plasma

$P_{Cl}$, concentration of chloride ions ($Cl^-$) in plasma

$P_{HCO_3}$, concentration of bicarbonate ions ($HCO_3^-$) in plasma

NKCC-1, $Na^+$, $K^+$, 2 $Cl^-$ cotransporter 1

NHE-3, sodium hydrogen cation exchanger-3

$P_{Albumin}$, concentration of albumin in plasma

$P_{Aldosterone}$, concentration of aldosterone in plasma

ANP, atrial natriuretic peptide

EABV, effective arterial blood volume

AQP, aquaporin water channel

GFR, glomerular filtration rate

PCT, proximal convoluted tubule

DtL, descending thin limb (of the loop of Henle)

AtL, ascending thin limb (of the loop of Henle)

mTAL, medullary thick ascending limb (of the loop of Henle)

cTAL, cortical thick ascending limb (of the loop of Henle)

DCT, distal convoluted tubule

CCD, cortical collecting duct

MCD, medullary collecting duct

CDN, cortical distal nephron, which consists of the late DCT, the connecting segment, and the CCD

NKCC-2, $Na^+$, $K^+$, 2 $Cl^-$ cotransporter 2

ROMK, renal outer medullary $K^+$ channel

NCC, $Na^+$, $Cl^-$ cotransporter

ENaC, epithelial $Na^+$ channel

Ca-SR, calcium-sensing receptor

SPAK, STE20-related proline-alanine-rich-kinase

OSR1, oxidative stress response kinase type 1

SGK-1, serum and glucocorticoid-regulated kinase-1

$K_{sp}$, solubility product constant for the activity of ions in a solution

It is important to understand the physiology of sodium ($Na^+$) and of water homeostasis to determine the pathophysiology that leads to alteration in the extracellular fluid (ECF) volume and/or the concentration of sodium ions ($Na^+$) in plasma ($P_{Na}$), and what is the optimal therapy to deal with these disorders.

This chapter is divided into four sections. The first section deals with the factors that determine the distribution of water between the ECF and intracellular fluid (ICF) compartments, and factors that determine the distribution of ECF volume between its vascular and interstitial subcompartments. The second and third sections deal with the physiology of how balances for $Na^+$ ions and water, respectively, are achieved. In the final section, we provide a more in-depth look at selected aspects of the integrative physiology of $Na^+$ ions and water homeostasis.

## OBJECTIVES

- To emphasize that the number of effective osmoles in the ECF and ICF compartments determines their respective volume.
- To emphasize that the hydrostatic pressure in capillaries and the concentration of albumin in plasma ($P_{Albumin}$) are the two major factors that determine the distribution of the ECF volume between its two subcompartments: the plasma volume and the interstitial fluid volume.
- To emphasize that, with some exceptions, the $P_{Na}$ determines the ICF volume. The ICF volume is expanded in patients with hyponatremia and is contracted in patients with hypernatremia.
- To point out that $Na^+$ ion homeostasis and water homeostasis are regulated by different control systems.
- To emphasize that the content of $Na^+$ ions in the ECF compartment is regulated by modulation of the rate of the reabsorption of $Na^+$ ions by the kidneys.
- To describe the mechanisms for $Na^+$ ion handling in the different nephron segments and how they are regulated.
- To emphasize that water balance is primarily the result of the interplay of thirst and renal actions of vasopressin. When vasopressin acts, the volume of urine is dependent on the rate of excretion of effective urine osmoles and the effective osmolality in the renal papillary interstitial compartment. When actions of vasopressin are absent, the urine volume is determined by the volume of distal delivery of filtrate and the volume of water reabsorbed in the inner medullary collecting duct (MCD) via residual water permeability.

# PART A
# BODY FLUID COMPARTMENTS

### CASE 9-1: A RISE IN THE $P_{NA}$ AFTER A SEIZURE

A 20-year-old man experienced a generalized tonic–clonic seizure one day prior to presenting to the hospital. He had been well before and had no history of seizures prior to this episode. The physical examination was normal, and all the results of blood tests performed, including the $P_{Na}$ (140 mmol/L), were in the normal range. A few hours later, he had another generalized tonic–clonic seizure. A brachial venous blood sample was drawn immediately after the seizure; the results revealed the expected metabolic acidosis with a large increase in the $P_{Anion\,gap}$ because of accumulation of L-lactic acid. To everyone's surprise, however, his $P_{Na}$ was 154 mmol/L after the seizure, but on a repeat measurement done on a brachial venous sample obtained few hours later, his $P_{Na}$ fell back to 140 mmol/L. Of note, there was no large increase in urine output prior to the development of hypernatremia, and he did not ingest a large volume of water nor was he given hypotonic fluids after the seizure.

### Question

What is the basis for the acute rise in the patient's $P_{Na}$?

## TOTAL BODY WATER

Water is the most abundant constituent of the body. Although it is said to constitute approximately 60% of body mass, the actual percentage of body weight due to water in any individual depends on the relative proportions of muscle and fat in the body. Skeletal muscle is the largest organ in the body, and about half of total body water is located in the ICF and ECF compartments of muscle. Because neutral fat does not dissolve in water, triglycerides are stored in fat cells without water. Accordingly, when relating total body water to body weight, one must consider the relative proportions of muscle and fat. For example, females tend to have a higher proportion of fat to body weight than males, and hence they have a lower percentage of water relative to body weight (typically 50% in females vs 60% in males). Obese individuals have less water per kg body weight. Similarly, older people have less water per kg body weight because they often have a relatively smaller proportion of muscle. Newborn infants, on the other hand, have less adipose tissue and therefore they have a higher proportion of water per kg body weight (~70%).

### DISTRIBUTION OF WATER ACROSS CELL MEMBRANES

Water crosses cell membranes rapidly through aquaporin (AQP) water channels to achieve osmotic equilibrium. Not all compounds and ions are distributed equally in the ICF and ECF compartments, however, because there are active pumps and transporters that affect the distribution of individual solutes between the ECF and ICF compartments (Table 9-1). Water distribution across cell membranes depends on the number of particles that are restricted to either the ICF or ECF compartment (Fig. 9-1); these particles account for the effective osmolality, or the tonicity, in these compartments. The particles restricted to the ECF compartment are largely $Na^+$ ions and their attendant anions (chloride [$Cl^-$] and bicarbonate [$HCO_3^-$] ions). In contrast, the major cation in the ICF compartment is potassium ions ($K^+$); electroneutrality is maintained primarily by the anionic charge on organic phosphate esters inside the cells (RNA, DNA, phospholipids, phosphoproteins, adenosine triphosphate [ATP], and adenosine diphosphate [ADP]). These are relatively large molecules and hence exert little osmotic force. Other organic solutes contribute to the osmotic force in the ICF compartment. The individual compounds, however, differ from organ to organ. The organic solutes that have the highest concentration in skeletal muscle cells are phosphocreatine and carnosine; each is present at ~25 mmol/kg. Other solutes include amino acids (e.g., glutamine, glutamate, taurine), peptides (e.g., glutathione), and sugar derivatives (e.g., myoinositol).

TABLE 9-1  **CONCENTRATION OF IONS IN THE EXTRACELLULAR FLUID AND INTRACELLULAR FLUID COMPARTMENTS**

|  | ECF | ICF |
|---|---|---|
| $Na^+$ | 150 | 10-20 |
| $K^+$ | 4.0 | 120-150 |
| $Cl^-$ | 113 | ~5 |
| $HCO_3^-$ | 25 | 10 |
| Phosphate | 2.0 (inorganic) | ~130 (organic in macromolecules) |

Data are expressed as mEq/kg of water. Concentrations of ions in the ICF compartment are not known with certainty, because some of the water in the ICF compartment is held in a "bound form" and there are regions of cytoplasm where there appears to be less "solvent water." Moreover, these concentrations differ from organ to organ. Values provided are approximations for the ICF in skeletal muscle. *ECF*, Extracellular fluid; *ICF*, intracellular fluid.

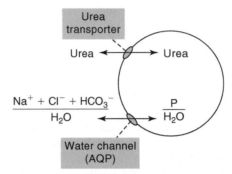

**Figure 9-1 Factors Regulating Water Distribution Across Cell Membranes.**
The *circle* represents the cell membrane. Water crosses this membrane rapidly through aquaporin (AQP) water channels to achieve equal sum of the concentrations of effective osmoles on both sides of the cell membrane. Effective osmoles are ones that are largely restricted to the extracellular fluid (ECF) compartment or the intracellular fluid (ICF) compartment. The major particles that are restricted largely to the ECF compartment are $Na^+$ ions and their attendant anions, $Cl^-$ and $HCO_3^-$ ions. The major particles (P) that are restricted to the ICF compartment are predominantly $K^+$ ions and a number of small organic compounds. Macromolecular organic phosphates and proteins make only a minor direct contribution to the effective osmolality in cells. Particles such as urea are transported across cell membranes rapidly via urea transporters; hence, urea molecules do not play a role in determining the distribution of water across cell membranes.

This difference in the concentrations of the major cations between the ECF and the ICF compartments is maintained because $Na^+$ ions that enter the ICF compartment are actively exported out of cells by the Na-K-ATPase, which are located in cell membranes. Particles such as urea are transported across cell membranes rapidly via urea transporters. Hence, the concentration of urea molecules is virtually equal in the ICF and ECF compartments, and therefore, urea molecules do not play a role in the distribution of water across cell membranes (i.e., urea is not an effective osmole).

The number of effective osmoles in each compartment determines that compartment's volume. It is commonly stated that the ICF volume is twice as large as the ECF volume, so that 67% of body water is in the ICF compartment whereas 33% is in the ECF compartment. Hence, a 70-kg, nonobese male subject with a total body water of 60% of body weight (42 L) will have an ECF volume of 14 L and an ICF volume of 28 L. The data to support this conclusion are not robust and vary depending on the method used to estimate ECF volume. It has also been suggested that only slightly more than half of body water (55%) is in the ICF compartment and 45% is in the ECF compartment. Changes in ECF and ICF volumes after administering isotonic saline or the administration of water are illustrated in Figure 9-2.

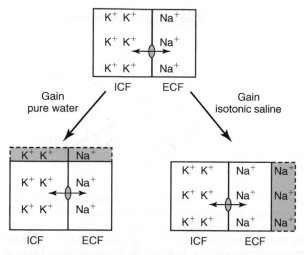

**Figure 9-2  Changes in Volumes of Body Fluid Compartments After Administering Water or Saline.** The normal volumes of the extracellular fluid (ECF) and intracellular fluid (ICF) compartments are shown in the *top rectangle*. Water moves across cell membranes through the aquaporin (AQP) water channel (represented by the *oval structure*) until the sum of the concentrations of effective osmoles are equal in both compartments. A surplus of water (*bottom left*) distributes in the ICF and the ECF compartments in proportion to their existing volumes (shown by the *horizontal pink rectangle* above the normal compartment sizes); this causes hyponatremia. In contrast (*bottom right*), when there is a positive balance of isotonic saline, only the ECF volume becomes expanded (shown in the *vertical pink rectangle*), and there is no change in the $P_{Na}$ or in the ICF volume in this setting.

The content of $Na^+$ ions and their attendant monovalent anions in the ECF compartment determine the ECF volume. Although macromolecular phosphate compounds in the ICF do not exert a large osmotic pressure (they do not represent a large number of particles), they nonetheless carry a large anionic net charge and as a result help retain a large number of cations (primarily $K^+$ ions) to achieve electroneutrality. Because particles in the ICF compartment are relatively "fixed" in number and charge, changes in the ratio of particles to water in the ICF compartment usually come about by changes in its content of water. The concentration of $Na^+$ ions in the ECF compartment is the most important factor that determines the ICF volume (except when the ECF compartment contains other effective osmoles [e.g., glucose in a patient with diabetes mellitus and relative lack of insulin, mannitol]). Hence, hyponatremia (because of a gain of water in or the loss of $Na^+$ ions from the ECF compartment) is associated with an increase in ICF volume; in contrast, hypernatremia (because of a loss of water from or the gain of $Na^+$ ions in the ECF compartment) is associated with a decrease in ICF volume.

## DEFENSE OF BRAIN CELL VOLUME

Defense of brain cell volume is necessary because the brain is contained in a rigid box: the skull (Fig. 9-3). When brain cells swell (as occurs when the $P_{Na}$ is low), the initial defense mechanism is to expel as much $Na^+$ and $Cl^-$ ions and water as possible from the interstitial space into the cerebrospinal fluid to prevent a large rise in intracranial pressure. If brain cells continue to swell, the intracranial pressure will rise, the brain will be pushed caudally, which may result in compression of the cerebral veins against the bony margin of the foramen magnum, and hence the venous outflow will be diminished. Because the arterial pressure is likely to be high enough to permit the inflow of blood to continue, the intracranial pressure rises further and abruptly.

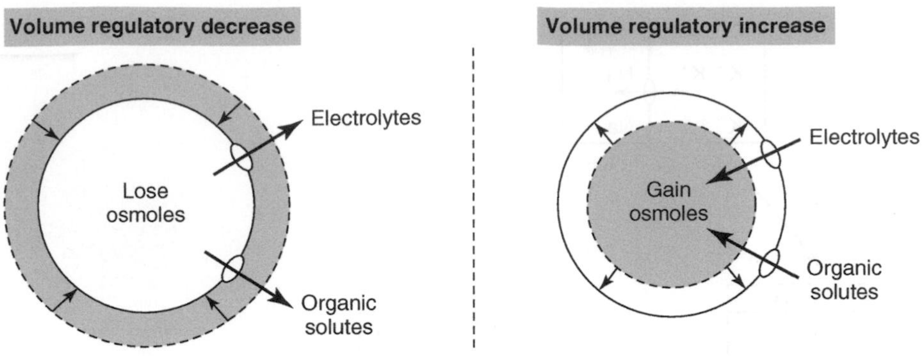

| Volume regulatory decrease | Volume regulatory increase |
|---|---|

**Figure 9-3  Regulation of Brain Cell Volume.** The *solid circle* represents the normal volume of a brain cell. In the *left portion*, brain cells have increased in size (*dashed circle*) during acute hyponatremia. To return their volume toward normal (*solid circle*), these cells export effective osmoles: $K^+$ ions with anions (other than organic phosphate) and organic osmoles. In the *right portion*, brain cells have decreased in size (*dashed circle*) during acute hypernatremia. To return their volume toward normal (*solid circle*), these cells must import effective osmoles: $Na^+$, $K^+$, and $Cl^-$ ions and organic osmoles.

This may lead to serious symptoms (seizures, coma) and eventually herniation of the brain through the foramen magnum, causing irreversible midbrain damage and death.

In contrast, excessive shrinkage of brain cell volume (as occurs when the $P_{Na}$ is high) stretches the vessels coming from the inner surface of the skull, which may cause their rupture, leading to focal intracerebral and subarachnoid hemorrhages.

Because the large intracellular macromolecular anions are essential compounds for cell structure and function, defense of brain cell volume requires that small ions or nonelectrolyte osmoles be exported from swollen brain cells or be imported into shrunken brain cells to return their cell sizes close to normal in either case.

### Regulatory decrease in brain cell volume

In patients with hyponatremia, primary mechanism to return swollen brain cells toward their original size is to decrease the number of effective osmoles inside the cells. Close to half of this decrease in the number of effective osmoles is the result of exporting $K^+$ cations with an accompanying anion (other than organic phosphate) to maintain electroneutrality (see margin note). Another mechanism to cause water to exit from cells is to have some intracellular effective ions "disappear" and thereby lower the osmolality in this compartment. This could occur if ions were to become bound to intracellular macromolecules and hence become osmotically inactive; this, however, is not known to occur in neuronal cells. Organic solutes are extruded from brain cells as part of the regulatory decrease in volume. The major organic osmoles that are lost from brain cells are the amino acids glutamine, glutamate, and taurine, and the sugar derivative myoinositol.

### Regulatory increase in brain cell volume

In patients with hypernatremia, the mechanism to return of shrunken cells toward their original volume begins with an influx of $Na^+$ and $Cl^-$ ions (see margin note), which usually occurs via the furosemide-sensitive $Na^+$, $K^+$, 2 $Cl^-$ cotransporter-1 (NKCC-1), but it is also possible that this may be achieved by parallel flux through the $Na^+/H^+$ cation exchanger and the $Cl^-/HCO_3^-$ anion exchanger. The second mechanism for increasing the size of shrunken brain cells is via an

**ANIONS EXPORTED FROM BRAIN CELLS WITH $K^+$ IONS**

- The authors are not clear on which anions are exported from brain cells with $K^+$ ions during this regulatory decrease in brain cell volume.
- One of these anions could be $Cl^-$ ions. The concentration of $Cl^-$ ions, however, is very low in the ICF compartment. Notwithstanding, it may be higher in nonneuronal brain cells (e.g., astrocytes).
- It is unlikely that this volume defense mechanism involves the export of $HCO_3^-$ ions because changes in their concentration alter the pH in cells and thereby the net charge on intracellular proteins.

**INCREASE IN THE INTRACELLULAR CONCENTRATION OF $Na^+$ IONS**

- To permit a rise in the intracellular $Na^+$ ion concentration, the Na-K-ATPase either must have a lower affinity for $Na^+$ ions or there must be fewer active pump units in the cell membrane.

increase in the number of organic compounds in brain cells (e.g., taurine and myoinositol), which seems to account for close to half of the increase in the number of effective osmoles in this adaptive process.

## DISTRIBUTION OF WATER IN THE ECF COMPARTMENT

The ECF compartment is subdivided into two subcompartments: the plasma fluid volume (~4% of body weight, ~3 L in a 70-kg nonobese male) and the interstitial fluid volume (i.e., fluid in tissues between the cells; ~16% of body weight, ~11 L in a 70-kg nonobese male). In certain disease states, fluid accumulates in the interstitial space of the ECF compartment to an appreciable degree, causing peripheral edema, ascites, or pleural effusion (see margin note). Because the interstitial fluid volume is much larger than the intravascular volume, whenever expansion of the interstitial space is detected (e.g., peripheral edema), the patient always has an expanded ECF volume even if the intravascular volume is reduced (e.g., in a patient with chronic hypoalbuminemia).

The major driving force for fluid movement from the intravascular space to the interstitial space is the hydrostatic pressure difference. The hydrostatic pressure at the venous end of the capillary is higher under conditions that lead to venous hypertension (e.g., venous obstruction, congestive heart failure).

The major driving force for inward flow of fluid (from the interstitial space to the intravascular space) is the colloid oncotic pressure difference. This difference is the result of a higher concentration of proteins in plasma than in the interstitial fluid. The osmotic pressure generated by plasma proteins (the plasma oncotic pressure) is attributed not only to the concentration of proteins in plasma (~0.8 mmol/L) but also to their net negative charge (Gibbs–Donnan equilibrium; see the following).

Interstitial fluid returns to the venous system via the lymphatic system.

### Gibbs–Donnan equilibrium

The net negative valence on plasma proteins causes ions to redistribute between the intravascular and interstitial spaces, because it attracts cations (largely $Na^+$ ions) into, and repels anions (largely $Cl^-$ and $HCO_3^-$ ions) out of, the capillaries. According to the Gibbs–Donnan equilibrium, the product of diffusible cations and diffusible anions in the fluid on either side of a semipermeable membrane must be the same. Therefore, the intravascular space ultimately has a slightly larger total concentration of ionic species than the interstitial space. Although this difference in the sum of the concentrations of ions is small in quantitative terms (~0.4 mmol/L), it is appreciable relative to the concentration of protein in plasma (~0.8 mmol/L); hence, it makes an appreciable contribution to the colloid osmotic pressure. In quantitative terms, according to the Van't Hoff factor, 1 mmol of a solute in a solution generates an osmotic pressure of 19.3 mm Hg. The plasma oncotic pressure with a normal plasma protein concentration is ~24 mm Hg. Hence, approximately one-third of the plasma oncotic pressure (7.7 mm Hg) is attributed to the Gibbs–Donnan effect.

It was suggested that changes in intravascular volume may lead, via a yet unknown mechanism, to conformational changes in albumin that lead to a change in its negative valence and hence the Gibbs–Donnan effect. A decrease in the effective arterial blood volume (EABV) is associated with an increase in the net negative valence on albumin (detected by a rise in the anion gap in plasma ($P_{Anion\ gap}$) that is not accounted for by changes in the concentration of albumin in plasma

**THIRD SPACE**
- This term is commonly used to refer to a space into which fluid may move and from which it is difficult to return to the intravascular space. Common situations in which this is said to occur include following abdominal surgery and in patients with pancreatitis.

($P_{Albumin}$), an increase in the negative valence on albumin due to a rise in plasma pH, or the gain of new anions). This increase in negative net valence on plasma albumin may help defend the intravascular volume by increasing the plasma oncotic pressure via the Gibbs–Donnan effect, which may cause fluid to move from the interstitial space to the intravascular volume.

## QUESTIONS

9-1  *Hypertonic saline is the treatment of choice to shrink brain cell size in a patient with acute hyponatremia. What is the major effect of hypertonic saline that reduces the risk of brain herniation?*

9-2  *What would happen acutely to the ICF volume if the permeability of capillary membranes to albumin were to increase?*

9-3  *What is the volume of distribution if 1 L of each of the following intravenous fluids is retained in the body: isotonic saline, half-isotonic saline, 300 mmol of NaCl/L, or 1 L of $D_5W$? What would the change in the $P_{Na}$ be in a normal 50-kg subject who has 30 L of total body water before the infusion of each of these solutions?*

# PART B
# PHYSIOLOGY OF SODIUM

### OVERVIEW

Although there is some evidence for stimulation of salt intake in humans when the ECF volume is low (salt craving), this is not an important element in the control of $Na^+$ ion homeostasis. Rather, $Na^+$ ion balance is regulated primarily by adjusting the rate of excretion of $Na^+$ ions in response to signals related to the degree of expansion of the EABV.

Our current understanding of $Na^+$ ion homeostasis is based on short-term balance studies in humans, in which there were large changes in salt intake. These studies suggested that a new steady state is achieved within a few days, in which $Na^+$ ion excretion matches its intake, with little change in total body $Na^+$ ion content. A number of studies, however, have challenged this accepted dogma. In two very long-term studies (105 and 520 days), $Na^+$ ion balance in healthy humans on a fixed $Na^+$ ion intake was examined, with daily urine collections for the entire duration of the study. The studies were meticulously conducted because they were done in the setting of a simulated flight to Mars; hence, subjects were confined to an enclosed, restricted environment. While these subjects remained in $Na^+$ ion balance, with the cumulative urinary excretion of $Na^+$ ions very closely matching the cumulative intake of $Na^+$ ions, there was considerable day-to-day variability in 24-hour $Na^+$ ion excretion. The subjects seem to accumulate or release $Na^+$ ions with regular periodicity of approximately 1 month independent of daily salt intake. These findings are in clear contradiction to the widely held view that the total body $Na^+$ ion content is maintained within a narrow limit. It also calls into question the validity of the 24-hour urine collection as a measure of $Na^+$ ion intake. In these studies, large amounts of $Na^+$ ions were retained or excreted without changes in body weight, indicating that $Na^+$ ions seemed to be stored in the body in an osmotically inactive form, without water retention. In fact, Na MRI measurements of $Na^+$ ion content suggested that large amounts of $Na^+$ ions are stored in the skin interstitium and in skeletal muscles bound to the highly sulfated, negatively charged glycosaminoglycans.

# CONTROL SYSTEM FOR SODIUM BALANCE

## NORMAL ECF VOLUME

To define what a normal ECF volume is, we start by emphasizing that control mechanisms were developed in Paleolithic times. There are no survival-related pressures in modern times that have enough control strength to negate this regulation. The diet of our ancient ancestors consisted mainly of fruit and berries and contained very little NaCl. Hence, control mechanisms were set for the kidneys to preferentially retain NaCl. Because the diet in modern times is rich in salt (subjects who consume a typical Western diet have an intake of NaCl that is in excess of 150 mmol/day), it is "physiologically not correct" to think of our ECF volume as being "normal." In fact, an expanded ECF volume is needed to provide the kidneys with a signal to prevent it from reabsorbing virtually all the filtered $Na^+$ ions. Hence, from a physiologic perspective, a "normal" ECF volume should be defined based on measurements of ECF volume in subjects who have a low intake of NaCl, because this represents the conditions in Paleolithic times, when important control mechanisms developed.

In order to understand the mechanisms regulating the ECF volume, it is important to appreciate that what is sensed is the EABV. EABV can be defined as the part of the ECF volume that is located in the arterial blood system and that effectively perfuses tissues. Changes in the EABV are sensed by baroreceptors located in the large arterial blood vessels (the carotid sinus and the aortic arch) and glomerular afferent arterioles. These are stretch receptors that detect changes in the pressure inside or the "filling" of these vessels.

The EABV is often, although not always, correlated with the ECF volume and is proportional to total body $Na^+$ ion content. $Na^+$ ion loading generally leads to EABV expansion, whereas $Na^+$ ion loss leads to EABV depletion. Hence, regulation of both $Na^+$ ion balance and the EABV are related functions. Nevertheless, there are several situations in which this correlation is lost. An example is the patient with congestive heart failure. A decrease in cardiac output leads to a decrease in the perfusion pressure of the baroreceptors (i.e., a reduced EABV is sensed). This leads to renal $Na^+$ ion retention and ECF volume expansion. The net result is a state of increased total ECF volume, but a reduced EABV. The increase in plasma volume is partially appropriate in that intraventricular filling pressure rises and, by increasing myocardial stretching, leads to improved ventricular contractility, thereby raising cardiac output and restoring blood pressure and the stretch of the baroreceptors toward normal. However, $Na^+$ ion retention and ECF volume expansion may lead to both peripheral and pulmonary edema.

## CONTROL OF THE EXCRETION OF SODIUM IONS

The regulation of $Na^+$ ion excretion is the most important factor that maintains the EABV. The major renal work that requires energy expenditure is the reabsorption of filtered $Na^+$ ions. With a glomerular filtration rate (GFR) of 180 L/day and $P_{Na}$ of 150 mmol/L of plasma water, the load of $Na^+$ ions that is filtered daily is enormous (27,000 mmol). In an adult who consumes a typical Western diet that contains 150 mmol of NaCl each day, only 150 mmol of NaCl need to be excreted to achieve balance for these electrolytes. The kidneys use a large amount of fuel to provide the ATP needed to reabsorb close to 99.5% of the filtered load of $Na^+$ ions (26,850 mmol/day). Depending on the properties of the nephron site where reabsorption of $Na^+$ ions occurs, the kidneys utilize this energy to reabsorb other valuable compounds or ions (e.g., glucose and $HCO_3^-$ ions in the proximal convoluted tubule [PCT]) or to secrete others (e.g., $K^+$ ions in the late cortical distal nephron [CDN]).

**ANOTHER BENEFIT FOR THE HIGH GFR**

• Having a high GFR permits more fuel oxidation because more work is being done (reabsorbing a larger filtered load of Na+ ions).

• During metabolic acidosis, one of the fuels that is consumed by the kidneys to provide the energy to reabsorb Na+ ions is glutamine. Thus, the kidneys can have a higher rate of production of ammonium ions ($NH_4^+$) and hence a higher rate of addition of new $HCO_3^-$ ions to the body (see Chapter 1).

Nevertheless, filtering and reabsorbing such a large quantity of Na+ ions may be thought of as a "waste of energy" at first glance. Filtering this large amount of Na+ ions is dictated by the high GFR. Although there are several hypotheses to explain why there is such a high GFR, the one favored by the authors is to think of the high GFR in energy or $O_2$ consumption terms. In more detail, to make the kidneys the ideal site for the production of erythropoietin, a central requirement is that the $PO_2$ at the site of release of erythropoietin should be influenced solely by the concentration of hemoglobin in blood. Because the kidney has a large blood flow, only a small amount of $O_2$ is extracted from each liter of blood. When the same amount of $O_2$ is extracted from blood that has a lower content of $O_2$ because of a lower hemoglobin concentration, the drop in $PO_2$ would be larger because one is operating on the flat part of the sigmoid-shaped oxygen-hemoglobin dissociation curve. In addition, because there is little variation in $P_{Na}$, renal work, which is largely the reabsorption of filtered Na+ ions ($O_2$ consumption) is directly related to the GFR. Because the ratio between the GFR ($O_2$ consumption) to renal plasma flow ($O_2$ delivery)—that is, the filtration fraction does not vary appreciably—the sensor for $PO_2$ should be exposed to near constant $PO_2$ unless hemoglobin concentration in blood falls (see margin note).

Before dealing with a detailed description of reabsorption of Na+ ions in individual nephron segments, the overall strategy for the reabsorption of Na+ ions will be considered. There are two elements: a driving force (a low concentration of Na+ ions and a negative voltage inside tubular cells) and a means (transporters or channels) to permit Na+ ions to cross the luminal membrane in each nephron segment. A diagrammatic illustration of the nephron segments is shown in Figure 9-4, and a quantitative estimate of the amount of Na+ ion reabsorbed in the different nephron segments is provided in Table 9-2. In the next several sections, we provide a detailed explanation for our estimates of the amount of Na+ ions that is reabsorbed in each segment of the renal tubule. Although a bit complex at times, we believe it provides the

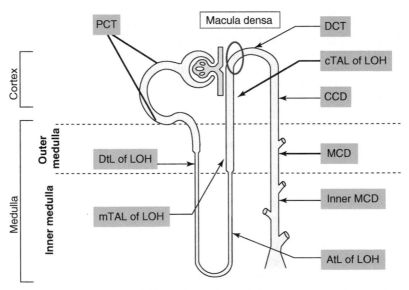

**Figure 9-4 Tubular Segments of Juxtamedullary Nephrons.** Juxtamedullary nephrons represent about 15% of all nephrons. Superficial nephrons (about 85% of all nephrons) have similar tubular segments, but their loops of Henle do not descend into the inner medulla. *PCT,* Proximal convoluted tubule; *DtL of LOH,* descending thin limb of the loop of Henle; *AtL of LOH,* ascending thin limb of the loop of Henle; *mTAL of LOH,* medullary thick ascending limb of loop of Henle; *cTAL of LOH,* cortical thick ascending limb of loop of Henle; *MCD,* medullary collecting duct; *CCD,* cortical collecting duct; *DCT,* distal convoluted tubule.

reader with a more clear picture of the role of each tubule segment in Na⁺ ion handling.

### Driving force

A low concentration of Na⁺ ions and a negative voltage in renal tubular cells are created by the electrogenic pumping of Na⁺ ions out of cells by the Na-K-ATPase in their basolateral membranes. This ion pump is electrogenic because it exports 3 Na⁺ ions out of the cell and imports only 2 K⁺ ions into the cell.

### Transport mechanism

The Na-K-ATPase generates an electrochemical gradient that favors the movement of Na⁺ ions into cells, but cell membranes are not permeable to Na⁺ ions. Therefore, specific transporters (cotransporters or antiporters) that bind Na⁺ ions and another ligand, or specific Na⁺ ion channels in the luminal membrane of cells, are required for the transport of Na⁺ ions in different nephron segments.

## Proximal convoluted tubule

The function of the PCT is to reabsorb most of the filtered Na⁺ ions in order to deliver only a small quantity of Na⁺ ions to downstream sites; these latter sites can then adjust their rate of reabsorption of Na⁺ ions to achieve balance for this cation in the steady state.

The mechanism for the reabsorption of Na⁺ ions in the PCT is active and is driven by the basolateral Na-K-ATPase. Virtually all the valuable water-soluble compounds and some ions (e.g., glucose, amino acids, HCO₃⁻) that are filtered have transport systems in PCT that are linked directly to the reabsorption of Na⁺ ions.

### Quantitative analysis

It was formerly thought that about 66% of the GFR is reabsorbed along the entire PCT. This is based on the measured ratio of the concentration of inulin in fluid samples obtained from the lumen of the PCT (TF), and its concentration in plasma (P) – (TF/P)$_{inulin}$ in micropuncture studies in rats in which inulin was infused. Because inulin is freely filtered at the glomerulus and is not reabsorbed or secreted in the tubules, a (TF/P)$_{inulin}$ value of around 3 suggests that approximately two-thirds

**TABLE 9-2    AMOUNT OF Na⁺ REABSORBED IN DIFFERENT SEGMENTS OF THE NEPHRON**

| NEPHRON SEGMENT | AMOUNT OF Na⁺ REABSORBED/DAY |
|---|---|
| • Proximal convoluted tubule | 22,650 |
| • Thin ascending limb of the loop of Henle of juxtamedullary nephrons | 360 |
| • Medullary thick ascending limb of the loop of Henle | 750 |
| • Cortical thick ascending limb of the loop of Henle | 1890 |
| • Distal convoluted tubule and cortical distal nephron | 1200 |
| • Medullary collecting duct | 0 |

The numbers in the table are approximations based on a filtered load of Na⁺ ions of 27,000 mmol/day (GFR 180 L/day × P$_{Na}$ 150 mmol/L) in a subject who consumes a typical Western diet and excretes 150 mmol of Na⁺ ions in his/her urine per day. A large amount of Na⁺ ions are reabsorbed in the medullary thick ascending limb of loop of Henle (about 3135 mmol/day), but only 750 mmol represent net reabsorption of Na⁺ ions. The remainder does not represent net reabsorption but rather recycling of Na⁺ ions because it is added back to the thin descending limbs of the loop of Henle of superficial nephrons. *GFR*, Glomerular filtration rate.

## CONCENTRATION OF Na⁺ IONS IN LUMINAL FLUID ENTERING THE LOOP OF HENLE

**CONCENTRATION OF $Na^+$ IONS IN LUMINAL FLUID ENTERING THE LOOP OF HENLE**

- The osmolality of the fluid entering the loop of Henle is about 300 mosmol/kg $H_2O$.
- Because the amount of urea filtered is about 900 mmol/day (GFR 180 mmol/day × plasma urea 5 mmol/L), and because about 500 mmol of urea are reabsorbed in the PCT, 400 mmol of urea/day are delivered to the loop of Henle. Because 30 L of fluid are delivered to the loop of Henle, the concentration of urea in this fluid will be close to 13 mmol/L.
- Therefore, the concentration of $Na^+$ ions in the luminal fluid entering the loop of Henle is close to 145 mmol/L ([300 − 13]/2).

(66%) of the filtrate was reabsorbed in the PCT. However, these measurements underestimate the actual volume of fluid reabsorbed in the PCT because in micropuncture studies, measurements are made at the last visible portion of the PCT that reaches the surface of the renal cortex and hence do not take into account additional volume that may be reabsorbed in the deeper part of the PCT, including its pars recta portion. An important recent observation is that AQP1 water channels are not present in the descending thin limbs (DtL) of the loop of Henle of superficial nephrons. Because superficial nephrons constitute about 85% of the total number of nephrons, the entire loop of Henle of the large majority of the nephrons is likely impermeable to water. Therefore, the volume of filtrate that enters their loops of Henle can be deduced using of the value for the $(TF/P)_{inulin}$ obtained from micropuncture studies in the early distal convoluted tubule (DCT) in rats. Because the minimum measured value is around 6, a reasonable estimate of the proportion of filtrate that is reabsorbed in the entire PCT of superficial nephrons is close to five-sixths (83%). This value is close to the estimate of fractional reabsorption in the PCT obtained with measurement of lithium clearance (which is thought to be a marker for fractional reabsorption in the PCT) in human subjects. Hence, a larger proportion of the filtered load of $Na^+$ ions is subject to regulation by mechanisms that influence the rate of $Na^+$ ion reabsorption in the PCT.

Based on this, with a GFR of 180 L/day and if five-sixths of the GFR is reabsorbed in the PCT, the volume of filtrate that exits the PCT into the loop of Henle is about 30 L/day (Table 9-3). If the concentration of $Na^+$ ions in this fluid is close to 145 mmol/L (see margin note), then 4350 mmol of $Na^+$ ions/day are delivered to the loop of Henle. Because 27,000 mmol of $Na^+$ ions are filtered per day, 22,650 mmol of $Na^+$ ions are reabsorbed in PCT per day.

### Process

AQP1 are constitutively present in the PCT. Hence, when $Na^+$ and $Cl^-$ ions are reabsorbed, water follows. Accordingly, the fluid reabsorbed is isotonic to plasma.

In the early PCT, the $Na^+/H^+$ exchanger-3 (NHE-3) is the main transporter for the entry of $Na^+$ ions into cells. This transporter mediates the indirect reabsorption of $NaHCO_3$ in the PCT. The

TABLE 9-3 **COMPARISON BETWEEN SUPERFICIAL NEPHRONS AND JUXTAMEDULLARY NEPHRONS**

| | SUPERFICIAL NEPHRONS | JUXTAMEDULLARY NEPHRONS |
|---|---|---|
| • % total | 85% | 15% |
| • GFR (L/day) | 153 | 27 |
| • Volume reabsorbed in the PCT (L/day) | 127 | 22.5 |
| • Volume exit from the PCT (L/day) | 26 | 4.5 |
| • Volume reabsorbed in the outer medulla (L/day) | 0 | 3.0 |
| • Volume reabsorbed in the inner medulla (L/day) | 0 | 0.2 |
| • Volume delivered to the DCT (L/day) | 26 | 1.3 |

The numbers are approximations. In contrast to juxtamedullary nephrons, thin descending limbs of superficial nephrons (the large majority of nephrons) lack aquaporin 1 (AQP1) in their luminal membranes and hence are largely water impermeable. Out of the 4.5 L of filtrate that are delivered to the descending thin limbs of the loop of Henle of the juxtamedullary nephron per day, 3 L/day are reabsorbed in the outer medulla as the osmolality in the medullary interstitial compartment rises from 300 to 900 mosmol/kg $H_2O$. The volume of water reabsorbed from the descending thin limbs of the juxtamedullary nephrons in the inner medulla was calculated at a medullary interstitial osmolality of 1050 mosmol/kg $H_2O$ (i.e., the midpoint between 900 and 1200 mosmol/kg $H_2O$) because descending thin limbs have their bends at different levels in the inner medulla. GFR, Glomerular filtration rate; PCT, proximal convoluted tubule; DCT, distal convoluted tubule.

reabsorption of $Na^+$ and $HCO_3^-$ ions in the early PCT results in the transport of water and thereby causes a rise in the concentration of $Cl^-$ ions in the remaining tubular fluid. The electrochemical gradient for $Na^+$ ions provides the driving force for the reabsorption of $Na^+$ ions with glucose and other filtered solutes (e.g., amino acids, phosphate, and organic anions) via $Na^+$ ion-dependent transporters. This electrogenic transport of $Na^+$ creates a small, lumen-negative, transepithelial potential difference of approximately $-2\,mV$. The rise in luminal fluid $Cl^-$ ion concentration and the small lumen-negative transepithelial voltage provide the driving force for the reabsorption of $Cl^-$ ions via the paracellular route (Fig. 9-5). This paracellular flux of $Cl^-$ ions causes reversal of the transepithelial voltage to a small lumen-positive voltage ($+2\,mV$), which drives the paracellular reabsorption of $Na^+$.

Transcellular reabsorption of $Cl^-$ ions coupled to reabsorption of $Na^+$ ions also occurs in the latter part of the PCT, mediated by NHE-3 (or by an $Na^+$-sulfate cotransporter) in tandem with a $Cl^-$/ $base^-$ exchanger (CFEX, SLC26A6) that is capable of transporting, in addition to $Cl^-$ ions, other anions such as formate, $HCO_3^-$, sulfate, and oxalate (Fig. 9-6).

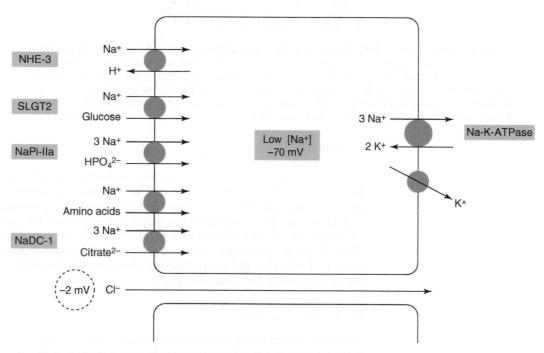

**Figure 9-5  $Na^+$-Coupled Transport in the PCT.** A low concentration of $Na^+$ ions and a negative voltage in proximal convoluted tubule (PCT) cells are created by the electrogenic pumping of $Na^+$ ions out of cells by the Na-K-ATPase. The $Na^+/H^+$ exchanger-3 (NHE-3) mediates the indirect reabsorption of $NaHCO_3$ in the PCT. The reabsorption of $Na^+$ and $HCO_3^-$ ions in the early PCT results in the transport of water and thereby causes a rise in the concentration of $Cl^-$ ions in the remaining tubular fluid. The electrochemical gradient for $Na^+$ ions is utilized to reabsorb a number of valuable compounds and ions that are filtered. Important examples include glucose, amino acids, phosphate, and citrate anions (transporter for urate anions is not shown in the figure). This electrogenic transport of $Na^+$ ions creates a small lumen-negative, transepithelial potential difference of approximately $-2\,mV$. The rise in luminal fluid $Cl^-$ ion concentration and the small luminal negative transepithelial voltage provide the driving force for the reabsorption of $Cl^-$ ions via the paracellular route. This paracellular flux of $Cl^-$ ions causes reversal of the transepithelial voltage to a small lumen-positive voltage ($+2\,mV$), which drives the paracellular reabsorption of $Na^+$ ions (not shown in the figure). *PCT*, Proximal convoluted tubule; *ATP*, adenosine triphosphate; *SLGT2*, sodium linked glucose cotransporter-2; *NaPi-IIa*, sodium- dependent phosphate cotransporter-IIa; *NaDC-1*, sodium dicitrate cotransporter-1.

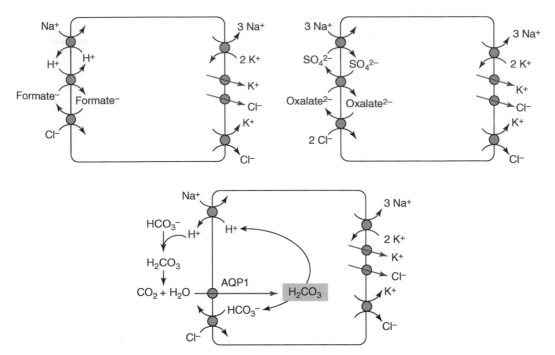

**Figure 9-6 Transepithelial NaCl Transport in the Proximal Convoluted Tubule.** Transcellular reabsorption of Cl⁻ ions coupled to the reabsorption of Na⁺ ions occurs in the latter part of the proximal convoluted tubule (PCT), mediated by Na⁺/H⁺ exchanger-3 (NHE-3) (or by an Na⁺-sulfate cotransporter) in tandem with a Cl⁻/base⁻ exchanger (CFEX, SLC26A6) that exchanges Cl⁻ anions for another anion such as formate, $HCO_3^-$, sulfate, or oxalate. Na⁺ ions exit the cell on the Na-K-ATPase, while Cl⁻ ions exit the cell via a Cl⁻ channel or a K⁺/Cl⁻ cotransporter. *AQP1*, Aquaporin 1.

### Control

Precise control of the excretion of Na⁺ ions cannot be exerted in the PCT because ~27,000 mmol of Na⁺ are filtered and ~22,650 mmol are reabsorbed daily in this nephron segment. Hence, it is extremely unlikely that the PCT could adjust its rate of reabsorption of Na⁺ ions to change the rate of excretion of Na⁺ ions by 100 or so mmol/day. This does not mean that there is no regulation of Na⁺ ion reabsorption in the PCT but rather that it is not the site where fine adjustment of the rate of excretion of Na⁺ ions takes place.

#### Glomerulotubular balance

Glomerulotubular balance refers to the phenomenon whereby changes in the GFR are matched by equivalent changes in tubular reabsorption so that fractional reabsorption of fluid and NaCl is maintained constant. The impact of changes in the GFR on the reabsorption of Na⁺ and Cl⁻ ions are particularly pronounced in the PCT.

In the PCT, both peritubular and luminal factors are thought to contribute to glomerulotubular balance. With regard to peritubular factors, an increase in the GFR without a rise in renal blood flow reflects an increase in filtration fraction and hence a higher concentration of albumin in peritubular capillary blood. The higher oncotic pressure in peritubular capillary blood can increase net reabsorption in the PCT. With regard to luminal factors, an increase in the GFR increases the filtered load of $HCO_3^-$ ions, glucose, and other solutes, the absorption of which is coupled to the reabsorption of Na⁺ ions by their respective Na⁺ ion-dependent cotransporters. The resultant rise in luminal Cl⁻ ion concentration drives its passive, paracellular reabsorption.

Changes in the EABV seem to alter this relationship between the GFR and fractional reabsorption in the PCT. For example, a decrease in the EABV leads to a fall in the GFR but an increase in fractional reabsorption in the PCT. This is likely mediated by activation of the sympathetic nervous system and the release of angiotensin II, both of which are known to enhance the reabsorption of NaCl in the PCT.

### Neurohumoral effects

NaCl reabsorption by the PCT is affected by a number of hormones and neurotransmitters. NaCl reabsorption in PCT is stimulated by renal sympathetic activation and angiotensin II, and inhibited by dopamine.

Epinephrine and norepinephrine stimulate proximal NaCl reabsorption via binding to α-adrenergic receptors at the basolateral membrane. Angiotensin II has a potent effect on NaCl reabsorption in the PCT. In addition to circulating angiotensin II, angiotensin II is also synthesized and secreted by the PCT; its effect is mediated via the AT1 receptor, both at the luminal and basolateral membrane. Dopamine is synthesized in the PCT and inhibits NaCl reabsorption via binding to its $D_1$ receptor.

NHE-3 is the primary target for these stimulatory and inhibitory effects. NHE-3 is regulated by the combined effects of its direct phosphorylation and interaction with scaffolding proteins, which affect its trafficking to the luminal membrane.

In addition to a direct effect on NHE-3, these effects on NaCl reabsorption may also be mediated by changes in glomerular hemodynamics. For example, angiotensin II is a potent vasoconstrictor, especially of the renal efferent arterioles (and to a lesser degree the afferent arterioles). Efferent arteriolar constriction increases the filtration fraction and hence the peritubular capillary plasma oncotic pressure. The latter promotes the uptake of fluid into capillaries and, as a result, an increase in the net reabsorption of NaCl in PCT.

### Disorders involving the PCT

The presence of excessive excretion of glucose, phosphate, organic anions, $HCO_3^-$, and/or urate in the presence of low values for their concentrations in plasma indicates a defect in PCT function. These defects may occur in isolation or as part of generalized proximal tubular dysfunction (Fanconi syndrome). The clinical diagnosis of proximal renal tubular acidosis can be confirmed by detecting a high fractional excretion of $HCO_3^-$ ions during $NaHCO_3$ loading and by the presence of a high rate of excretion of citrate anions in the urine in the presence of metabolic acidosis (see Chapter 4 for more discussion).

The only important pharmacologic diuretic that acts on the PCT is acetazolamide, which inhibits the luminal carbonic anhydrase, carbonic anhydrase IV, and hence diminishes the reabsorption of $NaHCO_3$ and thus of NaCl in PCT.

## Descending thin limb of the loop of Henle

The traditional view of the physiology of this nephron segment is that it has AQP1 and is therefore permeable to water. This means that, for example, when the interstitial osmolality doubles, half of the volume of water reaching the descending thin limb is reabsorbed. An important finding is that AQP1 are not present in the descending thin limbs of the loop of Henle of superficial nephrons, which constitute ~85% of all nephrons. Hence, in contradiction to the traditional view, with the exception of descending thin limbs of juxtamedullary nephrons

(~15% of all nephrons), the vast majority of the descending thin limbs of the loop of Henle are likely to be largely impermeable to water.

Of note, the concentration of $Na^+$ ions rises progressively in the luminal fluid in the descending thin limb of the loop of Henle of superficial nephrons as they descend down into the medulla. It is necessary to have a high concentration of $Na^+$ ions in the luminal fluid that reaches the medullary thick ascending limb (mTAL) of the loop of Henle to allow for the voltage-driven, paracellular $Na^+$ ion reabsorption (which represents 50% of $Na^+$ ion reabsorption in this nephron segment) to occur in the face of a high medullary interstitial concentration of $Na^+$ ions. Because AQP1 are not present in the descending thin limb of the loop of Henle of the majority of the nephrons, and hence they are likely to be largely impermeable to water, the rise in $Na^+$ ion concentration in their luminal fluid is unlikely to be caused by water exit. Accordingly, entry of $Na^+$ ions (via $Na^+$ ion channels) and $Cl^-$ ions (via $Cl^-$ ion channels) is likely to be the mechanism responsible for the bulk of this rise in the luminal concentrations of $Na^+$ and $Cl^-$ ions. The quantitative implications of this process of addition of $Na^+$ and $Cl^-$ ions to the luminal fluid in the descending thin limbs of the loop of Henle of the superficial nephrons are further discussed when events in the mTAL of the loop of Henle are considered.

### Ascending thin limb of the loop of Henle

Reabsorption of $Na^+$ ions in the ascending thin limb of the loop of Henle of the juxtamedullary nephrons in the inner medulla is a passive process, occurring down a concentration difference for $Na^+$ ions between the tubular fluid (higher) and the interstitial compartment (lower). In more detail, actions of vasopressin cause the insertion of both AQP2 and urea transporters in the luminal membrane of cells in the inner MCD. The addition of water (with urea) into the interstitial compartment lowers the concentration of $Na^+$ and $Cl^-$ ions in the interstitial compartment in the inner medulla. This creates a driving force for the passive movement of $Na^+$ and $Cl^-$ ions from the luminal fluid in the water impermeable, ascending thin limbs of the loop of Henle into the interstitial compartment in the inner medulla. As the osmolality in the interstitial compartment in the inner medulla rises (because of the addition of urea and NaCl), water will be reabsorbed from the thin descending limbs of the loop of Henle because they possess AQP1, and therefore are water permeable. This movement of water raises the concentration of $Na^+$ and $Cl^-$ ions in the luminal fluid in the descending thin limbs of the loop of Henle, and therefore in the ascending limbs, which will further facilitate the diffusion of $Na^+$ and $Cl^-$ ions into the medullary interstitial compartment.

### Quantitative analysis

If juxtamedullary nephrons represent ~15% of the total number of nephrons and hence receive 27 L of GFR/day (180 L/day × 15%), and because about five-sixths of the filtrate is reabsorbed in the PCT, ~4.5 L/day will enter the loop of Henle of these nephrons. Because the concentration of $Na^+$ ions in the luminal fluid is about 145 mmol/L, ~650 mmol of $Na^+$ per day (4.5 L × 145 mmol/L) will be delivered to their loops of Henle. Our best estimate of the amount of $Na^+$ ions reabsorbed in the thin ascending limbs of the loop of Henle of the juxtamedullary nephrons is approximately 360 mmol/day (see Part D for details of our calculation).

## Medullary thick ascending limb of the loop of Henle

### *Quantitative analysis*

There are four important issues to consider to estimate the amount of $Na^+$ ions that are reabsorbed in the loop of Henle (Table 9-4). First, the volume of fluid delivered to the loops of Henle, of both superficial and juxtamedullary nephrons, is close to one-sixth of the GFR, or 30 L/day ($1/6 \times 180$ L/day = 30 L/day). Second, the concentration of $Na^+$ ions in the fluid delivered to the loop of Henle is about 145 mmol/L. Therefore, approximately 4350 mmol of $Na^+$ ions are delivered to the loop of Henle each day (145 mmol/L $\times$ 30 L/day). Third, the volume of filtrate delivered to the early DCT is about 27 L/day (see Table 9-3). Fourth, to estimate how many $Na^+$ ions are reabsorbed in the loop of Henle, one needs to know the concentration of $Na^+$ ions in the fluid that is delivered to the DCT. The $Na^+$ ion concentration measured in fluid obtained from the early accessible part of the DCT in micropuncture studies in rats is close to 50 mmol/L. If applicable to humans, then 1350 mmol of $Na^+$ ions/day exit the loop of Henle (27 L $\times$ 50 mmol/L). Because ~4350 mmol/day of $Na^+$ ions entered the loop of Henle and 360 mmol/day are reabsorbed in the ascending thin limbs (see Part D), we estimate that close to 2640 mmol of $Na^+$ ions are reabsorbed daily in both the medullary and cortical segments of the thick ascending limb of the loop of Henle.

There are two functions of the process of reabsorption of $Na^+$ and $Cl^-$ ions into the mTALs of the loop of Henle.

1. *Add $Na^+$ ions to water reabsorbed in the renal medulla to make it into an isotonic solution.*

   The volume of water that is reabsorbed in the medulla and added to the blood that exits the medulla via the ascending vasa recta is approximately 7.4 L per day. This includes 3.3 L of water/day that are reabsorbed from the MCD in the outer medulla (Table 9-5), 3 L of water/day that are reabsorbed from the descending thin limbs of the loop of Henle of juxtamedullary nephrons (those with AQP1) in the outer medulla, and 1.1 L of water/day that are reabsorbed in the inner medulla from the inner MCD and from the descending thin limbs of the loops of Henle (see Table 9-6 and Part D for a detailed analysis). Because every liter of this water must exit the renal medulla via the as-

---

TABLE 9-4    **CALCULATION OF THE AMOUNT OF $Na^+$ IONS THAT ARE REABSORBED IN THE MEDULLARY AND CORTICAL SEGMENTS OF THE THICK ASCENDING LIMB OF THE LOOP OF HENLE**

| | |
|---|---|
| • Volume of filtrate that enters the loop of Henle (L/day) | 30 |
| • $Na^+$ concentration in luminal fluid that enters the loop of Henle (mmol/L) | 145 |
| • Amount of $Na^+$ delivered to the loop of Henle (mmol/day) | 4350 (30 × 145) |
| • Amount of $Na^+$ reabsorbed in the ascending thin limbs of the loop of Henle of juxta medullary nephrons (mmol/day) | 360 |
| • Amount of $Na^+$ delivered to the mTAL of the loop of Henle (mmol/day) | 3990 (4350 − 360) |
| • Volume of filtrate delivered to the early DCT (L/day) | 27 |
| • $Na^+$ concentration in luminal fluid in the early DCT (mmol/L) | 50 |
| • Amount of $Na^+$ delivered to the early DCT (mmol/day) | 1350 (27 × 50) |
| • Amount of $Na^+$ reabsorbed in the mTAL and cTAL of the loop of Henle (mmol/day) | 2640 (3990 − 1350) |

For details, see text. *mTAL,* Medullary thick ascending limb; *cTAL,* cortical thick ascending limb; *DCT,* distal convoluted tubule.

cending vasa recta with the same $Na^+$ ion/$H_2O$ ratio as the fluid that entered the medulla via the descending vasa recta (~150 mmol/kg $H_2O$), about 1110 mmol of $Na^+$ ions are required to be added to these 7.4 L of water. We estimated that 360 mmol of $Na^+$ ions are reabsorbed from the ascending thin limbs of the loop of Henle of juxtamedullary nephrons; hence, about 750 mmol of $Na^+$ ions need to be reabsorbed from the mTAL of the loop of Henle to serve this function. This is the only component of $Na^+$ ion reabsorption in the mTAL of the loop of Henle that represents a net reabsorption of filtered $Na^+$ ions.

2. *Replace $Na^+$ ions that entered the descending thin limbs of the loop of Henle of superficial nephrons from the medullary interstitial compartment.*

As mentioned earlier, the descending thin limbs of the loop of Henle of the majority of the nephrons do not have AQP1, and therefore are likely water impermeable. Therefore, the rise in $Na^+$ ion concentration in their luminal fluid is likely to be because of entry of $Na^+$ ions from the medullary interstitial compartment. This component of $Na^+$ reabsorption from the mTAL simply restores the interstitial concentration of $Na^+$ ions to its original hypertonic value. We estimate that about 2530 mmol of $Na^+$ ions per day are reabsorbed from the mTAL of loop of Henle for this purpose (for a detailed calculation, see Part D). Notwithstanding, this considerable amount of $Na^+$ ion reabsorption does not represent a net reabsorption of $Na^+$ ions, but rather a recycling of $Na^+$ ions. This is because these $Na^+$ ions are

---

**TABLE 9-5    VOLUME OF WATER REABSORBED IN THE CORTICAL AND MEDULLARY COLLECTING DUCTS**

| | |
|---|---|
| • Volume delivered to collecting ducts (L/day) | 27 |
| • Volume reabsorbed in the CCD (L/day) | 22 |
| • Volume delivered to the MCD (L/day) | 5 |
| • Volume reabsorbed in the outer medulla (L/day) | 3.3 |
| • Volume reabsorbed in the inner medulla (L/day) | 0.4 |

We estimated that 5 L exit the terminal CCD based on: (1) when vasopressin acts, the osmolality in the terminal CCD is equal to the plasma osmolality (300 mosmol/kg $H_2O$), and (2) the number of osmoles in the terminal CCD is 1500 mosmol (1000 mosmol of urea and 500 mosmol of electrolytes [$Na^+ + K^+$ ions with their accompanying anions]). In the outer medulla, the osmolality in the interstitial compartment rises from 300 to 900 mosmol/kg $H_2O$, hence two-thirds of the volume of water delivered will be reabsorbed (i.e., 3.3 L out of 5 L). In the inner medulla, the osmolality in the interstitial compartment rises from 900 to 1200 mosmol/kg $H_2O$; hence, one-quarter of the volume of water delivered will be reabsorbed ( i.e., 0.4 L out of 1.7 L). *CCD*, Cortical collecting duct; *MCD*, medullary collecting duct.

---

**TABLE 9-6    CALCULATION OF VOLUME OF WATER REABSORBED IN THE INNER MEDULLA**

| | |
|---|---|
| • Volume of water reabsorbed from the inner MCD with 600 mmol of urea (L/day) | 0.5 |
| • Volume of water reabsorbed from the inner MCD as interstitial osmolality rises from 900 to 1200 mosmol/kg $H_2O$ (L/day) | 0.4 |
| • Volume of water reabsorbed from the descending thin limbs of juxtamedullary nephrons (L/day) | 0.2 |
| • Total volume of water reabsorbed in the inner medulla (L/day) | 1.1 |

About 600 mmol/day of urea are reabsorbed in the inner MCD and added to the interstitial compartment at an osmolality of 1200 mosmol/kg $H_2O$ (see Figure 9-21). Therefore, 0.5 L of water is reaborbed in the inner MCD with this amount of urea. As medullary interstitial osmolality rises from 900 to 1200 mosmol/kg $H_2O$, one-quarter of the volume of water in the MCD (1.7 L) will be reabsorbed (0.4 L). The volume of water in the descending thin limbs of juxtamedullary nephrons as they enter the inner medulla is 1.5 L (see Table 9-3). Because the descending thin limbs of the loop of Henle have their bends at different levels in the inner medulla, the volume of water reabsorbed from the descending thin limbs of the juxtamedullary nephrons was calculated at medullary interstitial osmolality of 1050 mosmol/L (i.e., the midpoint between 900 and 1200 mosmol/kg $H_2O$). Therefore, if 1.5 L of fluid with osmolality of 900 mosmol/L enter the inner medulla in the descending thin limbs of the loop of Henle, because the interstitial osmolality in the inner medulla rises to 1050 mosmol/kg $H_2O$, 0.2 L of water will be reabsorbed. *MCD*, Medullary collecting duct.

reabsorbed from the mTAL of the loop of Henle and are added back
to the thin descending limb of the loop of Henle.

Therefore, out of a total amount of ~3990 mmol of $Na^+$ ions
that are delivered to the mTAL of the loop of Henle per day (see
Table 9-4), there is net reabsorption of 750 mmol of $Na^+$ ions, and
3240 mmol of $Na^+$ ions are delivered to the cortical thick ascending
limb (cTAL) of the loop of Henle.

### Process

Because of the action of Na-K-ATPase at the basolateral membrane,
$Na^+$ ions enter cells in the mTAL from the lumen down its concentration gradient on the electroneutral $Na^+$, $K^+$, 2 $Cl^-$ cotransporter-2
(NKCC-2). This transporter requires the presence of all three ions and
hence is limited by the quantity of $K^+$ ions in the lumen of this nephron
segment. Hence, $K^+$ ions must re-enter the lumen via the renal outer
medullary $K^+$ (ROMK) ion channel. $Cl^-$ ions exit from the cell in an
electrogenic fashion via the $Cl^-$ ion channel (ClC-Kb) at the basolateral
membrane. This entry of $K^+$ ions into the lumen and the electrogenic
exit of $Cl^-$ ions at the basolateral membrane generate a transepithelial,
lumen-positive voltage (Fig. 9-7). The transepithelial, lumen-positive
voltage drives the electrogenic reabsorption of $Na^+$ ions, as well as of

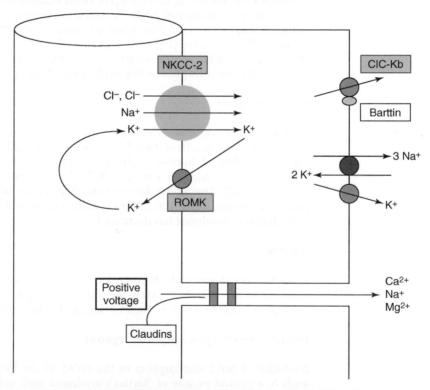

**Figure 9-7  Transport of $Na^+$ and $Cl^-$ Ions in the mTAL of the Loop of Henle.** A low concentration of
$Na^+$ ions and a negative voltage are created in the mTAL of the loop of Henle cells by the electrogenic pumping of $Na^+$ ions out of cells by the Na-K-ATPase. $Na^+$ ions enter cells in the medullary
thick ascending limb (mTAL) from the lumen down their concentration gradient on the electroneutral $Na^+$, $K^+$, 2 $Cl^-$ cotransporter 2 (NKCC-2) in their luminal membrane, which transports 1
$Na^+$, 1 $K^+$, and 2 $Cl^-$ ions. $Cl^-$ ions exit the cell via a basolateral $Cl^-$ channel (ClC-Kb). $K^+$ ions must
re-enter the lumen via the renal outer medullary $K^+$ ion channel (ROMK) to supply the needed $K^+$
ions for the continued operation of this transporter. This also generates a positive voltage in the
lumen that "pushes" $Na^+$, $Ca^{2+}$, and $Mg^{2+}$ ions between cells of the mTAL of the loop of Henle.
This accounts for 50% of $Na^+$ reabsorption in this nephron segment.

ionized calcium ($Ca^{2+}$) and ionized magnesium ($Mg^{2+}$), through the paracellular pathway, which expresses the tight junction proteins, claudin 16 (paracellin-1) and claudin 19. About 50% of the amount of $Na^+$ ion reabsorbed by the mTAL occurs via the paracellular pathway.

### Control

Because regulation of NaCl reabsorption is likely to be mediated by inhibitory control (see Part C), this process is not likely to be regulated by activation of NKCC-2 or the quantity of NKCC-2 in the luminal membrane.

The signal to increase the reabsorption of $Na^+$ ions in the mTAL of the loop of Henle is likely to be mediated by a fall in the concentration of an inhibitor in the medullary interstitial compartment. This fall in concentration of the inhibitor may begin with the addition of water from the water-permeable nephron segments that traverse the medullary interstitial compartment. One possible candidate that seems to have ideal properties for this function is the activity of ionized $Ca^{2+}$ ions in the medullary interstitial compartment. In more detail, when the concentration of ionized calcium rises, it binds to the calcium-sensing receptor (Ca-SR) at the basolateral membrane of cells of the mTAL of the loop of Henle. This generates a signal (an arachidonic acid metabolite, 20-hydroxyeicosatetraenoic acid) that leads to inhibition of the ROMK. This latter step is critical for the process of NaCl reabsorption in the mTAL of the loop of Henle because it supplies the $K^+$ ions for the function of NKCC-2 and also generates the lumen-positive voltage required for the passive reabsorption of $Na^+$ ions via the paracellular pathway (Fig. 9-8). Hence, a fall in the concentration of ionized $Ca^{2+}$ in the medullary interstitial compartment will lead to increased NaCl reabsorption in the mTAL of the loop of Henle.

### Role of hormones

A number of hormones, which increase cyclic adenosine monophoshate (cAMP) in cells of the mTAL of the loop of Henle (e.g., vasopressin, parathyroid hormone, glucagon, calcitonin, $\beta_2$ adrenergic activation), are thought to activate NKCC-2 and increase the reabsorption of NaCl. These probably act to facilitate faster rates of transport once the interstitial concentration of the inhibitor of the ROMK in the luminal membrane has decreased.

### Inhibitors

Loop diuretics (furosemide, bumetanide, ethacrynic acid) inhibit the reabsorption of $Na^+$ and $Cl^-$ ions in the thick ascending limb of the loop of Henle by competing with luminal $Cl^-$ ions for binding to NKCC-2.

### Disorders involving this nephron segment

Inhibition of NaCl reabsorption in the mTAL of the loop of Henle leads to a clinical picture of Bartter's syndrome with urinary wasting of $Na^+$, $K^+$, and $Cl^-$ ions: a contracted EABV, hypokalemia, metabolic alkalosis, a renal concentrating defect, hypercalciuria, and less commonly renal $Mg^{2+}$ wasting with hypomagnesemia (for more discussion, see Chapter 14). Mutations that cause Bartter's syndrome have been identified in five separate genes (see Fig. 14-1). The first two abnormalities lead to antenatal Bartter's syndrome and include mutations in the gene encoding NKCC-2 and the gene encoding the ROMK channel. A third lesion involves the basolateral $Cl^-$ channel (ClC-Kb); this may also affect the functions of the DCT. Mutations in

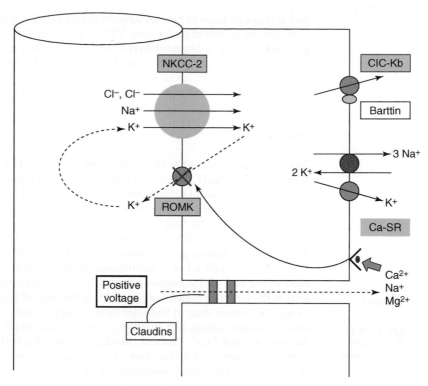

**Figure 9-8 Control of NaCl Reabsorption in the mTAL by Interstitial Ionized Calcium.** When the concentration of ionized calcium (Ca²⁺) in the medullary interstitial compartment rises, it binds to the calcium-sensing receptor (Ca-SR) at the basolateral membrane of cells of the mTAL of the loop of Henle. This generates a signal that leads to inhibition of the renal outer medullary K⁺ channel (ROMK). This latter step is critical for the process of NaCl reabsorption in the medullary thick ascending limb (mTAL) of the loop of Henle because it supplies the K⁺ ions for the Na⁺, K⁺, 2 Cl⁻ cotransporter 2 (NKCC-2) and it also generates the lumen-positive voltage for the passive paracellular reabsorption of 50% of the amount Na⁺ ions reabsorbed in the mTAL of the loop of Henle. *ClC-Kb,* Chloride channel.

the gene that encodes for an essential β-subunit of this Cl⁻ channel, called Barttin, have been reported in patients with Bartter's syndrome and sensorineural deafness, which suggests that Barttin is involved in the function of the Cl⁻ channels in the inner ear. Patients with Bartter's syndrome and hypocalcemia have been reported; the basis of this disorder is an activating mutation in the gene encoding the Ca-SR.

There are also acquired disorders that lead to loop diuretic-like effects and hence a Bartter's-like clinical picture. Examples include hypercalcemia and cationic drugs that bind to the Ca-SR (e.g., gentamicin, cisplatin). It is also possible that cationic proteins may bind to Ca-SR and lead to a Bartter's-like clinical picture, as may be the case in some patients with multiple myeloma or autoimmune disorders.

### Cortical thick ascending limb of the loop of Henle

#### *Quantitative analysis*

We estimated that about 3990 mmol of Na⁺ ions are delivered to the mTAL of the loop of Henle per day, and that there is net reabosrption of about 750 mmol of Na⁺ ions in this nephron segment per day. Therefore, about 3240 mmol of Na⁺ ions per day exit the mTAL of the loop of Henle. To obtain a quantitative estimate of the amount of Na⁺ ions that are reabsorbed in cTAL of the loop of Henle per day, we use data from micropuncture studies in the early accessible part of DCT in rats and extrapolate them to human subjects to estimate the amount of $Na^+$ ions that are delivered to the early DCT. Extrapolated to human subjects, the volume of filtrate delivered to the early DCT is about 27 L/day (see Table 9-3), and the measured $Na^+$ ion concentration is close to 50 mmol/L. Therefore, about 1350 mmol of $Na^+$ ions per day are delivered to the early DCT. Therefore, ~1890 mmol of $Na^+$ ions (3240 - 1350) are reabsorbed in the cTAL of loop of Henle per day.

### Process

This nephron segment has the same major transporters for the reabsorption of $Na^+$ and $Cl^-$ ions as the mTAL of the loop of Henle (luminal NKCC-2 and ROMK; basolateral Na-K-ATPase, $Cl^-$ ion channels, $K^+$ ion channels; paracellular pathway for the reabsorption of $Na^+$ ions and ionized $Ca^{2+}$). Its function is to reabsorb a large proportion of the $Na^+$ ions that are delivered from the mTAL of the loop of Henle. Hence, a larger lumen-positive voltage is needed to achieve this function and have such a low concentration of $Na^+$ ions in the luminal fluid at the end of this nephron segment (i.e., concentration of $Na^+$ ions in the lumen at the end of the cTAL of the loop of Henle is three- to fourfold lower than in the interstitial compartment). This higher lumen-positive voltage will, however, cause the reabsorption of a large amount of ionized $Ca^{2+}$. Notwithstanding, because the cortical plasma flow rate is large (~900 L/day) (see margin note), this will cause only a tiny rise in the interstitial concentration of ionized $Ca^{2+}$.

### Control

The major difference between the cTAL and the mTAL is the relative lack of an inhibitory effect of the activity of interstitial ionized $Ca^{2+}$ on the reabsorption of $Na^+$ and $Cl^-$ ions because of the enormous renal blood flow rate in the cortex. Accordingly, the limit for the reabsorption of $Na^+$ and $Cl^-$ ions in this nephron segment could be set either by the maximum lumen-positive voltage or by the affinity of its NKCC-2 for the concentration of $Cl^-$ ions in the lumen ($K_m$ ~40 mmol/L). Hence, a large quantity of $Na^+$ and $Cl^-$ ions are reabsorbed in this nephron segment.

### Reabsorption of $Na^+$ and $Cl^-$ ions in the macula densa

The macula densa cells are a small subset of approximately 20 cells per nephron at the distal end of the cTAL of the loop of Henle. These cells are in close approximation to the juxtaglomerular vascular smooth muscle cells of the afferent arterioles of their glomeruli, and together they form what is known as the juxtaglomerular apparatus. Cells of the macula densa share the same transporters as the other cells in the cTAL of the loop of Henle, though they express a high-affinity isoform of NKCC-2 in their apical membrane. Increased NaCl delivery and its uptake through NKCC-2 in macula densa cells is coupled to the generation of a signal that causes vasoconstriction of the afferent arterioles, which lowers the GFR and returns the distal delivery of NaCl to close to its usual levels. This response is known as tubuloglomerular feedback. The signal relates to the release of ATP from the basolateral membrane of macula densa cells into the juxtaglomerular interstitium. Subsequently, adenosine is formed, which through activation of $A_1$ adenosine receptors causes vasoconstriction of afferent arterioles. Furosemide and other NKCC-2 inhibitors (bumetanide, ethacrynic acid) inhibit NKCC-2 and the tubuloglomerular feedback mechanism.

**RENAL CORTICAL PLASMA FLOW RATE**

- With a GFR of 180 L/day and a filtration fraction of ~20%, the renal plasma flow rate is close to 900 L/day.

### Early distal convoluted tubule

#### Quantitative analysis

About 1350 mmol of $Na^+$ are delivered to the early DCT per day (see Table 9-4). Subjects who consume a typical Western diet eat and excrete about 150 mmol of $Na^+$ ions daily. Because there is little reabsoption of $Na^+$ ions in the MCD, about 1200 mmol of $Na^+$ are reabsorbed in the early DCT and the CDN. The latter segment includes the late DCT, the connecting segment, and the cortical collecting duct (CCD).

Na$^+$ and $Cl^-$ ions are reabsorbed in an electroneutral fashion via a $Na^+$ and $Cl^-$ cotransporter (NCC). Because this nephron segment has low luminal concentrations of $Na^+$ and $Cl^-$ ions, only a relatively small quantity of $Na^+$ and $Cl^-$ ions can be reabsorbed. Regulation of $Na^+$ and $Cl^-$ ion reabsorption in this nephron segment must also allow for a large enough delivery of $Na^+$ and $Cl^-$ ions (~400 mmol/day) to the CDN to permit the secretion of a large $K^+$ ion load if needed, as might have been the case in Paleolithic times, when the human diet consisted of a very large amount of fruit such as berries and therefore provided large, intermittent loads of $K^+$ ions.

#### Process

Because of the action of the Na-K-ATPase in the basolateral membrane, the concentration of $Na^+$ ions in cells of the DCT is ~10 to 15 mmol/L; hence, there is a chemical driving force for the entry of $Na^+$ and $Cl^-$ ions into these cells, which is mediated by an electroneutral NCC. This transporter has a high affinity for $Na^+$ and $Cl^-$ with a concentration of $Na^+$ ions required for the NCC to operate at half of its maximum velocity of ~7.5 mmol/L and a concentration of $Cl^-$ ions of ~6.5 mmol/L. $Cl^-$ ions exit the cell via a basolateral $Cl^-$ channel (ClC-Kb) (Fig. 9-9).

#### Control

A long-term increase in $Na^+$ and $Cl^-$ ion delivery to the early DCT is associated with hypertrophy of this nephron segment, increased Na-K-ATPase activity, an increased number of NCC, and enhanced reabsorption of NaCl. In contrast, chronic inhibition of NCC by thiazide diuretics may be associated with apoptosis of DCT cells and tubular atrophy.

A complex network of With-No-Lysine kinases (WNKs), WNK4 and WNK1, modulate the reabsorption of $Na^+$ and $Cl^-$ ions in the

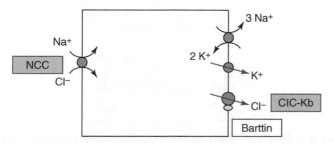

**Figure 9-9 Transport of Na$^+$ and Cl$^-$ Ions in the Early DCT.** A low concentration of $Na^+$ ions and a negative voltage are created in distal convoluted tubule (DCT) cells by the electrogenic pumping of $Na^+$ out of cells by the Na-K-ATPase. $Na^+$ ions enter the cells from the lumen down its concentration gradient on the electroneutral $Na^+$/$Cl^-$ cotransporter (NCC). $Cl^-$ ions exit the cell via a basolateral $Cl^-$ channel (ClC-Kb).

early DCT via an effect on the quantity of active NCC inserted into the luminal membrane. WNK4 is thought to diminish NCC activity by reducing its abundance in luminal membranes by diverting post-Golgi NCC to the lysosome for degradation. Angiotensin II is released in response to a low EABV (or low salt intake). Angiotensin II signaling through its AT1 receptor converts WNK4 from an NCC-inhibiting to an NCC-activating kinase. The activated form of WNK4 phosphorylates members of the STE20 family of serine/threonine kinases, specifically the STE20-related proline-alanine-rich-kinase (SPAK) and the oxidative stress response kinase type 1 (OSR1). Phosphorylated SPAK/OSR1 in turn phosphorylates and activates NCC (Fig. 9-10).

WNK1 is another member of the WNK kinase family that is involved in modulating the activity of NCC. Alternative promoter usage of the WNK1 gene produces a kidney-specific, truncated form of WNK1, called KS-WNK1, and a more ubiquitous long form, called L-WNK1. The KS-WNK1 isoform inhibits the L-WNK1. When the ratio of KS-WNK1 to L-WNK1 is low, L-WNK1 exerts its effect to upregulate NCC either by blocking the inhibitory form of WNK4 or directly by phosphorylating SPAK/OSR1 (Fig. 9-11).

The role of WNK kinases as part of a switch system to change the response of the kidneys to either conserve $Na^+$ ions or excrete $K^+$ ions, depending on whether the release of aldosterone is induced by a reduction in dietary $Na^+$ ion intake or an increase in dietary $K^+$ ion intake, is discussed in detail in Chapter 13.

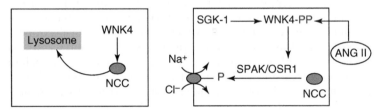

**Figure 9-10  Effects of WNK4 on the NCC.** As shown on the part of the figure, with-no-lysine kinase 4 (WNK4) inhibits $Na^+/Cl^-$ cotransporter (NCC) activity by reducing its abundance in luminal membranes by diverting NCC to the lysosome for degradation. As shown in the part of the figure on the right, angiotensin II (ANG II) signaling through its AT1 receptor converts WNK4 from an NCC-inhibiting to an NCC-activating kinase. The activated form of WNK4 phosphorylates STE20-related proline-alanine-rich-kinase (SPAK) and oxidative stress response kinase type 1 (OSR1). Phosphorylated SPAK/OSR1 in turn phosphorylates and activates NCC. *SGK-1,* Serum and glucocorticoid regulated-kinase-1.

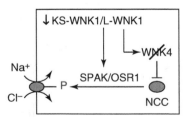

**Figure 9-11  Effects of WNK1 on the NCC.** Alternative promoter usage of the with-no-lysine kinase 1 (WNK1) gene produces a kidney-specific, truncated form of WNK1, called KS-WNK1, and a more ubiquitous long form, called L-WNK1. The KS-WNK1 isoform inhibits L-WNK1. When the ratio of KS- WNK1 to L-WNK1 is low, L-WNK1 exerts its effect to upregulate $Na^+/Cl^-$ cotransporter (NCC) either by blocking the inhibitory form of WNK4 or directly by phosphorylating STE20-related proline-alanine-rich-kinase/oxidative stress response kinase type 1 (SPAK/OSR1).

Aldosterone increases the abundance of phosphorylated active NCC in the luminal membrane of cells in early DCT and the reabsorption of NaCl by this nephron segment. The effect seems to be mediated by the WNK/SPAK (OSR1) pathway.

### Inhibitors

Thiazide diuretics (e.g., hydrochlorothiazide) and thiazide-like diuretics (e.g., chlorthalidone, indapamide) inhibit NCC by competing with $Cl^-$ ions for their binding site on NCC. The natriuretic effect of these diuretics is diminished when the EABV is low because there is more avid reabsorption of $Na^+$ and $Cl^-$ ions in upstream nephron sites.

### Disorders involving NCC

There is a decreased activity of this cotransporter in patients with Gitelman's syndrome (see Chapter 14) and an increase in its activity in patients with the syndrome of familial hyperkalemia with hypertension (see Chapter 15).

## Cortical distal nephron

This nephron segment includes the late DCT, the connecting tubule, and the CCD. Reabsorption of $Na^+$ ions in this nephron segment can be electrogenic (i.e., without its accompanying anion, which is usually $Cl^-$ ions) or electroneural. Electrogenic reabsorption of $Na^+$ ions generates a lumen-negative voltage, which allows for the secretion of $K^+$ ions by principal cells in the CDN if open ROMK are present in their luminal membrane.

### Electrogenic reabsorption of $Na^+$ ions in the CDN

This occurs via the amiloride sensitive, epithelial $Na^+$ channel (ENaC) in the luminal membrane of principal cells in the CDN. The driving force for $Na^+$ ion reabsorption via the ENaC is a higher concentration of $Na^+$ ion in the lumen of the CDN than in principal cells (~10 to 15 mmol/L) and a negative cell interior voltage caused by the actions of the Na-K-ATPase at the basolateral membrane in these cells (Fig. 9-12).

Aldosterone is the major hormone that causes an increase in the number of open ENaC units in the luminal membrane of principal cells. The steps involved include binding of aldosterone to its receptor in the cytoplasm of principal cells, entry of this hormone–receptor complex into the nucleus, and then the synthesis of new proteins including the serum and glucocorticoid-regulated kinase-1 (SGK-1). SGK-1 increases the expression of the ENaC in the apical membrane of principal cells. The mechanism seems to be related to the effect of SGK-1 to phosphorylate and inactivate the ubiquitin ligase Nedd4-2. Nedd4-2 ubiquinates ENaC subunits, leading to their removal from the cell membrane and degradation in proteasomes. Therefore, inhibition of the Nedd4-2 leads to diminished endocytosis and hence increased expression of the ENaC in the luminal membrane (Fig. 9-13). Another mechanism by which aldosterone activates ENaC involves proteolytic cleavage of the channel by serine proteases. Aldosterone induces production of "channel activating proteases" 1–3. These proteases activate ENaC by increasing its open probability rather than by increasing the expression of ENaC units at the luminal membrane.

### Inhibitors

The $K^+$ ion sparing diuretics amiloride and triamterene, and the antibiotic trimethoprim in its cationic form, block the ENaC. The aldosterone antagonists spironolactone and eplerenone compete with aldosterone for binding to its receptor in principal cells.

### Disorders involving the ENaC

In addition to renal salt wasting, hyperkalemia with a low rate of excretion of $K^+$ ions in the urine may be present if the activity of the ENaC is diminished or if ENaC is blocked (e.g., by amiloride or trimethoprim). The diagnostic approach in these patients is discussed in Chapter 15.

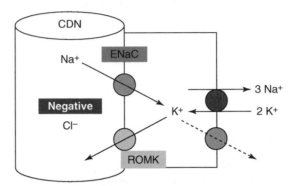

**Figure 9-12 Electrogenic Reabsorption of Na+ Ions in the CDN.** A low concentration of $Na^+$ ions and a negative voltage are created in principal cells in the cortical distal nephron (CDN) by the electrogenic pumping of $Na^+$ ions out of cells by the Na-K-ATPase. Electrogenic reabsorption of $Na^+$ ions in the CDN (i.e., reabsorption of $Na^+$ ions without their accompanying anion [usually $Cl^-$ ions]) occurs via the amiloride-sensitive ENaC in the luminal membrane of principal cells in the CDN. $K^+$ ions preferentially leaves the cell across the apical membrane via the renal outer medullary $K^+$ ion channel (ROMK) because the electrochemical gradient for apical $K^+$ ions exit is more favorable than across the basolateral membrane. This is because of the electrogenic movement of $Na^+$ ions across the apical membrane through ENaC, which depolarizes the apical membrane and creates a lumen-negative transepithelial potential. *ENaC*, Epithelial $Na^+$ channel.

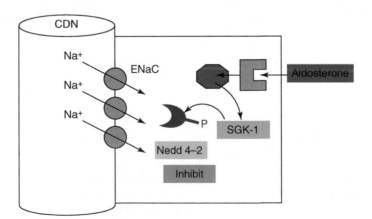

**Figure 9-13 Mechanism of Action of Aldosterone.** Aldosterone binds to its receptor in the cytoplasm of principal cells; this hormone–receptor complex enters the nucleus and causes the synthesis of new proteins including the serum and glucocorticoid regulated kinase-1 (SGK-1). SGK-1 phosphorylates and inactivates the ubiquitin ligase Nedd4-2, which leads to diminished endocytosis and hence increased expression of epithelial Na+ channel (ENaC) in the luminal membrane. *CDN*, Cortical distal nephron.

In contrast, conditions associated with an increased number of open ENaC in the luminal membrane of principal cells in the CDN can lead to hypertension and hypokalemia. The diagnostic approach in these patients is discussed in Chapter 14.

### Electroneutral reabsorption of Na⁺ ions in the CDN

If the reabsorption of $Na^+$ in the CDN is electroneutral (i.e., $Na^+$ ions are reabsorbed with their accompanying anions, usually $Cl^-$ ions), a negative lumen voltage will not be generated. Hence, this component of $Na^+$ ion reabsorption will result in NaCl retention but not $K^+$ ion secretion. Recently, an electroneutral, thiazide-sensitive, amiloride-resistant $Na^+$ and $Cl^-$ transport mechanism was identified in the β-intercalated cells of the CCD in rats and mice. This seems to be mediated by the parallel activity of the $Na^+$-independent $Cl^-/HCO_3^-$ exchanger (pendrin) and the $Na^+$-dependent $Cl^-/HCO_3^-$ exchanger (NDCBE) (Fig. 9-14). This transport mechanism is apparently responsible for as much as 50% of transport of NaCl in the CCD of the mouse in response to mineralocorticoids.

Because the $HCO_3^-$ ion gradient provides the driving force for the activity of the $Cl^-/HCO_3^-$ exchanger (pendrin), it was suggested that an increase in luminal $HCO_3^-$ ion concentration in the CDN may inhibit pendrin and hence the NDCBE and the electroneutral NaCl reabsorption. This may lead to a higher rate of electrogenic reabsorption of $Na^+$ ions and hence a higher rate of secretion of $K^+$ ions. The role of modulation of delivery of $HCO_3^-$ ions to the CDN in switching the renal response from NaCl retention to $K^+$ ion secretion when faced with a large $K^+$ ion load is discussed in Chapter 13.

### Medullary collecting duct

The MCD is the site where final adjustments are made to determine the rate of excretion of NaCl. All the $Na^+$ ions delivered to the MCD are reabsorbed there, unless the MCD receives a message that leads to the inhibition of the reabsorption of $Na^+$ ions. The message is related to atrial natriuretic peptide (ANP), which is released in response to increased right atrial volume. As discussed previously, our "normal" ECF volume is in fact an expanded ECF volume. Therefore our diet,

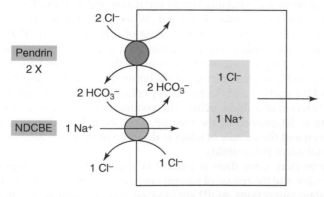

**Figure 9-14  Electroneutral Reabsorption of Na⁺ Ions in the Cortical Collecting Duct.** The exchange of two $Cl^-$ ions for two $HCO_3^-$ ions via two cycles of pendrin, with the subsequent uptake of two $HCO_3^-$ ions and one $Na^+$ ion in exchange for one $Cl^-$ ion via one cycle of the $Na^+$-dependent $Cl^-/HCO_3^-$ exchanger (NDCBE) results in net electroneutral transport of one $Na^+$ ion and one $Cl^-$ ion across the luminal membrane.

which is rich in NaCl, leads to further expansion of ECF volume and an increase in right atrial volume sufficient to release ANP to inhibit the reabsorption of NaCl in MCD to permit the excretion of the dietary NaCl load.

### Process

The entry of $Na^+$ ions into the MCD cells is primarily via an amiloride-sensitive, cation-selective channel at their apical membrane. This is driven by the electrochemical gradient generated by the Na-K-ATPase at their basolateral membrane. Reabsorption of $Cl^-$ ions seems to be passive, driven by the lumen-negative voltage generated by the electrogenic reabsorption of $Na^+$ ions.

### Role of hormones

ANP is primarily released from the right atrium of the heart in response to stretch caused by a high central venous volume. ANP is both a peripheral vasodilator, which may lower the systemic blood pressure, and a natriuretic hormone. This latter effect is mediated by increasing the GFR and decreasing the reabsorption of $Na^+$ ions in the MCD. ANP increases the GFR without raising the renal blood flow, suggesting that it causes efferent arteriolar constriction.

### Inhibitors

ANP directly inhibits reabsorption of $Na^+$ ions in the MCD via activation of guanylate cyclase and the production of cyclic guanosine monophosphate (cGMP). cGMP seems to diminish $Na^+$ ion reabsorption by decreasing the number of the open amiloride-sensitive, cation-selective channels in the luminal membrane of MCD cells.

# PART C
# PHYSIOLOGY OF WATER

## OVERVIEW

Regulation of water balance has an input arm and an output arm. The input of water is stimulated by thirst. When enough water is ingested to cause a fall in the $P_{Na}$ and swelling of cells of the hypothalamic osmoreceptor (tonicity receptor), there is a decrease in thirst and an inhibition of the release of vasopressin. In the absence of vasopressin actions, AQP2 are not inserted in the luminal membranes of principal cells of the cortical and the medullary collecting ducts, which leads to the excretion of a dilute urine. The volume of urine excreted in this setting is determined by the volume of filtrate delivered to the distal nephron and the volume of water reabsorbed in the inner MCD via its residual water permeability.

Conversely, when there is a deficit of water and thereby a high $P_{Na}$, both thirst and the release of vasopressin are stimulated. In the presence of vasopressin actions, AQP2 are inserted into the luminal membranes of principal cells of the cortical and the medullary collecting ducts. Water is reabsorbed until the effective osmolality of the fluid in the lumen of each of the late distal nephron segments is equal to the effective osmolality in its surrounding interstitial compartment. This results in the excretion of a small volume of concentrated urine.

# CONTROL OF WATER BALANCE

The components of the control system for water balance are shown in Figure 9-15. The goal of this system is to return the $P_{Na}$ to a normal value of 140 mmol/L.

## SENSOR

The main osmosensory cells appear to be located in the organum vasculosum laminae terminalis and the supraoptic and paraventricular nuclei of the hypothalamus. The mechanism of osmosensing appears to be at least in part caused by activation of nonselective calcium-permeable cation channels of the transient receptor potential vanilloid (TRPV), which can serve as stretch receptors. The osmoreceptor is linked to both the thirst center and the vasopressin release center via nerve connections.

Because $Na^+$ ions and their accompanying anions are the major effective osmoles in the ECF compartment, changes in $P_{Na}$ provide the main input for the osmoreceptor. Particles such as urea, which achieve equal concentrations in the ICF and ECF compartments, do not cause swelling or shrinkage of the cells of the osmoreceptor, and hence are not effective osmoles. Glucose is also not an effective osmole for the cells of the osmoreceptor. Stimulation of thirst and the release of vasopressin in patients with severe hyperglycemia are likely caused by the release of angiotensin II because of the low EABV, the result of the associated osmotic diuresis and natriuresis.

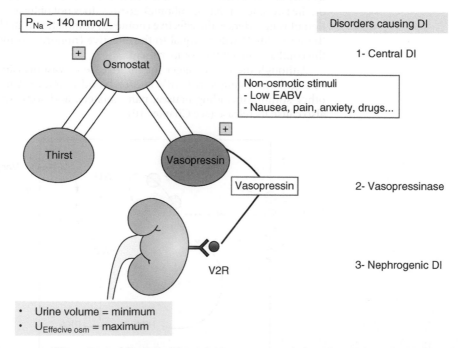

**Figure 9-15 Water Control System.** The primary sensor is the osmoreceptor (*top circle*), which detects a change in $P_{Na}$ via an effect on its cell volume. The osmoreceptor is linked to the thirst center (*lower left circle*) and to the vasopressin release center (*lower right circle*). Nonosmotic stimuli (e.g., nausea, pain, anxiety) also influence the release of vasopressin. Vasopressin release is also stimulated when there is a large decrease in the effective arterial blood volume (EABV); a lower $P_{Na}$ is needed to suppress the release of vasopressin in this setting. When vasopressin acts, the urine flow rate depends on the number of effective osmoles to be excreted and the effective osmolality in the inner medullary interstitial compartment. The clinical disorders associated with a water diuresis (i.e., diabetes insipidus [DI]) and the sites of these lesions are listed on the *right*.

## THIRST

Thirst is stimulated by an increase in the tonicity of plasma (high $P_{Na}$). Contraction of the EABV is another stimulus for thirst; an elevated level of angiotensin II may mediate this effect. Other factors unrelated to a need for a positive water balance may lead to a higher intake of water (e.g., dryness of the mouth, habit, culture, psychological conditions).

## VASOPRESSIN

Vasopressin is synthesized by the magnocellular neurons in the supra-optic and paraventricular nuclei of the hypothalamus and transported down the axons of the supraoptic–hypophyseal tract to be stored in and released from the posterior pituitary (neurohypophysis). Binding of vasopressin to its V2-receptor (V2R) in the basolateral membrane of principal cells in collecting ducts stimulates adenylyl cyclase to produce cyclic adenosine monophosphate (cAMP), which in turn activates protein kinase A (PKA). PKA phosphorylates AQP2, which causes their shuttling from an intracellular store to the luminal membrane of principal cells (Fig. 9-16). In the presence of AQP2 in their luminal membrane, principal cells in the collecting ducts become highly permeable to water. Water is reabsorbed until the effective osmolality in the lumen of the collecting duct is equal to that in the surrounding interstitial compartment. Therefore, when vasopressin acts, the osmolality of the fluid at the end of the CCD will be equal to the plasma osmolality. Because cells in the inner MCD have urea transporters (UTA-1 and UTA-3) in their luminal membranes when vasopressin acts, urea is usually an ineffective osmole (the concentration of urea is nearly equal on the two sides of that membrane), so urea does not obligate the excretion of water. Hence, the effective (nonurea) osmolality in the lumen of the inner MCD will be equal to the effective (nonurea) osmolality in the papillary interstitial compartment.

Although the main trigger for the release of vasopressin is a rise in $P_{Na}$, large changes in EABV and/or blood pressure, a number of other stimuli, including nausea, pain, anxiety, and some drugs, can also cause its release (see Chapter 10).

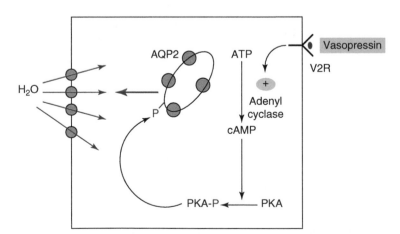

**Figure 9-16 Vasopressin Actions on the Distal Nephron.** Binding of vasopressin to its vasopressin 2 (V2)-receptor (V2R) in the basolateral membrane of principal cells in collecting ducts stimulates adenylyl cyclase to produce cyclic adenosine monophosphate (cAMP), which in turn activates protein kinase A (PKA). PKA phosphorylates aquaporin 2 (AQP2), which causes their shuttling from an intracellular store to the luminal membrane of principal cells. *AQP2,* Aquaporin 2 water channels; *ATP,* adenosine triphosphate; *PKA-P,* phosphorylated protein kinase A.

## Excretion of a Large Volume of Dilute Urine

Three steps are needed to excrete a large volume of water with low concentration of electrolytes in the urine.

1. Delivery of a large volume of filtrate to the distal nephron.
2. Generation of electrolyte-free water by reabsorption of $Na^+$ and $Cl^-$ ions from nephron segments that are impermeable to water.
3. Absence of vasopressin to prevent the insertion of AQP2 into the luminal membrane of principal cells in the late distal nephron.

### 1. Distal delivery of filtrate

The volume of filtrate delivered to the early DCT is estimated to be about 27 L/day (see Table 9-3). Because the descending thin limbs of the loop of Henle of the majority of nephrons lack AQP1, and hence are largely water impermeable, the volume of distal delivery of filtrate is determined by the GFR and the volume of filtrate that is reabsorbed in the PCT. As discussed earlier, close to 83% of the GFR is reabsorbed in the entire PCT. In the presence of a low EABV, a larger fraction of the GFR is reabsorbed in the PCT, as a result of sympathetic nervous system activation and the release of angiotensin II. Hence, the absence of a contracted EABV is needed for maximal excretion of water. Conversely, when there is both a low GFR and an enhanced reabsorption of filtrate in PCT caused by a low EABV, the volume of distal delivery of filtrate may not be large enough to exceed the volume of water that can be absorbed in inner MCD via its residual water permeability by an amount sufficient to allow for the excretion of the daily intake of water. Hyponatremia may develop, even when there is only a modest water load in the absence of vasopressin actions.

### 2. Reabsorption of $Na^+$ and $Cl^-$ ions without water: desalination of luminal fluid

The major nephron segments where reabsorption of $Na^+$ and $Cl^-$ ions occurs without water (i.e., diluting segments) are the thick ascending limb of the loop of Henle (with its medullary and cortical portions) and the early DCT, because these nephron segments lack AQP channels. As mentioned earlier, control of NaCl reabsorption in the mTAL of the loop of Henle seems to be under inhibitory control by the concentration (or more precisely the activity) of ionized $Ca^{2+}$ in the medullary interstitial compartment. In more detail, to reabsorb $Na^+$ and $Cl^-$ ions in the mTAL of the loop of Henle, $K^+$ ions reaborbed via NKCC-2 must be recycled into the lumen via the ROMK to provide the $K^+$ ions for the NKCC-2 and also to generate the lumen-positive voltage required for the passive reabsorption of $Na^+$ ions via the paracellular pathway. This lumen-positive voltage also drives the paracellular reabsorption of ionized $Ca^{2+}$. Because the concentration of ionized $Ca^{2+}$ in the medullary interstitial compartment rises, it binds to the Ca-SR, and a signal is generated to inhibit the flux of $K^+$ ions via the ROMK and hence both the transcellular and paracellular reabsorption of $Na^+$ ions (Fig. 9-17).

To lower the concentration of ionized $Ca^{2+}$ in the medullary interstitial compartment and hence remove its inhibition of $Na^+$ and $Cl^-$ ion reabsorption requires the addition of a calcium-poor solution to this interstitial compartment (see Fig. 9-17). This process occurs both when water is conserved (i.e., during antidiuresis) and also during water diuresis. The mechanism during antidiuresis consists of a high interstitial osmolality to draw water out of those nephron segments that have AQP in their luminal membranes. Hence, water is reabsorbed from the MCD when actions of vasopressin lead to the

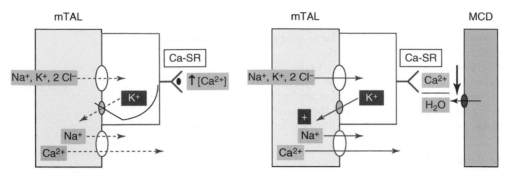

**Figure 9-17 Control of the Concentrating Process in the Renal Medulla by Interstitial Ionized Calcium.** As shown in the left part of the figure, the concentration of ionized $Ca^{2+}$ in the medullary interstitial compartment rises, it binds to the calcium-sensing receptor (Ca-SR), and a signal is generated to inhibit the flux of $K^+$ ions via renal outer medullary $K^+$ channel (ROMK) and hence both the transcellular and paracellular reabsorption of $Na^+$ ions. As shown in the right part of the figure, to lower the concentration of ionized $Ca^{2+}$ in the medullary interstitial compartment and hence remove its inhibition of the reabsorption of $Na^+$ and $Cl^-$ ions, requires the addition of a calcium-poor solution to the interstitial compartment. This process occurs both when water is conserved (i.e., during antidiuresis) and also during water diuresis. The mechanism during antidiuresis consists of a high interstitial osmolality to draw water out of those nephron segments that have luminal aquaporin (AQP). Water is absorbed from the medullary collecting duct (MCD) when actions of vasopressin lead to the insertion of AQP2 into the luminal membrane of principal cells. Water is also removed from the descending thin limb of juxtamedullary nephrons because they always have AQP1 (not shown in figure). During water diuresis, water is added to the medullary interstitial compartment from the inner MCD via its residual water permeability (not shown in figure). *mTAL*, Medullary thick ascending limb.

insertion of AQP2 into their luminal membranes. Water is also reabsorbed from the descending thin limb of juxtamedullary nephrons because they always have AQP1. Notwithstanding, the mechanisms are different during water diuresis because in this setting, vasopressin actions are absent; therefore, the MCD is impermeable to water. During water diuresis, water is reabsorbed in the inner MCD via its residual water permeability. This calcium-poor solution enters the ascending vasa rectae in the inner medulla, and is delivered to the outer medullary interstitial compartment, where it causes the concentration of ionized $Ca^{2+}$ to fall. As a result, its effect to inhibit the reabsorption of $Na^+$ and $Cl^-$ ions in the mTAL of the loop of Henle is removed, which allows for desalination of the luminal fluid in the mTAL of the loop of Henle.

The CDN is another major diluting site that contributes to the excretion of the maximum volume of electrolyte-poor urine during water diuresis by enhancing the reabsorption of $Na^+$ and $Cl^-$ ions, because a high flow rate activates ENaC and increases the rate of reabsorption of $Na^+$ ions in this nephron segment.

### Residual water permeability

There are two pathways for transport of water in the inner MCD: a vasopressin-responsive system via AQP2 and a vasopressin-independent system called residual water permeability. Although the mechanism for water reabsorption is not clear, two factors may affect the volume of water reabsorbed by residual water permeability. The first is the driving force, which is the enormous difference in osmotic pressure between the luminal fluid and the interstitial fluid compartment in the inner MCD during a water diuresis. The second factor is contraction of the renal pelvis. Each time the renal pelvis contracts, some of the fluid in the renal pelvis travels in a retrograde direction up toward the inner MCD, and some of that fluid may be reabsorbed via residual water permeability after it enters the inner MCD for a second (or a third) time. This would be especially be the case if there is some turbulence, which aids diffusion and prolongs contact time.

From a quantitative perspective, recall that as calculated earlier 27 L/day are delivered to the distal nephron in a normal subject with a GFR of 180 L/day and normal EABV. The peak urine flow rate during water diuresis (when vasopressin is fully suppressed) in an adult human is around 10 to 15 mL/min. If this flow rate could be maintained for 24 hours, the urine volume will be about 14 to 22 L/day. Therefore, somewhat more than 5 L of water would be reabsorbed per day in the inner MCD by residual water permeability during water diuresis. Hence, the volume of water reabsorbed in the MCD during water diuresis (in the absence of vasopressin actions) is similar to the volume reabsorbed during antidiuresis (presence of vasopressin actions) (see Table 9-5). Although it seems somewhat counterintuitive, as discussed earlier, reabsorption of water in the inner MCD via residual water permeability lowers the concentration of ionized $Ca^2$ in the medullary interstitial compartment and hence removes its inhibition of the reabsorption of $Na^+$ and $Cl^-$ ions in the mTAL of the loop of Henle. As such, it should be viewed as an investment: reabsorbing water in the inner MCD will generate more electrolyte-free water in the lumen of the mTAL of the loop of Henle, which in turn facilitates the excretion of a larger volume of free water.

## 3. Absence of actions of vasopressin

When vasopressin fails to act, the distal nephron becomes impermeable to water, and almost all of the volume of water delivered to the DCT minus the volume of water that is reabsorbed in the inner MCD via its residual water permeability is excreted in the urine. For a water diuresis to occur, it requires a low $P_{Na}$ and also the absence of nonosmotic stimuli for the release of vasopressin.

### Retain "nondangerous" water load

A rapid ingestion of a water load (e.g., 20 mL/kg body weight) may cause a large water diuresis. Nevertheless, if the same water load is consumed slowly (i.e., sipped rather than gulped), a water diuresis does not immediately ensue, and a large proportion of this water load is retained for a period of time. The explanation for this is that immediately following the rapid ingestion and absorption of water, there is an appreciable fall in $P_{Na}$ in portal venous blood and hypotonic plasma is delivered to the heart, and ultimately to the brain, where this fall in $P_{Na}$ in arterial blood is sensed by the osmoreceptor and the release of vasopressin is suppressed. A water diuresis ensues to excrete this dangerous water load. This fall in $P_{Na}$ in arterial blood may not be detected by measurement of $P_{Na}$ in brachial venous blood because large muscles "suck up" water quickly, causing the venous $P_{Na}$ to rise (Fig. 9-18). In quantitative terms, the brain receives such a large portion of the cardiac output (~20%), yet its weight is relatively small. In contrast, while the bulk of water in the body is in skeletal muscle, on a per kg basis the rate of blood flow to muscle is only one-twentieth the rate of the blood flow to the brain (Fig. 9-19).

On the other hand, if this water load is sipped slowly, a large fall in arterial $P_{Na}$ is prevented, and a large proportion of the water load is temporarily retained. Water intake is needed primarily to permit evaporative heat loss during periods of exercise. Because exercise and drinking water are not synchronous events, one must be able to store the ingested water for future loss in sweat during exercise in a hot

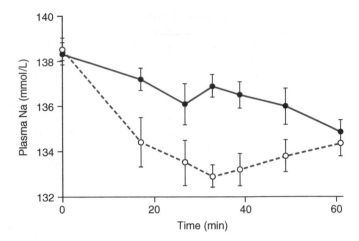

**Figure 9-18 Fall in the $P_{Na}$ in Arterial and Venous Plasma During a Water Load of 20 mL/kg.** The time in minutes after beginning to ingest the water, which takes about 15 min, is shown on the x-axis and the $P_{Na}$ in mmol/L is shown on the y-axis. The *dashed line* depicts the arterial $P_{Na}$ and the *solid line* depicts the $P_{Na}$ in the brachial vein. All the arterial $P_{Na}$ values, except the zero time and the 60-min time, are significantly lower than the venous $P_{Na}$ values.

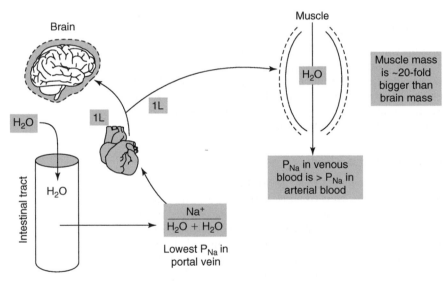

**Figure 9-19 Mechanism to Explain Why $P_{Na}$ in Venous Blood Might Not Reflect the Degree of Brain Cell Swelling Shortly After "Gulping" Water.** When water is ingested rapidly, it will be absorbed from the intestinal tract and enter the portal vein. If the volume is large and the rate of stomach emptying is rapid, there will be a large fall in the arterial $P_{Na}$. When arterial blood is delivered to the brain and skeletal muscle cells, the initial swelling in individual brain cells is much greater than in individual muscle cells because the mass (water content) of muscle is much larger than that of the brain and their blood flow rates are similar at rest (~1 L/min). As a result, the $P_{Na}$ in venous blood draining muscle cells will be appreciably higher than the arterial $P_{Na}$ (to which the brain is exposed) before equilibrium is reached, and the danger of brain swelling may be underestimated.

## EVAPORATIVE WATER LOSS: A QUANTITATIVE ANALYSIS

- Heat loss (about 2500 kcal of heat per day) occurs by multiple mechanisms: convection, conduction, radiation, and evaporation.
- When 1 L of water evaporates on the skin surface, 500 to 600 kcal are lost.

environment (e.g., hunting in Paleolithic times). Hence, a moderate volume of water (~1 L in an adult) needs to be retained for possible future loss as sweat for heat dissipation (see margin note). As the $P_{Na}$ falls toward 136 mmol/L, the release of vasopressin is diminished and excess water is excreted to return the $P_{Na}$ back toward 140 mmol/L.

## EXCRETION OF CONCENTRATED URINE

The urinary concentrating mechanism achieves two functions. The first is to excrete the minimum volume of water when there is a deficit of water. The second is to excrete urine with the highest possible concentration of electrolytes when there is a large hypertonic load of salt.

### 1. Conserve water when there is a deficit of water

The usual description of the renal concentrating process focuses primarily on conservation of water when there is a deficit of water. The first step in this process is to sense that there is a deficit of water, which is detected by the osmoreceptor when the $P_{Na}$ rises to just above 140 mmol/L. This stimulates the release of vasopressin, which causes the insertion of AQP2 channels into the luminal membranes of principal cells in the cortical and medullary collecting ducts. As soon as luminal fluid reaches the nephron segments that have AQP2 in their luminal membrane, water will be absorbed untill the effective osmolality of the luminal fluid is nearly equal to the effective osmolality in the surrounding interstitial fluid compartment. The net result is the excretion of a small volume of urine that has a high effective osmolality.

### 2. Excrete a large hypertonic load of Na⁺ and Cl⁻ ions

When there is a large intake of salt with little water, this salt load must be excreted in the smallest possible volume of urine. Vasopressin is released because of a higher $P_{Na}$. An expanded EABV caused by the positive balance for Na⁺ and Cl⁻ ions leads to inhibition of the reabsorption of NaCl and water in the PCT. Therefore, a larger number of effective osmoles (Na⁺ and Cl⁻ ions) is delivered to the terminal CCD. Because the volume of filtrate that exits the terminal CCD is determined by the number of osmoles and the osmolality of the fluid in the terminal CCD (which is equal to the plasma osmolality when vasopressin acts [i.e., ~300 mosmol/kg $H_2O$]), a larger volume of filtrate with an osmolality of 300 mosmol/kg $H_2O$ will be delivered to the MCD. When this larger volume of filtrate reaches, for example, the level in the MCD where the interstitial osmolality is 600 mosmol/ kg $H_2O$, half of its water will be absorbed, and therefore a larger volume of water will be added to the medullary interstitial compartment. Accordingly, there will be a greater degree of dilution of an inhibitor (possibly ionized $Ca^{2+}$) in the medullary interstitial compartment for the reabsorption of Na⁺ and Cl⁻ ions from the mTAL of the loop of Henle. The reabsorption of more Na⁺ and Cl⁻ ions from the mTAL of the loop of Henle will restore the osmolality in the medullary interstitial compartment back to its original value, and therefore hypertonicity in the medullary interstitial compartment is maintained. The urine will have the highest effective osmolality, but its volume will not be very low because there will be a large natriuresis and thereby a salt-induced osmotic diuresis. If this load of NaCl could not be excreted with the highest possible concentration of Na⁺ and Cl⁻ ions in the urine, hypernatremia would develop.

### *Overview of the renal concentrating process*

Three major factors permit the kidneys to conserve water and/or excrete Na⁺ and Cl⁻ ions in a hypertonic form.

1. *The presence of a unique blood supply, the vasa recta, which functions as a countercurrent exchanger.* This minimizes the washout of osmoles from the medullary interstitial compartment.

2. *Insertion of AQP2 water channels into the luminal membranes of the late distal nephron. This is the result of actions of vasopressin.*
3. *Generation of a high medullary interstitial osmolality. This occurs when Na⁺ and Cl⁻ ions are reabsorbed without water from the mTAL of the loop of Henle.*

### The vasa recta functions as a countercurrent exchanger

There is a progressive rise in the concentration of solutes in the interstitial compartment as one descends into the medulla from its junction with the renal cortex to the papillary tip. The unique blood supply to this area avoids "washing" solutes out of the medullary interstitial compartment. In addition to a slow rate of blood flow, its architecture is such that it functions as a countercurrent exchanger because the vessels that run down to the medullary tip (descending limbs) bend back and travel upward (ascending limbs). Some vasa recta vessels bend at more superficial levels while others bend at deeper levels in the medulla. These blood vessels are very permeable to electrolytes and urea (they have a urea transporter in their luminal membranes). In fact, there are twice as many ascending as compared to descending limbs of the vasa recta, and the ascending limbs have large holes (called fenestra) to accelerate this diffusion process. The concentration of solutes becomes progressively lower in the lumen of the ascending vasa recta limbs as well as in the interstitial fluid compartment as one proceeds from the papillary tip to the junction of the renal medulla with the renal cortex.

### Insertion of AQP2 when vasopressin acts

The major stimulus for the release of vasopressin is a $P_{Na}$ that is greater than $140 \, mmol/L$ (the exact threshold will vary depending on the presence of nonosmotic stimuli for the release of vasopressin).

Vasopressin binds to its V2-receptors on the basolateral membrane of principal cells of the collecting ducts and leads to the insertion of AQP2 into the luminal membrane of these cells (acute effect) and the synthesis of more AQP2 (chronic effect). In the presence of AQP2 in their luminal membrane, principal cells in the collecting ducts become highly permeable to water. Water is reabsorbed until the effective osmolality in the lumen of that nephron segment is equal to that in its surrounding interstitial compartment in the same horizontal plane.

Although the difference in osmolality between the luminal fluid and the interstitial compartments in the CDN is relatively small, there is a very large osmotic driving force to reabsorb water in this region (see margin note). In fact, the majority of water that is reabsorbed in the collecting duct occurs in the cortex (about 22 L, see margin note and Table 9-5) even though the rise in the osmolality is only two- to threefold in the cortex and almost fourfold in the renal medulla. While a large amount of water is reabsorbed and added rapidly to the cortical interstitial compartment each day when vasopressin acts, this does not pose a danger, for two reasons. First, we calculated that about 3090 mmol of Na⁺ ions are reabsorbed in the cTAL of the loop of Henle, the early DCT, and the CDN (see Table 9-2), which makes this addition of water into virtually an isotonic solution. Second, the plasma flow rate in the cortex is enormous.

### Generation of a high interstitial osmolality in the outer medulla

The rise in the interstitial osmolality in the outer medulla occurs when Na⁺ and Cl⁻ ions are reabsorbed actively without water from the

---

**OSMOTIC FORCE FOR WATER REABSORPTION IN THE CORTEX**

- Each $mosmol/kg \, H_2O$ in a solution exerts an osmotic pressure of 19.3 mm Hg (one can approximate this as 20 mm Hg for easy arithmetic).
- In the cortex, the interstitial osmolality is similar to the plasma osmolality (~300 mosmol/ $kg \, H_2O$ for easy arithmetic), and the osmolality in luminal fluid that arrives at the early DCT is ~150 $mosmol/kg \, H_2O$. Multiplying the difference between the interstitial and luminal osmolalities (150 $mosmol/kg \, H_2O$) by 20 mm Hg per mosmol reveals that the osmotic pressure exerted is ~3000 mm Hg, a value that is equivalent to the mean arterial blood pressure generated by 30 beating hearts.

**VOLUME OF WATER REABSORBED IN THE CORTICAL COLLECTING DUCT**

- The volume of filtrate delivered to the early DCT is ~27 L.
- The volume of fluid that exits the CCD is about 5 L. This is based on the fact that about 1500 mosmol/day are delivered to the CCD (~1000 mmol of urea and ~500 mmol of Na⁺ and K⁺ ions with their accompanying anions), and that when vasopressin acts, the osmolality of the fluid in the terminal part of the CCD will be equal to the plasma osmolality (~300 $mosmol/kg \, H_2O$).
- Therefore, about 22 L of water are reabsorbed in the CCD.

water-impermeable mTAL of the loop of Henle. While the traditional view is that reabsorption of NaCl from the mTAL is the initial step in the process to reabsorb water out of the MCD when this nephron segment is permeable to water (i.e., when vasopressin acts), we favor an alternative view. In our opinion, the first step is the reabsorption of water from the MCD, which initiates signals to augment the reabsorption of $Na^+$ and $Cl^-$ ions from the mTAL of the loop of Henle (see the following discussion).

### Regulation of the urine concentrating process in the outer medulla

There are two possible generic mechanisms for control of the concentrating process in the renal medulla: a substrate driven control or an inhibitory control. A critique of the two models of control using the example of heating a house in the Canadian winter is provided in Figure 9-20.

#### Substrate-driven control

In this model, which is the most popular interpretation of the control of the medullary concentrating mechanism, primary regulation is in the mTAL of the loop of Henle. The primary event is reabsorption of $Na^+$ and $Cl^-$ ions in the mTAL of the loop of Henle, which raises the medullary interstitial osmolality to drive the reabsorption of water from the MCD. Hence, the mTAL must reabsorb just enough $Na^+$ and $Cl^-$ ions to determine the volume of water to reabsorb from the MCD. This raises a disquieting question, "How can the mTAL of the loop of Henle 'know' just how much $Na^+$ and $Cl^-$ ions to reabsorb at any one moment in time?" For example, if too much $Na^+$ and $Cl^-$ ions were

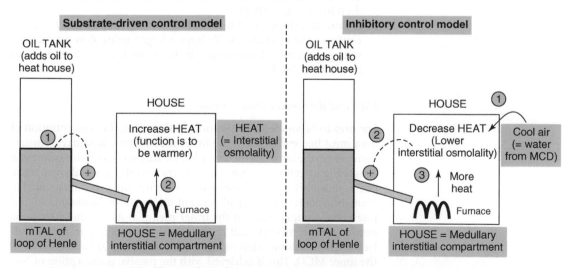

**Figure 9-20  Models of Control Mechanisms.** A substrate-driven model is shown on the *left*, and an inhibitory control model is shown on the *right*. The *oil tank* represents the medullary thick ascending limb (mTAL) of the loop of Henle, the *house* represents the medullary interstitial compartment, and the rise in temperature represents an increase in osmolality in the medullary interstitial compartment. In the inhibitory control model, the thermostat detects the temperature of the house (which represents the osmolality in the medullary interstitial compartment). If the temperature rises, a message is sent to stop the inflow of oil from the oil tank to the furnace. This message should persist as long as the temperature of the house is at or above the desired level. It is also noteworthy that the "single effect" in the renal medulla is to dilute the medullary interstitial compartment, and the response is to restore its composition to the original value very quickly by releasing the inhibition exerted on the mTAL of the loop of Henle. *MCD,* Medullary collecting duct.

reabsorbed from the mTAL, too much water will be reabsorbed from the MCD, the urine volume will be too low, and urinary precipitates (and eventually stones) may form.

### Inhibitory control

In this model, the volume of water reabsorbed from the MCD signals the loop of Henle to reabsorb the correct amount of $Na^+$ and $Cl^-$ ions to maintain a steady state. To achieve this goal, there must be an inhibitor of the reabsorption of $Na^+$ and $Cl^-$ ions in the mTAL of the loop of Henle in the medullary interstitial compartment—its concentration will fall when more water is added to the interstitial compartment, which then removes the inhibition of the reabsorption of $Na^+$ and $Cl^-$ ions in this nephron segment, such that more $Na^+$ and $Cl^-$ ions are reabsorbed and added to the medullary interstitial compartment. A possible candidate for this inhibitor is ionized $Ca^{2+}$ because cells of the mTAL of the loop of Henle have a receptor for ionized $Ca^{2+}$ on their basolateral membrane (see margin note). When ionized $Ca^{2+}$ binds to its receptor, a signal is generated that causes inhibition of the ROMK and thereby inhibition of the reabsorption of $Na^+$ and $Cl^-$ in the mTAL of the loop of Henle via both NKCC-2 and the paracellular route for $Na^+$ ion reabsorption. When the concentration of ionized $Ca^{2+}$ falls, more $Na^+$ and $Cl^-$ ions are reabsorbed from the mTAL of the loop of Henle (see Fig. 9-17).

### Regulation of the urine concentrating process in the inner medulla

There are two major functions of the inner medulla in the urinary concentrating mechanism:
1. **Excrete urea without obligating the excretion of extra water.** For this to occur, urea must be an ineffective osmole in the luminal fluid in the inner MCD.
2. **Ensure that the urine volume is large enough even when the urine contains few electrolytes.** To have a larger urine flow rate in this setting, urea must become an effective osmole in the luminal fluid in the inner MCD.

### Urea and the conservation of water

For urea to be an ineffective osmole in the urine, the concentration of urea must become equal in the inner medullary interstitial compartment and in the lumen of the inner MCD. This occurs when vasopressin causes the insertion of urea transporters into the luminal membrane of the inner MCD. These transporters permit urea to diffuse quickly enough to achieve near equal concentrations in the luminal fluid and interstitial compartment in the inner medulla. Also, a mechanism is needed to minimize the fall in the effective osmolality in the medullary interstitial compartment when urea and water are absorbed from the inner MCD. This is achieved with the passive reabsorption of $Na^+$ and $Cl^-$ ions from the water-impermeable, ascending thin limbs of the loop of Henle in the inner medulla, as described earlier.

**Intrarenal urea recycling:** Intrarenal recycling of urea serves a number of important functions. First, this is a critically important component of the function of the inner medulla to allow urea to be excreted without obligating the excretion of water. Second, reabsorption of urea and water in the inner medulla lowers the concentration of $Na^+$ and $Cl^-$ ions in the interstitial compartment in the inner medulla, which allows for the passive reabsorption of $Na^+$ and $Cl^-$ ions from the ascending thin limbs of the loop of Henle. This diminishes the requirement for active reabsorption of $Na^+$ and $Cl^-$ ions in the mTAL of the loop of Henle deep in the renal outer medulla (see

### SIGNAL RELATED TO IONIZED CALCIUM

- Although it is common to say that receptors "see" the concentration of ligands that bind to them, this is not technically true for the Ca-SR. Rather than concentration, one must think of activity when ions are concerned. This is because the activity of an ion in a solution is not necessarily the same as its concentration in the solution, because it depends on the concentration of other ions in the solution. This is especially true for divalent ions such as $Ca^{2+}$.
- In the renal medullary interstitial compartment, the high concentration of electrolytes increases the ionic strength, which lowers the activity of ionized $Ca^{2+}$ at any given concentration of this electrolyte.

Part D). Third, this process also aids the excretion of K⁺ ions, as will be discussed in detail in Chapter 13.

***Process:*** For simplicity, we shall begin with the absorption of urea in the inner MCD (Fig. 9-21). This absorption requires the presence of urea transporters in the luminal membrane of cells of the inner MCD and a higher concentration of urea in the luminal fluid in the inner MCD than that in the interstitial fluid compartment in the inner medulla. Vasopressin phosphorylates and causes the insertion of urea transporters: UT-A1 and UT-A3 in the luminal membrane of cells in the inner MCD. A high concentration of urea in the luminal fluid in the inner MCD is achieved because all nephron segments upstream of the inner MCD are impermeable to urea, but most of the water delivered to the early DCT is reabsorbed in the CCD and MCD because they are highly permeable to water when vasopressin causes the insertion of AQP2 in the luminal membrane of their principal cells. Therefore, the concentration of urea rises to greater than 600 mmol/L in the luminal fluid that is delivered to the inner MCD.

The bulk of the urea that is reabsorbed in the inner MCD leaves the inner medulla via the ascending vasa recta because it has UT-A2, so it is permeable to urea. Once in the deep outer medulla, most urea will enter the luminal fluid of the descending thin limbs of the loop of Henle of superficial nephrons that have their bends deep in the outer medulla, because they possess the UT-A2 and the concentration of urea is higher in the interstitial compartment than in the luminal fluid of the descending thin of the loop of Henle. This allows for a high rate of delivery of urea to the early DCT.

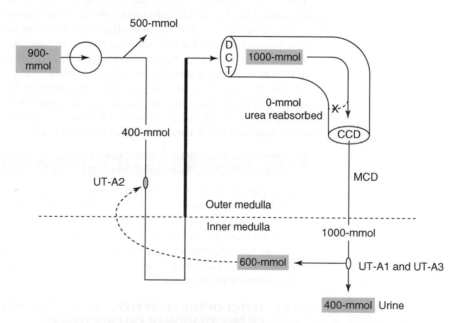

**Figure 9-21 Intrarenal Recycling of Urea.** Vasopressin phosphorylates and causes the insertion of urea transporters UT-A1 and UT-A3 in the luminal membrane of cells in the inner medullary collecting duct (MCD). The bulk of the urea that is reabsorbed in the inner MCD leaves the inner medulla via the ascending vasa recta because it has UT-A2. Most of this urea will enter the luminal fluid of the descending thin limbs of the loop of Henle of superficial nephrons that have their bends deep in the outer medulla, because they possess the UT-A2. This allows for a high rate of delivery of urea to the early distal convoluted tubule (DCT). Extrapolated to an adult human with a glomerular filtration rate of 180 L per day and a plasma urea of 5 mmol/L, approximately 1000 mmol of urea would be delivered to the early DCT per day. Because approximately 400 mmol of urea are excreted daily in an adult human who consumes a typical Western diet, approximately 600 mmol of urea are reabsorbed downstream from the DCT and recycled to the DCT. *CCD,* Cortical collecting duct.

**QUANTITATIVE ESTIMATE OF INTRARENAL RECYCLING OF UREA**

• This calculation does not take into account the relatively small amount of urea that exits the medulla via the ascending vasa recta.

*Quantities:* To obtain a quantitative estimate of the amount of urea that is recycled, one needs an estimate of the amount of urea that is delivered to the early DCT and the amount of urea that is excreted in the urine over a given period of time. Because the amount of urea delivered to the early DCT cannot be measured in human subjects, we use data from experiments with the micropuncture technique in the early DCT in fed rats. In these studies, the amount of urea delivered to the early DCT was 1.1 times the amount of urea that was filtered. Extrapolated to a human adult with a GFR of 180 L/day and a plasma urea concentration of 5 mmol/L, and therefore a filtered load of 5 mmol/L × 180 L/day = 900 mmol/day, a reasonable estimate of the daily delivery of urea to the early DCT is approximately 1000 mmol/day. Because subjects eating a typical Western diet excrete close to 400 mmol of urea per day, the amount of urea that recycles would be approximately 600 mmol per day (see margin note).

*Avoiding oliguria when the urine is electrolyte poor*

Water conservation must be achieved when there is a water deficit. On the other hand, the urine volume must be high enough to decrease the risk of precipitation of poorly soluble constituents in the urine and thereby the formation of kidney stones (Table 9-7). To have a large enough volume of urine when vasopressin acts, the number of effective osmoles in the urine must increase.

Experimental data in rats show that the inner MCD is not sufficiently permeable to urea when few electrolytes are being excreted and vasopressin actions are present. Hence, urea becomes an effective osmole in the inner MCD in this setting and it obligates the excretion of water.

During prolonged starvation, the urine does not contain its usual effective osmoles ($Na^+$ and $K^+$ salts) and it also contains little urea. Therefore, there is a need to generate new effective osmoles in the urine to have a sufficient urine volume to avoid formation of precipitates. This is accomplished by excreting ammonium ($NH_4^+$) and β-hydroxybutyrate ions, which are effective osmoles in the urine. Because each molecule of urea has two nitrogens, and the excretion of 2 mmol of $NH_4^+$ ions is accompanied by the excretion of 2 mmol of β-hydroxybutyrate anions, excreting nitrogen wastes as $NH_4^+$ salts adds four times as many osmoles than the excretion of the same amount of nitrogen as urea.

## QUESTION

9-4 Two patients have a maximum urine osmolality of 600 mos/kg $H_2O$ when vasopressin acts. One of them has sickle cell anemia and papillary necrosis, whereas the other has a lesion that affects his outer medulla, but he has an intact papilla. Both patients eat the same diet and excrete 900 mosmol/day (urine osmoles are half urea and half electrolytes). Why do they not have the same minimum urine flow rate?

TABLE 9-7 **EFFECT OF THE URINE FLOW RATE ON THE LIKELIHOOD OF PRECIPITATION OF CALCIUM OXALATE**

| FLOW RATE (mL/min) | Ca²⁺ (mmol/L) | OXALATE (mmol/L) | Ca²⁺ × OXALATE |
|---|---|---|---|
| 1.2 | X | Y | XY |
| 0.6 | 2 X | 2 Y | 4 XY |
| 0.3 | 4 X | 4 Y | 16 XY |

For ease of illustration, the concentrations of Ca²⁺ and oxalate are assigned values of X and Y mmol/L, respectively, at a urine flow rate of 1.2 mL/min. Their ion product rises 4- and 16-fold when the urine flow rate goes down by half to 0.6 mL/min and down again by half to 0.3 mL/min, assuming that the excretion rates for these ions remain constant. The point is that only a small increase in urine flow rate is needed to decrease the risk of precipitation of calcium-containing stones.

# PART D
# INTEGRATIVE
# PHYSIOLOGY

## INTEGRATIVE PHYSIOLOGY OF THE RENAL MEDULLA

### LACK OF AQP1 IN THE MAJORITY OF THE DESCENDING THIN LIMBS OF THE LOOP OF HENLE

A recent study suggested that the descending thin limbs of the loop of Henle of superficial nephrons (those nephrons that do not enter the inner medulla [~85% of all nephrons]) lack AQP1. Accordingly, the entire loop of Henle of these nephrons is likely to be impermeable to water. This finding has a number of physiological implications.

### 1. About five-sixths of the GFR is reabsorbed in the PCT

As discussed earlier, the $(TF/P)_{inulin}$ in luminal fluid in the early DCT reveals the volume of filtrate delivered to the loops of Henle of superficial nephrons. Because this value is close to 6, about five-sixths of the GFR (and not two-thirds as was previously thought) is reabsorbed in the PCT. Quantitatively, 150 L out of a GFR of 180 L/day (instead of 120 L/day) are reabsorbed in the PCT. Hence, a larger proportion of the GFR is subject to factors that modulate the reabsorption of $Na^+$ ions (and water) in the PCT. In addition, there is a much smaller delivery of ionized $Ca^{2+}$ to the loop of Henle. The importance of this will become evident when the risks for deposition of calcium salts in the renal medullary interstitial compartment (nephrocalcinosis) and the initiation of calcium-containing kidney stone formation are considered.

### 2. During water deprivation, the inhibitory signals that modulate the reabsorption of $Na^+$ and $Cl^-$ in the mTAL of the loop of Henle can only be influenced by the volume of water that is reabsorbed from the MCD

The absence of AQP1 in the descending thin limbs of the loop of Henle of the majority of the nephrons improves the inhibitory controls on reabsorption of $Na^+$ and $Cl^-$ ions in the mTAL of the loop of Henle. This is because there is no large addition of water from the descending thin limbs of the loop of Henle to obfuscate the new "single effect," the volume of water reabsorbed from the MCD.

### 3. The rise in the concentrations of $Na^+$ and $Cl^-$ ions in the descending thin limb of the loop of Henle in superficial nephrons is via addition of $Na^+$ and $Cl^-$ and not via water reabsorption

It is necessary to have a high concentration of $Na^+$ ions in the luminal fluid that reaches the mTAL of the loop of Henle to allow for the voltage-driven, paracellular $Na^+$ ion reabsorption (which represents 50% of $Na^+$ ion reabsorption in this nephron segment) to occur in the face of a high medullary interstitial concentration of $Na^+$ ions. Because the descending thin limbs of the loop of Henle of the superficial nephrons are likely impermeable to water, this rise in luminal fluid Na⁺ ion concentration occurs because of addition of Na⁺ ions and not because of reabsorption of water. This addition of Na⁺ ions requires an increased reabsorption of Na⁺ ions from the mTAL of the loop of Henle (which is in essence a recycling of Na⁺ ions). This seems to be a problem because it occurs in a region of the kidneys with a low blood flow and a low hematocrit and hence has a precarious delivery of oxygen. Nevertheless, as we shall see in the following section, the bulk of this reabsorption of Na⁺ ions occurs in the outer part of the outer medulla, which has a more favorable delivery of oxygen than the deeper part of the outer medulla.

## Minimizing the Dangers for the Renal Medulla

The process of concentrating the urine must be accomplished while preserving the integrity of the renal medulla. There are two important potential dangers, particularly in the deeper areas of the renal medulla. First, there is a risk of forming precipitates of calcium salts in the lumen of the nephron (nephrolithiasis) and in the interstitial compartment (nephrocalcinosis). Second, there is a risk of developing hypoxia because this region has a marginal delivery of oxygen.

### Preventing the precipitation of calcium salts in the deeper part of the renal medulla

Two anions are most likely to form a precipitate with ionized $Ca^{2+}$: divalent phosphate $(HPO_4^{2-})$ and carbonate $(CO_3^{2-})$. The concentration of $HPO_4^{2-}$ and $CO_3^{2-}$ in a solution rises when its pH becomes more alkaline. The relevant pH range for $HPO_4^{2-}$ is close to its $P_K$ (~6.8) whereas even higher pH are needed to raise the concentration of $CO_3^{2-}$ sufficiently to form a precipitate with ionized $Ca^{2+}$. In contrast to the descending thin limbs of the loop of Henle of superficial nephrons, the descending thin limbs of the loop of Henle of juxtamedullary nephrons have AQP1 in their luminal membranes. The concentrations of all solutes in a solution rise when water is removed. Hence, the ion product of ionized $Ca^{2+}$ and $HPO_4^{2-}$ or $CO_3^{2-}$ may exceed their solubility product constant (Ksp) and thus form a precipitate in the luminal fluid in the deeper part in the renal medulla.

### *Conundrum 1*

A high luminal pH is a major risk factor for the formation of $CaHPO_4$ and $CaCO_3$ precipitates. There is a major risk of forming luminal precipitates of $CaHPO_4$ and $CaCO_3$ in the juxtamedullary nephrons if the fractional reabsorption of $NaHCO_3$ in the PCT of these nephrons is similar to that in the PCT of superficial nephrons.

In micropuncture studies in the PCT in the fed rat, the pH of the luminal fluid was considerably less than 7.4. If the pH at the end of the PCT were 7.1 the concentration of $HCO_3^-$ ions in luminal fluid would be approximately 12 mmol/L. Because only one-sixth of the GFR of superficial nephrons or 26 L/day reaches their loops of Henle (see Table 9-3), if the concentration of $HCO_3^-$ ions in luminal fluid that exits the PCT was 12 mmol/L, a total of 312 mmol/day of $HCO_3^-$ ions escape reabsorption in the PCT. Because superficial nephrons are ~85% of the total nephrons, they receive about 150 L/day of GFR, and their filtered load of $HCO_3^-$ ions is about 3750 mmol/day. Hence, more than 90% of filtered $HCO_3^-$ ions must be reabsorbed for the concentration of $HCO_3^-$ in luminal fluid that exits the PCT in these nephrons to be approximately 12 mmol/L.

The descending thin limbs of the loop of Henle of juxtamedullary nephrons have AQP1 in their luminal membranes and thus water is reabsorbed while they traverse the hyperosmolar medullary interstitial compartment. In quantitative terms, as the interstitial osmolality rises from 300 to 900 mosmol/kg $H_2O$, two-thirds of the filtrate will be reabsorbed. Therefore, the concentration of $HCO_3^-$ ions in the luminal fluid at the 900 mosmol/kg $H_2O$ level will be threefold higher (i.e., 36 mmol/L), and the pH will be 7.65 if the interstitial $PCO_2$ is 40 mm Hg. The concentration of $HCO_3^-$ ions and the pH will be even higher at the bend of the loop of Henle of those juxtamedullary nephrons that descend down into the renal papilla where the osmolality of the medullary interstitial compartment reaches 1200 mosmol/kg $H_2O$ as more water is absorbed. At this high pH, the activities of $HPO_4^{2-}$ and $CO_3^{2-}$ along with that of $Ca^{2+}$ will exceed the Ksp for $CaHPO_4$ and for $CaCO_3$.

### Resolution

Because appreciable precipitation of these calcium salts must not occur, it is likely that more $HCO_3^-$ ions are reabsorbed in the PCT of juxtamedullary nephrons. In quantitative terms, because the volume of fluid remaining in the lumen of the descending thin limbs of the juxtamedullary nephrons at the 900 mosmol/kg $H_2O$ level is about 1.5 L (see Table 9-3), to have a luminal fluid pH of 7.1 (concentration of $HCO_3^-$ ions of 12 mmol/L), the quantity of $HCO_3^-$ in the luminal fluid of these nephrons must be only 18 mmol. If these nephrons constitute 15% of the total nephrons and hence receive 27 L of GFR per day, their filtered load of $HCO_3^-$ ions would be about 675 mmol/day (27 L × 25 mmol $HCO_3^-$/L). Hence, 97% of the filtered load of $HCO_3^-$ ions must be reabsorbed in the PCT of these nephrons.

In addition to avoiding a high pH in luminal fluid in the descending thin limbs of the loops of Henle, having such a high fraction reabsorption of $HCO_3^-$ ions in the PCT of juxtamedullary nephrons could also lead to a decrease in the quantity of ionized $Ca^{2+}$ in the their luminal fluid at the bend of their loops of Henle. In more detail, when $Na^+$ and $HCO_3^-$ ions are reabsorbed in the PCT, water follows. As a result, the concentration of $Cl^-$ ions in the luminal fluid rises, which provides a larger driving force for its paracellular reabsorption, leaving the lumen with a small positive voltage. This in turn drives the reabsorption of $Na^+$ ions through the paracellular pathway. The increased rate of reabsorption of NaCl (and water) raises the concentration of ionized $Ca^{2+}$ in the luminal fluid, which drives its reabsorption through the paracellular pathway. Therefore, a smaller quantity of ionized $Ca^{2+}$ is delivered to the descending thin limbs of the loops of Henle of these nephrons.

### Conundrum 2

The activity of $Ca^{2+}$ and of $HPO_4^{2-}$ in the luminal fluid at the 900 mosmol/kg $H_2O$ level could be high enough that, without another defense mechanism, $CaHPO_4$ would precipitate in this location. The risk of precipitation is even higher at the bend of the loop of Henle of those juxtamedullary nephrons that descend down into the renal papilla where the osmolality of the medullary interstitium reaches 1200 mosmol/kg $H_2O$, as more water is absorbed, and hence the concentrations of ionized $Ca^{2+}$, $HPO_4^{2-}$, and $CO_3^{2-}$ will be appreciably higher.

*Resolution*

A compound or an ion should be present in luminal fluid to minimize the risk of $CaHPO_4$ precipitate formation. We shall speculate that the differential renal handling of $Ca^{2+}$ and $Mg^{2+}$ ions in the PCT and in the mTAL of the loop of Henle may be important with respect to minimizing the risk of formation of precipitates of $CaHPO_4$ and $CaCO_3$ in the luminal fluid and in the medullary interstitial compartment in the deeper part of the medulla.

### Minimizing the risk of precipitation of calcium salts: role of magnesium

Because $Mg^{2+}$ ions form ion complexes with both $HPO_4^{2-}$ and $CO_3^{2-}$ ions that have a Ksp that is at least three orders of magnitude higher than for their respective calcium salts, $Mg^{2+}$ ions could diminish the risk of formation of these precipitates.

The concentration of ionized $Ca^{2+}$ in plasma is more than twofold higher than that of ionized $Mg^{2+}$ (~1.1 vs ~0.5 mmol/L, respectively), because about 40% of the total content of $Mg^{2+}$ ions in plasma is also bound to albumin. Nevertheless, by the time luminal fluid in the loop of Henle reaches the inner medulla, the concentration of $Mg^{2+}$ ions becomes higher than that of $Ca^{2+}$ ions. This is because most of the filtered ionized $Ca^{2+}$, but only a small proportion of filtered ionized $Mg^{2+}$, is reabsorbed in the PCT. In quantitative terms, as juxtamedullary nephrons receive 27 L of GFR, their filtered load of ionized $Ca^{2+}$ is about 27 mmol, while that of ionized $Mg^{2+}$ is about 13.5 mmol. Because approximately 70% of filtered ionized $Ca^{2+}$, but only approximately 20% of filtered ionized $Mg^{2+}$, is reabsorbed in the PCT, 8.9 mmol of ionized $Ca^{2+}$ and 10.8 mmol of ionized $Mg^{2+}$ exit the PCT of these nephrons. Because close to 83% of the GFR is reabsorbed in PCT, 4.5 L/day exit the PCT of these nephrons. Because these nephrons descend deep in the medulla to the 900 mosmol/kg $H_2O$ level, only about 1.5 L of water will be left in their luminal fluid. Hence, the concentration of ionized $Ca^{2+}$ rises to about 5.9 mmol/L, while that of ionized $Mg^{2+}$ rises to about 7.2 mmol/L. As described earlier, even more ionized $Ca^{2+}$ may be reabsorbed in the PCT of juxtamedullary nephrons.

There is another benefit for the preferential reabsorption of $Mg^{2+}$ in deep regions of the outer medulla. In more detail, $HCO_3^-$ ions are added to this interstitial fluid compartment in the deeper part of the outer medulla secondary to the reabsorption of $K^+$ ions by the $H^+/K^+$-ATPase in the MCD. This leads to a higher concentration of $CO_3^{2-}$ ions in this location. Hence, the presence of a high concentration of ionized $Mg^{2+}$ in the interstitial compartment will decrease the likelihood of precipitation of $CaCO_3$ in the medullary interstitial compartment when ionized calcium is also reabsorbed in the mTAL of the loop of Henle. After much of the ionized $Mg^{2+}$ is reabsorbed in the mTAL, preventing the precipitation of $CaHPO_4$ in the luminal fluid becomes the task of Tamm Horsfall proteins that are secreted in this nephron segment.

### Minimizing work in the deep part of the outer medulla

The rate of blood flow to the deeper region of the outer medulla should be high enough to deliver sufficient oxygen to permit the required rate of active transport of electrolytes (primarily $Na^+$ and $Cl^-$ ions). On the other hand, it should be low enough to prevent washout of reabsorbed osmoles and maintain a high osmolality in the medullary interstitial compartment. Blood delivered to the medulla has a low hematocrit. Although this improves the blood flow rate because of a reduction in viscosity, it may also lead to a decrease in oxygen carrying capacity and hence a low delivery of oxygen to deeper areas in the outer medulla. There is another limiting factor for the delivery of oxygen to these deeper areas: the shunting of oxygen from descending vasa recta to their ascending limbs in the more superficial regions of the medulla because of its countercurrent exchange property.

### Conundrum 3

There may not be enough oxygen delivered to the deeper part of the outer medulla to permit active reabsorption of the requisite quantity of $Na^+$ and $Cl^-$ ions. Although glycolysis permits ATP to be regenerated without the consumption of oxygen, it is unlikely to be a useful strategy for two reasons. First, there is also a low rate of delivery of glucose, and second, $H^+$ ions formed as a product of glycolysis may cause extensive local damage.

*Resolution*

Having passive reabsorption of $Na^+$ and $Cl^-$ ions in the inner medulla will decrease the requirement for the active reabsorption of $Na^+$ and $Cl^-$ ions in the mTAL of the loop of Henle in the deeper part of the outer medulla, where delivery of oxygen may be limited. For this passive reabsorption of $Na^+$ and $Cl^-$ ions in the inner medulla to occur, a lower concentration of $Na^+$ and $Cl^-$ ions in the interstitial compartment in the inner medulla is required. This is achieved with the addition of urea, and therefore water, to the interstitial compartment in the inner medulla in the process of urea recycling. The addition of water lowers the interstitial concentrations of $Na^+$ and $Cl^-$ ions and creates the driving force for the passive addition of $Na^+$ and $Cl^-$ ions into this compartment from the water-impermeable ascending thin limbs of the loop of Henle, which are permeable to both $Na^+$ and $Cl^-$.

For a quantitative analysis of how much $Na^+$ ions are reabsorbed from the ascending thin limbs in the inner medulla, we start by estimating the amount of water that is added to the interstitial compartment in the inner medulla (see Table 9-6). There are three sources of addition of water to the interstitial compartment in the inner medulla. First, 0.5 L of water is added with 600 mmol of urea to the interstitial compartment at an osmolality of 1200 mosmol/kg $H_2O$. Second, as the osmolality in the interstitial compartment in the inner medulla rises from 900 to 1200 mosmol/kg $H_2O$, one-quarter of the volume of water in the descending thin limbs of the loop of Henle of juxtamedullary nephrons will be reabsorbed. Because 1.5 L are delivered, about 0.4 L will be reabsorbed. Not all the descending thin limbs of the loop of Henle, however, reach the 1200 mosmol/kg $H_2O$ level, because loops of Henle have their bends in the inner medulla at different levels, therefore, this number should be adjusted downward. For simplicity, we will assume that half of the loops of Henle of these nephrons will have their bends above the midpoint between 900 and 1200 mosmol/kg $H_2O$ (i.e., at the 1050 mosmol/kg $H_2O$ level), and the other half will have their bends below this midpoint. Therefore, 0.2 L of water will be added to the interstitial compartment in the inner medulla from the descending thin limbs of the loop of Henle. Third, as the osmolality in the interstitial compartment in the inner medulla rises from 900 to 1200 mosmol/kg $H_2O$, one-quarter of the volume of water delivered to the inner MCD will be absorbed (i.e., 0.4 L out of 1.7 L; see Table 9-5). Therefore, a total of ~1.1 L of water is added to the interstitial compartment in the inner medulla per day.

For the osmolality of the interstitial compartment in the inner medulla to be kept at 1200 mosmol/kg $H_2O$, 1300 mosmol need to be added with this 1.1 L of water. Because 600 mmol of urea are added to the interstitial compartment in the inner medulla in the process of urea recycling, 360 mmol of Na$^+$ ions (and 360 mmol of Cl$^-$ ions) will need to be added by their passive reabsorption in the ascending thin limbs of the loop of Henle.

To realize the quantitative importance of this process, consider the following calculation. Approximately 7.4 L of fluid per day are added to the blood that exits the medulla via the ascending vasa recta. This represents 3.3 L of water/day that are reabsorbed from the MCD in the outer medulla, 3 L of water/day that are reabsorbed from the descending thin limbs of the loop of Henle of juxtamedullary nephrons (those with AQP1) in the outer medulla, and 1.1 L of water/day added to the interstitial compartment in the inner medulla (see Tables 9-3, 9-5, and 9-6). Because every liter of this water must exit the renal medulla via the ascending vasa recta with the same Na$^+$/H$_2$O ratio as the fluid that entered the medulla via the descending vasa recta (~150 mmol/L), about 1110 mmol of Na$^+$ ions need to be added to these 7.4 L of water. Hence, the passive reabsorption of Na$^+$ in the ascending thin limbs of the loop of Henle contributes about 30% (360/1110) to the total amount of Na$^+$ ion reabsorption in the medulla to make water reabsorption into a solution with a concentration of Na$^+$ ions of 150 mmol/L.

As there is "no free lunch," work is needed to achieve a high concentration of urea in the inner medulla. This requires the active reabsorption of Na$^+$ and Cl$^-$ ions and thereby of water without urea in nephron segments upstream from the inner medulla. This work, however, occurs in the renal cortex and in the renal medulla near the cortex, areas where there is an abundant supply of oxygen.

### Conundrum 4

A high concentration of Na$^+$ ions at the bend of the loop of Henle is required for the renal concentrating process to operate. Because descending thin limbs of the loop of Henle of the superficial nephrons lack AQP1, the rise in the concentrations of Na$^+$ and Cl$^-$ ions in the descending thin limb of the loop of Henle of the large majority of the nephrons is via addition of Na$^+$ and Cl$^-$ ions and not water reabsorption. This addition of Na$^+$ ions requires an increased active reabsorption of Na$^+$ ions from the mTAL of the loop of Henle.

### Resolution

One strategy to handle the energy demand this places on the mTAL is to have as little as possible of this process occurring in the deeper part of the outer medulla, where oxygen supply is more precarious. A quantitative analysis reveals that this is likely the case.

For this analysis, we start with the following assumption: superficial nephrons are 85% of total nephrons, so they receive 85% of GFR (150 L/day). Furthermore, five-sixths of this volume (127 L) is reabsorbed in their PCTs and hence 26 L are delivered to the descending thin limbs of their loops of Henle. Because descending thin limbs of loops of Henle have their bends at different levels in the renal medulla, we will assume that 75% have their bends in the 300 to 600 mosmol/kg H$_2$O area and only 25% descend down in the renal medulla to the 600 to 900 mosmol/kg H$_2$O area. For simplicity, we calculate the amount of Na$^+$ ions added at the midpoint of each of the two areas (i.e., at the 450 mosmol/kg H$_2$O level and at the 750 mosmol/kg H$_2$O level) (Table 9-8).

As calculated previously, the concentration of Na$^+$ ions in the fluid that exits the loop of Henle is 145 mmol/L; because the concentration of Na$^+$ ions in the medullary interstitial compartment at the 450 mosmol/kg H$_2$O level rises to 225 mmol/L, a total of 2080 mmol of Na$^+$ (26 L × 80 mmol of Na$^+$/L) will diffuse from the medullary interstitial compartment into the lumen of the descending thin limbs.

TABLE 9-8   **CALCULATION OF THE AMOUNT OF Na⁺ THAT RECYCLES FROM THE MTAL OF THE LOOP OF HENLE TO THE DESCENDING THIN LIMBS OF THE LOOP OF HENLE**

|  | VOLUME (# LITERS) | [Na⁺] AT ENTRY (mmol/L) | [Na⁺] AT LEVEL (mmol/L) | DIFFERENCE (mmol/L) | AMOUNT OF Na⁺ ADDED |
|---|---|---|---|---|---|
| At 450 mosmol/kg H₂O | 26 | 145 | 225 | 80 | 2080 |
| At 750 mosmol/kg H₂O | 6.5 | 300 | 375 | 75 | 450 |

For simplicity, we calculate the amount of Na⁺ added at the midpoint of the area of the medullary interstitium between the 300 and the 600 mosmol/kg H₂O levels (i.e., at the 450 mosmol/kg H₂O level), and at the midpoint of the area of the medullary interstitium between the 600 and the 900 mosmol/kg H₂O (i.e., at the 750 mosmol/kg H₂O) levels. We assumed that only 25% of thin descending limbs descend in the renal medulla to the 600–900 mosmol/kg H₂O area. A total of 2530 mmol of Na⁺ ions per day recycle between the medullary thick ascending limb (mTAL) of the loop of Henle and the descending thin limbs of superficial nephrons.

We assumed that only 6.5 L (25% of 26 L) of fluid will reach the deeper part of the outer medulla to the 600 to 900 mosmol/kg H₂O area. Because the concentration of Na⁺ ions in the medullary interstitial compartment at the 750 mosmol/kg H₂O level rises to 375 mmol/L from 300 mmol/L (because the concentration of Na⁺ ions in all the descending thin limbs of the loop of Henle that reached the 600 mosmol/kg H₂O level was 300 mmol/L), a total of about 450 mmol of Na⁺ ions (6.5 L × 75 mmol of Na⁺/L) will diffuse from the medullary interstitium into the lumen of the descending thin limbs. Hence, the total amount of Na⁺ ions that is recycled is 2530 mmol/day; less than 20% occurs in the deeper portion of the outer medulla.

When oxygen delivery to the renal medulla declines, the maximum urine osmolality falls appreciably. This is initially because of diminished recycling of Na⁺ ions, which is a way to diminish work performed in the medulla. The fall in urine osmolality may also be caused by a release of a vasopressinase from the hypoxic renal medulla. This may have the benefit of degrading vasopressin and diminishing its effect of causing vasoconstriction, and hence may increase blood flow to the renal medulla.

# DISCUSSION OF CASE 9-1

## CASE 9-1: A RISE IN THE $P_{Na}$ AFTER A SEIZURE

### What is the basis for the acute rise in the patient's $P_{Na}$?

Because there was no gain of Na⁺ ions to explain this rise in $P_{Na}$, its basis is a loss of water from the ECF compartment. Nevertheless, there is no site for water loss, and hypernatremia resolved without administration of water. Therefore, the most likely explanation for the water loss from the ECF compartment is a shift of water into cells or into the lumen of the intestinal tract. Because of the history of a recent seizure, the most likely site of water shift is into skeletal muscle cells. The driving force for this shift is a rise in the number of effective osmoles in skeletal muscle cells. Quantitatively, the breakdown of phosphocreatine$^{2-}$ to creatine and inorganic phosphate $(HPO_4^{2-})$ provides most of these osmoles. In addition, the breakdown of the macromolecule glycogen into many small molecules of L-lactic acid will also generate new osmoles, but only if their H⁺ ions do not react with $HCO_3^-$ ions, because if they do, there will be no gain of osmoles (L-lactate anions replace intracellular $HCO_3^-$ ions). Conversely, if some of these H⁺ ions bind to proteins in these cells, there is an increase in the number of osmoles in the form of L-lactate anions in muscle cells. Because there is vigorous muscle activity and hence a large rate of production of $CO_2$ and a low blood supply during a seizure, there is a high tissue $PCO_2$, and this promotes H⁺ ion binding to proteins rather than reacting with $HCO_3^-$ ions (Fig. 9-22).

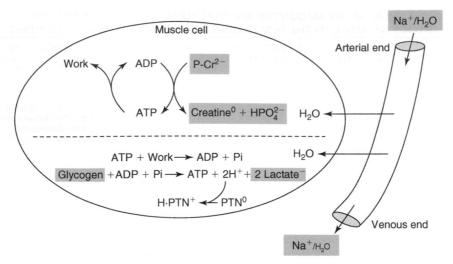

**Figure 9-22 Effect of a Seizure to Cause a Rise in the $P_{Na}$.** The *oval* is a skeletal muscle cell. During a seizure, phosphocreatine (P-Cr²⁻) is converted to creatine plus inorganic phosphate ($HPO_4{}^{2-}$) (above the *dashed horizontal line*) and glycogen is converted to many molecules of L-lactic acid. In each of these processes, there are more molecules of the products than of the substrates. With regard to L-lactic acid, because there is a high production of $CO_2$ and a relatively low blood flow rate, the tissue $P_{CO_2}$ is high, and hence many of the H⁺ ions formed bind to proteins instead of titrating intracellular $HCO_3{}^-$. This increase in number of particles causes water to be drawn into cells from their capillary blood, which raises the capillary $P_{Na}$ and thereby the venous $P_{Na}$. *ADP*, Adenosine diphosphate; *ATP*, adenosine triphosphate; *H.PTN⁺*, proteins with bound H⁺ ions; *PTNᵒ*, proteins with less bound H⁺ ions.

## DISCUSSION OF QUESTIONS

9-1 *Hypertonic saline is the treatment of choice to shrink brain cell size in a patient with acute hyponatremia. What is the major effect of hypertonic saline to reduce the risk of brain herniation?*

When the $P_{Na}$ is low, brain cells swell. Because brain cells occupy two-thirds of the volume in the skull and there is a small volume of fluid to squeeze out from the interstitial space into the cerebrospinal fluid, a point comes when intracranial pressure rises. Hence, therapy must be directed at removing water out of the skull (not just shifting water from the ICF to the ECF compartments of the brain). Because the capillaries of the brain form tight junctions (called the blood–brain barrier), hypertonic saline acts like albumin when infused rapidly, and therefore water moves from the brain into the capillaries faster than Na⁺ ions move in the other direction across the barrier. After this emergency therapy with the administration of a bolus of hypertonic saline, measures must be taken to create a negative water balance.

9-2 *What would happen acutely to the ICF volume if the permeability of capillary membranes to albumin were to increase?*

There will be no change in the ICF volume because there is no change in the $P_{Na}$. Rather there will be a fall in the intravascular volume and a rise in the interstitial fluid volume.

9-3 *What is the volume of distribution if 1 L of each of the following intravenous fluids is retained in the body: isotonic saline, half-isotonic saline, 300 mmol of NaCl/L, or 1 L of $D_5W$? What would the change in the $P_{Na}$ be in a normal 50-kg subject who has 30 L of total body water before the infusion of each of these solutions?*

The volumes of distribution are shown in the following table. The first step in this calculation is to assign the quantity of electrolytes into a solution of isotonic saline. The second step is to determine whether, after that is done, there is extra water or extra $Na^+$ ions. If there is extra water, it will distribute in the body in proportion to the original compartment volumes. On the other hand, if there are extra $Na^+$ ions they will be retained in the ECF compartment and one must obtain a volume of water from the ICF compartment to make it become an isotonic solution. The glucose infused is assumed to be metabolized into $CO_2 + H_2O$ or be converted into storage compounds. In either case, the infused water that remains after the metabolism of glucose distributes in body compartments based on their original volumes (see margin note for sample calculation for the addition of 300 mmol NaCl with 1 L of water).

| SOLUTION (1 L) | ECF VOLUME CHANGE | ICF VOLUME CHANGE | NEW $P_{Na}$ |
|---|---|---|---|
| Isotonic NaCl | +1.0 L | 0 L | 140 |
| Half-isotonic NaCl | +0.67 L | +0.33 L | 138 |
| 300 mmol/L NaCl | +1.70 L | −0.7 L | 145 |
| $D_5W$ | +0.33 L | +0.67 L | 136 |

9-4 *Two patients have a maximum urine osmolality of 600 mosmol/ kg $H_2O$ when vasopressin acts. One of them has sickle cell anemia and papillary necrosis, whereas the other has a lesion that affects his outer medulla, but he has an intact papilla. Both patients eat the same diet and excrete 900 mosmol/day (urine osmoles are half urea and half electrolytes). Why do they not have the same minimum urine flow rate?*

There are two factors that influence the urine flow rate when vasopressin acts: the number of effective osmoles in the luminal fluid of the inner MCD and the effective osmolality of the fluid in the medullary interstitial compartment. To illustrate the importance of each of these factors, consider the patient who has sickle cell anemia. In this disorder, there is obstruction of the blood vessels that descend into the inner medulla by sickled cells. As a result, there is necrosis of the renal papilla. Because the inner MCD is the nephron site where vasopressin causes the insertion of urea transporters, urea cannot be reabsorbed in the inner MCD at appreciable rate in this patient when vasopressin acts. Therefore, urea becomes an effective osmole in this setting and it obligates the excretion of water. In addition, if urea cannot be reabsorbed as an iso-osmotic solution in the inner MCD, this prevents the passive reabsorption of $Na^+$ and $Cl^-$ ions from the ascending thin limb of the loop of Henle. Accordingly, the maximum medullary interstitial osmolality is likely to be close to 750 mosmol/kg $H_2O$. The patient in this example has a maximum urine osmolality of 600 mOsm/kg $H_2O$ and an osmole excretion rate of 900 mosmol/day (all of them are effective osmoles). Therefore, the minimum urine volume would be close to 1.5 L/day.

Contrast these numbers with the second subject who has a similar osmole excretion rate of 900 mosmol/day (half urea, half electrolytes), a similar maximum urine osmolaity of 600 mosmol/kg $H_2O$, but no lesion involving the renal papilla. After vasopressin acts, urea transporters are present in the inner MCD and the concentration of urea is equal in the lumen of the inner MCD and in the papillary interstitial compartment. Because urea is not an effective urinary osmole in this setting, the rate of excretion of effective osmoles is only half of 900 mosmol/day or 450 mosmol/day. Accordingly, the daily urine volume would be 0.75 L, which is half the urine volume in the patient with sickle cell anemia and papillary necrosis at the same osmole excretion rate and maximum urine osmolality.

**ADDITION OF 300 MMOL NACL AND 1 L OF WATER TO A 50-KG PERSON**

- Before the addition of 300 mmol of NaCl, this person had total body water of 30 L, an ECF volume of 10 L and an ICF volume of 20 L.
- The quantity of osmoles added to the body is 600 mosmol (2 × 300 mmol NaCl per liter of water).
- The total number of effective osmoles in the body is equal to 2 $P_{Na}$ + $P_{Glucose}$ in mmol/L terms (285 mosmol/kg $H_2O$) × total body water (30 L) = 8550 mosmol, because the osmolality is equal in the ICF and ECF compartments.
- After adding 600 mosmol, the new total number of osmoles is 9150 mosmol. The new total body water is 31 L. Therefore, the new osmolality in the body is 295 mosmol/kg $H_2O$ (9150 mosmol ÷ 31 L).
- The number of osmoles in the ICF compartment does not change (20 L × 285 mosmol/kg $H_2O$ = 5700 mosmol). Hence, the new ICF volume is 19.3 L (5700 mosmol ÷ 295 mosmol/kg $H_2O$).
- The number of osmoles in the ECF compartment was 2850 mosmol. After the addition of 600 mosmol of NaCl, the number of osmoles in the ECF compartment becomes 3450 mosmol. Because the body osmolality now is 295 mosmol/kg $H_2O$, the new ECF volume is 11.7 L.
- The original quantity of $Na^+$ ions in the ECF compartment was 1400 mmol (140 mmol/L × 10 L). Because 300 mmol of $Na^+$ ions were added to the ECF compartment, the current content of $Na^+$ ions in the ECF compartment is 1700 mmol. The new $P_{Na}$ is 145 mmol/L (1700 mmol ÷ 11.7 L).

# Hyponatremia

# Introduction

Hyponatremia is defined as a concentration of sodium (Na$^+$) ions in plasma (P$_{Na}$) that is less than 135 mmol/L. Hyponatremia is the most common electrolyte disorder encountered in clinical practice. It can be associated with considerable morbidity and even mortality. The initial step in the clinical approach to the patient with hyponatremia must focus on what the danger is to the patient rather than on the cause of hyponatremia. Regardless of its cause, acute hyponatremia may be associated with swelling of brain cells and increased intracranial pressure and the danger of brain herniation, necessitating inducing a rapid rise in P$_{Na}$ to shrink brain cell size. In contrast, in a patient with chronic hyponatremia, the danger is a too rapid rise in P$_{Na}$, which may lead to the development of osmotic demyelination syndrome (ODS). Hence, the clinician must be vigilant to avoid a rise in P$_{Na}$ that exceeds what is considered a safe maximum limit.

It is also important to recognize that hyponatremia is not a diagnosis but rather is the result of diminished renal excretion of electrolyte-free water because of a number of disorders. Hyponatremia may be the first manifestation of a serious underlying disease such as adrenal insufficiency or small cell carcinoma of the lung. Hence, a cause of hyponatremia must always be sought.

Hyponatremia has been associated with increased mortality, morbidity, and length of hospital stay in hospitalized patients with a variety of disorders. Whether these associations reflect the severity of the underlying illness, a direct effect of hyponatremia, or a combination of both remains unclear.

## ABBREVIATIONS

P$_{Na}$, concentration of sodium ions (Na$^+$) in plasma

P$_K$, concentration of potassium ions (K$^+$) in plasma

P$_{Cl}$, concentration of chloride ions (Cl$^-$) in plasma

P$_{HCO_3}$, concentration of bicarbonate ions (HCO$_3^-$) in plasma

P$_{Glucose}$, concentration of glucose in plasma

P$_{Albumin}$, concentration of albumin in plasma

P$_{Osm}$, osmolality in plasma

BUN, blood urea nitrogen

P$_{Urea}$, concentration of urea in plasma

P$_{Creatinine}$, concentration of creatinine in plasma

U$_{Osm}$, urine osmolality

ADH, antidiuretic hormone

AQP, aquaporin water channels

EABV, effective arterial blood volume

dDAVP, desmopressin (1-deamino 8-D-arginine vasopressin), a synthetic long acting vasopressin

TRPV, transient receptor potential vanilloid

SIADH, syndrome of inappropriate antidiuretic hormone

PCT, proximal convoluted tubule

ECF, extracellular fluid

ICF, intracellular fluid

MDMA, 3,4-methylenedioxy-methamphetamine

DCT, distal convoluted tubule

CRH, corticotropin-releasing hormone

CCD, cortical collecting duct

MCD, medullary collecting duct

CDN, cortical distal nephron, which consists of nephron segments in the cortex, the late DCT, the connecting segment, and the CCD

U$_{Na}$, concentration of Na$^+$ ions in the urine

U$_{Cl}$, concentration of Cl$^-$ ions in the urine

U$_K$, concentration of K$^+$ ions in the urine

TURP, transurethral resection of prostate

## OBJECTIVES

- To emphasize that a low effective plasma osmolality (P$_{Osm}$) implies that the intracellular fluid (ICF) volume is expanded. Brain cells adapt to swelling by extruding effective osmoles, and if the time course is greater than 48 hours, brain cells have had time to export a sufficient number of effective osmoles to return their size toward normal.

- To emphasize that, from a clinical perspective, hyponatremia is divided into acute hyponatremia (<48 hour duration), chronic hyponatremia (>48 hour duration), and chronic hyponatremia with an acute component. The importance of this classification is that the danger to the patient, and hence the design of therapy, is different in the three groups. In the patient with acute hyponatremia, the danger is brain cell swelling with possible brain herniation. In the patient with chronic hyponatremia, the danger is development of osmotic demyelination syndrome due to a large rise of P$_{Na}$. In the patient who develops an acute component on top of chronic hyponatremia, the danger is twofold. There is the danger of brain cell swelling and brain herniation due to the acute component of the hyponatremia, and there is the danger of development of osmotic demyelination if the rise of P$_{Na}$ exceeds what is considered a maximum safe limit. In many patients, the duration of hyponatremia is not known with certainty and therefore, the design of therapy is based on the presence of symptoms that may suggest an increased intracranial pressure.

- To emphasize that hyponatremia is a diagnostic category and not a single disease; rather, it is the result of diminished renal excretion of electrolyte-free water caused by a number of disorders. A cause of hyponatremia must always be sought and treatment in patients with chronic hyponatremia should be directed to the specific pathophysiology in each patient.

## CASE 10-1: THIS CATASTROPHE SHOULD NOT HAVE OCCURRED!

A 25-year-old woman (weight 50 kg) developed central diabetes insipidus 18 months ago. There was no obvious cause for the disorder. Treatment consisted of desmopressin (dDAVP) to control her polyuria and maintain her $P_{Na}$ close to 140 mmol/L. Her current problem began after she developed the flu, with low-grade fever, cough, and runny nose, which started about 1 week ago. To alleviate her symptoms, she sipped ice-cold liquids. Because she felt progressively unwell over time, she visited her physician yesterday afternoon. She was noted to have gained close to 3 kg (7 lb) in weight. Accordingly, her $P_{Na}$ was measured and it was 125 mmol/L. Although she was advised by her physician not to drink any fluids and to go to the hospital immediately, she waited until the next morning before acting on this advice. On arrival in the emergency department, she complained of nausea and a moderately severe headache. There were no other new findings on physical examination; unfortunately, her weight was not measured. Her laboratory data are summarized in the following table:

|  |  | PLASMA | URINE |
| --- | --- | --- | --- |
| Na+ | mmol/L | 112 | 100 |
| K+ | mmol/L | 3.9 | 50 |
| Cl- | mmol/L | 78 | 100 |
| BUN (urea) | mg/dL (mmol/L) | 6 (2.0) | 120 mmol/L |
| Creatinine | mg/dL (μmol/L) | 0.6 (50) | 0.6 g/L (5 mmol/L) |
| Glucose | mg/dL (mmol/L) | 90 (5.0) | 0 |
| Osmolality | mosmol/kg H$_2$O | 230 | 420 |

### Questions

What dangers to the patient are there on presentation?

What dangers should be anticipated during therapy, and how can they be avoided?

## CASE 10-2: THIS IS FAR FROM ECSTASY!

A 19-year-old woman suffers from anorexia nervosa. She went to a rave party, where she took the drug Ecstasy (MDMA). Following advice from others at the party, she drank a large volume of water that night to avoid dehydration from excessive sweating. As time passed, she began to feel unwell, with her main symptoms were lassitude and an inability to concentrate. After lying down in a quiet room for 2 hours, her symptoms did not improve and she developed a severe headache. Accordingly, she was brought to the hospital. In the emergency department, she had a generalized tonic-clonic seizure. Blood was drawn immediately after the seizure and the major electrolyte abnormality was a $P_{Na}$ of 130 mmol/L; a metabolic acidemia (pH 7.20, $P_{HCO_3}$ 10 mmol/L) was also present.

### Questions

Is this acute hyponatremia?

Why did she have a seizure if the $P_{Na}$ was only mildly reduced at 130 mmol/L?

What role might anorexia nervosa have played in this clinical picture?

What is your therapy for this patient?

## CASE 10-3: HYPONATREMIA WITH BROWN SPOTS

A 22-year-old woman has myasthenia gravis. In the past 6 months, she has noted a marked decline in her energy and a weight loss of 7 lb, from 110 to 103 lb (50 to 47 kg). She often felt faint when she stood up quickly. On physical examination, her blood pressure was 80/50 mm Hg, her pulse rate was 126 beats per minute, her jugular venous pressure was below the level of the sternal angle, and there was no peripheral edema. Brown pigmented spots were evident on her buccal mucosa. The electrocardiogram was unremarkable. The biochemistry data on presentation are shown in the following table:

|  |  | PLASMA | URINE |
|---|---|---|---|
| $Na^+$ | mmol/L | 112 | 130 |
| $K^+$ | mmol/L | 5.5 | 20 |
| BUN (urea) | mg/dL (mmol/L) | 28 (10.0) | (130 mmol/L) |
| Creatinine | mg/dL ($\mu$mol/L) | 1.7 (150) | 0.7 g/L (6 mmol/L) |
| Osmolality | mosmol/kg $H_2O$ | 240 | 430 |

### Questions

What is the most likely basis for the very low effective arterial blood volume (EABV)?

What dangers to the patient are present on presentation?

What dangers should be anticipated during therapy, and how can they be avoided?

## CASE 10-4: HYPONATREMIA IN A PATIENT ON A THIAZIDE DIURETIC

A 71-year-old woman was started on a thiazide diuretic for treatment of hypertension. She had ischemic renal disease with an estimated glomerular filtration rate (GFR) of 28 mL/min (40 L/day). She consumed a low salt, low protein diet and drank eight cups of water a day to remain hydrated. A month after starting the diuretic, she presented to her family doctor feeling unwell. Her blood pressure was 130/80 mm Hg, her heart rate was 80 beats per minute, there were no postural changes in her blood pressure or heart rate, and her jugular venous pressure was about 1 cm below the level of the sternal angle. Her $P_{Na}$ was 112 mmol/L. Her other laboratory data are summarized in the following table:

|  |  | PLASMA | URINE |
|---|---|---|---|
| $Na^+$ | mmol/L | 112 | 22 |
| $K^+$ | mmol/L | 3.6 |  |
| $HCO_3^-$ | mmol/L | 28 |  |
| BUN (urea) | mg/dL (mmol/L) | 28 (10.0) |  |
| Creatinine | mg/dL ($\mu$mol/L) | 1.3 (145) | 0.7 g/L (6 mmol/L) |
| Osmolality | mosmol/kg $H_2O$ | 240 | 325 |

### Questions

What is the most likely basis for the hyponatremia in this patient?

What dangers should be anticipated during therapy, and how can they be avoided?

# PART A
# BACKGROUND

## REVIEW OF THE PERTINENT PHYSIOLOGY

### THE PLASMA Na$^+$ CONCENTRATION REFLECTS THE ICF VOLUME

Water crosses cell membranes rapidly through aquaporin (AQP) water channels to achieve equal sum of concentration of effective osmoles in the extracellular fluid (ECF) compartment and ICF compartment. Effective osmoles are particles that are largely restricted to either the ECF compartment or the ICF compartment. The effective osmoles in the ECF compartment are largely Na$^+$ ions and their attendant anions (Cl$^-$ and HCO$_3^-$ ions). The major cation in the ICF compartment is potassium (K$^+$) ions; electroneutrality of the ICF compartment is achieved by the anionic charge on organic phosphate esters inside the cells (RNA, DNA, phospholipids, phosphoproteins, adenosine triphosphate [ATP], and adenosine diphosphate [ADP]). These are relatively large molecules, and hence exert little osmotic pressure. Other organic solutes contribute to the osmotic force in the ICF compartment. The individual compounds differ from organ to organ. The organic solutes that have the highest concentration in skeletal muscle cells are phosphocreatine and carnosine; each is present at ~25 mmol/kg. Other solutes include amino acids (e.g., glutamine, glutamate, taurine), peptides (e.g., glutathione), and sugar derivatives (e.g., myoinositol).

Because particles in the ICF compartment are relatively fixed in number and charge, changes in the concentration of particles in the ICF compartment usually come about by changes in its content of water. Water enters cells when the tonicity in the ICF compartment exceeds that in the ECF compartment. Because the *concentration* of Na$^+$ ions in the ECF compartment is the major determinant of ECF tonicity, the *concentration* of Na$^+$ ions in the ECF compartment is the most important factor that determines the ICF volume (except when the ECF compartment contains other effective osmoles, e.g., glucose [in conditions of relative lack of insulin actions], mannitol). Hence, hyponatremia (whether caused by the loss of Na$^+$ ions or the gain of water) is associated with an increase in the ICF volume (Fig. 10-1).

### THE CONTENT OF Na$^+$ IONS DETERMINES THE ECF VOLUME

The number of effective osmoles in each compartment determines that compartment's volume because these particles attract water

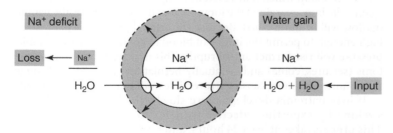

**Figure 10-1 Cell Swelling During Hyponatremia.** The *circle with the solid line* represents the normal intracellular fluid (ICF) volume. Whether the basis for hyponatremia is a deficit of Na$^+$ ions (*left*) or a gain of water (*right*), the ICF volume is increased (*circle with a dashed line*). The *ovals* represent aquaporin (AQP) water channels in the cell membrane.

molecules via osmosis. The most abundant effective osmoles in the ECF are $Na^+$ ions and their attendant monovalent anions, and therefore they determine the ECF volume. However, the concentration of $Na^+$ ions in the ECF compartment depends on the ratio between the content of $Na^+$ ions and the volume of water in the ECF compartment. Hyponatremia may be seen in patients with a reduced ECF volume, normal ECF volume, or increased ECF volume.

A reduced concentration of $Na^+$ ions (i.e., hyponatremia) may be present in a patient with reduced ECF volume, in which case the content of $Na^+$ ions is reduced and so is the volume of water, but the reduction of the content of $Na^+$ ions is proportionally larger. For instance, consider a patient who starts with an ECF volume of 10 L and $P_{Na}$ of 140 mmol/L, and so a content of $Na^+$ ions in the ECF compartment of 140 mmol/L × 10 L or 1400 mmol. If this patient develops a reduced ECF volume of 8 L and a $P_{Na}$ of 120 mmol/L, then the content of $Na^+$ ions in her ECF compartment would now be 960 mmol. This means the patient's ECF volume has fallen by 20%, but content of $Na^+$ ions in her ECF compartment would have fallen by $(1400 - 960)/1400 = 440/1400 = 31\%$. A patient may have a normal ECF volume of 10 L but a reduced $P_{Na}$ of 120 mmol/L, in which case the content of $Na^+$ ions in the ECF compartment is reduced by 200 mmol. Finally, a patient may have an expanded ECF volume and an increased content of $Na^+$ ions in the ECF compartment, yet the concentration of $Na^+$ ions in the ECF compartment may be reduced if the increase in the content of $Na^+$ ions in the ECF compartment is proportionally smaller than the increase in the ECF volume. Consider a patient with congestive heart failure who may have an increase in ECF volume from 10 to 14 L (an increase of 40%), who has a fall in $P_{Na}$ from 140 mmol/L to 120 mmol/L. The content of $Na^+$ ions in her ECF compartment is now 14 L × 120 mmol/L = 1680 mmol, which is an increase of $(1680 - 1400)/1400 = 280/1400 = 20\%$.

Hence, hyponatremia can be associated with low, normal, or increased ECF volume. Stated another way, one cannot make conclusions about the ECF volume simply by looking at the patient's $P_{Na}$.

## REGULATION OF BRAIN VOLUME

Defense of brain cell volume is necessary because the brain is contained in the skull, a rigid box (Fig. 10-2). When hyponatremia develops quickly over several hours, brain cells swell. The initial defense is to expel as much NaCl and water as possible from the interstitial space in the brain into the cerebrospinal fluid to prevent a large rise in intracranial pressure. If brain cells continue to swell, this defense mechanism will be overcome. Hence, the intracranial pressure will rise, and because of the physical restriction imposed by the rigid skull, the brain will be pushed caudally, which may result in compression of the cerebral veins against the bony margin of the foramen magnum. Therefore, the venous outflow will be diminished. Because the arterial pressure is likely to be high enough to permit the inflow of blood to continue, the intracranial pressure will rise further and abruptly. This may lead to serious symptoms (seizures, coma) and eventually herniation of the brain through the foramen magnum, causing irreversible midbrain damage and death.

If hyponatremia develops more slowly, the brain cells adapt to swelling by exporting effective osmoles to shrink their volume. This process takes at least 24 hours, and by approximately 48 hours, these adaptive changes have proceeded sufficiently to shrink the volume of brain cells back toward their normal size. Approximately half of the particles exported are electrolytes ($K^+$ ions and accompanying anions *see* Chapter 9), and the other half is organic solutes of

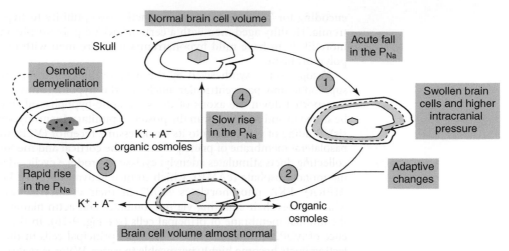

**Figure 10-2 Changes in Brain Cell Volume in a Patient With Hyponatremia.** The structure represents the brain; its ventricles are depicted as *hexagons* and the *bold line* represents the skull. When the $P_{Na}$ falls, water enters brain cells, and there is a rise in intracranial pressure (ICP; *site 1*). This rise in ICP squeezes some of the extracellular fluid of the brain out into the cerebrospinal fluid. As the $P_{Na}$ approaches 120 mmol/L, the danger of herniation mounts enormously. If, however, the fall in $P_{Na}$ has been more gradual (*site 2*), adaptive changes have time to occur (export $K^+$ salts and organic molecules), and brain cell size is now close to normal despite the presence of hyponatremia. If the $P_{Na}$ rises too quickly at this stage, osmotic demyelination may develop (*site 3*). This complication can be prevented if the rise in the $P_{Na}$ occurs over a long period of time sufficient for brain cells to reaccumulate the lost $K^+$ ions and their anions and the lost organic osmolytes. (*site 4*).

diverse origin. The major organic osmoles that are lost from brain cells are the amino acids glutamine, glutamate, taurine, and myo-inositol, which is a sugar derivative. If hyponatremia is corrected too rapidly in this setting, brain cells may not have sufficient time to regain their lost organic osmolytes, and this may lead to osmotic demyelination. The pathophysiology of this very serious neurological complication is not well understood but seems to be related to the osmotic stress caused by a rapid rise in $P_{Na}$, causing shrinkage of cerebral vascular endothelial cells. This leads to a disruption of the blood–brain barrier, allowing lymphocytes, complement, and cytokines to enter the brain, damage oligodendrocytes, and cause demyelination. Microglial activation also seems to contribute to this process.

## SYNOPSIS OF WATER PHYSIOLOGY

Regulation of water balance has an input arm and an output arm. The ingestion of water is stimulated by thirst. When enough water is ingested to cause a fall in the $P_{Na}$ and swelling of cells of the hypothalamic osmoreceptor (which is really a tonicity receptor), the release of vasopressin is inhibited. In the absence of vasopressin actions, AQP2 are not inserted in the luminal membranes of principal cells of the cortical and medullary collecting ducts, which leads to the excretion of a hypotonic urine.

The main osmosensory cells appear to be located in the organum vasculosum laminae terminalis and the supraoptic and paraventricular nuclei of the hypothalamus. The mechanism of osmosensing appears to be at least in part caused by activation of nonselective calcium-permeable cation channels of the transient receptor potential vanilloid (TRPV), which can serve as stretch receptors. The osmoreceptor is linked to both the thirst center and the vasopressin release center via nerve connections. Polymorphism in the gene encoding for TRPV4 may confer genetic susceptibility to hyponatremia. Healthy aged men with a certain TRPV4 polymorphism are more likely to have mild hyponatremia than are men without this polymorphism.

Vasopressin is synthesized by the magnocellular neurons in the supraoptic and paraventricular nuclei of the hypothalamus and is transported down the axons of the supraoptic-hypophyseal tract to be stored in and released from the posterior pituitary (neurohypophysis). Binding of vasopressin to its vasopressin 2 receptor (V2R) in the basolateral membrane of principal cells in the cortical and medullary collecting ducts stimulates adenylyl cyclase to produce cyclic adenosine monophosphate (cAMP), which in turn activates protein kinase A(PKA). PKA phosphorylates AQP2 in their endocytic vesicles, which causes their shuttling via microtubules and actin filaments to the luminal membrane of principal cells (see Fig. 9-16). In the presence of AQP2 in their luminal membrane, principal cells in the collecting ducts become highly permeable to water. Water is reabsorbed until the effective osmolality in the lumen of the collecting duct is equal to that in the surrounding interstitial compartment at any horizontal plane.

Although the main trigger for the release of vasopressin is a rise in $P_{Na}$, large changes in the EABV and/or the blood pressure can also cause its release. Baroreceptors located in the carotid sinus and aortic arch are stretch receptors that detect changes in EABV. When EABV is increased, afferent neural impulses inhibit the secretion of vasopressin. In contrast, when EVAB is decreased, this inhibitory signal is diminished, leading to vasopressin release. Notwithstanding, acutely decreasing EABV by 7% in healthy adults had little effect on plasma vasopressin level; a 10% to 15% decline in EABV is required to double the plasma vasopressin level. Furthermore, even a larger degree of decreased EABV is required for this baroreceptor-mediated stimulation of vasopressin release to override the inhibitory signals related to hypotonicity.

Nausea, pain, stress, and a number of other stimuli, including some drugs (e.g., carbamazepine, selective serotonin reuptake inhibitors, and 3,4-methylenedioxy-methamphetamine [ecstasy]) can also cause the release of vasopressin.

Once a water load leads to a fall in the arterial $P_{Na}$ and the absence of circulating vasopressin, principal cells of the cortical and the medullary collecting ducts lose their luminal AQP2 channels. As a result, a large water diuresis ensues. The limiting factors for the excretion of water in this setting are the volume of filtrate delivered to the distal nephron and the amount of water reabsorbed in the inner MCD by pathways that are independent of vasopressin (called residual water permeability).

### Distal delivery of filtrate

The volume of filtrate delivered to the early distal convoluted tubule (DCT) is estimated to be about 27 L/day in a healthy young adult (see Table 9-3). Because the descending thin limb of the loop of Henle of the majority of nephrons lacks AQP1 and therefore is largely water impermeable, the volume of distal delivery of filtrate is determined by the volume of glomerular filtration (GFR) less the volume of filtrate that is reabsorbed in the proximal convoluted tubule (PCT). As discussed in Chapter 9, close to 83% of the GFR is reabsorbed in the entire PCT. In the presence of a low EABV, a larger fraction of the GFR is reabsorbed in the PCT as a result of sympathetic nervous system activation and the release of angiotensin II. Therefore, the absence of a contracted EABV is needed for maximal excretion of water. Conversely, when there is both a low GFR and an enhanced reabsorption of filtrate because of a low EABV, the volume of distal delivery of filtrate may be very low. If the volume of distal delivery of filtrate is not sufficiently large to exceed the volume of water that is reabsorbed via residual water permeability in the inner MCD to allow for the excretion of the daily water load, chronic hyponatremia may develop, even when the daily water load is modest and in the absence of vasopressin actions.

### RESIDUAL WATER PERMEABILITY

There are two pathways for transport of water in the inner MCD: a vasopressin-responsive system via AQP2 and a vasopressin-independent system called residual water permeability. Two factors may affect the volume of water reabsorbed by residual water permeability. First, the driving force that is the enormous difference in osmotic pressure between the luminal and the interstitial fluid compartments in the inner MCD during a water diuresis. Second, contraction of the renal pelvis. In more detail, each time the renal pelvis contracts, some of the fluid in the renal pelvis travels in a retrograde direction up toward the inner MCD; some of that fluid may be reabsorbed via residual water permeability after it enters the inner MCD for a second (or a third) time. From a quantitative perspective, we estimate that in an adult, somewhat in excess of 5 L of water would be reabsorbed per day in the inner MCD by residual water permeability during water diuresis (see Chapter 9).

The appropriate renal response to hyponatremia (i.e., to an excess of water in the body) is to excrete the largest possible volume (~10 to 15 mL/min or ~ 15 to 21 L/day) of maximally dilute urine (urine osmolality [$U_{Osm}$] ~ 50 mosmol/kg $H_2O$; *see margin note*). If this response is not observed, one should suspect that either vasopressin is acting and/or that the volume of distal delivery of filtrate is low.

## BASIS OF HYPONATREMIA

In patients with acute hyponatremia, vasopressin is commonly present and acting. One must, however, look for a reason why so much water was ingested, because normal subjects have an aversion to drinking large amounts of water when the thirst center is intact and mental function is normal (Table 10-1). In fact, most cases of acute hyponatremia occur in a hospital setting, particularly in the perioperative period, and hence this defense mechanism of aversion to drinking large amounts of water is bypassed with the intravenous administration of fluids.

In a patient with chronic hyponatremia, the major pathophysiology is a defect in the excretion of water (Table 10-2). The traditional approach to the pathophysiology of hyponatremia centers on a reduced electrolyte-free water excretion caused by actions of vasopressin. In some clinical settings, release of vasopressin is thought to be caused by decreased EABV. Notwithstanding, at least in some patients, the degree of decreased EABV does not seem to be large enough to cause the release of vasopressin. We suggest that hyponatremia may develop in some patients even in the absence of vasopressin action. Two important factors in this regard are diminished volume of filtrate

**URINE OSMOLALITY DURING A WATER DIURESIS**

- In the absence of vasopressin actions, the $U_{Osm}$ depends on the number of osmoles to excrete and the urine volume. The latter is determined by the volume of distal delivery of filtrate and the volume of water that is reabsorbed in the inner MCD via its residual water permeability.
- Consider two subjects who excrete urine with an $U_{Osm}$ that is much less than the $P_{Osm}$, indicating that vasopressin is not acting.
- Each patient excretes 600 mosmol/day. Subject 2 has a lower volume of distal delivery of filtrate because of a lower GFR and an enhanced reabsorption in the PCT due to a low EABV. Notice the difference in the values for their $U_{Osm}$.

| SUBJECT | URINE VOLUME | $U_{Osm}$ |
|---|---|---|
| 1 | 10 L/day | 60 |
| 2 | 5 L/day | 120 |

TABLE 10-1    **SOURCES OF A LARGE INPUT OF WATER IN A PATIENT WITH HYPONATREMIA**

**Ingestion of a Large Volume of Water**
- Aversion to a large water intake is suppressed by mood-altering drugs (e.g., MDMA)
- Drinking too much water during a marathon to avoid dehydration
- Beer potomania
- Psychotic state (e.g., paranoid schizophrenia)

**Infusion of a Large Volume of 5% Dextrose in Water Solution ($D_5W$)**
- During the postoperative period (especially in a young patient with a low muscle mass)

**Infusion of a Large Volume of Hypotonic Lavage Fluid**
- Input of water and organic solutes, with little or no $Na^+$ ions (e.g., hyponatremia following transurethral resection of the prostate)

**Generation and Retention of Electrolyte-Free Water ("Desalination")**
- Excretion of a large volume of hypertonic urine caused by a large infusion of isotonic saline in a setting where vasopressin is present

In these patients, look for a reason why the aversion to drink water was "ignored." Also, look for a reason for a decreased rate of excretion of water (e.g., release of vasopressin and/or a low distal delivery of filtrate [see Table 10-2]). *MDMA*, 3,4-Methylenedioxy-methamphetamine.

TABLE 10-2    **CAUSES OF A LOWER THAN EXPECTED RATE OF EXCRETION OF WATER**

**Lower Rate of Water Excretion Because of Low Volume of Distal Delivery of Filtrate**
- States with a very low GFR
- States with enhanced reabsorption of filtrate in the PCT caused by low EABV:
  - Loss of $Na^+$ and $Cl^-$ in sweat (e.g., patients with cystic fibrosis, a marathon runner)
  - Loss of $Na^+$ and $Cl^-$ via the gastrointestinal tract (e.g., diarrhea)
  - Loss of $Na^+$ and $Cl^-$ via the kidney (diuretics, aldosterone deficiency, renal or cerebral salt wasting)
  - Conditions with an expanded ECF volume but low EABV (e.g., congestive heart failure, liver cirrhosis)

**Lower Rate of Excretion of Water Because of Vasopressin Actions**
- Baroreceptor-mediated release of vasopressin because of markedly low EABV
- Nonosmotic stimuli including pain, anxiety, nausea
- Central stimulation of vasopressin release by drugs, including MDMA, nicotine, morphine, carbamazepine, tricyclic antidepressants, serotonin reuptake inhibitors, antineoplastic agents such as vincristine and cyclophosphamide (probably via nausea and vomiting)
- Pulmonary disorders (e.g., bacterial or viral pneumonia, tuberculosis)
- Central nervous system disorders (e.g., encephalitis, meningitis, brain tumors, subdural hematoma, subarachnoid hemorrhage, stroke)
- Release of vasopressin from malignant cells (e.g., small-cell carcinoma of the lung, oropharyngeal carcinomas, olfactory neuroblastomas)
- Administration of dDAVP (e.g., for urinary incontinence, treatment for diabetes insipidus)
- Glucocorticoid deficiency
- Severe hypothyroidism
- Activating mutation of the V2R (nephrogenic syndrome of inappropriate antidiuresis)

*GFR*, Glomerular filtration rate; *PCT*, proximal convoluted tubule; *EABV*, effective arterial blood volume; *MDMA*, 3,4-methylenedioxy-methamphetamine; *V2R*, vasopressin 2 receptor.

delivered to the distal nephron and enhanced water reabsorption in the inner MCD through its residual water permeability.

In the absence of a low distal delivery of filtrate in a patient with chronic hyponatremia, the diagnosis is the syndrome of inappropriate antidiuretic hormone secretion (SIADH). A rare cause of SIADH is a genetic disorder in which there is a gain of function mutation in the gene encoding V2R, causing its constitutive activation. This disorder is called nephrogenic syndrome of inappropriate antidiuresis. The diagnosis is suspected in a patient with chronic SIADH of undetermined etiology in whom vasopressin levels are undetectable and who does not respond with a water diuresis to the administration of V2R antagonist (e.g., tolvaptan).

# PART B
# ACUTE HYPONATREMIA

## CLINICAL APPROACH

The clinical approach to patients with hyponatremia has three steps:
1. Deal with emergencies.
2. Anticipate and prevent dangers that may develop during therapy.
3. Proceed with diagnostic issues.

### DEAL WITH EMERGENCIES

The danger in a patient with acute hyponatremia (duration <48 hours) is brain cell swelling with a rise in intracranial pressure and the risk of brain herniation. The symptoms that develop when brain cells swell are often mild at an early stage (e.g., mild headache, decrease in attention span). When the rise in intracranial pressure is somewhat greater, the patient may become drowsy, mildly confused, and may complain of nausea. At a later stage, there may be a major degree of confusion, decreased level of consciousness, vomiting, seizures, or even coma. Notwithstanding, the time period for the transition between early mild symptoms and later severe symptoms may be very brief. In many patients the duration for the development of hyponatremia is not known, though acute hyponatremia is more likely in certain settings as will be discussed later.

If the patient has hyponatremia and severe symptoms (e.g., seizures, coma), we would treat it as an emergency and aim to induce a rapid rise in $P_{Na}$ (see Flow Chart 10-1). In our view, the risk of severe neurological damage and possibly death due to cerebral edema is a more important consideration than the risk of osmotic demyelination. Furthermore, based on data from the neurosurgical literature, an increase in $P_{Na}$ of 5 mmol/L (which does not exceed what is considered the maximum daily limit for a rise in $P_{Na}$ in patients with chronic hyponatremia; see later) is sufficient to promptly reverse clinical signs of herniation and reduce intracranial pressure by 50% in these patients who in fact did not have hyponatremia. Notwithstanding, the percentage rise in $P_{Na}$ from an increase of 5 mmol/L will be appreciably higher in a patient with hyponatremia than in a normonatremic patient. In addition, with the rapid infusion of hypertonic saline, the initial rise in arterial $P_{Na}$ will be appreciably higher than what is detected by simultaneous measurement of $P_{Na}$ in brachial venous blood. Therefore, in patients with hyponatremia and severe symptoms, our goal of therapy is to raise the $P_{Na}$ rapidly by 5 mmol/L with the administration of 3% hypertonic saline (within 60 minutes), with at least 50% of the required volume of 3% hypertonic saline administered in the first 30 minutes. The dose of 3% hypertonic saline required for this is discussed in the following. In patients with severe symptoms whose symptoms persist despite raising the $P_{Na}$ by 5 mmol/L, if hyponatremia is definitely known to be acute, we would raise the $P_{Na}$ rapidly by another 5 mmol/L by administering 3% hypertonic saline. If the symptoms subside after the initial rise in $P_{Na}$ by 5 mmol/L, and if the hyponatremia is definitely known to be acute, we continue the infusion of 3% hypertonic saline to bring the $P_{Na}$ close to ~135 mmol/L over a few hours. We monitor the arterial $P_{Na}$ because it is the $P_{Na}$ to which the brain is exposed, especially if there is a suspicion that a large volume of water may have been ingested and retained in the lumen of the gastrointestinal tract.

In a patient with hyponatremia and moderately severe symptoms (e.g., nausea, confusion) who has a clear history of acute hyponatremia, our goal of therapy is the same as outlined earlier. In a patient with

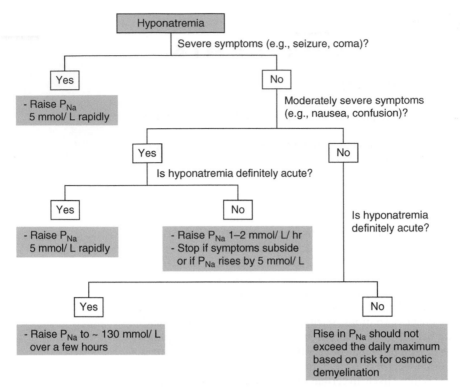

**Flow Chart 10-1  Initial Steps in the Clinical Approach to the Patient With Hyponatremia.** The initial steps in the clinical approach to the patient with hyponatremia focus on dealing with dangers and preventing threats that may arise during therapy. Acute hyponatremia (<48 hours) may be associated with swelling of brain cells and increased intracranial pressure and the danger of brain herniation, In contrast, in a patient with chronic hyponatremia (>48 hours), the danger is a rapid rise in $P_{Na}$, which may lead to the development osmotic demyelination syndrome (ODS). The duration of hyponatremia is not known in many patients. If the patient has severe symptoms (e.g., seizures, coma), we would treat as an emergency and aim to induce a rapid rise in $P_{Na}$. In our view, the risk of severe neurological damage and possibly death is a more important consideration than the risk of osmotic demyelination in this setting.

hyponatremia and moderately severe symptoms in whom it is not clear whether the symptoms are caused by an acute component of hyponatremia or by conditions other than hyponatremia, our goal of therapy is to raise the $P_{Na}$ by 1 to 2 mmol/L/hr until the symptoms disappear, but not to exceed a rise in $P_{Na}$ of 5 mmol/L. This is because a rise in $P_{Na}$ of 5 mmol/L is sufficient to relieve the symptoms if they were caused by increased intracranial pressure; meanwhile, by limiting the rise in $P_{Na}$ to 5 mmol/L, the risk of causing osmotic demyelination is likely to be minimal.

If a patient clearly has acute hyponatremia and the $P_{Na}$ is <130 mmol/L (this cutoff is an arbitrary one), without severe or moderately severe symptoms, our recommendation is to treat this patient with 3% hypertonic saline to raise the $P_{Na}$ to close to 130 mmol/L over a few hours. Our rationale is that it is unlikely that adaptive changes in the brain have proceeded sufficiently and hence, there is little risk of osmotic demyelination with a rise in $P_{Na}$, whereas the patient may be in danger because of a further drop in $P_{Na}$ for the following reasons:

**1.** The $P_{Na}$ in capillaries of the brain (reflected by the arterial $P_{Na}$) may be much lower than $P_{Na}$ drawn from a brachial vein, which is what is usually measured in clinical practice. Therefore, even mild symptoms (e.g., nausea, mild headache) may be manifestations of an increased intracranial pressure, which is not suspected from the level of $P_{Na}$ measured in venous blood.

2. There may be a recent, large intake of water that is retained in the stomach and may be absorbed in a short period of time and cause an appreciable additional fall in the arterial $P_{Na}$.

3. If the patient has a small muscle mass, a smaller subsequent gain of water can create a larger fall in the arterial $P_{Na}$ and thereby a greater degree of brain cell swelling, which may result in a large rise in the intracranial pressure.

4. If a patient has a space-occupying lesion inside the skull (e.g., because of a tumor, infection [meningitis, encephalitis], a subarachnoid hemorrhage, or edema following recent neurosurgery), even a very small degree of brain cell swelling can lead to a dangerous rise in the intracranial pressure.

5. If a patient has an underlying seizure disorder, even a small degree of an acute fall in the $P_{Na}$ may provoke a seizure.

### Caution

In the initial phase during the use of hypotonic lavage solutions, an acute and large fall in the $P_{Na}$ may not be associated with a significant degree of brain cell swelling if the solute involved remains largely in the ECF. This is suggested by the absence of a significant fall in the $P_{Osm}$. The topic of acute hyponatremia following retention of hypotonic lavage fluid is discussed later in this chapter.

### Calculation of the volume of hypertonic 3% saline

For calculation of the dose of hypertonic 3% saline to be administered, we use the following formula (Eqn 1):

$$\text{Desired rise in } P_{Na} \text{ (mmol/L)} \times \text{total body water (L)} \times 2 \quad (1)$$

The amount of NaCl to be administered is calculated based on the assumption that NaCl will distribute as if it were mixing with total body water (TBW). TBW is estimated from body weight, assuming that TBW is approximately 50% of body weight in kilograms. If one is using a previously obtained body weight, this is likely to be an underestimation of TBW because patients with acute hyponatremia are likely to have a large positive water balance (*see margin note*). The factor 2 in this calculation is because hypertonic 3% saline has 513 mmol of $Na^+$ ions per 1 L of water, hence there is ~0.5 mmol of $Na^+$ ions per mL. Based on this, to raise $P_{Na}$ by 1 mmol/L requires the infusion of 1 mL of 3% saline per kg of body weight.

The $P_{Na}$ should be followed closely because it may fall again if there is an addition of water that was hidden, for example, in the gastrointestinal tract or in skeletal muscle after seizures (see discussion of Case 9-1).

### DIAGNOSTIC ISSUES

Acute hyponatremia is almost always caused by a large positive balance of water. The emphasis in the diagnostic process is to identify the source of the water. Look for a reason why the usual aversion to drink a large volume of water was ignored or bypassed. A low rate of excretion of water must also be present because of a nonosmotic cause for the release of vasopressin (e.g., pain, anxiety, nausea, drugs).

Patients with a smaller muscle mass develop a greater degree of hyponatremia for a given volume of retained water (*see margin note*). Young patients have more brain cells per volume of the cranium; therefore, a larger rise in the intracranial pressure because of brain cell swelling may develop with a smaller fall in $P_{Na}$ than in older patients. Also, patients with a disease causing increased brain volume such as

**POSITIVE WATER BALANCE IN PATIENTS WITH ACUTE HYPONATREMIA**

The volume of water that must be retained to cause acute hyponatremia is large:
- Assuming TBW is 50% of body weight in kg, a 60-kg person has 30 L of TBW.
- If the $P_{Na}$ falls from 140 mmol/L to 120 mmol/L because of a gain of water, TBW has increased by 14%. 14% of 30 L = 4.2 L.

**IMPACT OF BODY SIZE ON THE DEGREE OF HYPONATREMIA**

- Muscles represent the majority of the ICF volume (close to two-thirds).
- Consider two patients: one has well-developed muscle mass (TBW 40 L) and the other has a very low muscle mass (TBW 20 L). If each were to retain 4 L of water, the fall in $P_{Na}$ will be 10% in the former ($P_{Na}$ now 126 mmol/L) but 20% in the latter ($P_{Na}$ now 113 mmol/L).

meningitis, encephalitis, or a brain tumor have less room inside the skull for brain cell swelling, so they are at greater risk of increased intracranial pressure with acute hyponatremia.

## SPECIFIC CAUSES

### CLINICAL SETTINGS IN WHICH ACUTE HYPONATREMIA OCCURS IN THE HOSPITAL

#### Perioperative hyponatremia

This is a common setting for the development of acute and potentially life-threatening hyponatremia. Premenopausal women are said to be at greater risk for the development of brain cell swelling from acute hyponatremia. This is thought to be caused by hormonal factors that lead to less efficient brain adaptation to changes in its cell volume. Although this may be the case, other factors, which include their younger age (more brain cells per volume of the skull) and smaller body size, may perhaps be more important. One should also note that the most common setting for the development of acute hyponatremia in older male patients is the infusion of hypotonic lavage fluid during a transurethral resection of the prostate (TURP). As explained later, the hyponatremia in this setting, at least in its early phase, is not usually associated with an appreciable degree of brain cell swelling.

In the perioperative setting, vasopressin is present for a number of reasons (e.g., underlying illness, anxiety, pain, nausea, and administration of drugs; see Table 10-2). These patients have two obvious sources of water. First, the most common is the intravenous administration of glucose in water (such as 5% dextrose in water, which is virtually always a mistake; *see margin note*) or hypotonic saline (virtually always a mistake as well in the perioperative period). Second, ice chips or sips of water may be a source of an unrecognized large water load. Another source of water that may not be obvious is when isotonic saline is administered but hypertonic urine is excreted. This leads to the retention of electrolyte-free water. We call this process desalination of a saline solution (Fig. 10-3). Several liters of isotonic saline are usually administered in the perioperative period of even simple surgical procedures to maintain blood pressure and ensure a good urine output. If the NaCl is excreted (because of the expanded EABV) in a hypertonic urine (as a result of presence of actions of vasopressin), electrolyte-free water is retained in the body. Patients with small body

### D$_5$W

- Each mmol of glucose (molecular mass of glucose is 180 g) binds 1 mmol of water (molecular mass of water is 18). Therefore, the molecular mass of dextrose is 198 g.
- A liter of D$_5$W contains close to 45 g or 250 mmol of glucose. Therefore, it has a lower osmolality than in body fluids, but there is a gain of 1 L of electrolyte-free water after all the glucose is metabolized (converted to glycogen or oxidized to $CO_2$ and water).

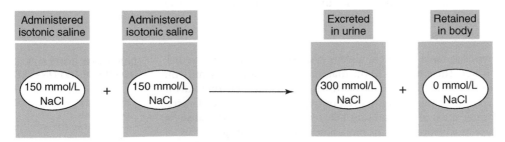

**Figure 10-3 Desalination: Making Saline Into Water.** The *two rectangles* to the *left* represent two 1-L volumes of infused isotonic saline. The concentration of Na$^+$ ions in each liter is 150 mmol/L. The fate of the infused isotonic saline is divided into two new solutions as shown to the *right*. Because of the actions of vasopressin, all of the NaCl that was infused (300 mmol) is excreted in 1 L of urine. Therefore, 1 L of electrolyte-free water is retained in the body.

size are particularly likely to develop a more serious degree of acute hyponatremia.

### Prevention of acute hyponatremia in the perioperative setting

There are cautions with regard to both the input and the output. The message concerning the input is this: Do not give water to a patient who has a defect in water excretion. The message concerning the output is this: A large urine output is a danger sign for development of acute hyponatremia if that urine is hypertonic.

In circumstance in which there is a large infusion of isotonic saline (e.g., patients with a subarachnoid hemorrhage) as well as the excretion of urine with a high concentration of $Na^+$ ions, one must prevent a fall in the $P_{Na}$ by maintaining a tonicity balance. That is, the volume of intravenous fluid infused should be equal to the urine volume, and the concentration of $Na^+ + K^+$ ions in the intravenous solutions should be equal to the concentration of $Na^+ + K^+$ ions in the urine (Fig. 10-4). One may achieve this goal by administering a loop diuretic (e.g., furosemide) which lowers the sum of the concentrations of $Na^+$ and $K^+$ ions in the urine to close to 150 mmol/L, and infusing isotonic saline at the same rate as the urine output.

### Hyponatremia caused by retained hypotonic lavage fluid

This type of acute hyponatremia occurs primarily in older men undergoing a transuretheral resection of the prostate (TURP). When a TURP is performed, the large venous plexus of the prostate is likely to be cut. Electrocoagulation is used to minimize blood loss. A large volume of lavage fluid is usually washed over the site of bleeding to permit better visualization. To make this safe, the lavage fluid must be electrolyte free (to avoid sparks when cautery is used to stop the bleeding), and therefore solutions that contain uncharged organic solutes are used. The lavage fluid may enter the venous blood because of the higher pressure in the urinary bladder. Glycine is a preferred solute for these lavage solutions because its solution is clear (nontranslucent). The molecular weight of glycine is 75 g. The solution commonly used is 1.5%, which contains 15 g or 200 mmol of glycine/L.

To understand the quantitative aspects of hyponatremia that may develop in this setting and its impact on brain cell volume, consider this example in which either 3 L of water or 3 L of 1.5% glycine are administered and retained in a person who has 30 L of TBW, an ECF volume of 10 L, an ICF volume of 20 L, and an initial $P_{Na}$ of 140 mmol/L (Table 10-3). For simplicity, we considered the effective $P_{Osm}$ to be equal to $2 \times P_{Na}$.

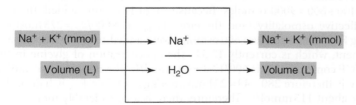

**Figure 10-4 Maintaining a Tonicity Balance.** To prevent a fall in the $P_{Na}$, a tonicity balance must be achieved. That is, the volume of water infused should be equal to the urine volume, and the concentration of $Na^+ + K^+$ ions in the intravenous solutions should be equal to the concentration of $Na^+ + K^+$ ions in the urine.

TABLE 10-3 **EFFECT OF ADDITION OF 3 L OF WATER OR 3 L OF 1.5% GLYCINE SOLUTION**

|  | WATER | GLYCINE 1.5% (200 mmol/L) |
|---|---|---|
| Added volume L | 3 | 3 |
| New ECF volume L | 11 | 12.3 |
| New ICF volume L | 22 | 20.7 |
| Initial total body osmoles | 8400 | 8400 |
| Added osmoles | 0 | 600 |
| New total body osmoles | 8400 | 9000 |
| New body osmolality mosmol/kg $H_2O$ | 254 | 273 |
| Added glycine osmoles to each liter of ECF volume | 0 | 49 |
| New $P_{Na}$ mmol/L | 127 | 115 |

In this example, either 3 L of water or 3 L of 1.5% glycine is administered and retained in a person who has 30 L of total body water, an extracellular fluid (ECF) volume of 10 L, an intracellular fluid (ICF) volume of 20 L, an initial $P_{Na}$ of 140 mmol/L, and an initial $P_{Osm}$ of 280 mosmol/kg $H_2O$. There is a considerably more severe degree of hyponatremia when the glycine solution is absorbed than when pure water is absorbed, but there is only a modest increase in ICF volume when glycine solution is added (0.7 L) as compared to the increase in ICF volume when water is added (2 L).

*Addition of 3 L of $H_2O$:* The 3 L of $H_2O$ will be distributed in the ECF and the ICF compartments in proportion to their initial volumes. Hence, the new ECF volume will be 11 L and the new ICF volume will be 22 L. Therefore, there is a 10% increase in ICF volume. Because the effective osmolality in the ECF compartment and the effective osmolality in the ICF compartment are equal, the initial total number of effective osmoles is $280 \times 30$ L = 8400. Because TBW now is 33 L, the new effective osmolality (and therefore $P_{Osm}$) is 254 mosmol/kg $H_2O$ and the new $P_{Na}$ is 127 mmol/L.

*Addition of 3 L of 1.5% glycine solution:* Because glycine does not cross cell membranes at an appreciable rate in the early time periods, it remains in the ECF compartment. Therefore, we should divide these 3 L of fluid into two parts: an iso-osmolal solution, which remains in the ECF compartment, and an osmole-free water, which will distribute between the ECF and the ICF compartments in proportion to their original volume. Because the 1.5% glycine solution has an osmolality of 200 mosmol/kg $H_2O$ (about two-thirds of body fluid osmolality), about two-thirds of each liter of fluid or 650 mL will be retained in the ECF compartment. The remaining 350 mL of each liter of fluid will be distributed between the ECF (one-third of or 115 mL) and the ICF (two-thirds of it or 235 mL). Because 3 L were absorbed, the increment in ICF volume will be ~700 mL ($3 \times 235$), and the remainder (2300 mL) will stay in the ECF compartment. Therefore, the new ECF volume will be 12.3 L and the new ICF volume will be 20.7 L. Hence, the ICF volume will increase by only 3%. Let us now calculate the new $P_{Osm}$ and the new $P_{Na}$. Because 600 osmoles of glycine were added, the new total number of effective osmoles in the body is $8400 + 600 = 9000$ osmoles. Because 3 L of $H_2O$ were added, the new effective osmolality (and therefore $P_{Osm}$) is $9000/33 = 273$ mosmol/kg $H_2O$. Because these 600 osmoles were added to the ECF compartment, which is currently 12.3 L, the concentration of glycine in the ECF compartment is $600/12.3 = 49$ mmol/L. The nonglycine osmolality is therefore $280 - 49 = 231$ mosmol/kg $H_2O$. The $P_{Na}$ is half of this or about 115 mmol/L. Therefore, there is a considerably more severe degree of hyponatremia when the glycine solution is absorbed than when pure water is absorbed, but there is only a modest increase in ICF volume (0.7 L) compared to the much greater rise when water is absorbed (2 L). This means absorption of the glycine-containing fluid is not associated with an appreciable degree of brain cell swelling, and it does not pose a threat of brain herniation.

These organic solutes are unmeasured osmoles in plasma; thus, the measured $P_{Osm}$ exceeds the calculated $P_{Osm}$ ($2 \times P_{Na} + P_{Urea} + P_{Glucose}$, all in mmol/L).

Glycine enters cells over several hours, and with its subsequent metabolism, all of the water that is administered with the glycine now becomes free water, and therefore hyponatremia is now associated with an increased risk of swelling of brain cells. A clinical clue that this may be the case is a fall in both the $P_{Osm}$ and the plasma osmolal gap while there is a rise in $P_{Na}$.

Metabolites of glycine (e.g., ammonium [$NH_4^+$] ions) may accumulate and cause neurotoxicity. Therefore, the clinical picture is complicated because development of neurological symptoms may be caused by increased intracranial pressure or neurotoxicity related to glycine metabolites.

Patients who develop hyponatremia and neurological symptoms post TURP should have their $P_{Osm}$ measured. For those patients in whom the $P_{Osm}$ is decreased, treatment with hypertonic saline is recommended because they are likely to have increased intracranial pressure. Because hyponatremia developed over a very short period of time, there is no concern if a rapid rise in $P_{Na}$ occurs because of the administration of hypertonic saline. For patients in whom $P_{Osm}$ is normal or near normal, urgent hemodialysis is suggested because it will rapidly correct the hyponatremia and also remove glycine and its toxic metabolites.

## CLINICAL SETTINGS IN WHICH ACUTE HYPONATREMIA OCCURS OUTSIDE THE HOSPITAL

If acute hyponatremia occurs outside the hospital, look for a reason why the normal aversion to drinking a large volume of water in the face of hyponatremia has been ignored. Examples include patients who have taken a mood-altering drug (e.g., 3,4-methylenedioxymethamphetamine [MDMA (ecstasy)]), patients who have a severe psychiatric disorder (e.g., schizophrenia), and patients who have followed advice to drink a very large volume of water to avoid dehydration (e.g., during a marathon race). It is also important to look for a reason why vasopressin may have been released despite the absence of the usual stimulus of its release, which is a high $P_{Na}$. The ingestion of a drug (e.g., MDMA) may cause the release of vasopressin despite the presence of hyponatremia (see Table 10-2). Alternatively, a low distal delivery of filtrate may diminish the ability to excrete a large volume of water. Hence, subjects who have a deficit of $Na^+$ ions and drink a large volume of water may develop a life-threatening degree of acute hyponatremia even in the absence of vasopressin actions.

In all of the aforementioned settings, there is an additional danger if the water load is ingested over a short time period and absorbed from the intestinal tract with little delay. In more detail, a larger degree of brain swelling may develop because there is a larger decline in the arterial $P_{Na}$ (which is the $P_{Na}$ to which the brain is exposed). This may not be revealed by measuring the brachial venous $P_{Na}$ because muscle cells take up a larger proportion of water as a result of their relatively larger mass per blood flow rate (see Chapter 9, Fig. 9-19) and hence venous $P_{Na}$ may be considerably higher than the arterial $P_{Na}$.

### Hyponatremia caused by the intake of MDMA

The most important reason for the development of acute hyponatremia in this setting is a positive balance of water. Notwithstanding, many of these patients may also have a modest deficit of $Na^+$ ions.

#### Positive balance for water

For this to occur there must be an intake of water that is larger than its output.

##### Large water intake

Drugs such as MDMA are often consumed at prolonged dance parties called raves. People attending such a party are usually advised to drink a large volume of water to prevent dehydration from excessive sweating and the development of rhabdomyolysis, which has been reported predominantly in men. Moreover, the relaxed feeling from the drug might permit them to overcome the aversion to drinking water in the presence of acute hyponatremia. It is possible that water may be stored in the lumen of the stomach and small intestine because of reduced gastrointestinal motility, so this occult water is not recognized by the hypothalamic osmostat and thus the thirst center. This overzealous consumption of water, however, creates a serious problem, the development of life-threatening acute hyponatremia, especially in people with a small muscle mass (usually females).

##### Low output of water

There are two reasons why the excretion of water may be decreased in this setting. First, MDMA may cause the release of vasopressin. Second, there may be a low delivery of filtrate to the distal nephron, which further decreases the rate of excretion of water. Decreased EABV may result from loss of NaCl in sweat. Furthermore, it is also possible that the drug may decrease the constrictor tone in venous capacitance vessels, and this could also cause a decrease in the EABV.

#### Negative balance for NaCl

At a rave party, subjects may have a loss of NaCl if they produce a large volume of sweat. The concentration of $Na^+$ ions in sweat in a normal adult human is ~25 mmol/L. Because this loss is hypotonic, the development of hyponatremia requires that the volume of water intake must be larger than the volume of sweat.

There is another possible way to lose $Na^+$ ions from the ECF compartment in this setting: $Na^+$ ions diffuse between the cells of the small intestine (this area is permeable to $Na^+$ ions) into its lumen, which contains a large volume of water because a large volume of water was ingested and is trapped there because of slow gastrointestinal motility.

### Hyponatremia caused by diarrhea in infants and children

Vasopressin is released in this setting in response to both the low EABV (i.e., the loss of near-isotonic solutions containing $Na^+$ ions during diarrhea) and the presence of nonosmotic stimuli caused by the acute illness. There is also decreased distal delivery of filtrate because of low EABV. This leads to the retention of ingested water. The ingestion of copious amounts of free water is common in this setting because these patients are often given water with sugar to rest their gastrointestinal tract and to prevent dehydration (*see margin note*).

### Exercise-induced hyponatremia (hyponatremia in a marathon runner)

Marathon runners are often advised to drink water avidly to replace sweat loss, which could be as large as 2 L/hr. A positive balance of water (reflected by weight gain; *see margin note*) is the most important factor leading to the development of acute hyponatremia in this setting. In addition, there is a deficit of $Na^+$ ions because of the large volume of sweat, which contains a concentration of $Na^+$ ions in a normal adult human of ~25 mmol/L.

The following factors may contribute to the development of a severe degree of hyponatremia in a marathon runner:

- The longer duration of the race, because there is more time to drink extra water. Hence, subjects who run more slowly may be at an increased risk.
- Participants with a smaller muscle mass (e.g., females) may have a greater risk.
- Women may be at a greater risk because they are said to be more likely than men to follow the advice to have a large intake of water.
- Participants who, near the end of the race, may gulp a large volume of water because they believe they are dehydrated. The reason this is dangerous is that rapid absorption of a large volume of water causes a large decline in the arterial $P_{Na}$ to which the brain is exposed, and hence it leads to a greater degree of acute swelling of brain cells.
- If water was retained in the stomach and/or the intestinal tract, this water may be absorbed later, causing a further fall in the arterial $P_{Na}$.
- If a participant is given a rapid infusion of isotonic saline because of suspected contraction of the ECF volume or to treat hyperthermia, this bolus of saline may alter Starling forces across capillary walls, including those in the blood–brain barrier. As a result, the volume of the interstitial compartment of the brain may increase. Recall that any further gain of volume inside the cranium may raise the intracranial pressure to a dangerous level once brain cells are swollen by an appreciable degree. Therefore, hypertonic saline rather than isotonic saline should be given if needed to expand the EABV, if the patient has even mild neurological symptoms.

**DEHYDRATION**

- The authors avoid using this term because it is ambiguous. To some, it means a lack of water, but to others, it means a decreased ECF volume.
- In a patient with acute hyponatremia, the ICF compartment is overhydrated rather than dehydrated. Therefore, using this term does not indicate the actual danger to the patient in this setting.

**WEIGHT GAIN IN MARATHON RUNNERS AND RISK OF HYPONATREMIA**

- Weight gain may underestimate the actual water gain in these subjects for the following reasons:
  - Fuels, including glycogen in muscle, are oxidized, and this could account for a weight loss of close to 0.5 kg.
  - Each gram of glycogen is stored with 2 to 3 g of bound water. Therefore, the addition of this water is not reflected as a gain of weight.

---

## QUESTIONS

**10-1**    *Calculation of electrolyte-free water is commonly used to determine the basis of a change in $P_{Na}$. We prefer to use the calculation of a tonicity balance for this purpose. How may these two calculations differ?*

**10-2**    *Does hypertonic saline reduce the intracranial pressure simply because it draws water out of brain cells?*

# PART C
# CHRONIC HYPONATREMIA

## OVERVIEW

Chronic hyponatremia ($P_{Na}$ <135 mmol/L; duration >48 hours) is the most common electrolyte abnormality in hospitalized patients. Hyponatremia is commonly recognized for the first time after routine measurement of electrolytes in plasma. Patients with chronic hyponatremia and no apparent symptoms may have subtle clinical abnormalities including gait disturbances and deficits of concentration and cognition, and may be at increased risk of falls. Patients with chronic hyponatremia are more likely than normonatremic patients to have osteoporosis and bone fractures. Hyponatremia has been associated with increased mortality, morbidity, and length of hospital stay in hospitalized patients with a variety of disorders. Whether this association reflects the severity of the underlying illness (e.g., heart failure, liver failure), a direct effect of hyponatremia, or a combination of these factors remains unclear.

### POINTS TO EMPHASIZE

1. Hyponatremia is a diagnostic category rather than a specific disease entity. Hyponatremia may be the first manifestation of a serious underlying disease such as adrenal insufficiency or small cell carcinoma of the lung. Hence, a cause of hyponatremia must always be sought.
2. In every patient with chronic hyponatremia, the central pathophysiology is an inability to excrete electrolyte-free water appropriately. In some patients, this is caused by the presence of vasopressin. In others, the major defect is a low rate of delivery of filtrate to the distal nephron.
3. A water diuresis may ensue if actions of vasopressin disappear (Table 10-4) and/or if the distal delivery of filtrate is increased. Examples include re-expansion of a low EABV (i.e., infusion of saline in a patient with a deficit of $Na^+$ ions). Osmotic demyelination may develop unless this water diuresis is reduced sufficiently to prevent a rapid rise in the $P_{Na}$.
4. Patients with chronic hyponatremia may also have an element of acute hyponatremia. In a patient with chronic hyponatremia who may also have a component of acute hyponatremia, the $P_{Na}$ must be raised quickly to lower intracranial pressure, but the rise in $P_{Na}$ should not exceed what is considered a safe maximum limit for a 24-hour period to avoid causing osmotic demyelination.

TABLE 10-4  **SETTINGS WHERE ACTIONS OF VASOPRESSIN MAY DISAPPEAR**

- Re-expansion of a contracted EABV
- Administration of corticosteriods to a patient with a deficiency of cortisol
- Disappearance of a nonosmotic stimulus for the release of vasopressin (e.g., decrease in anxiety, nausea, phobia, or discontinuation of certain drugs)
- Stopping the administration of dDAVP (e.g., children with enuresis, the elderly with urinary incontinence, patients with central diabetes insipidus)

*EABV*, Effective arterial blood volume.

5. Osmotic demyelination is the major danger in patients with chronic hyponatremia, which, when severe, can lead to quadriplegia, coma, and/or death. Its major risk factor is a rapid and large rise in the $P_{Na}$. This is usually the result of water diuresis, which occurs if the distal delivery of filtrate is increased or the actions of vasopressin disappear. Patients who are at high risk for the development of osmotic demyelination include patients with $P_{Na}$ <105 mmol/L, who are malnourished, who are $K^+$ ion depleted, with chronic alcoholism, and with advanced liver cirrhosis. In most patients, the rate of rise in $P_{Na}$ should not exceed 8 mmol/L/day, but in patients who are considered to be at high risk for the development of osmotic demyelination, we aim to limit the rate of rise of $P_{Na}$ to 4 mmol/L/day and consider a rate of rise of 6 mmol/L/day a maximum that should not be exceeded. These limits for the rise in $P_{Na}$ should be viewed as maximums not to be exceeded rather than targets to achieve. If a water diuresis occurs, the $P_{Na}$ should be measured promptly and followed frequently; if there is a risk that the rate of rise in the $P_{Na}$ may exceed what is considered maximum, further water loss should be halted. To achieve this, we suggest the administration of 2 to 4 μg of dDAVP via the intravenous route.

6. If overcorrection occurs, relowering of the $P_{Na}$ is recommended. This recommendation is based largely on data from experimental studies in animals with chronic hyponatremia, which showed that reinduction of hyponatremia after rapid overcorrection substantially reduced the incidence of osmotic demyelination and mortality. Relowering of $P_{Na}$ can be achieved by the intravenous administration of $D_5W$. Ongoing water diuresis must be stopped with the administration of dDAVP. For patients who are at low risk of osmotic demyelination, we would relower the $P_{Na}$ if the rate exceeds 10 mmol/L/day. For patients who are at high risk of osmotic demyelination, we would relower the $P_{Na}$ if the rate of rise exceeds 6 mmol/L/day. Because most reported cases of osmotic demyelination occurred in patients with $P_{Na}$ <120 mmol/L, in patients with chronic hyponatremia who have a $P_{Na}$ of >120 mmol/L and no risk factors for osmotic demyelination, we do not think it is necessary to relower $P_{Na}$ if the rise exceeds the maximum limit.

## CLINICAL APPROACH

### IDENTIFY EMERGENCIES ON ADMISSION

There are no dangers on admission that are specifically related to chronic hyponatremia. Nevertheless, there could be dangers if there are symptoms suggestive of a component of acute hyponatremia causing brain cell swelling or if there is a hemodynamic emergency when there is a large deficit of NaCl.

### ANTICIPATE RISKS DURING THERAPY

Osmotic demyelination may develop if there is a large and rapid rate of rise in $P_{Na}$. This is most commonly the result of a water diuresis. Water diuresis ensues if the actions of vasopressin disappear and/or if distal delivery of filtrate increases. The clinician must determine why vasopressin is being released to anticipate conditions in which its release may disappear (see Table 10-4). If a disappearance of actions of vasopressin and/or an increase in rate of distal delivery of filtrate is anticipated, particularly in a patient who is considered to be at high risk for the development of osmotic demyelination, prophylactic use of dDAVP to prevent a water diuresis may be considered. It is important to appreciate that a relatively small volume of water diuresis may result in a large rise in $P_{Na}$ in a patient with a small muscle mass. Strict water restriction must be imposed if dDAVP is administered.

## Determine Why the Excretion of Water Is Too Low

After pseudohyponatremia and hyponatremia caused by hyperglycemia are excluded, the next step is to determine why there is a reduced capability to excrete water (Flow Chart 10-2). The issues to resolve are to determine why vasopressin actions may be present or if the main reason for the diminished capacity to excrete water is a diminished distal delivery of filtrate and enhanced water reabsorption in the inner MCD via residual water permeability (see Table 10-2). As shown in the flow chart, the diagnosis of the syndrome of inappropriate secretion of antidiuretic hormone (SIADH) is one of exclusion.

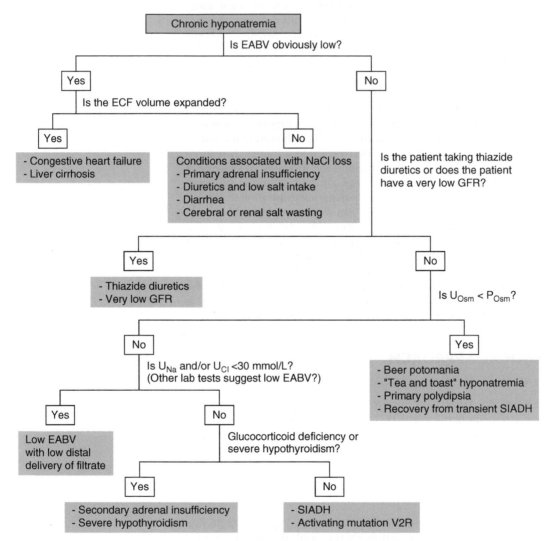

**Flow Chart 10-2  Diagnostic Approach to the Patient With Chronic Hyponatremia.** The issues to resolve are to determine why vasopressin actions may be present or if the main reason for the diminished capacity to excrete water is a diminished distal delivery of filtrate and enhanced water reabsorption in the inner medullary collecting duct via residual water permeability. In patients with a marked degree of decreased effective arterial blood volume (EABV), decreased renal excretion of water may be caused by a baroreceptor-mediated release of vasopressin. Syndrome of inappropriate antidiuretic hormone (SIADH) is a diagnosis of exclusion. Detecting a mild degree of decrease in EABV, which is sufficient to decrease distal delivery of filtrate, may be difficult by clinical assessment. At times, EABV expansion with infusion of saline may be required to rule out low distal delivery of filtrate as the cause of hyponatremia. Absence of water diuresis in response to expansion of the EABV with the administration of saline confirms the diagnosis of SIADH. *ECF*, extracellular fluid; *GFR*, glomerular filtration rate.

## PSEUDOHYPONATREMIA

Pseudohyponatremia is present when the $P_{Na}$ measured by the laboratory is lower than the actual ratio of $Na^+$ ions to plasma water in the patient. This occurs when the method used requires dilution of the plasma sample. This is because 7% of the plasma volume is a nonaqueous volume (i.e., lipids and proteins). When adjusting for the volume of the diluent, this nonaqueous plasma volume is not taken into consideration; therefore, the volume of plasma water is overestimated by 7% and the concentration of $Na^+$ ions in plasma water is underestimated by 7% (i.e., although the concentration of $Na^+$ ions in plasma water is 150 mmol/L, $P_{Na}$ measured by flame photometry is 140 mmol/L). If the nonaqueous volume of plasma increases by 14% because of hypertriglyceridemia or hyperproteinemia, adjusting for the volume of diluent, the volume of plasma water is overestimated by 14% and the concentration of $Na^+$ ions in plasma water is underestimated by 14% (i.e., although the concentration of $Na^+$ ions in plasma water is 150 mmol/L, $P_{Na}$ measured by flame photometry is 129 mmol/L). With the use of an ion-selective electrode, the activity of $Na^+$ ions in the aqueous plasma volume is measured; nevertheless, because of the use of automatic aspirators and dilutors to prepare the plasma samples, the $P_{Na}$ in plasma with a large nonaqueous volume will still be incorrectly reported as low. This error in measurement of $P_{Na}$ is detected by the finding of a normal $P_{Osm}$ value (in the absence of high concentration of other osmoles, e.g., urea, glucose, alcohol). Another way to detect pseudohyponatremia is to perform the analysis with an ion-selective electrode in an undiluted blood sample, for example, using a blood gas analyzer.

## HYPONATREMIA CAUSED BY HYPERGLYCEMIA

In conditions with relative lack of insulin actions, glucose is an effective osmole for skeletal muscle because skeletal muscle cells require insulin for the transport of glucose. Therefore, if hyperglycemia is associated with a rise in the plasma effective osmolality, water will shift out of skeletal muscle cells. This, however, occurs only when the addition of glucose to the body is as a hyperosmolar solution. When glucose is added as part of an iso- or a hypo-osmolar solution, water does not exit cells. Because patients with hyperglycemia have variable fluid intake and also variable loss of water and of $Na^+$ ions in the urine because of the glucose-induced osmotic diuresis and natriuresis, one cannot assume a fixed relationship between the rise in $P_{Glucose}$ and the fall in $P_{Na}$. This relationship is derived from theoretical calculations that were based on the addition of glucose without water, and different correction factors were proposed based on assumptions made about the ECF volume and the volume of distribution of glucose in the absence of insulin actions (see Chapter 16).

## CLASSIFICATION

The traditional approach to the pathophysiology of chronic hyponatremia focuses on a reduced electrolyte-free water excretion caused by the actions of vasopressin. In some clinical settings, release of vasopressin is thought to be caused by decreased EABV. Notwithstanding, at least in some patients, the degree of decreased EABV does not seem to be large enough to cause the release of vasopressin. We suggest that hyponatremia caused by impaired urinary excretion of electrolyte-free water may develop in some patients in the absence of vasopressin action. Two important factors are relevant in this regard: diminished volume of filtrate that is delivered to the distal nephron and enhanced water reabsorption in the inner MCD through its residual water permeability.

The volume of distal delivery of filtrate is reduced if the GFR is decreased and/or if the fractional reabsorption of NaCl in the PCT is increased. The fractional reabsorption of NaCl in the PCT is increased in response to a decreased EABV. This can be caused by a total body deficit of NaCl (e.g., diuretic use in a patient who consumes little salt, NaCl loss in diarrhea fluid or in sweat) or a disorder that causes a low cardiac output. Because there is an obligatory loss of $Na^+$ ions in each liter of urine during a water diuresis (albeit a small amount), a deficit of $Na^+$ ions can develop during the polyuria induced by a large intake of water in a subject who consumes little NaCl (e.g., a patient with beer potomania).

The driving force for water reabsorption via residual water permeability is the osmotic pressure gradient generated by the difference in osmolality between the luminal fluid in the inner MCD and that in the medullary interstitial compartment. As discussed previously, we estimate that somewhat more than 5 L of water is reabsorbed per day in the inner MCD via residual water permeability during water diuresis.

In some patients, hyponatremia is caused by reduced electrolyte-free water excretion because of the actions of vasopressin, but the release of vasopressin is not caused by a decreased EABV. This category is called the syndrome of the inappropriate secretion of antidiuretic hormone (SIADH). SIADH, however, is a diagnosis of exclusion, which cannot be made if the patient has a low volume of distal delivery of filtrate. The importance of differentiating between patients whose impaired free water excretion is caused by vasopressin actions and those in whom it is caused by diminished volume of distal delivery of filtrate is that the risks associated with therapy are different between both groups (see Table 9-2).

The common clinical approach to patients with hyponatremia is based on assessment of the ECF volume. Patients with hyponatremia are classified into those with hypovolemia, normovolemia, or hypervolemia. Nevertheless, detecting a mild degree of decrease in EABV, which is sufficient to decrease the volume of distal delivery of filtrate and diminish the rate of excretion of electrolyte-free water, may be difficult by clinical assessment. In addition, the pathophysiology of hyponatremia in patients with hypervolemic hyponatremia (e.g., patients with congestive heart failure or liver failure) is related to decreased EABV.

### Tools to detect a decreased EABV

The following laboratory tests may be helpful to suggest that hyponatremia is caused by a low EABV. At times, however, EABV expansion with infusion of saline may be required to rule out low distal delivery of filtrate as the cause of hyponatremia. Absence of water diuresis in response to volume expansion confirms the diagnosis of SIADH. If this test is to be performed, dDAVP should be available to stop a water diuresis if it occurs and prevent a rapid rise in $P_{Na}$ that may exceed the safe maximum limit.

#### Concentrations of $Na^+$ and $Cl^-$ ions in the urine

The expected renal response when the EABV is contracted is the excretion of urine with a very low concentration of $Na^+$ ions ($U_{Na}$) and of $Cl^-$ ions ($U_{Cl}$) (i.e., <15 mmol/L). A $U_{Na}$ >30 mmol/L is thought to be in keeping with euvolemia and the diagnostic category of SIADH. If the cause of the low EABV is the use of diuretics, the excretion of $Na^+$ and $Cl^-$ ions might be intermittently high. Electrolyte measurements in multiple spot urine samples are helpful if the patient denies the intake of diuretics. There are conditions, however, in which the $U_{Na}$ may be high despite the presence of a low EABV because of the presence of an anion in the urine that obligates the excretion of $Na^+$ (e.g., organic anions and/or $HCO_3^-$ anions in a patient with recent vomiting). In other conditions, the $U_{Cl}$ may be high despite the presence of a low EABV if there is a cation in the urine that obligates the excretion of $Cl^-$ (e.g., $NH_4^+$ ions in a patient with metabolic acidosis caused by the loss of $NaHCO_3$ in diarrheal fluid). Patients who have a low intake of NaCl can have low $U_{Na}$ and $U_{Cl}$ without an appreciable degree of EABV contraction. Said in another way, their EABV is not as expanded as in other subjects, rather than actually being contracted. Hence, $U_{Na}$ and $U_{Cl}$ can be low in patients with SIADH who consume a diet that is low in NaCl.

### Concentrations of urea and urate in plasma

Expansion of the EABV diminishes the rate of reabsorption of urea and urate in the PCT and therefore their plasma levels will be decreased. Because the excretion rates of urea and urate are equal to their production rates in steady state, it is therefore useful to examine their fractional excretions because this adjusts their excretion rates to their filtered loads. A low plasma level of urea ($P_{Urea}$ <3.6 mmol/L, blood urea nitrogen [BUN] <21.6 mg/dL), a low plasma level of urate (<0.24 mmol/L [<4 mg/dL]), a high fractional excretion of urea (>55%), and a high fractional excretion of urate (>12%) are more in keeping with the diagnostic category of SIADH because these patients are likely to have an expanded EABV.

### Other laboratory tests

A low concentration of $K^+$ ions in plasma ($P_K$), a rise in the concentration of creatinine in plasma ($P_{Creatinine}$), and a high concentration of $HCO_3^-$ ions in plasma ($P_{HCO_3}$) may suggest that EABV is low.

Because the reabsorption of urea in PCT is strongly influenced by the EABV, the relative rise in the $P_{Urea}$ is usually larger than the relative rise in $P_{Creatinine}$ in patients with a low EABV. Therefore, the ratio of $P_{Urea}/P_{Creatinine}$ is likely to be high (>100; where $P_{Urea}$ and $P_{Creatinine}$ are in mmol/L, and BUN/$P_{Creatinine}$ >20, where BUN and $P_{Creatinine}$ are in mg/dL) in patients with hyponatremia as a result of a deficit of $Na^+$ ions, causing a low distal delivery of filtrate. This, however, may not be the case if protein intake is low.

## SPECIFIC DISORDERS

### DIURETIC-INDUCED HYPONATREMIA

Diuretics, particularly thiazides, are a common cause of hyponatremia. The traditional explanation for the development of hyponatremia in these patients is that renal loss of $Na^+$ ions causes reduced EABV, which stimulates the release of vasopressin. In most patients, however, the degree of decreased EABV does not seem to be large enough to cause the release of vasopressin. Acutely decreasing EABV by 7% in healthy adults has been found to have little effect on plasma vasopressin levels; in fact, a 10% to 15% decline in EABV is required to double the plasma vasopressin level. Furthermore, an even larger degree of decreased EABV is required for this baroreceptor-mediated stimulation of vasopressin release to override the inhibitory signals related to hypotonicity. We suggest that the pathophysiology of hyponatremia that occurs in some patients taking diuretics may instead be related to decreased volume of distal delivery of filtrate and enhanced water reabsorption in the inner MCD via its residual water permeability. The decreased distal delivery of filtrate is a consequence of a low GFR (e.g., a patient with chronic renal dysfunction due to ischemic renal disease) and an increased fractional reabsorption of filtrate in PCT because of reduced

EABV due to a deficit of $Na^+$ ions caused by their loss in the urine in a patient who has a low intake of NaCl. The enhanced water reabsorption in the inner MCD via residual water permeability may be caused by a low rate of excretion of osmoles in patients who have a low intake of salt and protein. In addition, thiazides have been shown to increase water reabsorption in the inner MCD in normal rats and in Brattleboro rats who lack vasopressin. This is coupled with increased water intake, perhaps because of habit, or it may be also that thiazides have a dipsogenic effect. The quantitative aspects of this pathophysiology and the implications for therapy are detailed in the discussion of Case 10-4.

## BEER POTOMANIA

In the early stages of development of beer potomania, the picture is dominated by a large intake of beer, which is a large intake of water, that leads to a very large water diuresis. A deficit of $Na^+$ ions develops over days if the patient has a low intake of NaCl because each liter of urine will still have some $Na^+$ ions, albeit at a small amount. For example, if the urine volume is 10 L/day and the $U_{Na}$ is 10 mmol/L, the excretion of $Na^+$ ions is 100 mmol/day. Hence, a deficit of $Na^+$ ions will develop over days if the daily intake of NaCl is appreciably less than 100 mmol. Chronic hyponatremia is usually seen after the patient develops a negative balance for $Na^+$ ions. In this setting, there are two reasons for the diminished ability to excrete water: a low volume of distal delivery of filtrate and water reabsorption via residual water permeability in the inner MCD. The effect of residual water permeability is even larger in these patients because of the very low osmole excretion rate as a result of the very poor dietary intake of protein and salt. This leads to a lower osmolality of the luminal fluid in the inner MCD and thereby a large osmotic driving force for water reabsorption. The $U_{Osm}$ at this stage is low, generally lower than $P_{Osm}$. At times, however, the $U_{Osm}$ may be higher and even close to 300 mosmol/kg $H_2O$, despite the absence of vasopressin actions, depending on the degree of the decrease in the volume of distal delivery of filtrate, the volume of water that is reabsorbed via residual water permeability in the inner MCD, and the concentration of ethanol in the urine. Vasopressin may be released because of the presence of nonosmotic stimuli for its release (e.g., pain and nausea caused by alcohol-induced gastritis) or a marked degree of decreased EABV (e.g., large $Na^+$ ion deficit, gastrointestinal bleed). There is a danger of acute hyponatremia if the patient continues to drink a large volume of beer (water) while there is a marked decrease in water excretion. Furthermore, if the patient has ingested a large volume of beer recently and some of it is retained in the stomach, there is an acute infusion of electrolyte-free water if this water is absorbed rapidly, causing a fall in the arterial $P_{Na}$ to which the brain is exposed, with the danger of a further increase in the intracranial pressure and the risk of brain herniation.

The clinical picture is complicated by the fact that neurological symptoms in a patient with chronic alcoholism may not be related to an acute component of hyponatremia, but may be caused by some other underlying pathology (e.g., alcohol withdrawal, subdural hematoma). These patients, who are also usually malnourished and hypokalemic, are at a high risk for osmotic demyelination, with rapid correction of hyponatremia. Therefore, we suggest that the rate of rise in $P_{Na}$ should not exceed 4 to 6 mmol/L/day. Nevertheless, if the symptoms are severe (e.g., seizures, coma), the administration of hypertonic saline is recommended because these symptoms may herald permanent brain damage and death. The rise in $P_{Na}$, however, should not exceed 5 mmol/L because this rise in $P_{Na}$ is sufficient to cause an appreciable reduction in the intracranial pressure, so frequent monitoring of $P_{Na}$ is necessary.

## Primary Polydipsia

Primary polydipsia is most often seen in patients with psychiatric illness, particularly those with acute psychosis secondary to schizophrenia. Although a large water intake is a major factor for the development of hyponatremia in these patients, they also have impaired ability to maximally excrete electrolyte-free water. This may be because of diminished distal delivery of filtrate and enhanced water reabsorption via residual water permeability in the inner MCD. The decreased distal delivery of filtrate is caused by enhanced reabsorption of NaCl in the PCT because of a mildly decreased EABV, as a deficit of $Na^+$ ions develops because of the loss of $Na^+$ ions in the large urine volume and the low intake of salt. The increased reabsorption of water in the inner MCD may be because of the low osmolality in the lumen of the inner MCD caused by the low osmole excretion rate (low intake of salt and protein) and the large volume of luminal fluid. In addition, vasopressin may be released during acute psychotic episodes or because of prescribed medications such as phenothiazines, carbamazepine, or serotonin reuptake inhibitors.

## "Tea and Toast" Hyponatremia

This may occur in elderly subjects who have a low GFR (e.g., because of ischemic renal disease) and consume a diet that is poor in salt and protein but have a large intake of water. This pattern of intake of food and fluid has been labeled a "tea and toast" diet. In these patients, distal delivery of filtrate may be quite low because of the low GFR and perhaps an increased reabsorption in the PCT, owing to a modest chronic $Na^+$ ion deficit. In addition, water reabsorption in the inner MCD is increased because of the low rate of excretion of osmoles. If the volume of water intake exceeds the renal capacity for its excretion (volume of distal delivery of filtrate minus the volume of water reabsorbed in the inner MCD), hyponatremia develops. Again, the $U_{Osm}$ is generally lower than $P_{Osm}$, but it is at times may be higher and even close to $300\,mosmol/kg\,H_2O$, despite absence of vasopressin actions, depending on the degree of diminished volume of distal delivery of filtrate and the volume of water that is reabsorbed via residual water permeability in the inner MCD (see discussion of Case 10-4).

Another example of this pathophysiology may be seen in subjects who exercise vigorously and reduce their dietary intake markedly to lose weight but maintain a large intake of water to avoid dehydration. Because of a loss of NaCl in sweat and the low intake of NaCl, they develop a deficit of NaCl. The deficit of NaCl, and hence the degree of reduction in the volume of the distal delivery of filtrate, are likely, however, to be modest if these subjects continue to exercise vigorously. To develop hyponatremia, in addition to a large water intake, they will need to reabsorb a large volume of water in the inner MCD via residual water permeability. Perhaps there is a larger osmotic driving force for water reabsorption in the inner MCD because of a high medullary interstitial osmolality in these generally young and healthy individuals. It is also possible that a larger proportion of potential urine may undergo retrograde flux back into the inner MCD because of renal pelvic contraction, with more opportunity to reabsorb water in this nephron segment.

## Primary Adrenal Insufficiency

Primary adrenal insufficiency is most commonly caused by an autoimmune disease. It can also be seen in patients with the human immunodeficiency virus (HIV) as a result of cytomegalovirus infection. Although uncommon nowadays, primary adrenal insufficiency may be caused by tuberculosis.

Patients with this disorder have mineralocorticoid deficiency leading to renal salt wasting and decreased EABV. Hyponatremia is the result of loss of $Na^+$ ions and diminished renal excretion of water caused by decreased volume of distal delivery of filtrate and/or baroreceptor-mediated release of vasopressin. In addition, lack of cortisol may cause the release of corticotropin-releasing hormone (CRH) and of vasopressin from the paraventricular nuclei of the hypothalamus (see later).

Hyponatremia, a low EABV with an inappropriately high concentration of $Na^+$ and $Cl^-$ ions in the urine and the presence of hyperkalemia, should raise suspicion of primary adrenal insufficiency. Notwithstanding, about one-third of the patients do not have hyperkalemia on presentation.

## CEREBRAL SALT WASTING

There are two components to this syndrome: a cerebral lesion (e.g., subarachnoid hemorrhage, head injury, neurosurgical procedure) and renal salt wasting resulting in low EABV. When hyponatremia develops, the explanation is that it is because of water retention caused by vasopressin release in response to decreased EABV. Nevertheless, while the presence of a cerebral lesion is obvious, in many cases where this condition is suspected, the presence of salt wasting and low EABV are not.

The assumption of salt wasting is usually based on the finding of a high rate of excretion of $Na^+$ ions in the urine at the time when hyponatremia is noted. This, however, may not represent a negative balance for $Na^+$ ions because these patients would have usually received large amounts of NaCl to prevent hypovolemia, which is thought to result in vasospasm of cerebral arteries and hence diminished cerebral perfusion. To document a negative balance of $Na^+$ ions, one must take into account all of the $Na^+$ ions that was administered throughout the patient's course. This includes treatment received in multiple settings, such as the ambulance, the emergency department, in the operating room, and on the ward. In fact, the negative balance for $Na^+$ ions would need to be even larger, because a normal baseline EABV is actually an expanded EABV to provide the signals for the kidney to excrete the daily dietary $Na^+$ ion load. Although a brain-derived natriuretic peptide and/or a digitalis-like compound were found to be present at elevated levels in some patients with the diagnosis of cerebral salt wasting, this was not the case in others. Furthermore, it is not clear that the criteria to establish the presence of a negative salt balance were present in these patients with high levels of these hormones.

For salt wasting to be present, patients must have a high rate of excretion of $Na^+$ ions while their EABV is contracted. Physical examination is not sensitive enough to detect decreased EABV unless it is substantially contracted. Furthermore, even if there is salt wasting the EABV may not be sufficiently decreased to elicit a baroreceptor-mediated release of vasopressin. This is because patients under marked stress may have a high adrenergic tone, which may cause constriction of the venous capacitance vessels and/or increased myocardial contractility; therefore, EABV may be maintained despite a negative balance for $Na^+$ ions.

Hyponatremia in the setting of an acute neurological disease may instead be caused by SIADH and desalination of administered saline. In more detail, vasopressin release may occur in response to a number of nonosmotic stimuli such as pain, nausea, perioperative state, or the administration of various drugs, which may be used in this setting. If the patient has a normal renal concentrating ability, the concentration of $Na^+$ ions in the urine may rise to 300 mmol/L. If the patient was given a large volume of isotonic saline (150 mmol of $Na^+$ ions/L), for every 150 mmol of $Na^+$ ions excreted in the urine, half a liter of electrolyte-free water is generated and retained in the body, leading to hyponatremia. In this setting, the administration of isotonic saline to correct presumed hypovolemia may lead to worsening hyponatremia because the administered NaCl may be excreted in the urine as a hypertonic solution.

Fractional reabsorption of urea and fractional reabsorption of urate are not reliable markers in this setting to distinguish hyponatremia because of baroreceptor-mediated release of vasopressin, and hyponatremia caused by SIADH. This is because the defect in $Na^+$ ion reabsorption in patients with cerebral salt wasting seems to involve the PCT; therefore, these patients have also diminished reabsorption of urea and of urate.

Hyponatremia is of particular danger in these patients who may have a space-occupying lesion inside the skull (e.g., hematoma, edema, or a tumor), because in this setting, a small degree of brain cell swelling can lead to a dangerous rise in intracranial pressure. If there are symptoms to suggest increased intracranial pressure that may be caused by hyponatremia, hypertonic saline should be administered to raise the $P_{Na}$ by 5 mmol/L rapidly.

Because hypovolemia may worsen cerebral injury, and the assumption that hyponatremia in these patients is caused by baroreceptor-mediated release of vasopressin because of hypovolemia, saline is usually administered to correct the hypovolemia. If saline is to be administered, it should be as hypertonic saline. If hyponatremia is chronic, the rise in $P_{Na}$ should not exceed what is considered the safe daily maximum. To avoid a further fall in $P_{Na}$, we use a calculation of a tonicity balance in which the volume and tonicity of the input matches the volume and tonicity of the output (see Fig. 10-4 and Chapter 11).

## SYNDROME OF INAPPROPRIATE ANTIDIURETIC HORMONE

SIADH is a diagnosis of exclusion. One must first exclude patients who may have a low volume of distal delivery of filtrate because of a low EABV, patients with "tea and toast" hyponatremia, patients with very low GFR, patients with cortisol deficiency, and those with severe hypothyroidism. In patients with SIADH, the $U_{Osm}$ exceeds the $P_{Osm}$, and the concentration of $Na^+$ ions in the urine should be appreciable (e.g., usually >30 mmol/L). In addition, these patients generally have low $P_{Urea}$ and low $P_{Urate}$ with high fractional excretion of urea and urate. The next step is to establish why vasopressin is being released in the absence of physiological stimuli for its release (i.e., hypertonicity, low EABV) (see Table 10-2).

It has been suggested to use the term syndrome of inappropriate antidiuresis rather than syndrome of inappropriate antidiuretic hormone to include patients who have genetic mutations in the V2R leading to its constitutive activation in the absence of vasopressin. We are reluctant to use this term because it does not separate those patients in whom the pathophysiology of the inappropriate antidiuresis is decreased volume of distal delivery of filtrate rather than the presence of actions of vasopressin.

In some patients, the stimulus for the release of vasopressin may not be permanent (e.g., secondary to a drug, pain, anxiety). If vasopressin disappears, a water diuresis may ensue, resulting in a rapid rise in the $P_{Na}$ and the risk of osmotic demyelination. In patients with persistently high vasopressin levels, the major danger is a further acute fall in $P_{Na}$, when there is a large intake of water, or the administration of a large volume of hypotonic or isotonic saline with its subsequent excretion in the urine as a hypertonic solution, leading to the generation of electrolyte-free water in the body (i.e., desalination). The presence of vasopressin may be caused by an underlying serious illness (e.g., small-cell carcinoma of the lung).

### Subtypes of syndrome of inappropriate antidiuretic hormone

#### Autonomous release of vasopressin

Vasopressin levels in these patients are consistently high and unregulated (e.g., release of vasopressin from malignant cells). This subtype is said to represent approximately one-third of the patients with SIADH, but clearly this may vary depending on the population of patients being studied.

#### Reset osmostat

This pathophysiology may account for approximately one-third of the patients with SIADH. These patients have normal regulation of vasopressin release but around a hypotonic threshold. This diagnosis hinges on documenting that the patient can excrete a dilute urine when the $P_{Na}$ is lowered further. The excretion of hypotonic urine, however, stops before the $P_{Na}$ rises to normal levels. These patients are not in danger of developing a large fall in $P_{Na}$ when ingesting a water load because the release of vasopressin will be suppressed. Nevertheless, one should not attempt to test if a reset osmostat is the underlying pathophysiology of SIADH if the degree of hyponatremia is severe, because administering a substantial water load may lead to a dangerous fall in $P_{Na}$.

One possible pathophysiology that may lead to the development of a reset osmostat is a sick-cell syndrome. This has been described in patients with chronic, catabolic illness. The proposed mechanism is that cells of the osmostat have fewer effective osmoles because of the catabolic illness. Therefore, the volume of these cells is decreased, even at a lower than normal $P_{Na}$, and therefore vasopressin is released. With a more severe degree of hyponatremia, these cells swell to exceed their original size, and thus the release of vasopressin is suppressed. Hence, they now defend a lower $P_{Na}$. It is also possible that patients with certain polymorphisms in the gene encoding for TRPV4, an osmosensitive calcium channel in osmosensing neurons, may be an example of this reset osmostat type of pathophysiology of SIADH.

#### Nonosmotic stimuli (afferent) overload

In this putative model, nonosmotic afferent signals are perceived by cells of the osmostat or of the vasopressin release center, which leads to the release of vasopressin despite low $P_{Na}$. Findings that may be in keeping with this model are that it may occur in patients who have lesions involving the lungs (e.g., pneumonia) and/or the brain (e.g., following trauma or an intracerebral hemorrhage that involve an area in the brain that is remote from the osmostat and the vasopressin release center).

### Subtype with absent vasopressin

A subset of patients who were thought to have SIADH (~7%) has undetectable vasopressin levels in plasma. A recent study using the measurement of copeptin, a stable and easily measured surrogate of vasopressin release, in patients who were thought to have SIADH reported that 12% of their patients have suppressed copeptin plasma levels. Perhaps some of these patients may have a gain of function mutation in the gene encoding for V2R, leading to a constitutively active receptor. Of note, mutations in the V2R gene were not found in this subset of patients in the study in patients with SIADH using the measurement of copeptin. It was also suggested that perhaps some of these patients may have an upregulated V2R expression. We think it is also possible that the defect causing diminished electrolyte-free water excretion at least in some of these patients may be caused by a vasopressin-independent mechanism, perhaps diminished volume of distal delivery of filtrate (because of a low GFR or an enhanced reabsorption in the PCT), and an enhanced water reabsorption via residual water permeability in the inner MCD.

### Barostat reset

A new subtype of SIADH was identified in the study mentioned earlier in patients with SIADH, using the measurement of copeptin. In this subset of patients (20% of the whole group), who did not appear to be EABV depleted, the infusion of hypertonic saline suppressed the release of copeptin. It was thought that these patients might have reduced sensitivity of the baroreceptor-mediated pathway (perhaps because of tumor infiltration or compression or other neuronal damage), which mimics decreased EABV and hence leads to the stimulation of the release of vasopressin. Volume expansion stimulates these stretch receptors and inhibits the release of vasopressin/copeptin. The study, however, did not examine the response to the infusion of saline solution that is isotonic to the patient, i.e., inducing volume expansion without a rise in $P_{Na}$.

## Glucocorticoid Deficiency

Isolated cortisol deficiency occurs in patients with pituitary disorders with diminished adrenocorticotropic hormone secretion (ACTH). Because aldosterone secretion is primarily under the control of the renin–angiotensin system, these patients do not have deficiency of aldosterone. Cortisol suppresses the release of corticotropin-releasing hormone (CRH) from the paraventricular nuclei of the hypothalamus. In the absence of cortisol, the release of both CRH and vasopressin is stimulated. In a patient who presents with glucocorticoid deficiency and hyponatremia, administration of glucocorticoids suppresses the release of vasopressin, leading to a water diuresis, which may result in a rapid rise in $P_{Na}$ and the risk of osmotic demyelination. In this setting, prophylactic administration of dDAVP concomitant with the administration of glucocorticoids is suggested to avoid a large water diuresis.

## Hypothyroidism

Hyponatremia secondary to hypothyroidism occurs only in elderly patients with severe hypothyroidism or even myxedema coma. The defect in water excretion seems to be caused by low cardiac output causing decreased EABV and low GFR.

## Heart Failure and Liver Cirrhosis

Hyponatremia usually develops in patients with advanced heart failure (New York Heart Association classes III and IV) and advanced liver cirrhosis (Child-Pugh B and C).

In both of these disorders, the EABV is reduced because of decreased cardiac output in patients with heart failure and systemic vasodilation in patients with liver cirrhosis. Decreased EABV leads to baroreceptor-mediated activation of the sympathetic nervous system and the renin–angiotensin–aldosterone system (causing Na⁺ ion retention) and vasopressin release (causing water retention). In addition, angiotensin II stimulates the osmoreceptor, leading to increased thirst. Hyponatremia develops because the proportional increase in TBW is larger than the increase in total body $Na^+$ ion content.

Hyponatremia is associated with worse outcomes in these patients, although it is not clear if this reflects the severity of their underlying disease or a direct effect of hyponatremia.

## TREATMENT OF PATIENTS WITH CHRONIC HYPONATREMIA

Issues related to the rate of correction of hyponatremia and relowering of $P_{Na}$ if the rise in $P_{Na}$ exceeds the maximum rate were discussed previously. In this section, we will address issues related to specific measures for treatment of hyponatremia based on its underlying pathophysiology.

### HYPONATREMIA CAUSED BY LOW EABV/LOW DISTAL DELIVERY OF FILTRATE

Expansion of the EABV will suppress the release of vasopressin and/or increase the distal delivery of filtrate (via increasing GFR and decreasing fractional reabsorption in the PCT), leading to a water diuresis and correction of hyponatremia.

Intravenous infusion of isotonic saline may be needed if the patient has a hemodynamically significant degree of decreased EABV. Infusion of isotonic saline on its own does not cause much of a rise in $P_{Na}$; however, an appreciable rise in $P_{Na}$ occurs if water diuresis ensues. For example, in a patient who has 30 L of TBW and a $P_{Na}$ of 120 mmol/L, the addition of 1 L of isotonic saline (154 mmol/L) will raise $P_{Na}$ by only 1 mmol/L. The $P_{Na}$ will rise, however, to 125 mmol/L if 1 L of isotonic saline is added and 1 L of electrolyte-free water is excreted.

It is important to emphasize that the administration of KCl to correct coexisting hypokalemia (e.g., in a patient with chronic hyponatremia caused by thiazide diuretics) will cause a rise in $P_{Na}$ similar to what occurs with the administration of an equivalent amount of NaCl. This is because, in terms of body tonicity, $Na^+$ ions (the main ECF cation) and $K^+$ ions (the main ICF cation) are equivalent. As hypokalemia develops, $K^+$ ions exit from cells and are replaced with $Na^+$ ions from the ECF compartment. When KCl is administered, $K^+$ ions enter cells and $Na^+$ ions exit. Therefore, the administration of KCl will cause a rise in body tonicity, which will be reflected by a rise in $P_{Na}$ similar to that with the administration of an equivalent amount of $Na^+$ ions if there is no change in TBW. Furthermore, because $Na^+$ ions are retained in the ECF compartment, EABV may become expanded and a water diuresis may ensue. This is of particular concern because patients with hypokalemia are at high risk for the development of osmotic demyelination. Therefore, the administration of $K^+$ ions should be in a solution that is isotonic to the patient. For example, if the patent has a $P_{Na}$ of 120 mmol/L, a solution of half normal saline (0.45% NaCl, or 77 mmol/L) with 40 mmol of KCl/L will have a concentration of $Na^+ + K^+$ ions that is reasonably close to the patient. Administration of dDAVP to prevent the occurrence of a water diuresis may also be considered.

In the absence of a hemodynamically significant degree of contraction of EABV, the design of therapy will depend on a quantitative analysis of the composition of the ECF and ICF compartments and total body balance. There are a number of assumptions made in these calculations; therefore, they are meant to provided rough estimates to guide the design of therapy. To illustrate this, consider a patient who has been on thiazide diuretics and was referred to the emergency room by her family physician after she was noted on routine blood work to have a $P_{Na}$ of 120 mmol/L and a $P_K$ of 3.6 mmol/L. Her $P_{Na}$ on previous measurements was 140 mmol/L. Her weight before she was started on the thiazide diuretic was 60 kg, and so her TBW was estimated to be 30 L (ECF volume = 10 L, ICF volume = 20 L). Her blood pressure was 110/70 mm Hg, pulse was 92 beats/min, and jugular venous pressure was 1 cm below the sternal angle, so she was judged to have a mild degree of contraction of her ECF volume.

*ECF analysis:* There is no accurate way to assign a value for the patient's ECF volume, other than to say that it is contracted. Based on clinical assessment, she was felt to have a mild degree of ECF volume contraction, based on a low jugular venous pressure. It is reasonable to assume that her ECF volume has decreased from its normal value of 10 L to approximately 9 L. Therefore, there is a deficit of 1 L of water in her ECF compartment. With regard to $Na^+$ ion content in her ECF compartment, her initial ECF $Na^+$ ion content was 10 L × 140 mmol/L = 1400 mmol. Using the estimated new ECF volume of 9 L, her current ECF $Na^+$ ion content is 9 L × 120 mmol/L = 1080 mmol. Therefore, she has a deficit of $Na^+$ ions in her ECF compartment of 1400 − 1080 = 320 mmol.

*ICF analysis:* The rise in ICF volume is proportional to the fall in $P_{Na}$. Because her $P_{Na}$ fell by 14%, the ICF volume is increased by ~3 L (20 L × 14%).

*Balance:* The patient has a gain of 2 L of water (3 L water gain in the ICF compartment and a 1 L water deficit in the ECF compartment) and a deficit of 320 mmol of $Na^+$ ions. Therefore, the design of therapy to raise the $P_{Na}$ will be to induce a positive balance of $Na^+$ ions. Water diuresis will ensue once the volume of distal delivery of filtrate is increased.

## Design of therapy

To prevent a further fall in $P_{Na}$, we would restrict water intake to ~800 mL/day. This degree of water restriction is tolerated by most patients. We would try to create a positive daily balance for $Na^+$ ions to raise her $P_{Na}$ by 5 mmol/L/day. If her TBW is currently 32 L, then to raise her $P_{Na}$ by 5 mmol/L would require a positive balance of $Na^+$ ions of 32 L × 5 mmol/L = 160 mmol. If administration of $K^+$ ions is needed, the amount of $K^+$ ions should be included as part of the 160 mmol positive balance of $Na^+$ ions. Her inputs and outputs must be monitored, and the $P_{Na}$ should be measured at frequent intervals to be sure that the maximum rate of rise of $P_{Na}$ is not exceeded. We repeat the same procedure on day 2 if a water diuresis does not occur.

If a water diuresis occurs, the administration of dDAVP may be needed to diminish the loss of water in the urine and prevent a rise in the $P_{Na}$ that exceeds the daily upper limit, based on assessment of risk for developing osmotic demyelination. A water diuresis, however, indicates that the EABV has been restored sufficiently to increase the volume of distal delivery of filtrate. If the patient still has hyponatremia, the plan for therapy is to allow a daily negative balance of water that is sufficient to achieve the desired rise in the $P_{Na}$ that day. For example, if her TBW is 32 L and $P_{Na}$ is 125 mmol/L, a rise in $P_{Na}$ of 5 mmol/L requires a negative water balance of 1.2 L (i.e., urine volume is larger than water intake by 1.2 L). We would give dDAVP to reduce the urine output if a water diuresis that would lead to a rise in $P_{Na}$ that would exceed the daily maximum limit for the rise in the $P_{Na}$ occurs.

If a water diuresis does not occur after EABV has been expanded, look for a cause for SIADH.

## Hyponatremia Caused by SIADH

Some of the causes of SIADH may be transient (e.g., pain, anxiety, nausea, acute pneumonia), and other causes of SIADH may be rapidly reversible with the administration of specific therapy (e.g., administration of glucocorticoids in patients with cortisol deficiency) or the discontinuation of drugs (e.g., dADVP, selective serotonin reuptake inhibitors). In either case, a water diuresis may ensue, leading to a rapid rise in $P_{Na}$ and the risk of osmotic demyelination.

In patients with mild chronic hyponatremia caused by SIADH ($P_{Na}$ 130 to 135 mmol/L), we do not think that correction of hyponatremia is necessary. In patients with moderate hyponatremia ($P_{Na}$ 125 to 129 mmol/L), it is argued that while these patients may appear clinically asymptomatic, they often have impaired attention and gait disturbances on neurological testing, and are at higher risk for falls and bone fractures. Furthermore, there is a risk of a further fall in $P_{Na}$ that may lead to acute symptoms if, for example, there is a significant increase in water intake or decrease in water excretion (e.g., less salt or protein intake). Hence, raising the $P_{Na}$ in these patients is recommended. Raising $P_{Na}$ is obviously also recommended in patients with a more severe degree of hyponatremia.

The pathophysiology of hyponatremia in patients with SIADH is primarily because of the effects of vasopressin to cause water retention. However, the ensuing EABV expansion results in natriuresis. Nevertheless, a degree of EABV expansion will still be present to provide the signal to excrete the daily salt load. To understand the design of therapy, consider this case example. A patient has SIADH because of the autonomous release of vasopressin from a cancer in her lung. She is seen because her $P_{Na}$ is 125 mmol/L. Her weight used to be 60 kg. For the following calculations, we assume that her TBW was 30 L, her ECF volume was 10 L, and her ICF volume was 20 L.

*ECF analysis:* It is likely that there is a modest degree of expansion of her ECF volume, say from 10 to 10.5 L. Hence, there is a gain of 0.5 L of water in her ECF compartment. With regard to the content of $Na^+$ ions in her ECF compartment, her initial ECF $Na^+$ ion content was 140 mmol/L × 10 L = 1400 mmol; her current ECF $Na^+$ ion content is 125 mmol/L × 10.5 L = 1312 mmol. The balance is a deficit of $Na^+$ ions in her ECF compartment of 88 mmol.

*ICF analysis:* Because there is a 10% fall in the $P_{Na}$, there is close to a 10% positive balance of water in the ICF compartment, which is a gain of 2 L of water.

*Balance:* There is a positive balance of 2.5 L of water and a small deficit of 88 mmol of $Na^+$ ions. Hence, the design of therapy to raise $P_{Na}$ will be mainly to induce a negative balance of water.

### Design of therapy

To understand the different options for therapy to raise the $P_{Na}$ in a patient with SIADH, it is important to emphasize that in the presence of vasopressin actions, the urine volume is determined by the rate of excretion of effective osmoles ($Na^+ + K^+$ ions and their accompanying anions) and the effective osmolality in the inner medullary interstitial compartment which is equal to the urine effective osmolality ($=2[U_{Na} + U_K]$). Because in patients with SIADH vasopressin is always present, the effective urine osmolality is relatively fixed. Hence, urine volume in these patients is determined by the rate of excretion of effective osmoles.

## Water restriction

To raise the $P_{Na}$ by 5 mmol/L from 125 mmol/L to 130 mmol/L in a patient with a TBW of 30 L requires a negative water balance of 1.2 L. As mentioned earlier, the urine volume in patients with SIADH is determined by rate of excretion of effective osmoles ($Na^+ + K^+$ ions and their accompanying anions). On a usual daily intake of 150 mmol of $Na^+$ ions and 50 mmol of $K^+$ ions, the rate of excretion of effective osmoles is 200 mmol from these cations, and another 200 mmol from their accompanying anions, for a total of 400 mosmol/day. If the effective osmolality in the inner medullary interstitial compartment is 600 mosmol/kg $H_2O$, which will also be the final urine effective osmolality, the urine volume will be 400 mosmol/600 mosmol/L = 0.67 L/day. Hence, to induce a negative water balance of 1.2 L requires no intake of water for almost 2 days. Therefore, water restriction alone (with the usual intake of $Na^+$ and $K^+$ ions) is not an effective means to raise $P_{Na}$, nor is it effective as the sole intervention to maintain $P_{Na}$ once it is raised to the desired level. One needs to increase the urine volume by increasing the rate of excretion of effective osmoles and/or decreasing the effective medullary interstitial osmolality (with the administration of a loop diuretic). Water intake, however, should be restricted along with these interventions because to raise $P_{Na}$, the tonicity of the input must be higher than the tonicity of the output.

## Loop diuretics and increasing salt intake

Loop diuretics (e.g., furosemide) decrease the reabsorption of $Na^+$ and $Cl^-$ ions in the thick ascending limb of the loop of Henle and hence decrease the effective medullary interstitial osmolality. A small dose of furosemide is needed to achieve this purpose, but because of its short duration of action, furosemide may need to be given twice daily. If as a result of this intervention the urine effective osmolality were to decrease to 300 mosmol/kg $H_2O$, and if the intake of NaCl were to be increased to 200 mmol/day, the number of effective osmoles to excrete would be 500 mosmol/day (400 mosmol of NaCl and 100 mosmol of $K^+$ ions with an anion); therefore, the urine volume will increase to 500 mosmol/300 mosmol/L = 1.7 L/day.

## Urea

When vasopressin acts, both AQP2 and urea transporters are inserted into the luminal membrane of the inner MCD. As a result, urea and water can be reabsorbed in this nephron segment and therefore urea is not an effective urine osmole. Notwithstanding, urea can become an effective osmole in the lumen of the inner MCD and cause the excretion of extra water if the distal delivery of urea is high enough to exceed the capacity for its reabsorption in the inner MCD. This may occur when urea is ingested as a large bolus. The effect may be even larger in an elderly patient with medullary interstitial disease and limited transport of urea in the inner MCD. The usual dose of urea given to patients with SIADH is about 30 g/day (500 mmol/day). Although used in Europe, its use in North America is rather limited because it is not readily available as a medicinal preparation. Furthermore, urea is not palatable, so patients may not tolerate using it for an extended period of time.

The effect of urea is not likely to be mimicked by the ingestion of a large load of protein. This is because with ingestion of protein, urea is produced at a slow, continuous rate. Hence, increasing protein intake does not provide a large bolus of urea, which would exceed the capacity of the urea transporters.

### Vasopressin receptor antagonists (Vaptans)

There are three receptors for vasopressin: V1A, V1B, and V2. V1A and V1B signal via an increase in intracellular calcium. Signaling via V1A, vasopressin causes vasoconstriction and the release of von Willebrand factor. Signaling via the V1B receptor, vasopressin is involved in the secretion of ACTH from the anterior pituitary. The V2R is present in the principal cells of the collecting duct. Binding to V2R, vasopressin increases intracellular levels of cyclic AMP, which causes the insertion of AQP2 channels into the luminal membranes of these cells.

Vaptans are nonpeptide antagonists of vasopressin. Although they do not bind the same locus in V2R, binding of vaptans to the receptor induces conformational changes that alter the binding of vasopressin to the receptor, leading to a water diuresis without natriuresis (hence their designation as aquaretics).

Conivaptan (which blocks both the V1A and the V2 receptors) is available for intravenous use. Tolvaptan (a more selective V2R blocker) is available in a tablet form for oral use. Both conivapatan and tolvaptan are approved for treatment of euvolemic and hypervolemic hyponatremia in the United States, and for treatment of euvolemic hyponatremia in Canada and in Europe. Both drugs are metabolized by the hepatic cytochrome P450 isoenzyme CYP3A4 system. Conivaptan is a potent inhibitor of this enzyme, which raises concern about drug interactions and therefore its use is limited to a 4-day intravenous course.

A number of clinical trials have reported efficacy of vaptans in increasing the $P_{Na}$ in patients with SIADH, congestive heart failure, and liver cirrhosis. In a recent meta-analysis by the European Clinical Guideline group of 20 randomized controlled trials involving 2900 patients with mild to moderate hyponatremia with a $P_{Na}$ of >125 mmol/L in most patients, patients who received vasopressin receptor antagonists had a mean rise in $P_{Na}$ of 4.3 mmol/L above that in the placebo group at 3 to 7 days, and of 3.5 mmol/L at 7 months.

There is concern, however, about overcorrection of hyponatremia and the risk for osmotic demyelination with the use of vaptans. In the Study of Ascending Levels of Tolvaptan in Hyponatremia 1 and 2 (SALT 1 and 2) trials, 4 out of 223 patients had a rise in $P_{Na}$ that exceeded 0.5 mmol/L/hr, and the $P_{Na}$ exceeded 146 mmol/L in a similar number of patients. In the Safety and sodium Assessment of the Long-term Tolvaptan (SALTWATER) study, 18 of 111 patients in the tolvaptan group had a $P_{Na}$ of more than 145 mmol/L at least once. Of note, the incidence of rapid overcorrection was likely higher if a maximum limit for a rise in $P_{Na}$ of 8 mmol/L was used. Furthermore, the risk for rapid overcorrection and hypernatremia is likely to be higher when the drug is used outside of a study setting that is conducted by expert physicians. Although osmotic demyelination did not develop or was not diagnosed in any of these patients, there is the concern that mild neurological deficits may not be readily recognized clinically.

Another concern is about the risk of liver injury with the use of tolvaptan. In a study that examined the effect of tolvaptan on disease progression in adult patients with polycystic kidney disease, use of tolvaptan (although at a dose that was four times higher than that used in patients with chronic hyponatremia) was associated more frequently than placebo with a greater than 2.5-fold increase in liver enzymes. Two patients who were receiving tolvaptan were withdrawn from the study because of liver injury that resolved after discontinuation of the drug. Based on these data the Food and Drug Administration (FDA) issued safety warnings regarding the use of tolvaptan, recommending that its use be limited to 30 days and that it is not to be used in patients with liver disease (including liver cirrhosis).

In view of possible harm, the lack of evidence of benefit in terms of patient survival or improved quality of life (using a measure of quality of life that is validated for patients with hyponatremia), we are not in favor of using these drugs in the management of patients with SIADH. The high cost of these drugs ($300 to $350 per 30 mg tablet) is also to be noted.

## Hyponatremia in Patients With Heart Failure

Despite the association of even mild hyponatremia with poor outcomes in patients with heart failure, it is not clear whether this association reflects the severity of the cardiac dysfunction or if hyponatremia itself contributes to the poor outcomes in these patients. There is no evidence that correction of hyponatremia ameliorates the hemodynamic abnormalities of cardiac dysfunction or improves clinical outcomes. It is also difficult to ascertain whether neurological symptoms, if present, are related to hyponatremia or to poor cardiac output. Considering the difficulty in management of hyponatremia in these patients, and the lack of evidence of benefit, it seems reasonable to suggest that one should only attempt to raise the $P_{Na}$ if it falls to <120 mmol/L. Even though evidence of benefit from correction in this setting is lacking, there may be a risk to the patient if there is further fall in $P_{Na}$.

Patients with heart failure and hyponatremia have an increase of TBW that is larger than the increase in total body $Na^+$ ion content. Vasopressin is present because of decreased EABV, although the ECF volume is expanded. Urine volume in this setting is determined by the rate of excretion of effective osmoles. Obviously, increasing the intake of salt is not an option in a patient with heart failure. It is commonly stated that water restriction is the main intervention to raise $P_{Na}$ in these patients. A quantitative analysis that is based on tonicity balance, however, shows the limitation of water restriction in this setting. Consider a patient with heart failure who is taking a loop diuretic. This patient has a TBW of 40 L and $P_{Na}$ of 125 mmol/L. The effective osmolality in his plasma is 250 mosmol/kg $H_2O$ (ignoring $P_K$ for the purpose of this calculation). Therefore, the total number of effective osmoles in his body is 250 mosmol/L × 40 L= 10,000 mosmol. As mentioned previously, in terms of body tonicity, $Na^+$ and $K^+$ ions are equivalent. Hence, if this patient is taking a loop diuretic that causes the excretion of 2 L of urine in a day with a concentration of $Na^+$ + $K^+$ ions of 150 mmol/L, and if he were to consume a diet that provides 150 mmol of $Na^+ + K^+$ ions, he will have a negative balance on that day of 150 mmol of $Na^+$ + $K^+$ ions (i.e., the total number of effective osmoles in his body decreases by 300 osmoles to 9700 mosmol). If his water intake is restricted to 500 mL/day (which many patients find intolerable), his water balance will be 2 L of excretion minus 0.5 L of intake or negative 1.5 L, so his TBW will fall to 38.5 L. As a result of these balance changes, the effective osmoality in his body will be 9700 mosmol/38.5 L = 250 mosmol/kg $H_2O$, and his $P_{Na}$ will rise by only 1 mmol/L to 126 mmol/L.

The limitations of using urea were discussed earlier.

The use of vaptans may provide an option to raise $P_{Na}$, if deemed necessary. Water diuresis in these patients is limited by the low volume of distal delivery of filtrate (low GFR and increased reabsorption in the PCT), so there is less risk of overly rapid correction of hyponatremia. There is, however, concern about the risk of liver injury and, as noted, there is a safety warning by the FDA that tolvaptan use should be limited to 30 days. In addition, the drug is rather costly. We do, however, think it is a reasonable option to raise $P_{Na}$ in patients who are admitted to hospital with acute exacerbation of heart failure who have $P_{Na}$ <120 mmol/L because its use will be for a very limited time period, provided the heart condition improves.

### HYPONATREMIA IN PATIENTS WITH LIVER CIRRHOSIS

Similar considerations to those discussed for patients with heart failure apply to patients with liver cirrhosis. Severe hyponatremia in these patients carries a poor prognosis, reflecting the severity of their disease. Raising $P_{Na}$ in these patients is difficult to achieve, and there is no evidence that it improves their outcome. The use of urea in these patients is not recommended in our view because of the risk of $NH_4^+$ production in the gut from breakdown of urea by gut bacteria, because the rise in the level of $NH_4^+$ in blood may worsen the hepatic encephalopathy. The FDA has issued a safety warning recommending that tolvaptan should not be used in patients with liver disease (including patients with liver cirrhosis). Patients with liver cirrhosis are also at high risk of osmotic demyelination, so the rate of rise of $P_{Na}$ in these patients should not exceed 4 mmol/L/day.

QUESTIONS

**10-4**    *What role might K$^+$ ion depletion play in determining the severity of hyponatremia?*

# PART D
# DISCUSSION OF CASES

### CASE 10-1: THIS CATASTROPHE SHOULD NOT HAVE OCCURRED!

**What dangers are there on presentation?**

Because the patient's $P_{Na}$ yesterday was 125 mmol/L and today is 112 mmol/L, there is an acute component to her hyponatremia. Of great importance, the new symptoms (nausea, headache) suggest the possibility of increased intracranial pressure and therefore urgent therapy with hypertonic saline is needed. The aim is to draw water out of the cranium quickly by giving a bolus of hypertonic saline to rapidly raise her $P_{Na}$ by 5 mmol/L. If symptoms disappear, we would stop the infusion of hypertonic saline. If she continues to have symptoms that suggest increased intracranial pressure, it is our view to continue with the infusion of hypertonic saline but to a maximum rise in $P_{Na}$ of 10 mmol/L. The reason for this fairly aggressive approach to correction of hyponatremia is that it is known with certainty that she has an acute component of hyponatremia. Furthermore, there is a danger of permanent neurological damage and even death caused by brain herniation if her symptoms reflect increased intracranial pressure. Lastly, with an increase in $P_{Na}$ of 10 mmol/L per day, the risk of osmotic demyelination is still low.

### What dangers should be anticipated during therapy, and how can they be avoided?

The first danger is the absorption of a large volume of previously ingested water from her gastrointestinal tract, which will lower her arterial $P_{Na}$. Measuring the $P_{Na}$ in arterial blood and comparing this value to the $P_{Na}$ in brachial venous blood will help reveal whether water is currently being absorbed in the intestinal tract (see Chapter 9). Also, one must be alert for even mild symptoms of raised intracranial pressure because they may herald danger.

The second risk is the development of osmotic demyelination with a rapid rise in $P_{Na}$ because she has an element of chronic hyponatremia. This is most likely to occur if she has a large water diuresis when the actions of dDAVP disappear. After the first 24 hours, we would limit the rate of rise in her $P_{Na}$ to no more than 8 mmol/L/day. Control of the urine output by giving dDAVP should prevent the $P_{Na}$ rising more than the maximum limit. If dDAVP is given, one must ensure that water restriction is imposed. The $P_{Na}$ should be closely monitored.

### CASE 10-2: THIS IS FAR FROM "ECSTASY"!

### Is this Acute Hyponatremia?

It is reasonable to presume that this is acute hyponatremia for two reasons. First, she has the recent ingestion of a large volume of water. Second, she had the intake of a drug, MDMA, which may cause the secretion of vasopressin. Importantly, in patients with acute hyponatremia, the situation can become very serious in a very short period, even if symptoms are initially mild (e.g., headache, drowsiness, mild confusion). Therefore, this patient needs urgent therapy with 3% hypertonic saline to shrink the size of her brain cells.

### Why did she have a seizure if the $P_{Na}$ was 130 mmol/L?

Generally, such a mild degree of hyponatremia should not lead to such severe symptoms. There are two possible explanations. First, she might have an underlying central nervous system lesion that makes her more susceptible to develop a seizure with a smaller degree of brain cell swelling. Second, her $P_{Na}$ was initially significantly lower than the value that was obtained after she had seizures. In more detail, because of the seizure, many new osmoles were generated in her skeletal muscle cells, which caused a shift of water from her ECF compartment to her ICF compartment, and hence her $P_{Na}$ measured now is significantly higher than what it was.

There are two major reasons why the number of osmoles in muscle cells may increase during a seizure (see Fig. 9-22). First, during muscle contraction, phosphocreatine is converted to creatine and inorganic divalent phosphate $(HPO_4^{2-})$, which increases the number of effective osmoles in these muscle cells. Second, the vigorous muscle contraction generates ADP in muscle cells that causes a rapid increase in flux in glycolysis with the production of L-lactic acid (see Chapter 6). Because intracellular $PCO_2$ rises in this setting, the new $H^+$ ions produced are forced to bind to proteins rather than to $HCO_3^-$ ions and hence there is a gain of L-lactate anions without a loss of $HCO_3^-$ ions and therefore an increase in the number of osmoles in cells because the source of glucose is from breakdown of large macromolecule: glycogen. In addition, these new L-lactate osmoles accumulate in muscle cells because the rate of exit of L-lactate anions from these muscle cells is not as fast as their rate of formation.

### What role might anorexia nervosa play in this clinical picture?

Approximately 50% of water in the body is located in skeletal muscles. This patient has a very small muscle mass, so a small positive water balance could cause a larger fall in her $P_{Na}$ compared with another subject with a larger muscle mass and the same gain in water.

### What is your therapy for this patient?

The aim of therapy is to draw water out of the cranium to decrease the intracranial pressure by raising the $P_{Na}$ by 5 mmol/L rapidly with the administration of hypertonic saline.

It is important to watch for addition of water from a reservoir in the intestinal tract or from the water that is retained in muscle cells because of the seizure. The $P_{Na}$ can be brought close to the normal range because in this patient, who clearly has acute hyponatremia, there is little concern about the risk of developing osmotic demyelination with a rapid rise in $P_{Na}$.

## CASE 10-3: HYPONATREMIA WITH BROWN SPOTS

### What is the most likely basis for the very low EABV?

In this case, the very contracted EABV (manifested by low blood pressure and tachycardia), the low $P_{Na}$, the high $P_K$ of 5.5 mmol/L, and the renal $Na^+$ ion wasting strongly suggest that the most likely diagnosis is primary adrenal insufficiency. This is likely caused by autoimmune adrenalitis because the patient has another autoimmune disorder: myasthenia gravis. The basis for the renal wasting of $Na^+$ ions is a lack of aldosterone. The low EABV is also caused in part by a lower degree of contraction of venous capacitance vessels because of glucocorticoid deficiency.

### What dangers to the patient are present on presentation?

There are two potential emergencies that dominate the initial management: a very contracted EABV and the lack of cortisol because of suspected primary adrenal insufficiency. To deal with the former to restore hemodynamic stability, the initial infusion can be given as 0.9% saline. Once the patient is hemodynamically stable, to further expand the EABV without changing the $P_{Na}$, the intravenous fluid therapy should be changed to a saline solution that is "isotonic to the patient". The patient's $P_{Na}$ is 112 mmol/L. The concentration of $Na^+$ ions in isotonic saline (0.9% NaCl) is 154 mmol/L, and in half-isotonic saline (0.45% NaCl) it is 77 mmol/L. Therefore, by alternating volumes of 0.9% NaCl with 0.45% NaCl, one can in effect administer fluids with an average concentration of $Na^+$ ions close to 112 mmol/L. The second emergency is related to lack of cortisol, and it can be dealt with by administering glucocorticoids.

There is one other possible emergency on admission: the presence of an acute element to her hyponatremia. This did not seem to be the case because the patient denied a recent large water intake and she did not have significant symptoms that could be related to an acute component of hyponatremia.

### What dangers should be anticipated during therapy, and how can they be avoided?

Re-expansion of the patient's EABV can lead to an increased urinary excretion of water because of an increased volume of distal delivery of filtrate and suppression of the release of vasopressin. In addition, the administration of cortisol will improve her hemodynamic state and also inhibit the release of CRH and hence of vasopressin. This may cause a large excretion of water and thereby a dangerous rise in the $P_{Na}$. Because the patient has a small muscle mass (and hence a small volume of TBW), the excretion of a relatively small volume of water can lead to a large rise in her $P_{Na}$. In addition, because of her poor nutritional state, which becomes even more evident if one interprets her weight loss in conjunction with a large gain of water in her ICF, one should set a much lower limit for the maximum rise in her $P_{Na}$ in the first day (i.e., $\leq 4$ mmol/L). Accordingly, we would administer dDAVP at the beginning of therapy to prevent a water diuresis. Water restriction must be imposed.

The major cause of hyponatremia in this patient is the $Na^+$ ion deficit because of the lack of aldosterone. Treatment with an exogenous mineralocorticoid was started. On the second day, our limit for the maximum rise in her $P_{Na}$ is 4 mmol/L because she is at high risk for the development of osmotic demyelination owing to her catabolic state. We would continue with water restriction and create a positive balance of $Na^+$ ions of 4 mmol per liter of TBW (TBW estimated as 50% of her body weight). On day 3, if a water diuresis did not occur on day 2, we continue with the administration of NaCl to raise $P_{Na}$, but not to exceed a maximum of 4 mmol/L. Once a water diuresis begins, we would administer dDAVP to prevent a further rise in the $P_{Na}$. Thereafter, we would create a further rise in the $P_{Na}$ by inducing a negative balance of water and allowing for a sufficient water diuresis to achieve the desired negative balance of water. We would administer dDAVP if needed to stop the water diuresis and control the rate of rise of $P_{Na}$. Once the $P_{Na}$ reaches 130 mmol/L, one can stop the administration of dDAVP.

### CASE 10-4: HYPONATREMIA IN A PATIENT ON A THIAZIDE DIURETIC

### What is the most likely basis for the chronic hyponatremia in this patient?

Although the patient was taking a thiazide diuretic, the degree of decreased EABV did not seem to be large enough to cause the release of vasopressin. The patient had a low baseline estimated GFR of 40 L/day. The use of diuretics and the low-salt diet led to a deficit of $Na^+$ ions and a mild reduction in her EABV. Even a relatively small decrease in EABV leads to sympathetic activation, and the $\beta$-adrenergic stimulation activates the renin–angiotensin–aldosterone system, both of which will increase reabsorption of

Na$^+$ ions and water in the PCT. If she were now to reabsorb 90% of her GFR (40 L/day, and may be even somewhat lower because of the mild reduction in her EABV) in the PCT instead of the normal rate of absorption of about 83% of GFR, less than 4 L/day will be delivered distally, and this is the maximum urine volume she can excrete. This volume exceeds the usual daily intake of water, but hyponatremia still can develop in such a patient because there is water reabsorption by residual water permeability along the inner MCD even in the absence of vasopressin action.

Because of the low intake of salt and protein, her rate of excretion of osmoles in the urine will be low. If her osmole excretion rate is 300 osmoles per day, and if 4 L are delivered to the inner MCD, the osmolality of the luminal fluid in the inner MCD will be 75 mosmol/kg H$_2$O. Even if the interstitial osmolality is substantially lower than normal, say only 375 mosmol/kg H$_2$O, there is still an enormous osmotic driving force for water reabsorption along the inner MCD because a difference of 1 mosmol/kg H$_2$O generates a pressure of ~19.3 mm Hg. It is also of interest that thiazides have been shown to induce water absorption in the inner MCD of normal rats and also of Brattleboro rats that lack vasopressin.

### What dangers should be anticipated during therapy, and how can they be avoided?

Understanding this pathophysiology has clinical implications for the management of patients with hyponatremia. Consider if this patient was thought to have hyponatremia because of stimulation of vasopressin release caused by decreased EABV, and hence was given isotonic saline to re-expand her EABV. A relatively small volume of saline (especially if it is given as a bolus) may be sufficient to reduce the fractional reabsorption of filtrate in the PCT and increase the volume of filtrate delivered to the distal nephron. If the fractional reabsorption in the PCT is decreased to say 83% of the GFR of 40 L/day, the volume of the distal delivery of filtrate will increase to ~7 L/day. This exceeds the volume of water reabsorption by residual water permeability, causing a water diuresis. Because of her small muscle mass, even a modest water diuresis may be large enough to cause a rapid rise in her P$_{Na}$ and hence the risk of osmotic demyelination, especially if she is malnourished or K$^+$ ion depleted.

The design of therapy for this patient was discussed earlier in this chapter.

### DISCUSSION OF QUESTIONS

10-1 *Calculation of electrolyte-free water is commonly used to determine the basis of a change in P$_{Na}$. We prefer to use the calculation of a tonicity balance for this purpose. How may these two calculations differ?*

The volume of electrolyte-free water in a solution is calculated by dividing the solution into a volume of isotonic saline, and if there is water left over, this is called electrolyte-free water. For example, if one has 3 L of a solution that each has 50 mmol of Na$^+$ ions, the total amount of Na$^+$ ions (150 mmol) with 1 L of water constitutes 1 L of isotonic saline; the other 2 L of water are therefore electrolyte-free. Thus, an infusion of hypotonic fluid adds electrolyte-free water to the body.

Electrolyte-free water can also be generated even if the infusate is isotonic saline. In more detail, if 1 L of fluid that contains 150 mmol of $Na^+$ ions is infused, and all of its $Na^+$ ions are excreted in 0.5 L of urine at a concentration of 300 mmol/L, one is left with 0.5 L of electrolyte-free water; we call this process desalination. For this desalination to occur, the concentration of $Na^+$ plus $K^+$ ions in the urine must be appreciably higher than that in the infusate (or in the patient if there are no infusions).

An analysis based on electrolyte-free water balance correctly predicts the change in the $P_{Na}$, but it does not determine its basis or its appropriate therapy. For example, if a patient has a positive balance of 300 mmol of $Na^+$, based on electrolyte-free water balance, this patient has a negative balance of 2 L of water. This is the same as another patient who has a net loss of 2 L of water.

Based on this analysis, therapy for both patients would be to induce a positive balance of 2 L of water. Although this therapy will lower the $P_{Na}$ in both patients, it is not the appropriate treatment to restore the volume and composition of the ECF and ICF compartments in each of them. Although it is the appropriate treatment for the second patient, for the first patient, the goal of therapy should be to induce the loss of 300 mmol of $Na^+$ ions. Therefore, the analyses based on electrolyte-free water balance terms do not reveal which of the two options is the correct way to treat an individual patient. This is why separate balances for $Na^+$ ions and water are needed to plan the ideal therapy for each of these two patients; we call this a tonicity balance (see Fig. 10-4).

**10-2** *Does hypertonic saline reduce the intracranial pressure simply because it draws water out of brain cells?*

Because water cannot be compressed, a gain of water in a closed box (the skull) causes a rise in intracranial pressure. Simply shifting water between the ICF and ECF compartments of the brain within the cranium does not lower the intracranial pressure. To lower this pressure, one must force water to leave the cranium. This is achieved when hypertonic saline is infused rapidly because water crosses the capillary membrane faster than $Na^+$ ions (Fig. 10-5).

**10-3** *What role might $K^+$ ion depletion play in determining the severity of hyponatremia?*

Ninety-eight percent of the amount of $K^+$ ions in the body is in cells. Therefore, when $K^+$ ions are lost from the body, the vast majority of them are lost from the ICF compartment. To determine the impact this loss of $K^+$ ions has on body tonicity, one needs to examine how electroneutrality is achieved when $K^+$ ions are lost from the body.

First, if $K^+$ ions left cells accompanied by intracellular anions, water would leave these cells and the $P_{Na}$ will fall. Second, if $K^+$ ions are lost from the cells, and these cells gain an equivalent amount of $Na^+$ ions, there is no change in the number of osmoles in cells. Now, if these $K^+$ ions are excreted with $Cl^-$ ions, the ECF compartment has lost effective osmoles ($Na^+$ and $Cl^-$ ions), and water will shift into cells. Because of the loss of $Na^+$ and $Cl^-$ ions, the EABV will become contracted, especially in a patient who has another cause for the loss of NaCl (e.g., intake of diuretics) and who is consuming a low salt diet. This decrease in the EABV diminishes the volume of distal delivery of filtrate and thereby the excretion of water, and therefore hyponatremia may develop if water intake is relatively large.

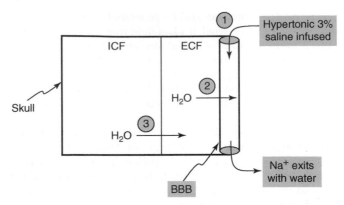

**Figure 10-5 Removal of Water From the Cranium Following an Infusion of Hypertonic Saline.** When hypertonic saline reaches the blood–brain barrier (BBB; *site 1*), water is drawn from the extracellular fluid (ECF) compartment (*site 2*) across the BBB into the capillary, because movement of Na+ ions out of the capillary blood is relatively slow. As a result, the concentration of Na+ ions rises in the interstitial fluid compartment of the brain, and this causes water to be drawn out of brain cells (*site 3*). The net effect is that the water that crossed the BBB is removed from the cranium. *ICF*, Intracellular fluid.

Another mechanism by which K+ ion depletion may affect the severity of hyponatremia is that patients who have a severe degree of hypokalemia may have decreased intestinal motility. As a result, ingested fluid may be retained in the lumen of the gastrointestinal tract. Na+ ions may be lost from the ECF compartment into this retained fluid in the lumen of the gastrointestinal tract, via the paracellular pathway that is permeable to Na+ ions, and this causes the $P_{Na}$ to fall further.

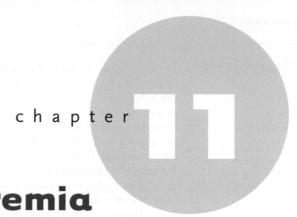

# Hypernatremia

# Introduction

**ABBREVIATIONS**

DI, diabetes insipidus
$P_{Effective\ osm}$, effective plasma
  osmolality
PCT, proximal convoluted tubule
DCT, distal convoluted tubule
MCD, medullary collecting duct
EABV, effective arterial blood
  volume
ENaC, epithelial sodium channel
ECF, extracellular fluid
ICF, intracellular fluid
$P_{Na}$, the concentration of sodium
  ($Na^+$) ions in plasma
dDAVP, 1-deamino 8-D-arginine
  vasopressin
BUN, blood urea nitrogen
$P_{Urea}$, concentration of urea in
  plasma
DKA, diabetic ketoacidosis
$P_K$, concentration of potassium
  ($K^+$) ions in plasma
$U_{Osm}$, urine osmolality
$U_{Na}$, concentration of $Na^+$ ions in
  the urine
$U_K$, concentration of $K^+$ ions in the
  urine
AQP, aquaporin water channel
$P_{Osm}$, plasma osmolality

Hypernatremia is defined as a concentration of sodium ($Na^+$) ions in plasma ($P_{Na}$) that is greater than 145 mmol/L. Hypernatremia is not a diagnosis; rather it is a laboratory finding that may be the result of a number of disorders of diverse etiology. Hence, one must determine its underlying cause. The first step in the clinical approach to the patient with hypernatremia is to deal with emergencies and to anticipate and prevent dangers that may arise because of therapy. Because the intracellular fluid (ICF) volume is inversely related to the $P_{Na}$, acute hypernatremia is associated with a decrease in the size of cells in the body. The organ that is most adversely affected is the brain, because as its volume shrinks, vessels coming from the inner surface of the skull become stretched and thus they may rupture, leading to focal intracerebral and subarachnoid hemorrhages. In patients with chronic hypernatremia, cells in the brain gain effective osmoles. Although it is uncertain when this adaptive response is completed, it is estimated that it takes about 48 hours for the brain to accumulate enough effective osmoles to return their volume close to their normal. After this occurs, the danger for the patient is a rapid decrease in the $P_{Na}$ because this may cause these cells to swell. This may result in a rise in intracranial pressure, which may lead to permanent neurological damage or even death caused by herniation of the brain.

The next step in the clinical approach is to examine for the presence of the expected responses in this setting, which are the sensation of thirst and the release of vasopressin leading to the excretion of the smallest volume of urine with the highest concentration of effective osmoles.

Hypernatremia that develops outside the hospital is usually caused by a large deficit of water. Although patients who develop hypernatremia in the hospital may also have a deficit of water, in many cases hypernatremia is caused in large part by a positive balance of $Na^+$ ions. In some patients with hypernatremia, there is a deficit of both $Na^+$ ions and water, with a proportionately larger deficit of water than of $Na^+$ ions.

The issues for therapy in the patient with hypernatremia are similar in principle to those that were discussed in patients with hyponatremia in Chapter 10. If the rise in the $P_{Na}$ has occurred over a time period of less than 48 hours, the $P_{Na}$ should be lowered rapidly if there are severe symptoms that could be related to hypernatremia. In patients with chronic hypernatremia, one should not permit the $P_{Na}$ to fall by more than 8 mmol/L/24 hr.

It is important to stress that there are times when the development of hypernatremia can be beneficial. For example, in children with diabetic ketoacidosis (DKA), it is important to prevent an appreciable fall in the effective osmolality in plasma ($P_{Effective\ osm}$) during the first 15 hours of treatment because a fall in $P_{Effective\ osm}$ may be a risk factor for the development of cerebral edema, and most cases occur 3-13 hours after therapy is instituted. Therefore, the design of therapy should be such that the $P_{Na}$ should rise by about one half the fall in the concentration of glucose in plasma ($P_{Glucose}$) because both $Na^+$ ions and their accompanying anions contribute to the $P_{Effective\ osmolality}$. Therefore, a degree of hypernatremia may develop, but it should be viewed as beneficial in this setting (see Chapter 5 for more discussion).

## OBJECTIVES

- To emphasize that hypernatremia represents an increase in the amount of $Na^+$ ions relative to the volume of water in the extracellular fluid (ECF) compartment. Hypernatremia can be primarily caused by a negative balance for water or a positive balance for $Na^+$ ions. For hypernatremia to develop, however, there must be a defect in sensing thirst, communicating the desire for water, and/or an inability to obtain water.

■ To emphasize that the danger to the patient with hypernatremia depends on whether the disorder is acute (duration for the development of hypernatremia <48 hours) or chronic (duration for the development of hypernatremia >48 hours).

■ To provide a diagnostic approach to the patient with hypernatremia based on understanding of its pathophysiology.

■ To provide an approach to the treatment of patients with hypernatremia based on whether the disorder is acute or chronic.

## CASE 11-1: CONCENTRATE ON THE DANGER

A 16-year-old young man who used to weigh 50 kg, had a craniopharyngioma resected. During surgery, his urine output was 3 L over 5 hours. His $P_{Na}$ rose from 140 to 150 mmol/L. During this time period, he received 3 L of isotonic saline. His urine osmolality ($U_{Osm}$) was 120 mosmol/kg $H_2O$, and the sum of the concentrations of $Na^+$ ions and potassium ($K^+$) ions in his urine ($U_{Na} + U_K$) was 50 mmol/L. Following the administration of desmopressin (dDAVP), his $U_{Osm}$ rose quickly to 375 mosmol/kg $H_2O$, and his $U_{Na}$ was 175 mmol/L.

### Questions

Why did hypernatremia develop (see margin note)?

What are the goals for therapy for his hypernatremia?

**NOTE**

• For a discussion of the basis for polyuria in this case, see the discussion of Case 12-2.

## CASE 11-2: WHAT IS "PARTIAL" ABOUT PARTIAL CENTRAL DIABETES INSIPIDUS?

A 32-year-old healthy man had a recent basal skull fracture. Since his head injury, his urine output has been consistently ~4 L/day and his $U_{Osm}$ is ~200 mosmol/kg $H_2O$ in multiple 24-hour urine collections. In blood samples drawn early in the morning, his $P_{Na}$ was ~143 mmol/L. Vasopressin was not detectable in his plasma from blood samples drawn at the same time. During the daytime, his $U_{Osm}$ was consistently ~90 mosmol/kg $H_2O$ and his $P_{Na}$ was ~137 mmol/L. When he was given dDAVP, his urine flow rate decreased to 0.5 mL/min and his $U_{Osm}$ rose to 900 mosm/kg $H_2O$. When he stopped drinking water after supper, his sleep was not interrupted by a need to void. In fact, his $U_{Osm}$ was ~425 mosmol/kg $H_2O$ in several first voided urine samples in the morning. Of interest, his urine flow rate fell to 0.5 mL/min and his $U_{Osm}$ rose to 900 mosmol/kg $H_2O$ after an infusion of hypertonic saline.

### Questions

What is the basis for the high urine flow rate in this patient?
What are the options for therapy?

## CASE 11-3: WHERE DID THE WATER GO?

A 55-year-old obese man who weighs 80 kg has had type 2 diabetes mellitus for the last 15 years. In the past several months, he complained of feeling very thirsty after eating a large meal. This usually lasted for a few hours and then subsided. This time, however, 12 hours after a large meal, which contained much more NaCl than his usual intake, he continued to have an intense feeling of thirst, despite drinking a large volume of water. He denied passing a large volume of urine. On arrival at the emergency room, he was alert and responded appropriately to questions. His blood pressure was 150/90 mm Hg, his pulse rate was 96 beats per minute (usual values for him), his weight was 1 kg higher than usual, and his ECF volume appeared to be normal. Fundoscopic examination showed changes consistent with diabetic retinopathy; he also had signs of peripheral neuropathy on clinical examination. Laboratory findings from a venous blood sample drawn when he presented to the emergency room are shown in the following table. Similar values were noted on another blood sample obtained 2 hours later. His arterial blood pH was 7.40. His hematocrit was similar to values from previous laboratory results.

| | | |
|---|---|---|
| $P_{Na}$ | mmol/L | 169 |
| $P_K$ | mmol/L | 5.2 |
| $P_{Glucose}$ | mg/dL | 180 |
| | mmol/L | 10 |
| $P_{Creatinine}$ | mg/dL | 1.8 |
| | µmol/L | 157 |
| $P_{Albumin}$ | g/dL | 3.8 |
| | g/L | 38 |
| Hematocrit | | 0.36 |
| $P_{Cl}$ | mmol/L | 133 |
| $P_{HCO_3}$ | mmol/L | 25 |
| BUN ($P_{Urea}$) | mg/dL | 22 |
| | (mmol/L) | (8) |
| Hemoglobin | g/dL | 12.5 |
| | g/L | 125 |

### Questions

What is the basis for the hypernatremia (in quantitative terms): a positive balance for $Na^+$ ions and/or a negative balance for water?

Why does he have such a severe degree of hypernatremia?

What is the therapy of hypernatremia in this patient?

# PART A
# BACKGROUND

## SYNOPSIS OF THE PERTINENT PHYSIOLOGY

### CONCENTRATION OF SODIUM IONS IN PLASMA

The $P_{Na}$ reflects the ratio of the amount of $Na^+$ ions to the volume of water in the ECF compartment. The actual concentration of $Na^+$ ions in plasma water is 152 mmol/kg $H_2O$. Measured per liter of plasma, however, the $P_{Na}$ is 140 mmol/L, because each liter of plasma has 6% to 7% nonaqueous volume (lipids and proteins). The normal range for the $P_{Na}$ is 136 to 145 mmol/L; thus, hypernatremia is defined as a $P_{Na}$ that is greater than 145 mmol/L.

Hypernatremia can be primarily caused by a negative balance for water or a positive balance for $Na^+$ ions (Figure 11-1). Hypernatremia is associated with a decrease in ICF volume unless its basis is a shift of water into cells secondary to a gain of effective osmoles in the ICF compartment (e.g., because of seizures or rhabdomyolysis; see Figure 9-22). The ECF volume, on the other hand, may be increased (because

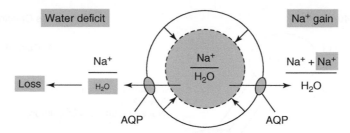

**Figure 11-1 Cell Size During Hypernatremia.** The *solid circle* represents the normal intracellular fluid (ICF) volume. Independent of whether the basis for hypernatremia is a deficit of water (*left side*) or a gain of Na⁺ ions (*right side*), the ICF volume shrinks (*dashed circle*). The *ovals* represent aquaporin (AQP) water channels in the cell membrane.

of positive balance of Na⁺ ions), normal, or decreased (because of a negative water balance, or because of a negative balance of both water and of Na⁺ ions, but with a larger negative balance of water than that of Na⁺ ions), depending on the basis for the rise in the $P_{Na}$.

## RESPONSES TO HYPERNATREMIA

When the $P_{Na}$ rises, the water control system elicits two responses that are designed to lower the $P_{Na}$ to prevent a further decrease in brain cell size: There is an input response (stimulation of thirst) and an output response (minimizing the loss of water in the urine).

The rise in the $P_{Na}$ is sensed in a group of cells in the hypothalamus (called the osmostat, or, better, the tonicity receptor). The main osmosensory cells appear to be located in the organum vasculosum laminae terminalis. In response to a high $P_{Na}$, this tonicity receptor sends messages to the thirst center to stimulate water intake and to the posterior pituitary to release vasopressin (Figure 11-2).

### Thirst

It is virtually impossible to have the $P_{Na}$ increase above the normal range if the thirst response is intact and water is available. In patients with a significant degree of hypernatremia, one must look for a reason why they cannot appreciate thirst or are unable to drink water. Examples include unconsciousness, disorders involving the osmostat or the thirst center (e.g., following a subarachnoid hemorrhage), inability to communicate the desire for water (e.g., infants, a patient with a stroke), inability to obtain water (e.g., inability to move), recurrent vomiting, or mechanical obstruction of the upper gastrointestinal tract (e.g., an esophageal tumor).

### Renal response

A rise in $P_{Na}$ triggers the release of vasopressin, which makes the cortical and medullary collecting ducts permeable to water. This results in conservation of water with the excretion of a small volume of urine with the highest concentration of effective osmoles (discussed in the following).

Vasopressin is synthesized by the magnocellular neurons in the supraoptic and paraventricular nuclei of the hypothalamus and is transported down the axons of the supraoptical–hypophyseal tract to be stored in and released from the posterior pituitary (neurohypophysis). Binding of vasopressin to its V2 receptors (V2R) in the basolateral membrane of principal cells in the collecting ducts stimulates adenylyl cyclase to produce cyclic adenosine monophoshate (cAMP), which in turn activates protein kinase A (PKA). PKA phosphorylates aquaporin 2 (AQP2) water channels, which causes their shuttling from an intracellular store to the luminal membrane of principal cells.

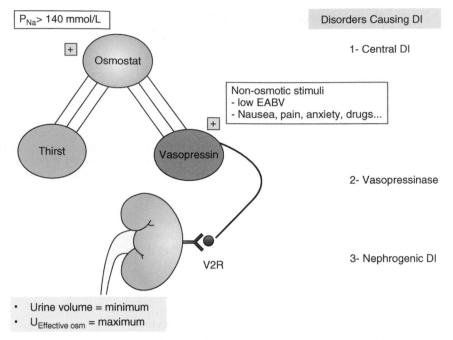

$P_{Na}$> 140 mmol/L

Osmostat

Thirst

Vasopressin

Non-osmotic stimuli
- low EABV
- Nausea, pain, anxiety, drugs...

V2R

Disorders Causing DI

1- Central DI

2- Vasopressinase

3- Nephrogenic DI

- Urine volume = minimum
- $U_{Effective\ osm}$ = maximum

**Figure 11-2 Water Control System.** The primary sensor is the osmostat, which consists of a group of cells that detect a change in their volume in response to a change in the $P_{Na}$. Thus *tonicity receptor* is a better description than *osmostat*. These cells are linked to a group of cells that control the intake of water (thirst center) and to others that are responsible for the release of vasopressin. Vasopressin binds to its vasopressin receptor 2 (V2R), resulting in the insertion of aquaporin 2 channels in the luminal membrane of principal cells in the distal nephron and the excretion of the smallest volume of urine with the highest concentration of effective osmoles. Other factors, such as a decrease in the effective arterial blood volume (EABV) and a number of afferent stimuli (e.g., pain, nausea, anxiety, drugs), also cause the release of vasopressin. The clinical disorders that may lead to water diuresis (i.e., diabetes insipidus) and the site of the lesions are shown on the *right side* of the figure. *DI*, Diabetes insipidus; $U_{Effective\ osm}$, urine effective osmolality; $U_V$, urine volume.

When vasopressin acts, the urine flow rate is determined by the rate of excretion of effective osmoles and the effective ("non-urea") osmolality in the inner medullary interstitial compartment. Because cells in the inner medullary collecting duct (MCD) have urea transporters (UTA-1 and UTA-3) in their luminal membranes when vasopressin acts, urea is usually an ineffective osmole (the concentration of urea is nearly equal on the two sides of that membrane), so urea does not obligate the excretion of water. Therefore, the effective osmoles in the urine are $Na^+$ and $K^+$ ions and their accompanying anions; thus, the excretion of effective osmoles in the urine is calculated as $2(U_{Na} + U_K)$. On a typical Western diet, the rate of excretion of effective osmoles is typically 450 mosmol/day, and the effective osmolality in the inner medullary interstitial compartment is close to 600 mosmol/kg $H_2O$. Hence, the minimum urine flow rate is close to 0.75 L/day or 0.5 mL/min. The urine flow rate is higher when the rate of excretion of effective osmoles rises.

The effective $U_{Osm}$ is virtually identical to the effective osmolalty in the inner medullary interstitial compartment when vasopressin acts. Notwithstanding, the effective osmolality in the inner medullary interstitial compartment can be lower because of several potential factors: diseases that cause medullary interstitial damage, drugs or disorders that compromise the function of the loop of Henle, or if the renal medulla is washed out by a prior water or osmotic diuresis.

If vasopressin is not present (e.g., in patients with central diabetes insipidus [DI]) or if it fails to act (e.g., in patients with congenital nephrogenic DI), the late distal nephron segments lack AQP2 in their luminal

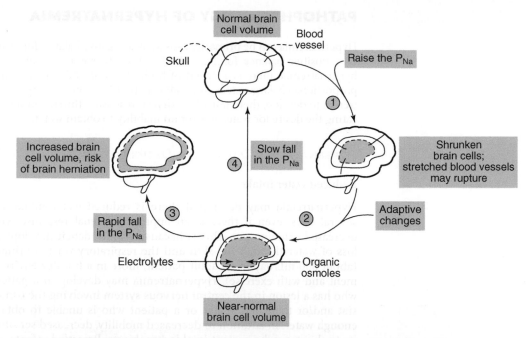

**Figure 11-3 Regulation of Brain Cell Volume During Hypernatremia.** The *dark outline* represents the skull and the *lighter line* represents brain cell volume. The *convoluted lines* from the skull to the brain represent blood vessels. When the $P_{Na}$ rises acutely (*site 1*), the brain cell volume decreases, which causes blood vessels to stretch and possibly rupture. Over a 48-hour period, adaptive changes are almost complete, and they return brain cell size toward normal—this involves the gain of electrolytes and effective osmoles in brain cells (*site 2*). If the $P_{Na}$ were to fall acutely at that time, brain cell volume will increase, and brain herniation may result (*site 3*). This danger is avoided if the $P_{Na}$ falls slowly (*site 4*).

membrane and therefore are impermeable to water. In this setting, the urine flow rate is determined by the volume of filtrate that is delivered to the distal nephron minus the volume of water reabsorbed via residual water permeability in the inner MCD. The volume of filtrate delivered to the distal nephron is a function of the glomerular filtration rate and the volume of fluid reabsorbed in the proximal convoluted tubule (PCT; see Chapter 9). In the absence of vasopressin actions, the rate of excretion of osmoles influences the $U_{Osm}$ but not the urine flow rate.

## REGULATION OF BRAIN CELL VOLUME

In response to chronic hypernatremia, cells in the brain gain effective osmoles. This begins with an influx of $Na^+$ and $Cl^-$ ions, which usually occurs via the furosemide-sensitive $Na^+$, $K^+$, 2 $Cl^-$ cotransporter-1 (NKCC-1), but it is also possible that this may be achieved by parallel flux through the $Na^+/H^+$ cation exchanger and the $Cl^-/HCO_3^-$ anion exchanger. The second mechanism for increasing the size of shrunken brain cells is via an increase in the number of organic compounds in brain cells (e.g., taurine and myoinositol), which seems to account for close to half of the increase in the number of effective osmoles in this adaptive process. As a result, water shifts from the ECF compartment into brain cells, which returns their volume toward normal (Figure 11-3). Although it is estimated that it takes 48 hours to accumulate enough effective osmoles, it is uncertain as to when this adaptive response is complete. Hence, the time frame that separates acute from chronic hypernatremia is not known with certainty and may differ from patient to patient. It is important to appreciate this adaptive change because if the $P_{Na}$ were to fall rapidly, brain cells would swell, and this could cause a dangerous rise in the intracranial pressure.

# PATHOPHYSIOLOGY OF HYPERNATREMIA

Hypernatremia can be primarily caused by a negative balance for water or a positive balance for $Na^+$ (Table 11-1). In some patients with hypernatremia, there is a deficit of both $Na^+$ ions and water, with a proportionately larger deficit of water than of $Na^+$ ions. For hypernatremia to develop, there must be a defect in sensing thirst, communicating the desire for water, and/or an inability to obtain water.

## HYPERNATREMIA CAUSED BY A DEFICIT OF WATER

### Reduced water intake

Hypernatremia may develop if there is reduced water intake for several days, even if there is an appropriate renal response with decreased urine output. This is because a water deficit develops as loss of water through the skin and the respiratory tract continues (about 800 mL/day in an adult patient, more in a hot dry environment and with exercise). Hypernatremia may develop in a patient who has a lesion in the central nervous system involving the osmostat and/or the thirst center or a patient who is unable to obtain enough water. In addition to decreased mobility, decreased sensitivity to thirst may be present in elderly subjects. Breastfed infants are completely dependent on their mothers for the intake of water. They may develop hypernatremia if they do not receive a sufficient number of feeds or if there are problems with breastfeeding. Infants also are at risk of hypernatremia from nonrenal water loss (e.g., caused by vomiting). In addition, infants in their first month of life have a reduced capacity to decrease their urine volume, a physiologic form of nephrogenic DI (see Part D for more discussion).

### Water loss

Water loss is the most frequent cause of hypernatremia; the sites of water loss are discussed below.

TABLE 11-1    **CAUSES OF HYPERNATREMIA**

**PRIMARY WATER DEFICIT**

**Reduced Water Intake for Many Days**
- Lack of water
- Inability to gain access to, or to drink, water
- Defective thirst caused by altered mental state, psychological disorder, or diseases involving the osmoreceptor and/or the thirst center

**Increased Water Loss**
- Renal loss: central DI, release of a vasopressinase from a necrotic tissue, nephrogenic DI, osmotic diuresis
- Gastrointestinal loss: vomiting, osmotic diarrhea
- Cutaneous loss: excessive sweating
- Respiratory loss: hyperventilation

**Shift of Water into Cells**
- Gain of effective osmoles in the intracellular fluid compartment (e.g., because of seizures, rhabdomyolysis)

**PRIMARY GAIN OF $Na^+$ IONS**
- Administration of intravenous fluid with a higher concentration of $Na^+ + K^+$ ions than their concentration in the urine during an osmotic or a water diuresis
- Infusion of hypertonic NaCl or $NaHCO_3$ in patients with oliguria
- Ingestion of sea water or replacing sugar by NaCl in feeding formula in infants

*DI*, Diabetes insipidus.

### Nonrenal water loss

#### Sweat

Sweat is important for thermoregulation because the evaporation of 1 L of water causes the loss of 500 to 600 kcal (heat of evaporation). Sweat is a hypotonic solution with a concentration of $Na^+$ ions that is close to 20 to 30 mmol/L. Because this water loss is derived from total body water rather than solely from the ECF compartment, and because the concentration of $Na^+$ ions in sweat is low, an appreciable degree of effective arterial blood volume (EABV) contraction does not usually develop because of excessive sweating. The usual volume of sweat is close to 0.5 L/day in an adult. Losses in sweat increase in febrile patients and can rise to 2 L per hour during exercise in a hot environment.

#### Respiratory tract

Because inspired air is not fully saturated with water, it gets humidified in the alveoli at normal body temperature. The source of this water, however, is from the oxidation of fuels (i.e., metabolic water). In more detail, oxidation of food yields $H_2O$ and $CO_2$ in a 1:1 proportion. Because the partial pressures of $H_2O$ and $CO_2$ in alveolar air are similar (47 and 40 mm Hg), $H_2O$ and $CO_2$ are also lost in almost a 1:1 proportion. Hence, there is no appreciable decrease in total body water as a result of loss of water in the alveolar air, unless the patient is hyperventilating (Figure 11-4).

Evaporation of water in the upper respiratory tract, however, results in loss of body water. The volume of this water loss is larger when the rate of ventilation is high.

#### Gastrointestinal tract

The loss of gastric secretions containing HCl is a loss of a hypotonic solution because at a pH of 1, the concentration of $Cl^-$ ions in gastric secretions is 100 mmol/L, and for every $Cl^-$ ion lost, one new $HCO_3^-$ ion is added to the body (see Figure 7-1). Loss of fluid containing both gastric and small intestinal secretions is also a loss of hypotonic solution. This is because if, for example, 1 L of isotonic HCl from gastric fluid were to react with 1 L of isotonic $NaHCO_3$ from the fluid secreted in the small intestine, the resulting solution will have 150 mmol of $Na^+$ ions and 150 mmol of $Cl^-$ ions in a total volume of 2 L. Therefore, the loss of this solution results in the loss of 2 L of half-isotonic NaCl.

Hypotonic fluid can be lost in osmotic diarrhea but not in secretory diarrhea. In osmotic diarrhea, the fluid lost is hypotonic to plasma because it contains organic osmoles (e.g., lactulose), and hence has a lower concentration of $Na^+$ ions.

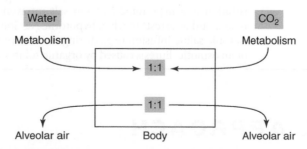

**Figure 11-4  Fate of Metabolic Water.** The body is depicted by the *large rectangle*. Events describing water are shown to the *left*, whereas events describing $CO_2$ are shown to the *right*. Both the production of water and $CO_2$ from the oxidation of fuels (*top arrows*) and their loss in alveolar air (*bottom arrows*) are close to a 1:1 proportion. Therefore, there is no net change in total body water balance as a result of water production in oxidation of fuels and its loss in alveolar air.

### Renal water loss

Renal water loss could be caused by a water diuresis (DI), an osmotic diuresis, or a renal concentrating defect (see Chapter 12 for more details).

DI could be caused by a lesion in the hypothalamic–posterior pituitary axis, which controls the production and release of vasopressin (central DI), the presence of a circulating vasopressinase that breaks down vasopressin, or a renal lesion that prevents the binding of vasopressin to its V2R or interferes with signaling to cause the insertion of AQP2 in the luminal membrane of principal cells in distal nephron (nephrogenic DI; see margin note).

In a patient with glucose- or urea-induced osmotic diuresis (see Chapter 12), the urine is hypotonic with a concentration of $Na^+ + K^+$ ions of typically 50 mmol/L. Hence, a water deficit and hypernatremia may develop.

Water loss could also be because of a renal concentrating defect. A low medullary interstitial effective osmolality could be because of diseases that cause medullary interstitial damage or because of drugs or disorders that compromise the function of the loop of Henle.

### Shift of water

In a setting where there is an acute rise in the number of effective osmoles in skeletal muscle cells (e.g., seizures, rhabdomyolysis), the hydrolysis of phosphocreatine to inorganic divalent phosphate and creatine can raise the number of effective osmoles in these cells. An acute shift of a large volume of water from the ECF compartment into muscle cells may occur for two reasons: the large size of that organ and its very high content of phosphocreatine (~25 mmol/kg). If L-lactic acid is produced in muscle cells during a seizure and the $H^+$ ions are titrated by intracellular proteins, accumulation of L-lactate anions increases the number of effective osmoles in muscle cells (see Discussion of Case 9-1).

An acute shift of water into the lumen of the intestinal tract may also occur, causing hypernatremia. To shift water into the lumen of the small intestine, there must be an accumulation of a large number of osmoles from the digestion of food because of a slow GI transit time or obstruction of the intestinal tract. An example of this pathophysiology is illustrated in Case 11-3.

#### HYPERNATREMIA CAUSED BY Na⁺ ION GAIN

Hypernatremia caused by a gain of $Na^+$ ions rarely occurs in an outpatient setting (e.g., ingestion of sea water, replacing sugar with salt in preparation of pediatric feeding formula, inducing abortion with hypertonic saline, suicide attempts). In contrast, hypernatremia because of a gain of $Na^+$ ions commonly occurs in a hospital setting as a result of the administration of a hypertonic $Na^+$ ion salt intravenously (e.g., $NaHCO_3$ to treat a cardiac arrest) or when hypotonic $Na^+$ ion losses are replaced with isotonic saline infusion (e.g., during the treatment of a patient with DI, or an osmotic diuresis caused by organic solutes such as glucose or urea).

**CLASSIFICATION OF NEPHROGENIC DI**

- We use the term nephrogenic DI to describe only the group of disorders in which there is diminished effectiveness of vasopressin to cause the insertion of AQP2 in the luminal membrane of principal cells in the distal nephron.
- We do not use the term nephrogenic DI to indicate a disorder in which there is a lesion that leads to a lower medullary interstitial osmolality, because from a pathophysiologic perspective, it is a different disorder. We prefer to use the term "renal concentrating defect" to describe this disorder.

# PART B
# CLINICAL APPROACH

## TOOLS IN THE CLINICAL APPROACH TO THE PATIENT WITH HYPERNATREMIA

### TOOLS TO DETERMINE THE BASIS OF HYPERNATREMIA

In patients with acute hypernatremia in a critical care setting, where balance data are usually available, calculating tonicity balance provides the data needed to determine the basis of hypernatremia and to define the appropriate therapy to restore the volume and the composition of the ICF and ECF compartments. Although we do not use electrolyte-free water balance for this purpose, we describe this approach first to illustrate its limitations.

### Electrolyte-free water balance

This calculation is based on how much water is needed to make all of the $Na^+ + K^+$ ions into a solution with a tonicity equal to the normal plasma tonicity (i.e., 150 mmol in 1 L of water). To perform this calculation, one must know the volume of and the concentrations of $Na^+ + K^+$ ions in the input and in the urine.

For example, a patient received 3 L of 0.9% saline ($Na^+$ ion concentration = 150 mmol/L) and excreted 3 L of urine with a concentration of $Na^+ + K^+$ ions of 50 mmol/L. There is no electrolyte-free water in the input. With regard to the output, one can divide it into 1 L of isotonic $Na^+$ ion solution (150 mmol/L) and 2 L of electrolyte-free water. Hence, he has a negative electrolyte-free water balance of 2 L, and his $P_{Na}$ will rise. Another patient received 3 L of 0.9% saline but excreted 3 L of urine; each liter has a concentration of $Na^+ + K^+$ ions of 200 mmol/L (a total of 600 mmol). There is no electrolyte-free water in the input. With regard to the output, because this patient would have needed to excrete 4 L (and not 3 L) of urine to make a total of 600 mmol of $Na^+ + K^+$ ions into an isotonic solution, this patient has a positive electrolyte-free water balance of 1 L, and hence her $P_{Na}$ will fall. This is because the excretion of 150 mmol of $Na^+ + K^+$ ions without water in the urine results in desalination of 1 L of body water, making it into 1 L of electrolyte-free water.

Table 11-2 shows the results of a similar analysis of three different cases. Although the balances for $Na^+ + K^+$ ions and for water are very different in the three examples used in the table, calculation of electrolyte-free water balance provided the same answer: a negative balance of 2 L of electrolyte-free water. Therefore, although calculation of electrolyte-free water balance correctly predicts the change in $P_{Na}$, it does not reveal whether its basis is a change in water balance or a change in $Na^+ + K^+$ ion balance. Hence, this calculation is not helpful to design the therapy needed to return the volume and composition of the ECF and ICF compartments to their normal values.

TABLE 11-2  **COMPARISON OF ELECTROLYTE-FREE WATER AND TONICITY BALANCE IN PATIENTS WITH HYPERNATREMIA**

| | $Na^+ + K^+$ (mmol) | WATER (L) | EFW (L) |
|---|---|---|---|
| **Infusion of 3 L of Isotonic Saline** | | | |
| Input | 450 | 3 | 0 |
| Output | 150 | 3 | 2 |
| Balance | +300 | 0 | −2 |
| **Infusion of 4 L of Isotonic Saline** | | | |
| Input | 600 | 4 | 0 |
| Output | 150 | 3 | 2 |
| Balance | +450 | +1 | −2 |
| **No Intravenous Fluid Infusion** | | | |
| Input | 0 | 0 | 0 |
| Output | 150 | 3 | 2 |
| Balance | −150 | −3 | −2 |

Three situations are illustrated in which the $P_{Na}$ rises from 140 to 150 mmol/L. The only difference is the volume of isotonic saline infused in each example. In all three examples, there is a negative balance of 2 L of electrolyte-free water (EFW). Notwithstanding, the balances for $Na^+$ ions and for water are very different in these three examples. From this comparison, it becomes clear that the basis of hypernatremia and the goals for therapy to correct the hypernatremia and restore the composition of the ECF and ICF compartments can be defined only when a tonicity balance is calculated.

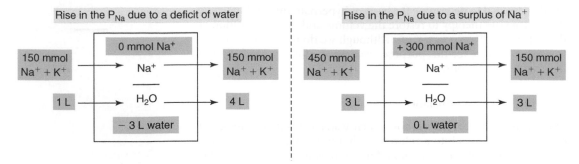

**Figure 11-5 Use of a Tonicity Balance to Determine the Basis for a Rise in the $P_{Na}$.** To perform a tonicity balance, the input and output volumes and the quantity of $Na^+$ and $K^+$ ions infused and excreted in the urine are required. Two examples of an acute rise in the $P_{Na}$ from 140 to 150 mmol/L in a patient who weighs 50 kg and has a total body water of 30 L are illustrated. In the example shown on the *left*, the rise in $P_{Na}$ is caused by a negative balance of 3 L of water. In the example shown on the *right*, the rise in $P_{Na}$ is caused by a positive balance of 300 mmol of $Na^+$ ions.

## Tonicity balance

To decide what the basis is for a change in the $P_{Na}$ and to define the proper therapy to return the volume and composition of the ECF and ICF compartments to their normal values, separate balances for water and for $Na^+ + K^+$ ions must be calculated. To perform a tonicity balance, the input and output volumes and the quantity of $Na^+$ and $K^+$ ions infused and excreted over the period when the $P_{Na}$ changed are examined (Figure 11-5). In practical terms, a tonicity balance can only be performed in a hospital setting in which inputs and outputs are accurately recorded. In a febrile patient, balance calculations will not be as accurate because sweat losses, which could be large, are not measured. Nevertheless, restricting the analysis of the output to the urine data is sufficient in an acute setting.

If the $P_{Na}$ at the beginning and the end of a certain time period, the volume of the urine, and the volume and amount of $Na^+ + K^+$ ions in the fluid that was infused during that time period are known, the clinician can calculate the quantity of $Na^+ + K^+$ ions that was excreted in the urine and determine why the $P_{Na}$ has changed (see answer to Question 11-1).

## QUESTION

11-1 *A 50-kg man receives 3 L of isotonic saline (150 mmol/L) and excretes 3 L of urine with an unknown concentration of $Na^+$ ions. In this period, his $P_{Na}$ rises from 140 to 150 mmol/L. If there is no other input or output during this period, what is the concentration of $Na^+$ ions in mmol/L in this urine?*

## TOOLS TO DETERMINE THE CAUSE OF HYPERNATREMIA

The most common cause of chronic hypernatremia is a negative balance of water. There are four possible routes for this water loss: sweat, the gastrointestinal tract, the respiratory tract in a patient who is hyperventilating; and, most commonly, the kidneys when a large volume of urine with a low concentration of $Na^+ + K^+$ ions is excreted (i.e., a large water diuresis or an osmotic diuresis caused by the excretion of glucose or urea). If the cause is a negative balance of water, the EABV volume is likely to be contracted and there should be a loss of weight in keeping with the magnitude of the water deficit. Conversely, if the cause of hypernatremia is a water shift (e.g., because of seizures or rhabdomyolysis), the ECF volume may be contracted, but a weight loss is not present. Although chronic hypernatremia in the outpatient setting is rarely caused by a positive balance of $Na^+$ ions, it should be suspected if there is an expanded ECF volume. In addition, if this is the sole cause for the hypernatremia, there should not be a loss of weight. One should look for the source of the addition of $Na^+$ ions.

In response to hypernatremia, vasopressin should be released and the urine output should be reduced to close to 0.5 mL/min (30 mL/hr) in an adult who consumes a typical Western diet, and the effective urine osmolality should be close to 600 mosmol/kg $H_2O$. These findings indicate that the cause of hypernatremia is reduced water intake, a nonrenal water loss, or a shift of water (into the ICF of muscle or maybe into the lumen of the intestinal tract).

In a patient with hypernatremia caused by a water loss, the assessment of $U_{Osm}$ and the osmole excretion rate help to determine whether the basis of the water loss is caused by a water diuresis or an osmotic diuresis. If the $U_{Osm}$ is <250 mosmol/kg $H_2O$ and the osmole excretion rate is <900 mosmol/day, water loss is caused by a water diuresis. On the other hand, if the $U_{Osm}$ is >300 mosmol/kg $H_2O$ and the osmole excretion rate is appreciably >1000 mosmol/day, water loss is caused by an osmotic diuresis (see Chapter 12).

The water deprivation test should not be performed in a patient who already has hypernatremia. Measurement of plasma vasopressin is technically challenging; there are only a few reliable and commercially available vasopressin assays. In addition, vasopressin is unstable in isolated plasma. Vasopressin is synthesized as prepro-hormone and consists of a signal peptide (vasopressin), neurophysin II (a carrier protein for vasopressin), and a C-terminal peptide named copeptin. Copeptin is much more stable than vasopressin and its measurement seems to be less complicated than that of vasopressin. In healthy individuals, copeptin and vasopressin levels are closely related over a wide range of plasma osmolalities. The clinical utility of measurement of copeptin in clinical diagnosis in patients with hypernatremia/polyuria is yet to be determined.

In a patient with central DI or water diuresis because of the release of a vasopressinase, $U_{Osm}$ should rise to a value higher than the osmolality in plasma ($P_{Osm}$) in response to the administration of dDAVP. If there is a reason to suspect the release of a vasopressinase, one should examine the response to the administration of vasopressin after the effect of dDAVP has worn off and the patient is having a water diuresis again. In contrast to the response to the administration of dDAVP, a patient in whom a vasopressinase is present will not show a response to the administration of a small dose of vasopressin. If $U_{Osm}$ does not rise to a value that is higher than the $P_{Osm}$ in response to the administration of dDAVP, the diagnosis is nephrogenic DI (see Chapter 12).

## STEPS IN THE CLINICAL APPROACH TO THE PATIENT WITH HYPERNATREMIA

The steps to take in the clinical approach to patients with hypernatremia are similar to those with all other fluid, electrolyte, and acid–base disorders. First, recognize whether there are emergencies prior to therapy; second, anticipate and prevent dangers that may arise during therapy; and third, proceed with therapy and the diagnosis of the cause of hypernatremia.

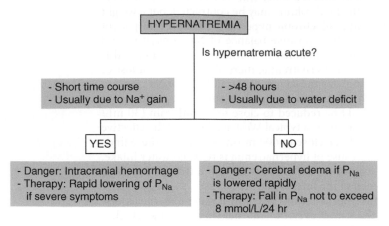

**Flow Chart 11-1  Emergencies Associated With Hypernatremia.** The emergencies in patients with acute hypernatremia are caused by brain cell shrinkage and resultant rupture of blood vessels, leading to focal intracerebral and subarachnoid hemorrhages. The danger in the patient with chronic hypernatremia is a rapid and large fall in the $P_{Na}$, which results in brain cell swelling and possibly brain herniation.

## IDENTIFY EMERGENCIES PRIOR TO THERAPY

To be succinct, we consider only those emergencies that are directly related to the presence of hypernatremia, independent of its cause. An emergency prior to therapy may be present in a patient who has acute hypernatremia (occurred in <48 hours; Flow Chart 11-1). In the patient with chronic hypernatremia who has a deficit of water and a deficit of $Na^+$ ions, there can be a hemodynamic emergency caused by a markedly reduced EABV. Our focus here will be on an emergency related to acute hypernatremia.

One typical setting for the development of a severe degree of acute hypernatremia in the hospital is in the patient who has DI (e.g., nephrogenic DI caused by lithium) who is undergoing surgery and is given a large infusion of isotonic saline, for instance to avoid a fall in blood pressure. In addition, this patient does not sense thirst or have the ability to drink water. Hypernatremia in this setting is largely because of gain of $Na^+$ ions.

The emergency in a patient with acute hypernatremia arises because the brain is confined in a rigid space and receives some of its blood supply from vessels that are attached to the inner surface of the skull. When the size of brain cells decreases, the brain shrinks, and this stretches these blood vessels and may cause them to rupture, leading to focal intracerebral and subarachnoid hemorrhages, with possible devastating results (see Figure 11-3).

If hypernatremia is acute and there are significant symptoms that could be caused by acute hypernatremia (e.g., decreased level of consciousness, convulsions), the $P_{Na}$ should be lowered rapidly, at least by 5% from its current level. The measures to lower $P_{Na}$ in this setting include inducing a rapid loss of $Na^+$ ions and/or a rapid gain of water. Both of these approaches may be difficult to achieve in a short time period. In some cases, hemodialysis may be the only option to cause a large and rapid fall in $P_{Na}$.

### Induce a negative balance of $Na^+$ ions

A rise in $P_{Na}$ from 140 to 155 mmol/L on the basis of a gain of $Na^+$ ions requires a positive balance of about 600 mmol of $Na^+$ ions in a

70-kg adult, with total body water of 40 L. It is almost impossible to induce a rapid and large loss of $Na^+$ ions in a hypertonic form by using diuretics alone. In more detail, the administration of a loop diuretic causes a high rate of excretion of $Na^+$ ions in the urine with water; this urinary loss, however, is hypotonic to the patient. To create a negative balance of $Na^+$ ions in a hypertonic form, one must replace all the water lost when the loop diuretic acts. Even with that, the loss of $Na^+$ ions in the urine is not likely to be large enough to cause a rapid fall in the $P_{Na}$.

### Induce a positive balance for water

To lower the $P_{Na}$ by 10% in a 70-kg patient who has 40 L of total body water by inducing a gain of water, one would need to give 4 L of water. Absorption of water from the gastrointestinal tract may be too slow to have a major decline in the $P_{Na}$ in a short time period using the oral route. It is not advisable to administer a large volume of water rapidly by the intravenous route as 5% dextrose in water solution ($D_5W$ [i.e.,~45 g of dextrose per liter]) because a limited amount of glucose can be oxidized in an ill patient (about 0.25 g/kg/hr). Hence, only close to 0.3 L of $D_5W$ can be given to a 70-kg person per hour. Administration of a larger amount of $D_5W$ may cause hyperglycemia, and the resulting osmotic diuresis and water loss could aggravate the degree of hypernatremia. The only way to lower $P_{Na}$ rapidly by inducing a gain of water is to infuse distilled water through a central vein. Distilled water should not be given via a peripheral vein, because it will mix with a small volume of plasma, which will be diluted sufficiently to cause hemolysis. Nevertheless, even with this drastic therapy, it is difficult to induce a large and rapid fall in the $P_{Na}$ (see discussion of Case 11-3).

### ANTICIPATE AND PREVENT DANGERS THAT MAY ARISE DURING THERAPY

There is no major emergency-related hypernatremia in the patient with chronic hypernatremia. When hypernatremia has been present for longer than 48 hours, brain cells may have gained sufficient number of effective osmoles to return their size to normal (see Figure 11-3). Thus, the danger in this setting is an error in the design of therapy that leads to a large, rapid fall in the $P_{Na}$, which may result in brain cell swelling, increased intracranial pressure, and possibly brain herniation. Hence, one should not permit the $P_{Na}$ to fall by more than 8 mmol/L per 24-hour period.

### DETERMINE THE APPROPRIATE RATE OF FALL IN THE $P_{Na}$

If hypernatremia is acute and there are significant symptoms that could be caused by acute hypernatremia (e.g., decreased level of consciousness, seizures), the $P_{Na}$ should be lowered rapidly, at least by 5% from its current level. If hypernatremia is acute but the patient is not very symptomatic, one should lower the $P_{Na}$ more slowly (e.g., by 1 to 2 mmol/L/hr). Because cerebral adaptation, with accumulation of organic osmolytes, is not likely to have proceeded to a sufficient degree, likely there is little risk for developing cerebral edema. Nevertheless, because the timeframe for this adaptive response is uncertain and may vary among patients, we prefer to limit the fall in $P_{Na}$ in this setting to 12 mmol/L in the first 24 hours.

    In patients with chronic hypernatremia, although there are no data from controlled trials, we recommend that the rate of fall in the $P_{Na}$

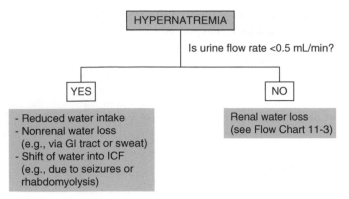

**Flow Chart 11-2 Hypernatremia: Assessing the Renal Response.** The objective is to assess whether vasopressin is present and acting on the kidney. If vasopressin is present and acting, the urine flow rate is expected to be <0.5 mL/min in an adult subject who consumes a typical Western diet (rate of excretion of effective osmoles (2 $U_{Na} + U_K$ is close to 450 mosmol/day), and the effective osmolality in the inner medullary interstitial compartment is close to 600 mosmol/kg $H_2O$. *GI,* Gastrointestinal; *ICF,* intracellular fluid.

should not exceed 8 mmol/L/24 hr. Specific issues related to the treatment of chronic hypernatremia are discussed later in this chapter.

### Recognize settings where the development of acute hypernatremia may be advantageous

Maintaining a degree of hypernatremia to minimize the rise in intracranial pressure may be beneficial in patients with other reasons for increased intracranial volume (e.g., cerebral edema fluid following recent neurosurgery or in patients with brain tumor, trauma, hemorrhage, or infection).

In patients with DKA, especially in children, it is essential to maintain a constant high $P_{Effective\ osm}$ during the first 15 hours of therapy to help prevent the development of cerebral edema. Therefore, when the $P_{Glucose}$ falls, the $P_{Na}$ must rise by half of the fall in $P_{Glucose}$ to keep the $P_{Effective\ osm}$ from decreasing. To achieve this aim, it is often necessary to create a degree of hypernatremia (see Chapter 5 for more discussion).

#### ASSESS THIRST AND THE APPROPRIATE RENAL RESPONSE TO HYPERNATREMIA

See Flow Chart 11-2.

#### DETERMINE THE CAUSE OF HYPERNATREMIA AND THE DESIGN OF THERAPY

A list of causes of hypernatremia is provided in Table 11-1. The tools used in the diagnostic approach to the cause of hypernatremia were discussed previously. The differential diagnosis of hypernatremia with a high urine flow rate is illustrated in Flow Chart 11-3.

The initial step in therapy in patients with central DI or DI due to a circulating vasopressinase is to stop ongoing water loss by giving dDAVP.

In patients with acute hypernatremia in a critical care setting, where balance data are usually available, calculating tonicity balance provides the optimal way to determine the basis of hypernatremia and to define the appropriate therapy to restore the volume and the composition of the ICF and ECF compartments.

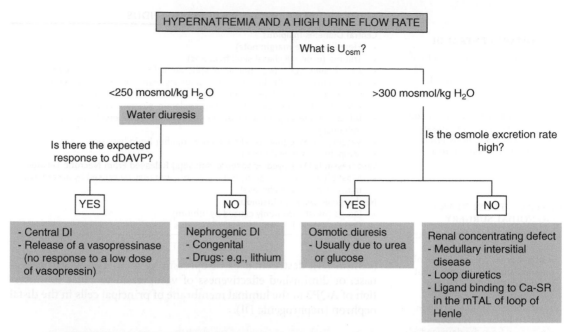

**Flow Chart 11-3  Hypernatremia With a High Urine Flow Rate.** The first step is to determine whether the water loss is caused by a water diuresis or an osmotic diuresis, or whether there is a renal concentrating defect. The principal tools are assessment of the $U_{Osm}$ and calculation of the osmole excretion rate. In a patient with central diabetes insipidus (DI) or a water diuresis caused by the release of a vasopressinase, $U_{Osm}$ should rise to a value that is higher than the $P_{Osm}$ in response to the administration of deamino-D-arginine vasopressin (dDAVP). If not, nephrogenic DI is the basis of the water diuresis. A value of the $U_{Osm}$ that is higher than 300 mosmol/kg $H_2O$ suggests that the basis of hypernatremia is an osmotic diuresis if the osmole excretion rate is appreciably higher than 1000 mosmol/day or a renal concentrating defect if the osmole excretion rate is not high. Examples of ligand binding to the calcium sensing receptor (Ca-SR) in the medullary thick ascending limb (mTAL) of the loop of Henle include calcium ions in a patient with hypercalcemia, cationic drugs (e.g., gentamicin, cisplatin).

Chronic hypernatremia that develops in an outpatient setting is most commonly caused by a deficit of water. Although patients who develop hypernatremia in the hospital may also have a deficit of water, in many, hypernatremia is caused in large part by a positive balance of $Na^+$ ions. In some patients with hypernatremia, there is a deficit of both $Na^+$ ions and water, with a proportionately larger deficit of water than of $Na^+$ ions. To determine the basis of hypernatremia and design therapy, one needs to perform a separate analysis of the balance for water and for $Na^+$ ions in the ICF and ECF compartments. We discuss this in detail in the section on therapy of hypernatremia.

# PART C
# SPECIFIC CAUSES OF HYPERNATREMIA

## DIABETES INSIPIDUS

DI is a group of disorders in which there is an inability of the kidneys to conserve water because of either decreased release of vasopressin

## HEREDITARY CENTRAL DI

- An autosomal dominant form of central DI can result from mutations in the gene that encodes neurophysin II, a carrier protein for vasopressin.
- These patients are asymptomatic at birth. Because of progressive decrease in vasopressin levels, polyuria and hypernatremia develop later in childhood.

## CENTRAL DI POST-TRANS-SPHENOIDAL SURGERY

- Although the incidence of central DI in the postoperative phase is about 20%, only about 2% of patients require long-term treatment with dDAVP.
- Syndrome of inappropriate antidiuretic hormone secretion (SIADH) because of vasopressin release from the damaged pituitary is observed in about 25% of patients. In a small number of patients, the clinical course follows a triphasic pattern, in which there is a transient initial phase of central DI, followed by a phase of SIADH, then permanent central DI.

TABLE 11-3  **ETIOLOGY OF DIABETES INSIPIDUS**

**Central Diabetes Insipidus**
- Hereditary (see margin note)
- Trauma (especially basal skull fractures)
- After brain surgery (e.g., post transspheniodal brain surgery; see margin note)
- Tumors involving the hypothalamic–pituitary region: primary (e.g., craniopharyngioma), secondary (e.g., lung cancer, leukemia, lymphoma)
- Infiltrative disorders involving the hypothalamic–pituitary region (e.g., sarcoidosis)
- Infections affecting the brain or the meninges (e.g., tuberculosis, histiocytosis, influenza)
- Vascular disease (e.g., cerebral aneurysm, after brain hypoxia)
- Idiopathic (may be familial)

**Vasopressin Is Destroyed by Vasopressinase(s) Released From Necrotic Tissues**
- Most often with retained necrotic placenta, but may be caused by other tissue injury (e.g., a large abscess)

**Nephrogenic Diabetes Insipidus**
- Drugs (most commonly caused by lithium)
- Congenital nephrogenic diabetes insipidus

(central DI), destruction of vasopressin by a circulating vasopressinase, or diminished effectiveness of vasopressin to cause the insertion of AQP2 in the luminal membrane of principal cells in the distal nephron (nephrogenic DI).

## CENTRAL DIABETES INSIPIDUS

In this disorder, there is decreased release of vasopressin because of an inborn error (hereditary central DI) or because of a lesion that compromises the osmostat, the site where vasopressin is synthesized (paraventricular and supraoptic nuclei in the hypothalamus), the neural pathway connecting the osmostat to these nuclei, the tracts connecting these nuclei to the posterior pituitary, and/or a lesion that involves the posterior pituitary. Clinically, a variety of infiltrative, neoplastic, vascular, and traumatic processes can be associated with abnormalities in vasopressin release (Table 11-3).

## CIRCULATING VASOPRESSINASE

The release of an enzyme (vasopressinase) that destroys vasopressin has been reported for the most part in patients with retained necrotic placenta, but it may also be seen with other diseases where there is extensive tissue injury (e.g., a large abscess). This group of peptidases targets the N-terminal amino group of vasopressin and/or its L-arginine. The hallmark of this diagnosis is that the kidney does not respond to a physiologic dose of vasopressin, but it does respond to a small dose of the vasopressin analog dDAVP because vasopressinase does not hydrolyze this compound.

## NEPHROGENIC DIABETES INSIPIDUS

This is a group of disorders in which there is diminished effectiveness of vasopressin to cause the insertion of AQP2 in the luminal membrane of principal cells in the distal nephron. The hallmark for the diagnosis of nephrogenic DI is a failure of dDAVP to cause an appreciable fall in the urine flow rate and a rise in the $U_{Osm}$ to a value that is $\geq P_{Osm}$.

### Congenital nephrogenic diabetes insipidus

Congenital nephrogenic DI is caused by mutations affecting the gene that encodes for the V2R or mutations affecting the gene that encodes for AQP2.

### Mutations in the V2R gene

The *V2R* gene is located on the X chromosome; thus, the disease follows an X-linked recessive inheritance pattern and affects males only. The vast majority of patients with congenital nephrogenic DI (~90%) have mutations in the *V2R* gene. These patients have a very large urine flow rate.

### Mutations in the AQP2 gene

Approximately 10% of patients with congenital nephrogenic DI have an autosomal dominant or autosomal recessive inherited disease. These families have mutations in the *AQP2* gene. In patients with the autosomal recessive form, mutations result in misrouting of the AQP2 and its retention within the endoplasmic reticulum. Patients with the autosomal dominant form have mutations in the carboxyl terminal of AQP2. The mutated AQP2 in this later group retains little capability of causing water permeability. Polyuria develops somewhat later in the first years of life rather than in the first months after birth. These patients may have lower urine volume (close to half that of patients with other types of congenital nephrogenic DI). They may also respond to large doses of dDAVP with a fall in the urine flow rate and a rise in the $U_{Osm}$.

## Lithium-induced nephrogenic diabetes insipidus

Lithium is used to treat bipolar disorders and is the most frequent cause of nephrogenic DI. Approximately 50% of patients on long-term lithium treatment develop nephrogenic DI. Lithium enters epithelial cells via the epithelial sodium channel (ENaC) on the apical membrane and leads to the inhibition of signaling pathways that involve glycogen synthase kinase-3 (GSK-3) (see margin note). Inhibition of GSK-3 reduces adenylate cyclase activity, cAMP generation, AQP2 phosphorylation, and their insertion into the luminal membrane of principal cells in the distal nephron. Inhibition of GSK-3 by lithium also leads to increased expression of cyclooxygenase-2 and the production of prostaglandin E2 by medullary interstitial cells. These prostaglandins then act on principal cells and decrease vasopressin-mediated generation of cAMP.

In addition to its effect on vasopressin signaling, lithium also causes nephrogenic DI by decreasing AQP2 protein abundance. Lithium causes a decrease in mRNA levels for AQP2 in cortical collecting duct cells, which suggests that lithium reduces *AQP2* gene transcription or mRNA stability.

It is interesting to note that lithium-induced nephrogenic DI often becomes irreversible even after the drug is discontinued, especially in patients who have been on the drug for more than 2 years. The mechanism for this irreversible nephrogenic DI is not clear (see margin note).

## Hypokalemia

Hypokalemia is often listed as a cause of nephrogenic DI. However, it is possible that chronic hypokalemia causes a renal concentrating defect rather than true nephrogenic DI.

Hypokalemia diminishes cAMP formation in response to vasopressin in MCD segments from rats in vitro. In addition, rats with hypokalemia have a decreased density of AQP2 in the luminal membrane of the distal nephron. To conclude, however, that the observed decreased expression of AQP2 is rate-limiting for the reabsorption of water, data are needed to show that the osmolality of the luminal fluid in the inner MCD is distinctly lower than the osmolality in the medullary interstitial compartment.

**GLYCOGEN SYNTHASE KINASE-3**

- GSK-3 was originally named for its ability to phosphorylate and inhibit glycogen synthase, a key regulator of glycogen synthesis.
- GSK-3 has been found to be ubiquitously expressed in cells, and has been identified as a critical enzyme that coordinates multiple signaling pathways that regulate cellular processes including gene transcription, cell cycle progression, and cell differentiation.

**IRREVERSIBLE NEPHROGENIC DI CAUSED BY LITHIUM**

- One possible explanation is that lithium may have an effect that modifies the gene encoding for AQP2 (e.g., methylation of cytosine bases or by another epigenetic mechanism) that causes a long-lasting inactivation of this gene.

On the other hand, patients with chronic hypokalemia may have a lower medullary interstitial osmolality resulting from the effect of chronic hypokalemia to cause medullary interstitial damage. In addition, potassium depletion has been shown to reduce the abundance of urea transporters in the renal medulla in mice. Therefore, urea may become an effective osmole in the inner MCD and obligate the excretion of water.

### Hypercalcemia

Hypercalcemia is thought to cause nephrogenic DI because it is associated with higher urine flow rates and $U_{Osm}$ values that are close to the $P_{Osm}$ when vasopressin acts. The finding that the calcium-sensing receptor (Ca-SR) colocalizes with AQP2 in vesicles derived from the inner MCD was thought to provide support for this conclusion. In addition, perfusion of inner MCD segments of the rat with a solution that has a high concentration of calcium ions resulted in a decrease in their water permeability. It is thought that nephrogenic DI caused by hypercalcemia and/or hypercalciuria would be beneficial because it would minimize the risk of precipitation of calcium-containing stones. As shown in Table 9-7, only a small increment in urine flow rate, which may be achieved by decreasing the number of AQP2 in the terminal nephron by endocytosis, is sufficient to diminish the risk of precipitation of calcium-containing stones in the terminal nephron without the need to develop nephrogenic DI that involves the entire late distal nephron.

There are clinical data to suggest that the observed higher urine flow rates and lower $U_{Osm}$ in subjects with hypercalcemia are not the result of true nephrogenic DI. First, the $U_{Osm}$ in patients with hypercalcemia is not lower than the $P_{Osm}$ when vasopressin acts. Second, in human subjects, the highest concentrations of calcium ions in the urine are observed in the urine of subjects with the lowest urine flow rate.

A more likely mechanism for the polyuria in patients with hypercalcemia is a saline-induced diuresis. This is caused by inhibition of NaCl reabsorption in the thick ascending limb of the loop of Henle. The mechanism begins with a high ionized calcium ($Ca^{2+}$) concentration in the renal medullary interstitial compartment; as a result, more ionized $Ca^{2+}$ binds to Ca-SR on the basolateral membrane of cells of the medullary thick ascending limb of the loop of Henle. This causes an effect akin to actions of a loop diuretic, with a higher rate of excretion of $Na^+$ and $Cl^-$ ions as well as a lower renal medullary interstitial effective osmolality (see Chapter 9).

### Renal concentrating defect

Water loss could be because of a renal concentrating defect caused by a low medullary interstitial effective osmolality. This could be because of medullary damage caused by medullary interstitial diseases including infections, infiltrations, or hypoxia (e.g., sickle cell disease); administration of loop diuretics; or occupancy of the calcium-sensing receptor in the thick ascending limb of the loop of Henle (e.g., by ionized $Ca^{2+}$ in a patient with hypercalcemia, by cationic drugs such as aminoglycosides, or by cationic proteins in patients with dysproteinemias).

Although the late distal nephron becomes permeable to water when vasopressin acts, the $U_{Osm}$ in these patients is not appreciably higher than the $P_{Osm}$ because the effective medullary interstitial osmolality is much lower than that in normal subjects. In addition, urea may become an effective osmole in the urine in these patients. In more detail, urea is not an effective urine osmole in normal subjects because vasopressin causes the insertion of urea transporters in the inner MCD, and therefore the concentration of urea in the lumen of the inner MCD and the inner medullary interstitial compartment are nearly equal. In patients with medullary interstitial disease involving the juxtamedullary nephrons, however, accumulation of urea in the medullary interstitial compartment is diminished. Hence, urea molecules in the lumen of the inner MCD become effective osmoles and obligate the excretion of water.

Therefore, if a patient were to excrete 450 mmol of urea and 450 mmol of electrolytes per day, and if this patient were to have a medullary interstitial osmolality of only 300 mosmol/kg H$_2$O, the urine volume will be 3 L/day. Thus, if the intake of water does not match this obligatory water loss, hypernatremia will develop.

## QUESTIONS

**11-2** *Why might the degree of polyuria be so much greater when the interstitial renal disease results from sickle cell anemia compared with other causes of renal medullary damage?*

11-3 *A patient with nephrogenic DI is treated with a loop diuretic to create a deficit of Na$^+$ ions. His $U_{Osm}$ rose from 100 to 200 mosmol/kg H$_2$O. Did his nephrogenic DI improve with this therapy?*

### Hypernatremia caused by a shift of water

In some circumstances, hypernatremia may be caused by a shift of water from the ECF compartment into cells. The basis for this water shift is a gain of effective osmoles in cells. The cells involved are almost always skeletal muscle cells because this is where most of the water in the body exists. The usual causes are seizures or mild rhabdomyolysis. A second example of this phenomenon is a shift of water into the lumen of the intestinal tract due to accumulation of a large number of osmoles from digestion of food in a patient with very slow intestinal motility (see discussion of Case 11-3).

The diagnosis is suspected from the clinical history, the absence of a change in body weight, and the presence of ECF volume contraction. Notwithstanding, the threat for brain cell shrinkage is just as important as when hypernatremia is caused by a gain of Na$^+$ ions or a total body water deficit.

### Hypernatremia and polyuria in geriatric patients

There are three settings where chronic hypernatremia may develop in geriatric patients. First, when there is a low intake of water; second, if urea-induced osmotic diuresis develops in a patient on protein supplements; and third, when a loop diuretic is given to a patient who has congestive heart failure.

#### Low water intake

Elderly patients may have the combination of a cause of water loss (e.g., fever), reduced sense of thirst, and an inability to communicate or complain of thirst and/or to gain access to water (e.g., because of a previous stroke). If this goes on for a period of time, hypernatremia may develop.

#### Urea-induced osmotic diuresis

When protein supplements are given to these patients, there is an increased production and excretion of urea. Nevertheless, the amount of urea excreted is less than that in subjects who consume a typical Western diet. Hence, there must be other reasons for the urea-induced osmotic diuresis and water loss to be large enough to lead to the development of hypernatremia. These patients often have medullary interstitial disease. Hence, accumulation of urea in the medullary interstitial compartment is diminished and urea becomes an effective osmole in the lumen of the inner MCD, which obligates the excretion of water. If water intake is also reduced, hypernatremia may develop.

### *Use of a loop diuretic in a patient who has congestive heart failure*

The basis for hypernatremia in this setting has two major components. First, there is the excretion of a large volume of urine with a relatively low concentration of $Na^+ + K^+$ ions. This results from the actions of the loop diuretic, which causes the excretion of a large quantity of $Na^+$ and $Cl^-$ ions, especially with mobilization of edema fluid. Because the $U_{Osm}$ is usually close to 350 mosmol/kg $H_2O$, the effective $U_{Osm}$ must be low. This is because of the actions of the loop diuretic to decrease the reabsorption of $Na^+$ and $Cl^-$ ions in the medullary thick ascending limb of the loop of Henle and also cause medullary washout by increasing medullary blood flow (see margin note). Hence, a large quantity of $Na^+$ and $Cl^-$ ions is excreted in hypotonic urine, which results in increased loss of electrolyte-free water. In addition, urea may become, at least in part, an effective urine osmole in this setting and obligate the excretion of water (see margin note).

Despite the increased water loss, most patients in this setting develop hyponatremia. This may be caused by increased thirst and the intake of water because of stimulation of the osmostat by angiotensin II, released because of decreased EABV. Hence, the second component for the development of hypernatremia in these patients is the failure to appreciate or communicate thirst and/or an inability to obtain water.

## TREATMENT OF PATIENTS WITH HYPERNATREMIA

### ACUTE HYPERNATREMIA

This topic was discussed earlier in this chapter.

### CHRONIC HYPERNATREMIA

Chronic hypernatremia may be associated with some symptoms such as generalized malaise. The danger to the patient, however, is brain swelling, which may result in increased intracranial pressure and the risk of brain herniation if there is a rapid fall in the $P_{Na}$. Although there are no data from controlled trials, we recommend that the rate of fall in the $P_{Na}$ should not exceed 8 mmol/L/24 hr.

Chronic hypernatremia is most commonly caused by a deficit of water. The initial step in therapy in these patients is to stop ongoing water loss by giving dDAVP to the patient with central DI or circulating vasopressinase. The design of therapy should be to restore the volume and composition of both the ICF and ECF compartments. This requires performing a separate analysis for the balance of water and of $Na^+$ ions in both the ICF and ECF compartments. Although there is a water deficit in the ICF that should be replaced, therapy for the ECF compartment depends on the status of the ECF volume. To illustrate these points, consider the example of two female patients who, before developing hypernatremia, weighed 60 kg each and had a total body water of 30 L. In each of them, the $P_{Na}$ rose from 140 mmo/L to 154 mmol/L. Based on clinical assessment, one patient was thought to have a normal ECF volume of 10 L, while the other patient was thought to have a contracted the ECF volume of 7 L (see Chapter 2 for a discussion on the use of hematocrit to obtain a quantitative assessment of

**FALL IN $U_{Osm}$ WITH ADMINISTRATION OF A LOOP DIURETIC**

- The concentration of urea may also decline in the inner medullary interstitial compartment because of urea washout caused by an increase in vasa recta blood flow because of the effect of loop diuretics. This may also explain the fall in $U_{Osm}$.

**EXALTATION OF UREA**

- The concentration of urea in the lumen of the inner MCD may become very low because of the large volume of luminal fluid caused by the effect of diuretics. Hence, a concentration difference for urea is created to permit the passive movement of urea from the interstitial compartment into the lumen of the inner MCD. Therefore, urea is actually secreted in this setting; this was called "exaltation of urea" in the older literature. Hence, urea may become, at least in part, an effective urine osmole and contribute to water loss in this setting.

the ECF volume). Clearly, a number of assumptions are made in these calculations; therefore, they are only meant to provide a rough guide to the design of therapy.

### Intracellular fluid analysis

A high $P_{Na}$ indicates that there is a water deficit in the ICF compartment with rare exceptions when hypernatremia is caused by a shift of water into the ICF of muscle (e.g., a patient with hypernatremia following a seizure or rhabdomyolysis). The amount of water needed to restore the ICF tonicity and volume can be estimated using the following calculation. For this calculation, we have made two assumptions: first, the normal ICF volume is two-thirds of the total body water; second, the number of particles in the ICF compartment does not change appreciably.

$$\text{ICF } H_2O \text{ deficit} = \text{Normal ICF volume} - \text{Current ICF volume}$$

$$\text{Current ICF volume} = \text{Normal } P_{Na} \text{ (140 mmol/L)} \times \text{Normal ICF volume (20 L)/Current } P_{Na} \text{ (154 mmol/L)}$$

Based on this calculation, there is a water deficit in the ICF in each of these two patients of 2 L.

### Extracellular fluid analysis

#### Patient 1 has a normal ECF volume (10 L)

With a $P_{Na}$ of 154 mmol/L and a normal ECF volume of 10 L, there is a positive balance of 140 mmol of $Na^+$ ions ($154 - 140$ mmol/L $\times$ 10 L) in the ECF compartment.

#### Patient 2 has an estimated ECF volume of 7 L

This patient has a water deficit in her ECF compartment of 3 L. Because the content of $Na^+$ ions in her ECF compartment now is 1078 mmol (154 mmol/L $\times$ 7 L) instead of 1400 mmol (140 mmol/L $\times$ 10 L), she has a deficit of about 320 mmol of $Na^+$ ions.

#### Therapy for patient 1

Overall, there is a negative balance of 2 L of water and a positive balance of 140 mmol of $Na^+$ ions. To lower the $P_{Na}$ by about 7 mmol/L (half of the rise in $P_{Na}$ of 14 mmol/L) on day 1, the goal of therapy is to create a positive balance of 1 L of water and a negative balance of 70 mmol of $Na^+$ ions. Depending on the actual fall in $P_{Na}$ on day 1, the plan of therapy on day 2 should be determined along the same goals.

#### Therapy for patient 2

This patient has a negative balance of 5 L of water (2 L from the ICF compartment and 3 L from the ECF compartment) and a negative balance of about 320 mmol $Na^+$ ions. There is also a significant degree of ECF and EABV contraction. If the patient were hemodynamically unstable, we would initially infuse isotonic saline to restore hemodynamic stability. Because this is an isotonic solution to the patient (and in fact could be a bit hypotonic in a patient with a more severe degree of hypernatremia), there will be little change in the $P_{Na}$. A positive balance of the remaining deficit of $Na^+$ ions and water can then be induced with the infusion of a hypotonic saline solution to lower the $P_{Na}$ by about 8 mmol/L/day.

# PART D
# INTEGRATIVE PHYSIOLOGY

## NEPHROGENIC DIABETES INSIPIDUS IN THE NEWBORN

Newborns have nephrogenic DI because they fail to insert a sufficient number of AQP2 into the luminal membrane of cells in the distal nephron when vasopressin is present (or after it is administered). To understand the integrative physiology of this process, one needs to examine it from the perspective of whether it was required for survival. In this context, survival depends on having enough adenosine triphosphate (ATP) to perform essential biologic work. The main (almost only) fuel that can be oxidized to regenerate ATP in the brain of the newborn is glucose. In fact, hypoglycemia poses a unique threat in the first month of life because the metabolic requirements of the brain are high, the availability of circulating ketoacids is low, and the size of storage pools of glucose is quite small. Therefore, the newborn needs a constant supply of sugar from the only source of exogenous caloric intake, mother's milk, to avoid neuroglycopenia. This source of brain fuel provides a large water load that the newborn must eliminate promptly (see margin note). Although some of this water is used for evaporative heat dissipation, a large volume of water must be excreted in the urine. Hence, a physiologic form of nephrogenic DI may provide a survival advantage because it permits rapid excretion of the large water load from milk. This could also lead to both thirst and a wet diaper and, hence, a cry for a source of sugar.

Having neonatal nephrogenic DI may provide another advantage. If the infant were to have a nonosmotic stimulus for the release of vasopressin (e.g., nausea, pain, distress), a severe degree of acute hyponatremia would not develop. Although a small degree of brain cell swelling can easily be accommodated by the large open fontanelles in the skull, there could be problems for two reasons: The daily intake of water is very large, and there could also be rapid absorption of water in the intestine, which lowers the arterial $P_{Na}$ (i.e., akin to gulping water; see Chapter 9 for more discussion).

### WATER LOAD FROM BREAST MILK

- A newborn drinks close to 150 mL of milk per kg of body weight per day (i.e., 15% of body weight). This is equivalent to 7.5 L/day in a 50-kg adult. Hence, this water must be excreted promptly to avoid a serious degree of acute hyponatremia (i.e., retention of this daily intake of water would cause the $P_{Na}$ to fall from 140 to 120 mmol/L).

## DISCUSSION OF CASES

### CASE 11-1: CONCENTRATE ON THE DANGER

#### Why did hypernatremia develop?

Several facts are obvious. This patient has DI because he is excreting dilute urine ($U_{Osm}$ was 120 mosmol/kg $H_2O$) despite the presence of hypernatremia ($P_{Na}$ was 150 mmol/L). This indicates that vasopressin either has not been released, has been destroyed by a vasopressinase released from damaged tissues, or has failed to act on principal cells in the distal nephron. The most likely diagnosis is central DI because the patient had neurosurgery there was a prompt response to the administration of dDAVP. Although it is tempting to conclude that the basis for hypernatremia is a deficit of water caused by the excretion of a large volume of dilute urine, data are available to calculate balances for $Na^+$ ion and for water (tonicity balance) to determine the basis

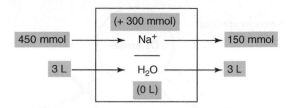

**Figure 11-6 Tonicity Balance in Case 11-1.** The patient received 3 L of isotonic saline (450 mmol of Na⁺ ions) and excreted 3 L of urine with a concentration of Na⁺+K⁺ ions of 50 mmol/L (150 mmol). Hence, there is a positive balance of 300 mmol of Na⁺ and nil balance for water.

of hypernatremia. As shown in Figure 11-6, the volumes of the input and output of water were equal. Therefore, the basis for hypernatremia is a positive balance for Na⁺ ions. The concentration of Na⁺ ions in the infusate was 150 mmol/L, whereas the concentration of Na⁺ ions in the urine was only 50 mmol/L, yielding a positive balance of 300 mmol of Na⁺ ions. Since his body weight was 50 kg, his total body water would be about 30 L. Therefore, the rise in his $P_{Na}$ should be 10 mmol/L (300 mmol/30 L), and, in fact, his $P_{Na}$ rose from 140 to 150 mmol/L.

### What are the goals for therapy of his hypernatremia?

Because hypernatremia was caused by a positive balance of 300 mmol of Na⁺ ions, efforts should be made to cause the patient to lose 300 mmol of Na⁺ ions while maintaining a nil balance for water. Although hypernatremia in this patient is acute, it is likely that there has been edema of the brain after surgery; therefore, it might be advisable to aim for a $P_{Na}$ that is close to 145 mmol/L for the next 24 hours. If intracranial pressure is being monitored, this may provide a useful guide to therapy.

To lower $P_{Na}$ by creating a negative balance of Na⁺ ions, the concentration of Na⁺ ions in the infusate should be lower than that in the urine while water balance is maintained by infusing fluid at a rate that is equal to the urine flow rate. After dDAVP was given, the patient's $U_{Na}$ was 175 mmol/L. Hence, infusion of 1.5 L half-isotonic saline (75 mmol/L) over the time period during which 1.5 liters of urine is excreted, would create a negative balance of 150 mmol of Na⁺ ions and lower his $P_{Na}$ to 145 mmol/L.

### CASE 11-2: WHAT IS "PARTIAL" ABOUT PARTIAL CENTRAL DIABETES INSIPIDUS?

### What is the basis for the high urine flow rate in this patient?

Because the patient's $U_{Osm}$ was 200 mosmol/kg $H_2O$ and the urine volume was 4 L/day, this was a water diuresis with the usual total osmole excretion rate for a subject consuming a typical Western diet (800 mosmol/day). The patient had an adequate renal response to dDAVP because his $U_{Osm}$ rose to 900 mosmol/kg $H_2O$. Hence, he had central DI. Because his urine volume was only 4 L/day and not 10 to 15 L/day, the diagnosis was partial central DI.

### *Central DI*

Although the diagnosis of central DI was straightforward, it remains unclear as to the site of the lesion that may cause a "partial" central

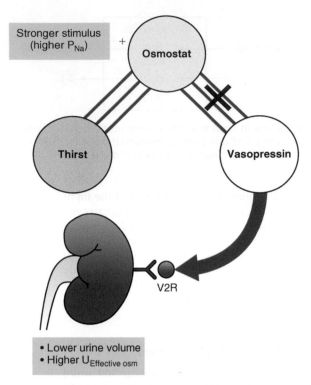

**Figure 11-7 Lesion Causing "Partial" Central Diabetes Insipidus.** The *upper circle* labeled "osmostat" is the sensor, the *lower left circle* is the thirst center, and the *lower right circle* is the vasopressin release center. The *X* represents a hypothetical lesion that causes severing of some but not all of the fibers connecting the osmostat to the vasopressin release center. A stronger stimulus (higher $P_{Na}$) causes the release of vasopressin, and hence a lower urine volume and a higher urine effective osmolality ($U_{Effective\ osm}$). *V2R*, Vasopressin receptor 2.

DI. Because he complained of thirst, the patient's osmostat, thirst center, as well as the fibers connecting them appeared to be functionally intact (see Figure 11-4). Similarly, because the $U_{Osm}$ was greater than the $P_{Osm}$ in the first-voided morning urine ($U_{Osm}$ was 425 mosmol/kg $H_2O$ when the $P_{Na}$ was 143 mmol/L), the vasopressin release center seemed to function but only when there was a relatively strong stimulus for the release of this hormone. In keeping with this hypothesis is the fact that the urine flow rate fell to 0.5 mL/min and the $U_{Osm}$ rose to 900 mosmol/kg $H_2O$ after an infusion of hypertonic saline. Therefore, a possible site for the lesion is destruction of some but not all of the fibers linking the osmostat to the vasopressin release center (Figure 11-7). Such a lesion might explain why polyuria was not present overnight if the patient stopped water intake several hours prior to going to sleep because this might have caused his $P_{Na}$ to rise sufficiently to stimulate the release of vasopressin.

### Primary polydipsia

The patient's $P_{Na}$ was high enough early in the morning (143 mmol/L) to stimulate the release of vasopressin. In contrast, during the daytime, his $P_{Na}$ was 137 mmol/L and his $U_{Osm}$ was consistently around 90 mosmol/kg $H_2O$, which suggest that primary polydipsia was present while he was awake. Its basis was likely a "learned behavior" to avoid the uncomfortable feeling of thirst.

This interpretation provides a rationale to understand the patho-physiology and, importantly, how to define the options for treatment of his partial central DI.

## What are the options for therapy?

A higher $P_{Na}$ in this patient could stimulate the release of vasopressin. There are two ways to raise the $P_{Na}$: a positive balance of $Na^+$ ions or a negative balance of water. The patient selected the intake of NaCl tablets to raise his $P_{Na}$ during waking hours. This therapy avoided the risk of acute hyponatremia, which may occur if he were given dDAVP and were to drink an excessive quantity of water by habit. In contrast, he selected water deprivation to raise his $P_{Na}$ overnight to permit him to have undisturbed sleep.

## CASE 11-3: WHERE DID THE WATER GO?

### What is the basis for the hypernatremia (in quantitative terms): a positive balance for $Na^+$ ions and/or a negative balance for water?

#### A gain of $Na^+$ ions

In quantitative terms, if a gain of $Na^+$ ions is the basis of hyperna-tremia, there should be a positive balance of more than 1100 mmol of NaCl (see margin note). It is highly unlikely that the patient has consumed this much NaCl. Both the physical examination and the unchanged value for his hematocrit (0.36), hemoglobin (125 g/L), and $P_{Albumin}$ (38 g/L) indicate that his ECF volume was not expanded as would be expected from this large gain of $Na^+$ ions. Therefore, it is unlikely that a large positive balance of $Na^+$ ions is the major cause of his hypernatremia.

#### A deficit of water

There was no obvious source of electrolyte-free water loss, and the EABV was not obviously contracted. In addition, he had a weight gain of 1 kg instead of a loss of 20% of total body water (~8 L or 8 kg) if the cause of hypernatremia was a water deficit (see mar-gin note). Therefore, a water deficit is not likely to be the cause of his hypernatremia.

### Why does he have such a severe degree of hypernatremia?

Because the sudden rise in the $P_{Na}$ cannot be explained simply by a gain of $Na^+$ ions or a deficit of water, there must be an internal shift of $Na^+$ ions or water to explain this acute and large rise in the $P_{Na}$.

#### A shift of water

There are two requirements for a large shift of water from the ECF compartment to another compartment.

1. This compartment must be large to accommodate about 8 L of wa-ter. Based on this consideration, the only organ in the body that is large enough is skeletal muscle. As discussed previously in this chapter, the driving force for a shift of water is a gain of effective osmoles in muscle cells during a seizure or because of rhabdomyol-ysis. Against this possibility, the patient did not have a seizure, and it is also unlikely that he had rhabdomyolysis because his plasma creatine kinase level was not elevated.

---

**GAIN OF $Na^+$ IONS AS A CAUSE OF A $P_{Na}$ OF 169 mmol/L**

- The calculation is based on total body water of 40 L (50% of 80 kg body weight because of a degree of obesity).
- With an acute rise in $P_{Na}$ of 29 mmol/L, his positive balance for $Na^+$ ions would have to be greater than 1000 mmol (40 L×29 mmol/L=1160 mmol). This is more than a 50% increase in the content of $Na^+$ ions in his ECF compartment (~14 L × 140 mmol/L=~2000 mmol).
- His ECF volume should be expanded by almost 5 L (content of $Na^+$ ions in ECF compartment = 3160 mmol, divided by the concentration of $Na^+$ in the ECF compartment = 169 mmol/L; there-fore, new ECF volume = 18.7 L. This is unlikely in view of the absence of overt signs of ECF volume expansion.

**WATER DEFICIT AS A CAUSE OF $P_{Na}$ OF 169 mmol/L**

- The rise in his $P_{Na}$ is 29 mmol/L, which is a 20% rise (29/140 mmol/L). Hence, the water deficit should be 20% of his total body water of 40 L, or 8 L.

2. This compartment must be able to "stretch" to accommodate this huge volume. Accordingly, another possible site for a large water shift is the lumen of the intestinal tract. The force to move water is a large rise in the number of effective osmoles in the lumen of the small intestine.

The fact that a shift of water into the lumen of the small intestine occurs in normal subjects after a meal has been demonstrated by measuring the $P_{Na}$ before and during the digestion of a meal containing a small amount of $Na^+$ ions. A typical rise in the $P_{Na}$ is about 3 mmol/L, even though there is secretion of $Na^+$ ions into the lumen of the intestine. To have a much larger rise in the $P_{Na}$, one would need a longer time period (e.g., because of low intestinal motility, perhaps the result of autonomic neuropathy secondary to long-standing type 2 diabetes mellitus) and a larger number of osmoles produced by digestion of dietary constituents (e.g., glucose and amino acids), which remain in the intestinal lumen. In this regard, the usual dietary intake of 270 g of carbohydrate (1500 mmol of glucose) and 1.5 g of protein per kg body weight (~1000 mmol of amino acids in an adult) are within the range of the number of osmoles needed to cause a sufficiently large and acute shift of water to be responsible for the very high $P_{Na}$.

Because there was no obvious contraction of the EABV, when water shifted into the lumen of the small intestine, it appears that some effective osmoles (i.e., $Na^+$ and $Cl^-$ ions) were absorbed from his dietary intake. Therefore, we suspect that the rise in $P_{Na}$ reflects the combination of water shift from the body into the lumen of the intestinal tract and the addition of $Na^+$ ions to the ECF compartment.

### What is the therapy of hypernatremia in this patient?

The major threat at this moment is intracranial hemorrhage caused by acute hypernatremia leading to shrinkage of brain cell volume, which stretches the blood vessels that come from the inner lining of the skull and may cause them to rupture.

It is important to recognize that we do not know whether his $P_{Na}$ will rise further as a result of a continuing shift of water into the lumen of his intestinal tract, or whether the opposite may happen because an increase in the gastrointestinal motility may lead to the absorption of glucose, amino acids, and water, and therefore cause a large fall in his $P_{Na}$. Hence, the most important initial therapy is to remove the contents of his stomach and upper intestinal tract by inserting a nasogastric tube and using suction. We would prefer to lower his $P_{Na}$ by close to 10 mmol/L and then re-evaluate the situation and determine further therapy, but this is just our opinion. Because the patient is not symptomatic, we would give water through the gastrointestinal tract. The volume of water needed to cause a fall in the $P_{Na}$ by 10 mmol/L is about 2.5 L. It is very unlikely that there is a large positive balance of $Na^+$ ions. In fact, a positive balance of $Na^+$ ions was valuable because it helped prevent a large degree of contraction of his EABV owing to the very large shift of water. Accordingly, we would not remove much of this $Na^+$ ion load by the administration of a natriuretic agent until a large volume of water has been added to his body, unless he develops symptoms related to an expanded EABV.

## DISCUSSION OF QUESTIONS

*11-1  A 50-kg man receives 3 L of isotonic saline (150 mmol/L) and excretes 3 L of urine with an unknown concentration of $Na^+$*

*ions. During this period, his $P_{Na}$ rises from 140 to 150 mmol/L. If there is no other input or output during this period, what is the concentration of $Na^+$ ions in mmol/L in this urine?*

To answer this question, examine the balances for water and for $Na^+$ and $K^+$ ions. Because water balance is neutral, and the $P_{Na}$ rose by 10 mmol/L, this patient retained 300 mmol of $Na^+$ ions (150 − 140 mmol/L = 10 mmol/L, multiplied by total body water of 30 L = 300 mmol). Because 450 mmol of $Na^+$ ions were infused (3 L × 150 mmol/L) and 300 mmol were retained, the urine must have contained 150 mmol of $Na^+$ ions. With a urine volume of 3 L, the concentration of $Na^+$ ions in the urine is 50 mmol/L (150 mmol ÷ 3 L).

*11-2  Why might the degree of polyuria be much greater when the interstitial renal disease results from sickle cell anemia compared with other causes of renal medullary damage?*

The volume of an osmotic diuresis is inversely proportional to the effective osmolality of the medullary interstitial compartment and directly proportional to the number of effective osmoles being excreted. With respect to the medullary interstitial effective osmolality, it makes no difference whether this osmolality is reduced because of sickle cell anemia or because of a different etiology. Conversely, in patients with sickle cell anemia, the number of effective urine osmoles may be increased without an increase in the total number of osmoles excreted. This occurs because red blood cells sickle in a hypoxic, hyperosmolar environment (e.g., in the inner medulla). As a result, this area may become damaged. Because this is the major site where urea transporters are present in the luminal membrane of cells in the MCD, less urea is reabsorbed; therefore, urea is now an effective urine osmole. This can cause the rate of excretion of effective osmoles to double because the number of urea osmoles are typically half of the total number of urine osmoles; the other half is electrolyte osmoles.

*11-3  A patient with nephrogenic DI is treated with a loop diuretic to create a deficit of $Na^+$ ions. His $U_{Osm}$ rose from 100 to 200 mosmol/kg $H_2O$. Did his nephrogenic DI improve with this therapy?*

When a loop diuretic acts, there is a large increase in the quantity of $Na^+$ ions delivered to the distal nephron. As a result of having more osmoles to excrete, the $U_{Osm}$ rises, but this rise in $U_{Osm}$ does not indicate that more water was reabsorbed in the late distal nephron. If the administration of a loop diuretic, however, leads to decreased EABV, the urine flow rate may decrease and the $U_{Osm}$ may rise as a result of decreased volume of distal delivery of filtrate. This, however, should not be interpreted to indicate that the administration of a loop diuretic led to an improvement in his nephrogenic DI because there was no increase in the number of AQP2 inserted into the luminal membrane of principal cells in the distal nephron.

chapter 12

# Polyuria

# Introduction

**ABBREVIATIONS**

DI, diabetes insipidus
RWP, residual water permeability
MCD, medullary collecting duct
$P_{Na}$, concentration of sodium
  ($Na^+$) ions in plasma
$U_{Osm}$, urine osmolality
$P_{Osm}$, plasma osmolality
AQP, aquaporin water channel
PCT, proximal convoluted tubule
DCT, distal convoluted tubule
DtL, descending thin limb
TAL, thick ascending limb
MCD, medullary collecting duct
EABV, effective arterial blood volume
V2R, vasopressin receptor 2
$P_{Glucose}$, concentration of glucose in
  plasma
$P_{Urea}$, concentration of urea in plasma

Polyuria is caused by either a water diuresis or an osmotic diuresis. Many patients who present with polyuria also have hypernatremia because they excrete a large volume of urine with a low concentration of sodium ($Na^+$) plus potassium ($K^+$) ions (e.g., patients with diabetes insipidus [DI] or patients with a urea-induced osmotic diuresis). Therefore, there are areas of overlap between this chapter and the previous one on hypernatremia. Nevertheless, there are a number of issues that are pertinent to polyuria, which are the focus of this chapter.

## OBJECTIVES

- To illustrate polyuria should not be defined based on a urine volume that is larger than the usual but on a urine volume that is larger than appropriate for the clinical setting.
- To illustrate that a large water diuresis can occur only if the distal nephron is virtually impermeable to water because of lack of actions of vasopressin. In this setting, the magnitude of the water diuresis depends on the volume of hypotonic fluid delivered to the distal nephron and on how much water is reabsorbed via residual water permeability (RWP) in the inner medullary collecting duct (MCD).
- To emphasize that because actions of vasopressin must be present during an osmotic diuresis, the urine flow rate is determined by the number of effective osmoles delivered to the distal nephron and the effective osmolality in the medullary interstitial compartment.
- To provide a clinical approach to the diagnosis and the management of the patient with polyuria.

### CASE 12-1: OLIGURIA WITH A URINE VOLUME OF 4 L PER DAY

This is a 22-year-old woman who runs 5 to 10 km each day to keep fit. She is very careful not to eat "unhealthy" foods, and restricts her salt intake. She lives in a hot climate and drinks a large volume of water to keep hydrated. Her urine volume is close to 4 L/day. On repeated measurements done on visits to the office of her physician, the concentration of $Na^+$ ions in her plasma ($P_{Na}$) was 130 mmol/L, and her urine osmolality ($U_{Osm}$) in multiple random urine samples was close to 80 mosmol/kg $H_2O$.

**Questions**

Does this patient have polyuria?
What dangers related to $Na^+$ and water issues may develop in this patient?

### CASE 12-2: MORE THAN JUST SALT AND WATER LOSS

A 70-kg man had a recent bone marrow transplant. His treatment included high doses of intravenous methylprednisolone. He developed sepsis over the past 24 hours. His 24-hour urine volume in this period was 6 L and the $U_{Osm}$ in a random urine sample was 500 mosmol/kg $H_2O$. He has not received mannitol. His $P_{Glucose}$ was 180 mg/dL (10 mmol/L) and his $P_{Urea}$ was 75 mmol/L (blood urea nitrogen 210 mg/dL).

**Questions**

Does this patient have an osmotic diuresis?
What is the source of urea? What are the implications for therapy?

# PART A
# BACKGROUND

## SYNOPSIS OF THE PHYSIOLOGY

### WATER DIURESIS

Following a large intake of water that lowered the $P_{Na}$ sufficiently to inhibit the release of vasopressin, aquaporin 2 water channels (AQP2) are not inserted into the luminal membranes of principal cells in the collecting ducts. Therefore, these nephron segments are now impermeable to water and the volume of filtrate delivered to the distal nephron will be excreted in the urine (except for the volume that is reabsorbed in the inner MCD via its residual water permeability, which does not require the presence of vasopressin) (Figure 12-1). Typical values for peak urine flow rates in a normal human adult are 10 to 15 mL/min, which occurs 60 to 90 minutes after the rapid ingestion of a large water load. Extrapolated to a 24 hour period, the urine volume would be ~15 to 22 L.

### Distal Delivery of Filtrate

The volume of distal delivery of filtrate is the volume of glomerular filtration minus the volume of filtrate that is reabsorbed in the nephron segments prior to the late cortical distal nephron. The volume of filtrate that is delivered to the distal nephron can be estimated in human subjects

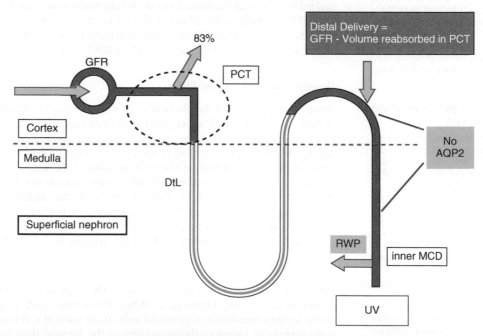

**Figure 12-1 Determinants of the Urine Volume During a Water Diuresis.** The stylized figure represents a superficial nephron. Aquaporin-1 channels are not present in the luminal membranes of the descending thin limb (DtL) of the loop of Henle of the superficial nephrons (about 85% of all the nephrons). Therefore, the entire loop of Henle of these nephrons is impermeable to water. In the absence of vasopressin actions, AQP2 water channels are not present in the luminal membrane of principal cells in the cortical and medullary collecting ducts. The urine flow rate in this setting is set by the volume of filtrate delivered to the distal nephron minus the volume of water reabsorbed via residual water permeability (RWP) in the inner medullary collecting duct. The volume of distal delivery of filtrate is the volume of glomerular filtrate minus the volume of filtrate that is reabsorbed in the entire proximal convoluted tubule (PCT), including its pars recta segment. This latter is about 83% of the glomerular filtration rate (GFR). *UV*, Urine volume.

## FRACTION OF GLOMERULAR FILTRATE REABSORBED IN PROXIMAL CONVOLUTED TUBULE

- It was thought that about 66% of the GFR is reabsorbed along the entire proximal convoluted tubule (PCT). This was based on the measured $(TF/P)_{inulin}$ of around 3 in micropuncture studies in rats.
- However, these micropuncture measurements underestimate the volume of fluid reabsorbed in the PCT because measurements were made at the last portion of the PCT at the surface of the renal cortex and therefore did not take into account that additional volume may be reabsorbed in the deeper parts of the PCT, including its pars recta portion.
- Findings now suggest that AQP1 are not present in the luminal membranes of the descending thin limbs (DtLs) of the superficial nephrons, which represent about 85% of all the nephrons. Therefore, the entire loop of Henle of the majority of nephrons is impermeable to water. Hence, the volume of filtrate that enters their loops of Henle can be deduced from the minimum value for the $(TF/P)_{inulin}$ obtained using the micropuncture technique from the early DCT. This value is around 6; therefore, a reasonable estimate of the proportion of filtrate that is reabsorbed in the rat PCT is close to five-sixths (83%).

## VOLUME OF DISTAL DELIVERY OF FILTRATE

- Juxtamedullary nephrons have AQP1 along their DtLs. If these nephrons are 15% of the total nephrons and receive 27 L of glomerular filtrate per day (15% of 180 L/day), and if 83% of the glomerular filtrate of these nephrons is reabsorbed along their PCTs, 4.5 L/day reach their DtLs.
- Because the interstitial osmolality rises threefold (from 300 to 900 mosmol/kg $H_2O$) in the outer medulla, two-thirds, or 3 L of the 4.5 L, is reabsorbed in the DtLs of these nephrons per day. Therefore, the volume of filtrate delivered to DCTs is likely to be 27 L/day (30 L/day exit the PCTs minus 3 L/day that are reabsorbed in DtLs of the juxtamedullary nephrons; see Table 9-3).

based on the measured ratio of concentration of inulin in tubular fluid (TF) from the late distal convoluted tubule (DCT) in comparison with that in plasma (P)—$(TF/P)_{inulin}$—in micropuncture studies in rats. Because inulin is freely filtered at the glomerulus and is not reabsorbed or secreted in the tubules, a $(TF/P)_{inulin}$ value of around 6 suggests that approximately 83% of the filtrate was reabsorbed prior to the last accessible part of the DCT for micropuncture. If these data can be extrapolated to human subjects with a glomerular filtration rate (GFR) of 180 L/day, then 30 L of filtrate would be delivered to the early cortical distal nephron daily. As detailed in Chapter 9 and described briefly here in the margin notes, the volume of distal delivery of filtrate in an adult human subject with a GFR of 180 L/day is likely about 27 L/day (*see margin note*).

### Residual Water Permeability

There are two pathways for transport of water in the inner MCD: a vasopressin-responsive system via AQP2 and a vasopressin-independent system called RWP. Two factors may affect the volume of water reabsorbed via RWP. The driving force is the enormous difference in osmotic pressure between the luminal fluid and the medullary interstitial compartment in the inner MCD during a water diuresis. The second factor is contraction of the renal pelvis. Each time the renal pelvis contracts, some of the fluid in the renal pelvis travels in a retrograde direction up toward the inner MCD, and some of that fluid may be reabsorbed via RWP after it enters the inner MCD for a second (or a third) time, especially if there is some turbulence, which aids diffusion and prolongs contact time.

We calculated that 27 L/day are delivered to the distal nephron in a normal subject. Because the urine flow rate during maximum water diuresis is around 10 to 15 mL/min (~15 to 22 L/day), if this maximum water diuresis could be maintained for 24 hours, somewhat more than 5 L of water would be reabsorbed per day in the inner MCD via RWP during water diuresis.

### Desalination of Luminal Fluid

Another component of the physiology of water diuresis is desalination of luminal fluid in nephron segments that can reabsorb $Na^+$ ions but lack a water channel. This desalination process occurs in the cortical and medullary thick ascending limbs (TALs) of the loop of Henle and the early DCT. Regulation of the reabsorption of $Na^+$ and $Cl^-$ ions in the medullary TAL of the loop of Henle seems to occur via dilution of the concentration of an inhibitor of this process in the medullary interstitial compartment (possibly ionized calcium, Fig. 9-17) by water that is reabsorbed from the water-permeable nephron segments in the renal medulla (i.e., the MCD and the DtLs of the juxtamedullary nephrons).

### OSMOTIC DIURESIS

For a high rate of excretion of osmoles to be the cause of polyuria, vasopressin must be acting (Figure 12-2). When this occurs, AQP2 are present in the luminal membrane of principal cells in the cortical and medullary collecting ducts, therefore the osmolality of the luminal fluid becomes equal to the medullary interstitial osmolality, and therefore the urine flow rate in this setting is determined by the rate of excretion of osmoles. Not all osmoles, however, are equal in their ability to increase the urine volume. Only osmoles that do not achieve equal concentrations in the lumen of the MCD and in the medullary interstitial compartment are effective osmoles. Hence, the urine flow rate during an osmotic diuresis is determined by the rate of excretion of effective osmoles and the effective osmolality in the medullary interstitial compartment.

Because cells in the inner MCD have urea transporters in their luminal membranes when vasopressin acts, urea is usually an

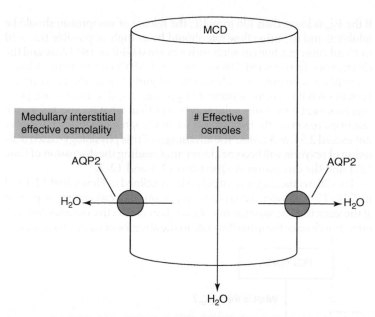

**Figure 12-2 Determinants of the Urine Volume During an Osmotic Diuresis.** The cylinder represents a medullary collecting duct (MCD). For a high rate of excretion of osmoles to be the cause of polyuria, vasopressin must be acting, leading to the insertion of aquaporin-2 (AQP2) water channels in the luminal membrane of principal cells in the MCD. The urine flow rate during an osmotic diuresis is determined by the rate of excretion of effective osmoles and the effective osmolality in the medullary interstitial compartment.

ineffective osmole (the concentration of urea is equal on the two sides of that membrane), so it does not cause water to be excreted. The net result of excreting some extra urea is a higher $U_{Osm}$ but not a higher urine flow rate. Urea, however, may become an effective urine osmole in some circumstances. When the rate of excretion of urea rises by a large amount, urea might not be absorbed fast enough to achieve equal concentrations in the lumen of the inner MCD and in the interstitium in the inner medulla. Hence, urea may become a partially effective osmole in the inner MCD and thereby obligate the excretion of water. Urea also may become an effective urine osmole if the concentration of electrolytes in the luminal fluid in the inner MCD is low.

The osmolality in the medullary interstitial compartment falls during an osmotic diuresis or when there has been a prior water diuresis because of medullary washout. During an osmotic diuresis, many liters of fluid are delivered to and reabsorbed in the MCD. Hence, medullary washout occurs and the osmolality in the medullary interstitial compartment falls. The expected effective osmolality in the medullary interstitial compartment is about 600 mosmol/kg $H_2O$ at somewhat high osmole excretion rates, and values close to the plasma osmolality ($P_{Osm}$) are observed at very high osmole excretion rates.

## DEFINITION OF POLYURIA

There are two different ways to define polyuria. The commonly used definition compares the urine volume in the patient to the usual urine volume in normal subjects who consume a typical Western diet. Therefore, polyuria is commonly defined as a 24-hour urine volume that is greater than 2.5 L or 3 L.

We prefer, however, to define polyuria based on the physiologic principles that determine the urine flow rate. In this case, polyuria is present if the urine volume is greater than what is expected for the clinical setting.

If the $P_{Na}$ is lower than 136 mmol/L, the release of vasopressin should be inhibited and the urine flow rate should be as high as possible (i.e., ~10 to 15 mL/min in a human adult with a normal GFR of 180 L/day and the absence of effective arterial blood volume [EABV] contraction). A lower urine flow rate in this case indicates that oliguria (rather than polyuria) is present even if the urine volume is larger than 3 L/day. In contrast, polyuria is present if the urine volume is higher than what is expected for the rate of excretion of effective osmoles when vasopressin acts, even if it does not exceed 2.5 L or 3 L/day. The advantages of this physiology-based definition of polyuria will become clearer after reading the discussion of Case 12-1 and the discussion of Questions 12-1 and 12-2.

The differential diagnosis of polyuria is outlined in Flow Chart 12-1 and in Table 12-1. A water diuresis and an osmotic diuresis cannot be present at the same time because the rate of excretion of effective osmoles does not directly influence the urine flow rate in the absence of vasopressin actions.

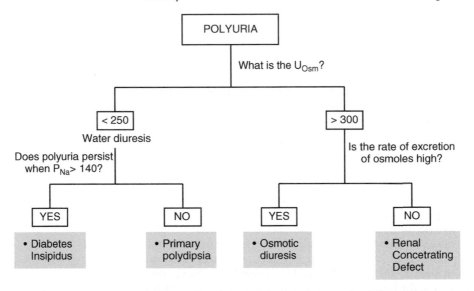

**Flow Chart 12-1 Approach to the Patient With Polyuria.** The initial step in the differential diagnosis of the cause of polyuria is to measure the $U_{Osm}$. A value of the $U_{Osm}$ that is less than 250 mosmol/kg $H_2O$ suggests that the basis of polyuria is a water diuresis. If polyuria persists when the $P_{Na}$ is >140 mmol/L, the diagnosis is diabetes insipidus. A value of the $U_{Osm}$ that is higher than 300 mosmol/kg $H_2O$ suggests that the basis of polyuria is an osmotic diuresis if the osmole excretion rate is appreciably higher than 1000 mosmol/day or a renal concentrating defect if the osmole excretion rate is not high.

TABLE 12-1    **DIFFERENTIAL DIAGNOSIS OF POLYURIA**

| BASIS | KEY FEATURE | DIAGNOSTIC TOOLS |
|---|---|---|
| **Water Diuresis** | | |
| • Primary polydipsia | • $P_{Na}$ <136 mmol/L | • ↑$U_{Osm}$ and ↓urine flow rate if water intake is stopped |
| • Central DI | • Central nervous system pathology | • ↑$U_{Osm}$ and ↓urine flow rate after dDAVP is given |
| • Vasopressinase | • Necrotic tissue | • Responds to dDAVP but not to "low-dose" vasopressin |
| • Nephrogenic DI | • Often caused by lithium | • No response to dDAVP |
| **Osmotic Diuresis** | | |
| • Organic compounds (e.g., urea, glucose) or electrolytes ($Na^+ + Cl^-$ ions) | • $U_{Osm}$ >300 mosmol/L and osmole excretion >1000 mosmol/day | • Calculate osmole excretion rate • Establish nature of the urine osmoles |
| **Renal Concentrating Defect** | | |
| • Low osmolality in the renal medulla | • Maximum $U_{Osm}$ is <600 mosmol/kg $H_2O$ • Osmole excretion rate is <1000 mosmol/day | • Diseases or drugs that affect the renal medulla |

*DI,* Diabetes insipidus; *dDAVP,* desmopressin.

# PART B

# WATER DIURESIS

## TOOLS USED IN ASSESSMENT OF A PATIENT WITH A WATER DIURESIS

### Urine Flow Rate

The peak urine flow rate during water diuresis is about 10 to 15 mL/min. Extrapolated to 24 hours, the urine volume would be 15 to 22 L. The maximum volume of urine during water diuresis is equal to the volume of distal delivery of filtrate minus the volume of filtrate reabsorbed in the inner MCD via RWP. If the urine volume is considerably less than 10 L/day, one should look for a reason for decreased distal delivery of filtrate (e.g., low GFR and/or enhanced reabsorption of filtrate in the PCT because of decreased EABV). Notwithstanding, the volume of the distal delivery of filtrate will ultimately fall, and this high urine flow rate is not likely to be sustained.

The urine flow rate declines when desmopressin (dDAVP) is given to a patient with central DI. The urine flow rate, however, will be higher than that observed in response to dDAVP in a normal subject who consumes a typical Western diet. The reason is that the medullary interstitial osmolality is likely to be lower because of medullary washout during the water diuresis (*see margin note*).

### $U_{Osm}$

The $U_{Osm}$ is equal to the number of excreted osmoles divided by the urine volume. Therefore, during a water diuresis, the $U_{Osm}$ reflects the osmole excretion rate and the volume of filtrate delivered to the distal nephron (which largely determines the urine volume in this setting). For example, if the rate of excretion of osmoles is 800 mosmol/day, the $U_{Osm}$ is 50 mosmol/kg $H_2O$ if the 24-hour urine volume is 16 L and 100 mosmol/kg $H_2O$ if the 24-hour urine volume is 8 L. In a patient with central DI or water diuresis caused by the release of a vasopressinase, $U_{Osm}$ should rise to a value that is higher than $P_{Osm}$ in response to the administration of dDAVP. A note of caution is needed: A rise in the $U_{Osm}$ following the administration of dDAVP may reflect a fall in the volume of the distal delivery of filtrate because of a fall in blood pressure and the GFR rather than a renal response to dDAVP with the insertion of AQP2 in the luminal membrane of principal cells. The effect of ethanol on the $U_{Osm}$ is described in the margin note.

### Osmole excretion rate

The osmole excretion rate is equal to the product of the $U_{Osm}$ and the urine flow rate (see Eqn 1). In subjects eating a typical Western diet, the rate of excretion of osmoles is 600 to 900 mosmol/day, with electrolytes and urea each accounting for close to half of the urine osmoles. During water diuresis, a change in the rate of excretion of osmoles does not directly affect the urine volume. This is because AQP2 are not present in the luminal membrane of principal cells in the late distal nephron; therefore, there is no reabsorption of water. Nevertheless, the rate of excretion of osmoles must be calculated in the patient with a water diuresis because if it is high, polyuria due to an osmotic diuresis may develop if dDAVP is administered and there is a renal response to its effect.

$$\text{Osmole excretion rate} = U_{Osm} \times \text{Urine flow rate} \qquad (1)$$

**EXPECTED RESPONSE TO dDAVP**

- Normal subjects have a medullary interstitial effective osmolality of 600 mosmol/kg $H_2O$ and they excrete 450 effective mosmol/day. Hence, in response to the administration of dDAVP, the average urine flow rate is close to 0.5 mL/min.
- Because the medullary interstitial osmolality falls to typically 400 mosmol/kg $H_2O$ during a water diuresis, the urine flow rate may be close to 0.8 mL/min when dDAVP acts, and even higher if the rate of excretion of effective osmoles is significantly elevated.
- On the other hand, a fall in the blood pressure after the administration of dDAVP may lead to a fall in the GFR and an enhanced reabsorption of NaCl and water in PCT. Therefore, the volume of the distal delivery of filtrate will fall and the urine flow rate will be much lower despite the absence of a renal response to dDAVP.

**ETHANOL AND THE $U_{Osm}$**

- Ethanol is not an effective osmole in plasma. It is also not an effective osmole in urine. The higher $U_{Osm}$ because of the presence of ethanol during a water diuresis should not be misinterpreted to reflect vasopressin action.

# CLINICAL APPROACH TO THE PATIENT WITH A WATER DIURESIS

The steps to take to determine the diagnosis in a patient with a water diuresis are outlined in Flow Charts 12-1 and 12-2.

## STEP 1: WHAT IS THE $U_{Osm}$?

A value of the $U_{Osm}$ that is less than 250 mosmol/kg $H_2O$ suggests that the basis of polyuria is a water diuresis. A large water diuresis is the expected physiologic response to a water intake that is large enough to cause the arterial $P_{Na}$ to fall below 136 mmol/L. In this case, the diagnosis is primary polydipsia. Once the $P_{Na}$ has returned to the normal range, the urine flow rate should decrease and the $U_{Osm}$ should rise appropriately. One must keep in mind that the prior water diuresis may have caused a lower medullary interstitial osmolality because of medullary washout. DI is present if a water diuresis persists when the $P_{Na}$ is higher than 140 mmol/L.

Calculate the osmole excretion rate (see Eqn 1)—the usual value is close to 0.5 mosmol/min (600 to 900 mosmol/day) in subjects consuming a typical Western diet. If the osmole excretion rate is appreciably higher, an osmotic diuresis will ensue once the patient has a renal response to the administration of dDAVP. This is important to recognize because an appreciable fall in the $P_{Na}$ that may lead to brain cell swelling may occur if a hypertonic urine is excreted while hypotonic or isotonic fluid is administered.

## STEP 2: EXAMINE THE RENAL RESPONSE TO VASOPRESSIN OR dDAVP (SEE FLOW CHART 12-2)

DI could be the result of a lesion in the hypothalamic–posterior pituitary axis, which controls the production and the release of vasopressin (central DI), the presence of a circulating vasopressinase that breaks down vasopressin, or a renal lesion that prevents the binding of vasopressin to its V2 receptor (V2R) or the insertion of AQP2 in the luminal membrane of principal cells (nephrogenic DI).

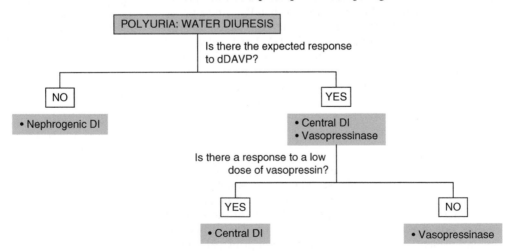

**Flow Chart 12-2 Approach to the Patient With Water Diuresis.** In a patient with central diabetes insipidus (DI) or a water diuresis because of the release of a vasopressinase, $U_{Osm}$ should rise to a value that is higher than the $P_{Osm}$ in response to the administration of desmopressin (dDAVP). If not, nephrogenic DI is the basis of the water diuresis. In contrast to the response to the administration of dDAVP, a patient in whom water diuresis is caused by the release of a vasopressinase does not show response to the administration of a small dose (5 units) of vasopressin.

In the diagnostic approach to the patient with polyuria, dDAVP should be given only if the $P_{Na}$ is elevated; water intake must be restricted if dDAVP is given. If there is the expected renal response to the administration of dDAVP (see previous), the diagnosis is central DI or the release of an enzyme that hydrolyzes vasopressin in plasma (vasopressinase). If there is a reason to suspect the latter, one should examine the response to the administration of vasopressin after the effect of dDAVP has worn off and the patient is having a water diuresis again. In contrast to the response to the administration of dDAVP, a patient in whom a vasopressinase is present will not show response to the administration of a small dose (5 units) of vasopressin. If the $U_{Osm}$ does not rise to a value that is equal to or higher than the $P_{Osm}$, the basis for the water diuresis is nephrogenic DI (see margin note).

### STEP 3: ESTABLISH THE BASIS FOR CENTRAL DI

The central water control system should be examined for a lesion that has caused the defect in vasopressin biosynthesis or release. An important part of this workup is to determine in a patient with hypernatremia whether the feeling of thirst is present. The absence of the feeling of thirst suggests that the defect involves the hypothalamic osmostat. The list of causes for central DI can be found in Chapter 11.

### STEP 4: ESTABLISH THE BASIS FOR NEPHROGENIC DI

Hereditary nephrogenic DI could be caused by an X-linked, recessive V2R mutation (more common) or an autosomal recessive or autosomal dominant AQP2 mutations. In the nonhereditary group of disorders, the most common cause of nephrogenic DI in an adult is the intake of lithium. The list of causes for nephrogenic DI can be found in Chapter 11.

## ISSUES IN THERAPY

Therapy should be individualized for each patient depending on the cause of the water diuresis. Hypernatremia is not common if the thirst response is intact. If a patient does not have a normal thirst response or does have a disorder that makes him or her unable to communicate the feeling of thirst or obtain water, he or she will need to be given a volume of water at frequent time intervals, and body weight should be monitored to provide an index of a significant change in total body water, and thereby the $P_{Na}$. If the cause of the water diuresis is central DI, the cornerstone of therapy is to administer the lowest possible dose of the long-acting preparation of vasopressin—dDAVP. The indicator of its effect is a decline in the urine flow rate to close to 1 mL/min (if the patient is consuming a typical Western diet). Early on, patients may be more sensitive to low doses of dDAVP because of upregulation of V2R in late distal nephron segments. The risk of this therapy is water retention, which would lead to the development of acute hyponatremia if the patient were to drink more water than can be excreted. To minimize this risk, daily water intake should be limited to close to 1 L/day, but compliance may be a challenge. To prevent the occurrence of hyponatremia, patients should check their weight each morning. If there is a weight gain of more than 1 kg, the $P_{Na}$ should be measured.

An example of how to treat a patient who has partial central DI is provided in the discussion of Case 11-2.

In a patient with nephrogenic DI, lowering the volume of distal delivery of filtrate decreases the urine flow rate. This requires a negative balance of $Na^+$ ions, which can be created by the combination of a low intake of NaCl and the intake of a diuretic. Thiazide diuretics are used

**NEPHROGENIC DI**

- We use the term nephrogenic DI only to indicate a disorder in which there is a failure to insert AQP2 in the luminal membrane of principal cells in the distal nephron in response to vasopressin.
- We do not use the term nephrogenic DI to indicate a disorder in which there is a lesion that leads to a lower medullary interstitial osmolality because, from a pathophysiologic perspective, it is a different disorder. We prefer to use the term renal concentrating defect to describe this disorder.
- In patients with nephrogenic DI, because actions of vasopressin are not present, the volume of distal delivery of filtrate (minus the volume of water reabsorbed by RWP in the inner MCD) determines the urine volume. In contrast, in patients with a renal concentrating defect, the rate of excretion of effective osmoles determines the urine volume.

because they do not lower the osmolality in the medullary interstitial compartment (see margin note). Nonsteroidal anti-inflammatory drugs may also decrease the volume of distal delivery of filtrate via a hemodynamic effect that reduces the GFR. The concern about their chronic use is the potential for the development of chronic renal insufficiency.

Amiloride has been suggested as a therapy in patients with lithium-induced nephrogenic DI. Amiloride blocks the epithelial sodium channel (ENaC) in principal cells in the distal nephron and hence may diminish further accumulation of lithium in these cells. Some data suggest an appreciable decrease in urine volume in patients with nephrogenic DI caused by lithium who were given amiloride, but the effect is likely to be more evident in patients with mild disease, who were started on amiloride early in the course of their disorder. Notwithstanding, to obtain a sufficiently high luminal concentration of amiloride for it to be an effective blocker of ENaC, high doses are needed. This is because of the high flow rate in the distal nephron. Serum lithium levels should be closely monitored as the natriuretic effect of amiloride may lead to a decreased EABV, which enhances the reabsorption of lithium in PCT. Polyuria, however, is likely to persist even after years of discontinuing lithium in patients who have taken lithium for more than 2 years (see Chapter 11). Many patients, however, are able to manage their disorder with increasing water intake as long as they can sense and communicate their feeling of thirst and are able to obtain water.

Patients with the autosomal dominant form of congenital nephrogenic DI have mutations in the carboxyl terminal of AQP2. The mutated AQP2 may retain little capability of causing water permeability. These patients may respond to the administration of large doses of dDAVP with a fall in the urine flow rate and a rise in the $U_{Osm}$.

# PART C
# OSMOTIC DIURESIS

## TOOLS USED IN THE ASSESSMENT OF A PATIENT WITH AN OSMOTIC DIURESIS

### $U_{Osm}$

The $U_{Osm}$ should be higher than the $P_{Osm}$.

### OSMOLE EXCRETION RATE

During an osmotic diuresis, the rate of excretion of osmoles should be appreciably greater than 1000 mosmol/day (>0.7 mosmol/min).

### NATURE OF THE URINE OSMOLES

The nature of the urine osmoles should be determined by measuring the rate of excretion of the individual osmoles in the urine. A large amount of mannitol is not usually given; hence, it is unlikely to be the sole cause of a large and sustained osmotic diuresis (see margin note). One can deduce which solute is likely to be responsible for the osmotic diuresis by measuring their concentrations in plasma (e.g., glucose, urea). A saline-induced osmotic diuresis may occur if the patient was given a large infusion of saline, or if she has cerebral or renal salt wasting. For a diagnosis of a state of salt wasting, there must be an appreciable excretion of $Na^+$ ions at a time when the EABV is definitely contracted.

## SOURCES OF THE URINE OSMOLES

In a patient with a glucose or urea-induced osmotic diuresis, it is important to decide whether these osmoles are derived from an exogenous source or from catabolism of endogenous proteins.

### Source of Urea

One can determine if the source of urea is from the metabolism of exogenous proteins or endogenous proteins by calculating the urea appearance rate and comparing it to the amount of urea that would have been produced from the metabolism of exogenous proteins if protein intake is known.

The rate of appearance of urea can be calculated from the amount of urea that is retained in the body plus the amount that is excreted in the urine over a given period of time. The former can be calculated from the rise in the concentration of urea in plasma ($P_{Urea}$), assuming a volume of distribution of urea equal to total body water (~60% of body weight in a nonobese patient).

Close to 16% of the weight of protein is nitrogen. Therefore, when 100 g of protein are oxidized, 16 g of nitrogen are formed. The atomic weight of nitrogen is 14; therefore, about 1140 mmol of nitrogen are produced. Because each mmol of urea contains two atoms of nitrogen, about 570 mmol of urea (1140 mmol of nitrogen/2) are produced from the oxidation of 100 g of protein or 5.7 mmol of urea per 1 g of protein. In terms of lean body mass, water is the main constituent in the body (~80% of weight); each kg of lean body mass has 800 g of water and 180 g of protein. Therefore, breakdown of 1 kg of lean body mass results in the production of about 5.7 mmol urea per g × 180 g = 1026 mmol of urea.

### Source of Glucose

The process of conversion of the carbon skeleton in amino acids to the gluconeogenic precursor, pyruvate, is obligatorily linked to the process of the conversion of their nitrogen to urea because they both share a common intermediate, argininosuccinate (see Chapter 16). The production of glucose from endogenous protein is relatively small. In more detail, only 60% of the weight of protein can be converted to glucose. This is because some of the amino acids cannot be metabolized in the gluconeogenesis pathway (e.g., the ketogenic amino acids leucine and lysine) and other amino acids must be partially oxidized in the citric acid cycle to be made into the gluconeogenic precursor pyruvate (e.g., the five-carbon skeleton in glutamine, the most abundant amino acid in proteins, is first converted to pyruvate, a three-carbon compound). Therefore, to produce enough glucose from protein to cause 1 L of osmotic diuresis (which has typically ~300 mmol of glucose), one would need the catabolism of 90 g of protein (equivalent to the catabolism of 1 lb of lean body mass; see margin note). Therefore, if there is a large glucose-induced osmotic diuresis, an exogenous source of glucose is most likely (e.g., the ingestion of a large amount of fruit juice or sugar-containing soft drinks).

## CLINICAL APPROACH TO THE PATIENT WITH AN OSMOTIC DIURESIS

The steps in the clinical approach to the patient with osmotic diuresis are illustrated in Flow Charts 12-1 and 12-3.

**GASTROINTESTINAL BLEED AND THE PRODUCTION OF UREA AND GLUCOSE**

- The stoichiometry of the process of the conversion of 100 g of protein to glucose and urea results in the production of 60 g (333 mmol) of glucose and 16 g of nitrogen (570 mmol of urea).
- There are about 180 grams of proteins in 1 L of blood (140 grams of hemoglobin and 40 grams of plasma proteins [concentration of proteins in plasma is 60 g/L, plasma volume is 60% of blood volume at a hematocrit of 40%]). Therefore, if a gastrointestinal bleed results in the loss of 1 L of blood, all this blood is retained in the lumen of the gastrointestinal tract, and all of its aminoacids are reabsorbed and metabolized, this will result in the formation of about 600 mmol of glucose and about 1026 mmol of urea.

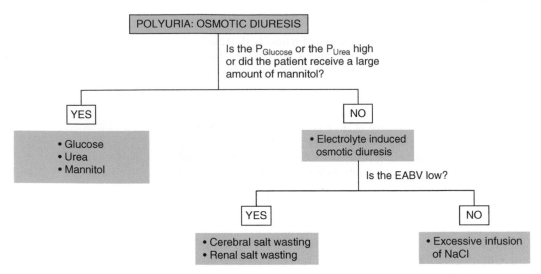

**Flow Chart 12-3 Approach to the Patient With Osmotic Diuresis.** During an osmotic diuresis, the rate of excretion of osmoles should be appreciably greater than 1000 mosmol/day (>0.7 mosmol/min). A large amount of mannitol is rarely given; hence, it is unlikely to be the sole cause of a large and sustained osmotic diuresis. One can deduce if glucose or urea is likely to be responsible for the osmotic diuresis by measuring their concentrations in plasma. A saline-induced osmotic diuresis may occur if there was a large infusion of saline or in a patient who has cerebral or renal salt wasting. For the diagnosis of salt wasting, the effective arterial blood volume (EABV) must be definitely contracted.

### Step 1: What Is the $U_{Osm}$?

**Calculate the osmole excretion rate**

In a patient with polyuria, if the $U_{Osm}$ is greater than the $P_{Osm}$ and the osmole excretion rate appreciably exceeds 1000 mosmol/day (or 0.7 mosmol/min), an osmotic diuresis is likely to be present. The caveat here, however, is that the $U_{Osm}$ from a spot urine sample may not be representative of the value of the $U_{Osm}$ throughout the 24-hour period if there are intermittent periods of water diuresis.

### Step 2: Define the Nature of the Excreted Osmoles

One should determine whether enough mannitol was administered to cause the observed degree of polyuria. One can make a reasonable assessment of the likelihood of a solute to cause polyuria if its concentration in plasma is measured, the GFR is estimated, and the renal handling of that solute is known (*see margin note*). A saline diuresis is the cause of polyuria if the rate of excretion $Na^+$ and $Cl^-$ ions is high and they represent the majority of the excreted osmoles.

### Step 3: Identify the Source of the Osmoles in the Urine

In a patient with glucose or urea-induced osmotic diuresis, it is important to determine whether these osmoles were derived from an exogenous source or from the catabolism of endogenous proteins. The clinician should be aware of hidden glucose in the lumen of the gastrointestinal tract, because it may soon be absorbed and contribute to the osmotic diuresis.

In a patient with a saline-induced osmotic diuresis, one must determine why so much NaCl is being excreted. Some potential causes are prior excessive saline administration (a common situation in a hospital setting), administration of a loop diuretic in a patient with significant edema, cerebral salt wasting, or renal salt wasting.

**QUANTITATIVE EXAMPLE**

- Consider a patient who has a $P_{Urea}$ of 50 mmol/L and a GFR of 100 L/day. The filtered load of urea the product of the $P_{Urea}$, and the GFR equals 5000 mmol/day.
- Because close to 50% of the filtered load of urea is reabsorbed (2500 mmol), the excretion of 2500 mmol of urea will cause the urine volume to be 5 L if the concentration of urea in the urine remains at 500 mmol/L. For this to occur, there must be a very high rate of input of urea.

A special example in which polyuria can be caused by multiple factors is postobstructive diuresis, which is discussed in the following paragraphs.

### Postobstructive Diuresis

In postobstructive diuresis, polyuria is caused by a constellation of abnormalities that occur as a result of an increase in intraluminal pressure in renal tubules for a sustained period of time:

- Saline diuresis. This may be caused by expansion of the EABV by prior intake of NaCl and water or infusion of saline or due to a distal defect in the reabsorption of $Na^+$ and $Cl^-$ ions (renal salt wasting). The urine volume may be higher than expected because of a low effective osmolality in the renal medullary interstitial compartment.
- Urea-induced osmotic diuresis. Because patients with a prolonged obstruction may have a low GFR, their $P_{Urea}$ could rise. Once the urinary tract obstruction is relieved and if the GFR rises, they could undergo a urea-induced osmotic diuresis if urea becomes an effective osmole in the lumen of the inner MCD. This may occur if the rate of delivery of urea is high enough to exceed the capacity of urea transporters in the inner MCD or if there is failure, because of prolonged obstruction, to insert urea transporters into the luminal membrane of the inner MCD.
- Nephrogenic DI. This may be due to the loss of AQP2 in the luminal membrane of principal cells in the distal nephron. In this setting, the urine volume is determined primarily by factors affecting the volume of the distal delivery of filtrate.

## ISSUES IN THERAPY

There are two important issues that should be considered in therapy in patients with an osmotic diuresis. First, one must determine the impact of the loss of solutes plus water on body tonicity (and hence brain cell volume) and the extracellular fluid (ECF) volume. Second, one must define the source of excreted osmoles.

### IMPACT OF THE URINE COMPOSITION ON BODY TONICITY AND ECF VOLUME

One must examine the volume and the concentration of $Na^+$ and $K^+$ ions in the urine, and the volume and the concentrations of $Na^+$ and $K^+$ ions in the input to perform a tonicity balance to determine the basis of a change in $P_{Na}$ and the appropriate therapy to restore the volume and tonicity of both the ECF and the ICF compartments (see Chapter 11). The concentrations of $Na^+$ and $K^+$ ions in the urine are low during an osmotic diuresis caused by high rates of excretion of glucose, urea, or mannitol. If the concentration of $Na^+$ and $K^+$ ions in the infusate is hypertonic to that of the urine, the $P_{Na}$ may rise, and hence the ICF volume (including brain cell volume) could shrink. Balance data for $Na^+$ and $K^+$ ions also indicate the changes in the ECF volume and $K^+$ ions balance. The latter may not be revealed by the $P_K$ because of other factors that may cause a shift of $K^+$ into cells.

### SOURCE OF EXCRETED OSMOLES

This is important during a urea or a glucose-induced osmotic diuresis because the source of these osmoles could be the breakdown of endogenous proteins. The impact of this catabolic state is illustrated in the discussion of Case 12-2.

## QUESTIONS

12-1    *An obese patient has been fasting for 2 weeks in a weight reduction program. His $P_{Na}$ is 145 mmol/L, his urine flow rate is 0.6 L/day, his $U_{Osm}$ is 700 mosmol/kg$H_2O$, and the concentration of urea in his urine is 100 mmol/L. Does this patient have a renal concentrating defect?*

12-2    *A patient with cirrhosis of the liver was placed on a diet that is low in protein and salt. While in the hospital, his urine flow rate was 0.4 L/day, his $U_{Osm}$ was 375 mosmol/kg$H_2O$, and his osmole excretion rate was 150 mosmol/day. Does this patient have oliguria, polyuria, and/or a renal concentrating defect?*

12-3    *A patient with central DI has polyuria, a low $U_{Osm}$ (50 mosmol/kg$H_2O$), and a $P_{Na}$ of 137 mmol/L. What does this imply for diagnosis and therapy?*

12-4    *A patient had a urine volume of 6 L in the past 24 hours. He was not receiving intravenous fluids. His $P_{Na}$ rose to 150 mmol/L. He did not complain of thirst. The last urine aliquot in this 24-hour period was sent for analysis; the $U_{Osm}$ was 500 mosmol/kg$H_2O$, $U_{Urea}$ was 250 mmol/L, and the concentration of $Na^+ + K^+$ ions in his urine was 125 mmol/L. His $P_{Glucose}$ and $P_{Urea}$ were in the normal range. Does the patient have a water diuresis and/or an osmotic diuresis?*

# PART D
# DISCUSSION OF CASES

## CASE 12-1: OLIGURIA WITH A URINE VOLUME OF 4 L PER DAY

### DOES THIS PATIENT HAVE POLYURIA?

**Conventional interpretation**

Polyuria is present because the urine volume is greater than 3 L/day. This is a water diuresis because the $U_{Osm}$ is considerably less than the $P_{Osm}$. The low $P_{Na}$ indicates that the patient has primary polydipsia.

**Physiology-based interpretation**

The observed urine flow rate (~3 mL/min) is much lower than what is expected during a water diuresis. In more detail, because of the low $P_{Na}$ of 130 mmol/L, vasopressin should be absent and the urine flow rate should be 10 to 15 mL/min. Hence, this patient does not have polyuria in physiologic terms.

The lower than expected urine flow rate could be due to the intermittent release of vasopressin because of the presence of nonosmotic stimuli for its release. Alternatively, there may be a low volume of delivery of filtrate to the distal nephron because of a mild degree of EABV contraction, resulting in a somewhat lower GFR and an enhanced reabsorption of filtrate in PCT (see Figure 12-1). There may also be an enhanced water reabsorption via RWP in the inner MCD. This is because of the low osmolality of the fluid in the lumen of the inner MCD duct as a result of her low rate of excretion of osmoles ($U_{Osm}$ 80 mosmol/kg$H_2O \times 4$ L/day or 320 mosmol/day instead of the usual rate of excretion of osmoles of 600 to 900 mosmol/day) (see Chapter 9).

## WHAT DANGERS RELATED TO Na⁺ AND WATER ISSUES MAY DEVELOP IN THIS PATIENT?

Understanding that this patient does not have polyuria, but rather diminished ability to excrete water, makes one realize that this patient is at risk for a substantial gain of water if she were to ingest more water and/or if her loss of water were to decrease. The latter may occur if she has a nonosmotic stimulus for the release of vasopressin (e.g., pain, nausea). Alternatively, her nonrenal loss of water in sweat would decrease if she fails to run for one or two days (sweat volume may be as large as 1 to 2 L/hr during vigorous exercise). The resulting acute fall in her $P_{Na}$ may place her at risk of developing acute brain cell swelling with possible brain herniation.

## CASE 12-2: MORE THAN JUST SALT AND WATER LOSS

### DOES THIS PATIENT HAVE AN OSMOTIC DIURESIS?

This high urine flow rate is the result of an osmotic diuresis because $U_{Osm}$ is greater than 300 mosmol/kg $H_2O$ and the calculated osmole excretion rate is 3000 mosmol/day. The next step in Flow Chart 12-3 is to define the nature of the urine osmoles. The patient did not receive mannitol. His $P_{Glucose}$ was 180 mg/dL (10 mmol/L); therefore, there would not have been enough glucose filtered to cause this osmotic diuresis. In contrast, because his $P_{Urea}$ was very high, he could have a urea-induced osmotic diuresis; this was confirmed by finding that the concentration of urea in his urine was 400 mmol/L.

### WHAT IS THE SOURCE OF UREA? WHAT ARE THE IMPLICATIONS FOR THERAPY?

In quantitative terms, he excreted approximately 2400 mmol of urea that day (6 L/day × 400 mmol of urea/L). As discussed previously, for every 100 g of protein oxidized, 16 g of nitrogen are converted to about 570 mmol of urea. Therefore, the amount of urea that was excreted represents the breakdown of close to 400 g of protein. On that day, the patient was given only 60 g of protein by the enteral route. Therefore, he catabolized approximately 340 g of endogenous protein.

Each kg of lean body mass has close to 180 g of protein. Therefore, the amount of urea excreted on that day represents the catabolism of close to 2 kg of lean body mass. Should this continue, he would undergo marked muscle wasting. This could compromise respiratory muscle function and lead to bronchopneumonia. Furthermore, this catabolic state could affect his immunologic defense mechanisms. One must look for the cause of this catabolic state (e.g., sepsis). Therapy should include a strong emphasis on nutrition. More exogenous calories and protein should be given to decrease catabolism of his lean body mass. Anabolic hormones (e.g., high-dose insulin with glucose to prevent hypoglycemia) or anabolic steroids and the provision of nutritional supplements such as the amino acid glutamine may minimize endogenous protein catabolism. In addition, one should reevaluate the need for continuing the use of high doses of drugs that can stimulate protein catabolism (e.g., high-dose glucocorticoids).

## DISCUSSION OF QUESTIONS

12-1     *An obese patient has been fasting for 2 weeks in a weight*
         *reduction program. His $P_{Na}$ is 145 mmol/L, his urine flow rate*
         *is 0.6 L/day, his $U_{Osm}$ is 700 mosmol/kg $H_2O$, and the concen-*
         *tration of urea in his urine is 100 mmol/L. Does this patient*
         *have a renal concentrating defect?*

If one considers only the $U_{Osm}$ of 700 mosmol/kg $H_2O$ when the $P_{Na}$
is 145 mmol/L, one might think that this patient has a concentrating
defect, but the control of the urine flow rate should be examined in
effective osmolality terms. Because the nonurea or effective $U_{Osm}$ is
600 mosmol/kg $H_2O$, the patient does not have a concentrating defect.
Rather, this is the expected $U_{Osm}$ because of the low rate of excretion
of urea (0.6 L/day × 100 mmol/L = 60 mmol/day). In addition, the low
urine flow rate (0.6 L/day) indicates that his medullary interstitial
effective osmolality is appropriately high.

12-2     *A patient with cirrhosis of the liver was placed on a diet that is*
         *low in protein and salt. While in the hospital, his urine flow rate*
         *was 0.4 L/day, his $U_{Osm}$ was 375 mosmol/kg $H_2O$, and his os-*
         *mole excretion rate was 150 mosmol/day. Does this patient have*
         *oliguria, polyuria, and/or a renal concentrating defect?*

Although the patient's urine flow rate appears to be low, a major factor that contributes to the low urine flow rate is his low rate of excretion of osmoles, which reflects his dietary intake (low protein, low
salt). Notwithstanding, his low $U_{Osm}$ while vasopressin is acting
(375 mosmol/kg $H_2O$) raises the suspicion that he has an underlying
lesion that compromises his ability to have a maximum effective medullary interstitial osmolality (~600 mosmol/kg $H_2O$). Therefore, this
patient may have a concentrating defect and hence polyuria (rather
than oliguria) in physiologic terms.

12-3     *A patient with central DI has polyuria, a low $U_{Osm}$ (50 mosmol/*
         *kg $H_2O$), and a $P_{Na}$ of 137 mmol/L. What does this imply for di-*
         *agnosis and therapy?*

The polyuria is a water diuresis because the $U_{Osm}$ is so low. Because the
$P_{Na}$ is 137 mmol/L, this indicates that the patient also has a high water
intake that is not driven by thirst. The usual basis for the excessive
water intake is to avoid the uncomfortable sensation of thirst. This
illustrates why the $P_{Na}$ cannot be relied on to determine if DI is the
basis of polyuria.

   To reach a final diagnosis, water intake should be curtailed and
the $P_{Na}$ and $U_{Osm}$ should be monitored. If the $P_{Na}$ rises to above
140 mmol/L and the $U_{Osm}$ remains low, the diagnosis of DI with
primary polydipsia is established. This is important to consider
because if this patient is treated with dDAVP and continues to have
a high water intake, acute hyponatremia may be a serious risk.

12-4     *A patient had a urine volume of 6 L in the past 24 hours. He was*
         *not receiving intravenous fluids. His $P_{Na}$ rose to 150 mmol/L.*
         *He did not complain of thirst. The last urine aliquot in this 24-hour*
         *period was sent for analysis; the $U_{Osm}$ was 500 mosmol/kg $H_2O$,*
         *$U_{Urea}$ was 250 mmol/L, and the concentration of $Na^+ + K^+$ ions in*
         *his urine was 125 mmol/L. His $P_{Glucose}$ and $P_{Urea}$ were in the normal*
         *range. Does the patient have a water diuresis and/or an osmotic*
         *diuresis?*

To decide whether this is really an osmotic diuresis, determine whether
the patient could have filtered enough nonelectrolyte osmoles (at least
3000 mosmol in 24 hours) to cause this marked degree of polyuria.
Because he did not have a high $P_{Glucose}$ or $P_{Urea}$ and did not receive
an infusion of mannitol, the only type of osmotic diuresis that could
be present is a saline-induced diuresis. Nevertheless, the sum of the

concentrations of $Na^+$ and $K^+$ ions in his urine is not high enough for this diagnosis. Moreover, he did not receive a large saline infusion and did not appear to have a significant degree of EABV contraction. Hence, all the causes for an osmotic diuresis are unlikely. As it turned out, he had a water diuresis for most of that day because of central DI but also had intermittent release of vasopressin resulting from nonosmotic stimuli (e.g., nausea, pain, anxiety). Thus, he has a defect involving his osmostat and possibly his thirst center, leaving enough capacity to secrete vasopressin if there are nonosmotic stimuli for its release. This illustrates that one can be misled if the findings from a spot urine sample are extrapolated to the entire 24-hour period. Therefore, one needs to examine multiple urine aliquots that are collected over short intervals during the 24-hour period to determine the basis of polyuria.

section three
# Potassium

Potassium

# Potassium Physiology

# Introduction

**ABBREVIATIONS**

$P_K$, concentration of potassium ($K^+$) ions in plasma

$U_K$, concentration of $K^+$ ions in the urine

$P_{Na}$, concentration of sodium ($Na^+$) ions in plasma

$U_{Na}$, concentration of $Na^+$ ions in the urine

$P_{Cl}$, concentration of chloride ($Cl^-$) ions in plasma

$U_{Cl}$, concentration of $Cl^-$ ions in the urine

$P_{HCO_3}$, concentration of bicarbonate ($HCO_3^-$) ions in plasma

$P_{Glucose}$, concentration of glucose in plasma

$P_{Urea}$, concentration of urea in plasma

$P_{Creatinine}$, concentration of creatinine in plasma

$U_{Creatinine}$, concentration of creatinine in the urine

$P_{Osm}$, osmolality in plasma

$U_{Osm}$, osmolality in the urine

CDN, cortical distal nephron, which includes the late distal convoluted tubule, connecting segment, and the cortical collecting duct

DCT, distal convoluted tubule

CCD, cortical collecting duct

RMP, resting membrane potential

$P_{Aldosterone}$, concentration of aldosterone in plasma

ECF, extracellular fluid

ICF, intracellular fluid

Na-K-ATPase, sodium-potassium-ATPase

ENaC, epithelial sodium ion channel

ADP, adenosine diphoshate

ATP, adenosine triphosphate

$K_{ATP}$, $K^+$ ion channel that is gated by intracellular nucleotides

ROMK, renal outer medullary potassium ion channel

Regulation of total body potassium ($K^+$) ion homeostasis is vital for survival. Changes in the concentration of $K^+$ ions in plasma ($P_K$) are associated with changes in the negative voltage across cell membranes and the resting membrane potential (RMP). This may have dangerous consequences (e.g., altered cardiac impulse conduction causing an arrhythmia).

The vast majority of $K^+$ ions in the body are located in cells. $K^+$ ions are retained in cells by an electrical force because the cell interior has a negative voltage caused by the negatively charged intracellular organic phosphates. Specific channels for $K^+$ ions in cell membranes permit $K^+$ ions to diffuse out of cells down their concentration difference. These chemical and electrical forces eventually come into balance, and an equilibrium potential for $K^+$ ions is achieved if there is sufficient $K^+$ ion channel conductance in the cell membranes. Because cell membranes have much higher permeability to $K^+$ ions than to sodium ($Na^+$) ions, the RMP is close to the equilibrium potential for $K^+$ ions.

Regulation of $K^+$ ion homeostasis has two main aspects: (1) control of the transcellular distribution of $K^+$ ions, which is vital for survival because it limits acute changes in the $P_K$, and (2) regulation of $K^+$ ion excretion by the kidney, which maintains whole body $K^+$ ion balance; this is, however, a much slower process.

The shift of $K^+$ ions into cells requires an increase in cell interior negative voltage. This can be achieved by increasing flux via the Na-K-ATPase, which results in net export of positive charges out of cells.

The major site where the renal excretion of $K^+$ ions is regulated is in the late cortical distal nephron (CDN), namely the late distal convoluted tubule (DCT), the connecting segment, and the cortical collecting duct (CCD). Two factors influence the rate of excretion of $K^+$ ions: (1) the rate of net secretion of $K^+$ ions by principal cells in the CDN and (2) the flow rate in the terminal CDN (i.e., the number of liters of fluid that exit the terminal CCD). To gain insights into the physiology of the regulation of $K^+$ homeostasis, it is helpful to examine this process from a Paleolithic perspective. The diet consumed by our ancient ancestors consisted mainly of fruit and berries, which provided a very small amount of $Na^+$ and chloride ($Cl^-$) ions but episodic and at times large loads of $K^+$ ions. Hence, there was a need for mechanisms to ensure renal conservation of sodium chloride (NaCl) to avoid a hemodynamic threat. To avoid the risk of dangerous hyperkalemia and cardiac arrhythmia, there was a need to have mechanisms to shift ingested $K^+$ ions rapidly into the liver before they could reach the heart and mechanisms to switch the renal response from NaCl conservation to $K^+$ ion excretion after ingested $K^+$ ions are released from liver cells.

It is important to realize that hyperkalemia and hypokalemia are not specific diseases; rather, they are the result of many disorders with different underlying pathophysiology. Therefore, an understanding of the physiology of $K^+$ ion homeostasis is critical to determine the underlying pathophysiology of each disorder and the appropriate therapy.

## OBJECTIVES

- To illustrate the common strategy used to control movement of $K^+$ ions across cell membranes. This requires a driving force (i.e., a more negative voltage in the area where $K^+$ ions must be retained) and regulation of the number of open $K^+$ channels in cell membranes.
- To illustrate how the voltage across cell membranes is regulated and its implications for the control of the shift of $K^+$ ions into cells.
- To illustrate how excretion of $K^+$ ions by the kidneys is regulated to maintain overall balance for $K^+$ ions.
- To illustrate that examining this process from a Paleolithic perspective provides insights into the control of $K^+$ ion homeostasis.

## CASE 13-1: WHY DID I BECOME SO WEAK?

A very fit, active, 27-year-old Caucasian woman was in excellent health until about 1 year ago. Her past medical history revealed mild asthma, for which she took a bronchodilator on an intermittent basis. In the past year, she had three episodes of extreme weakness. Each episode lasted for about 12 hours, and she felt perfectly well between attacks. On more detailed questioning, she said that she had ingested a large amount of sugar before the first attack. Each subsequent attack, however, was not preceded by the use of a bronchodilator, performance of exercise, or the ingestion of a large amount of sugar or caffeinated beverages. She denied the use/abuse of diuretics or laxatives, symptoms of bulimia, glue sniffing, substance abuse, or the ingestion of licorice or over-the-counter drugs. She did not seem to be overly concerned about her body weight. There was no family history of hypokalemia, hypertension, or paralytic episodes. On each of these occasions, other than the paralysis, the only findings of note were tachycardia (130 beats per minute) and mild systolic hypertension with a wide pulse pressure (150/70 mm Hg). There were no signs of hyperthyroidism. Because of the very low $P_K$ (~2.1 mmol/L), an intravenous infusion of KCl was started, and, as on the other occasions, she recovered promptly with the administration of a relatively small amount of $K^+$ ions. The laboratory data are provided below. In addition, all tests of thyroid function were in the normal range and investigations for a pheochromocytoma were negative. During the last admission, the insulin concentration in plasma was measured and it was in the normal range. The level of C-peptide in her blood was not elevated.

| $P_{Na}$ | mmol/L | 141 | $P_{Glucose}$ | mg/dL (mmol/L) | 133 (7.4) |
| $P_K$ | mmol/L | 2.1 | $P_{Creatinine}$ | mg/dL (μmol/L) | 0.9 (77) |
| $P_{HCO_3}$ | mmol/L | 22 | BUN ($P_{urea}$) | mg/dL (mmol/L) | 10 (3.4) |
| Arterial pH | | 7.38 | Arterial $PCO_2$ | mm Hg | 38 |
| $U_K$ | mmol/L | 8 | $U_{Creatinine}$ | (g/L) (mmol/L) | 0.8 (7) |

### Questions

What is the most likely basis for the repeated episodes of acute hypokalemia?
Was an adrenergic effect associated with the acute hypokalemia?
Are there any clues in her laboratory results to suggest what the cause of acute hypokalemia might be?

# PART A
# PRINCIPLES OF PHYSIOLOGY

Close to 98% of the total body $K^+$ ions is inside cells. The concentration of $K^+$ ions in cells is very high relative to its concentration in the ECF compartment. This is because $K^+$ ions in cells balance the charge on intracellular anions; these intracellular anions cannot exit from cells because they are macromolecules, and moreover, they are essential for cell functions (DNA, RNA, phospholipids, compounds for energy provision such as ATP and phosphocreatine). Hence, the vast majority of $K^+$ ions are is retained in cells, and only 2% of the total body $K^+$ ions are in the ECF compartment. Changes in the concentration of $K^+$ ions in the ECF compartment are, however, extremely important because they are proportionately much larger than changes in the concentration of $K^+$ ions in cells and it is the ratio of concentrations of $K^+$ ions across cell membranes that determines the RMP.

Acute $K^+$ ion homeostasis is achieved by control of the distribution of $K^+$ ions between the intracellular fluid (ICF) and ECF compartments (i.e., acute internal $K^+$ ion balance). Long-term $K^+$ homeostasis is achieved by control of the renal excretion of $K^+$ ions (external $K^+$ ion balance). Therefore, there must be sensitive regulatory mechanisms to minimize transient changes in the $P_K$ before renal excretion of $K^+$ ions occurs.

# GENERAL CONCEPTS FOR THE MOVEMENT OF K+ IONS ACROSS CELL MEMBRANES

There are two conditions that are required for the movement of $K^+$ ions across cell membranes to occur. First, a sufficient electrochemical driving force across that membrane; and, second, a sufficient number of open $K^+$ ion channels in that membrane.

## DRIVING FORCE FOR THE SHIFT OF K+ IONS ACROSS CELL MEMBRANES

The driving force for a shift of $K^+$ ions across cell membranes is a more negative voltage in the compartment in which $K^+$ ions will be located. There are two ways to generate a negative voltage across a cell membrane: (1) the import of anions or (2) the export of cations. A more negative voltage inside cells is generated by electrogenic exit of $Na^+$ ions via the sodium-potassium-ATPase (Na-K-ATPase) (Figure 13-1). Because the Na-K-ATPase extrudes $3\,Na^+$ ions out of cells and imports only $2\,K^+$ ions into cells, and because export of intracellular macromolecular phosphate anions out of cells does not occur, the net result is the generation of a more negative voltage inside cells. This increase in intracellular negative voltage limits the exit of $K^+$ ions from cells down their chemical concentration difference.

In the kidney, a transepithelial, lumen-negative electrical voltage drives the net secretion of $K^+$ ions by principal cells in the CDN (see Figure 13-1). This is generated when $Na^+$ ions are reabsorbed in an electrogenic fashion (i.e., reabsorption of $Na^+$ ions without their accompanying anions, which are usually $Cl^-$ ions). Reabsorption of $Na^+$ ions occurs via the epithelial $Na^+$ ion channel (ENaC) and is driven by the low concentration of $Na^+$ ions and the negative voltage inside principal cells, both of which are created by the activity of the Na-K-ATPase in their basolateral membranes.

## PATHWAYS FOR THE MOVEMENT OF K+ IONS ACROSS CELL MEMBRANES

$K^+$ ion channels are composed of a diverse family of membrane-spanning proteins that selectively conduct $K^+$ ions across cell membranes. $K^+$ ion channels have a pore that permits $K^+$ ions to cross the cell membrane and a selectivity filter that specifies $K^+$ ion as the ion species to move through the channel (see margin note). There are several different types of $K^+$ ion channels that permit $K^+$ ions to cross cell membranes. Some of these channels are regulated by voltage, others are regulated by ligands such as ionized calcium ions, and others are regulated by metabolites such as adenosine diphosphate (ADP) (these channels are called $K_{ATP}$ channels). In the presence of a driving force, movement of $K^+$ ions through the specific $K^+$ ion channels

**BASIS FOR THE SELECTIVITY OF THE K+ ION CHANNEL FOR K+ IONS**

- $Na^+$ ions are much smaller than $K^+$ ions, yet the $K^+$ ion channels are specific for $K^+$ ions.
- Ions in solution have layers of water surrounding them; therefore, one must think in terms of their hydrated size.
- Because of the chemical structure at the mouth of the $K^+$ ion channels, water shells surrounding $K^+$ ions are stripped off; therefore, $K^+$ ions become smaller than $Na^+$ ions and can pass through the channel, whereas $Na^+$ ions cannot.

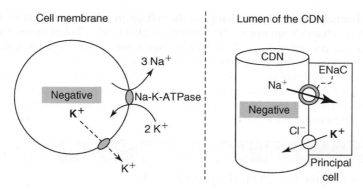

**Figure 13-1  Concept for the Movement of K⁺ Ions Across Cell Membranes.** The *circle on the left* represents a cell membrane and the *cylinder on the right* represents the cortical distal nephron (CDN). There is a much higher concentration of K⁺ ions in cells than in the extracellular fluid compartment because of the negative voltage inside cells, which is generated in part because more Na⁺ ions are extruded from than K⁺ ions are imported into cells by the Na-K-ATPase. To cause a redistribution of K⁺ ions across cell membranes, there must be a change in either the magnitude of the negative voltage inside cells or in the number, open probability, and/or conductance of K⁺ ion channels (because the concentration of K⁺ ions in cells is higher than the predicted value from the electrochemical equilibrium). K⁺ ions will enter the lumen of the CDN when it has a negative voltage and if there are open renal outer medullary K⁺ ion channels in the luminal membrane of principal cells in the CDN. A lumen negative voltage is generated when Na⁺ ions are reabsorbed in an electrogenic fashion (i.e., reabsorption of Na⁺ ions without their accompanying anions, which are usually Cl⁻ ions). Reabsorption of Na⁺ ions occurs via the epithelial Na⁺ ion channel (ENaC).

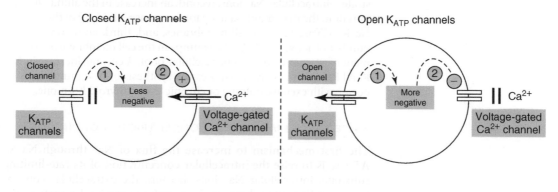

**Figure 13-2  Regulatory Roles for K_ATP Channels in Cell Function.** As shown on the *left*, when the K_ATP channels are closed, positive voltage (K⁺ ions) cannot exit from cells and the interior of the cells becomes less negative. As a result, the voltage-gated ionized calcium channels open, and the concentration of ionized calcium (Ca²⁺) in cells rises. In contrast, as shown on the *right*, when the K_ATP channels are opened, positive voltage (K⁺ ions) can exit from cells, and the interior of the cells becomes more negative. As a result, the concentration of Ca²⁺ ions in cells falls.

depends on the number of K⁺ ion channels, whether they are in an open or a closed configuration (their gating), and how quickly K⁺ ions can move through them (their conductance).

When K⁺ ions move out of cells, there is an increase in the net negative voltage inside cells. Because the concentration of K⁺ ions in cells is higher than that predicted from its electrochemical equilibrium, control of the open probability of K⁺ ion channels in cell membranes or their number is critical to regulate the magnitude of cell voltage, which in turn influences many essential cell functions. As illustrated in Figure 13-2, regulation of K_ATP channels influences the gating of calcium ion channels as a result of a change in the voltage in cells (more negative if $K_{ATP}$ channels are open—the converse is also true). Clinical examples where control of $K_{ATP}$ channels has important effects on physiologic functions are discussed in the answers to Question 13-1.

From a renal perspective, secretion of $K^+$ ions in principal cells of the CDN requires that open $K^+$ ion channels, primarily the renal outer medullary $K^+$ ion channel (ROMK), must be present in the luminal membrane of these cells.

## QUESTION

13-1   Is the $K_{ATP}$ channel regulated by ATP?

# PART B
# SHIFT OF POTASSIUM IONS ACROSS CELL MEMBRANES

## INCREASING THE NEGATIVE VOLTAGE IN CELLS

To shift $K^+$ ions into cells and retain them inside cells, a more negative cell voltage is required. This is generated by increasing flux through Na-K-ATPase. There are three ways to acutely increase ion pumping by Na-K-ATPase: first, a rise in the concentration of its rate-limiting substrate—intracellular $Na^+$ ions; second, an increase in the affinity for $Na^+$ ions or in the maximum capacity for ion transport ($V_{max}$) of the existing Na-K-ATPase units in cell membranes; and, third, an increase in the number of active Na-K-ATPase pumps in the cell membrane by recruitment of new units from an intracellular pool. A chronic increase in Na-K-ATPase pump activity requires the synthesis of new pump units, as occurs with exercise training or chronic excess thyroid hormone.

### RAISE THE INTRACELLULAR CONCENTRATION OF $NA^+$ IONS

The first mechanism to increase the flux of $Na^+$ through Na-K-ATPase is to raise the intracellular concentration of its rate-limiting substrate, intracellular $Na^+$ ions, because the extracellular concentration of $K^+$ ions is always high enough for maximal activity of the Na-K-ATPase. The impact of this increase in $Na^+$ ion pumping out of cells on the net cell voltage, however, depends on whether the $Na^+$ ion entry step into cells is electrogenic or electroneutral.

### Electrogenic entry of $Na^+$ ions into cells

The $Na^+$ ion channel in cell membranes is normally closed by the usual magnitude of the negative intracellular voltage. If the $Na^+$ ion channel in skeletal muscle cell membranes were to open (e.g., by the release of acetylcholine in response to neuronal stimulation), the cell interior voltage becomes less negative. This is because one positive charge enters the cell per $Na^+$ ion transported into the cell, but only one-third of a positive charge exits the cell per $Na^+$ ion pumped out of the cell via Na-K-ATPase (Figure 13-3). This decrease in intracellular negative voltage promotes the entry of ionized calcium ($Ca^{2+}$) via the voltage gated calcium ion channel, leading to muscle contraction. It also causes exit of $K^+$ ions from cells through open $K^+$ ion channels in

**ABBREVIATIONS**

$P_{Glucose}$, concentration of glucose in plasma

$P_{L-lactate}$, concentration of L-lactate in plasma

NHE-1, sodium hydrogen exchager-1

SLGT, sodium linked glucose transporter

EABV, effective arterial blood volume

DKA,diabetic ketoacidosis

MCT, monocarboxylic acid transporter

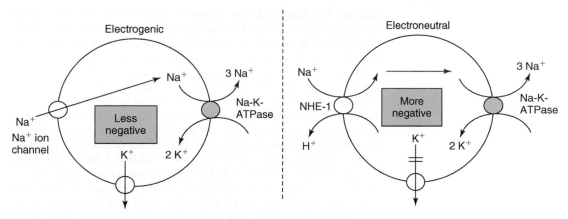

**Figure 13-3 Effect of Electroneutral Versus Electrogenic Entry of Na+ Ions on the Negative Voltage in Cells.** As shown on the *left* side of the figure, if the source of Na+ ions pumped out of cells is Na+ ions that entered cells via the Na+ ion channel, the voltage in cells becomes less negative (count the charges), and K+ ions exit the cells if a sufficient number of open K+ ion channels are present in the cell membrane. In contrast, a more negative voltage in cells is generated by Na-K-ATPase, if the source of Na+ ions pumped out is either Na+ ions that exist in cells or Na+ ions that entered the cells in an electroneutral fashion via the Na+/H+ exchanger (NHE-1); K+ ions are retained in cells (*right* side of the figure).

the cell membrane and thus a rise in the concentration of K+ ions in the ECF compartment.

### Clinical implications

An abnormally large increase in the entry of Na+ ions via Na+ ion channels in cell membranes of skeletal muscle and its subsequent exit via Na-K-ATPase diminishes the magnitude of the intracellular negative voltage. This is the underlying pathophysiology of hyperkalemia in some patients with hyperkalemic periodic paralysis.

### Electroneutral entry of Na+ into cells

This occurs when Na+ ions enter cells in exchange for H+ ions via the sodium-hydrogen cation exchanger-1 (NHE-1) (see Figure 13-3). The subsequent electrogenic exit of these Na+ ions out of cells via the Na-K-ATPase results in a more negative voltage inside cells. NHE-1 in cell membranes is normally inactive. This can be deduced from the fact that it is an electroneutral exchanger and that the concentrations of its substrates (Na+ ions in the ECF compartment and H+ ions in the ICF compartment) are considerably higher than the concentrations of ions that reflect its transport activity (Na+ ions in the ICF compartment and H+ ions in the ECF compartment) in the steady state. There are two major activators of NHE-1: a spike in insulin level in the interstitial fluid compartment and a higher concentration of H+ ions in the ICF compartment.

One major physiologic setting in which there is a need to shift K+ ions into cells and to do so quickly is when there is a large dietary intake of K+ ions (see margin note). Fruit and berries were the major sources of calories in the Paleolithic diet. Accordingly, this diet provided a large quantity of sugar (fructose and glucose) and K+ ions. To prevent this K+ ion load from entering the systemic circulation where it can be dangerous if it reaches the heart, the first line of defence is to induce a shift of this dietary load of K+ ions into liver cells.

It is well known that there is a rise in the plasma L- lactate anions ($P_{L\text{-lactate}}$) level in portal venous blood after absorption of dietary

**MAJOR SETTINGS IN WHICH A RAPID SHIFT OF K+ INTO CELLS IS NEEDED**

- *After the ingestion of a large K+ load*: The major hormone involved is insulin; the major site for the shift of K+ ions is into the liver.
- *After vigorous sprint*: The major hormones involved are β₂-adrenergics, which are released in the "fight-or-flight" response.

glucose. We suggested that a possible function of this high portal $P_{L\text{-lactate}}$ is to prevent hyperkalemia in hepatic venous blood following the absorption of $K^+$ ions from the diet. The process begins by increasing the rate of glycolysis in enterocytes as a result of performing more metabolic work. This extra metabolic work occurs because the sodium linked glucose transporter (SLGT) in this location is SLGT-1. Hence, when 1 mmol of glucose is absorbed, 2 mmol of $Na^+$ ions must be absorbed. Therefore, more adenosine triphosphate (ATP) must be regenerated to absorb a given quantity of glucose than if the stoichiometry of the transporter was the absorption of 1 mmol of $Na^+$ ions per 1 mmol of glucose. Should glycolysis occur at a faster rate than pyruvate oxidation, L-lactic acid will be released into the portal vein. In the liver, the uptake of L-lactic acid on the monocarboxylic acid cotransporter and its subsequent dissociation inside the hepatocytes into $H^+$ ions and L-lactic acid anions could raise the concentration of $H^+$ ions in the submembrane region of the hepatocytes adjacent to NHE-1 and hence activate NHE-1 by binding to its modifier site. The electroneutral entry of $Na^+$ ions into hepatocytes and their subsequent exit via the Na-K-ATPase in an electrogenic fashion will lead to a higher negative intracellular voltage and hence the retention of $K^+$ ions in hepatocytes (Figure 13-4). This mechanism requires the presence of insulin, which is released in response to the dietary sugar load with the ingestion of fruit and berries. This high concentration of insulin activates NHE-1 and also causes the translocation of more Na-K-ATPase units to the cell surface of hepatocytes.

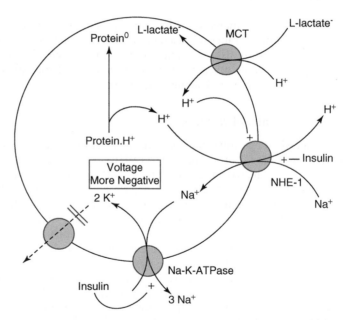

**Figure 13-4 Combined Actions of Insulin and L-Lactic Acid on a Shift of K⁺ Ions into Hepatocytes.** The *circle* represents the cell membrane of hepatocytes. When L-lactic acid enters hepatocytes on the monocarboxylic acid transporter (MCT), this may lead to the release of H⁺ ions immediately adjacent to the NHE-1. NHE-1 is activated when H⁺ ions bind to its modifier site. As a result, Na⁺ ions enter cells in exchange for H⁺ ions. The source of H⁺ ions is H⁺ ions that are bound to intracellular proteins (Protein.H⁺). The resulting higher concentration of Na⁺ ions in these cells drives the exit of Na⁺ ions through the Na-K-ATPase. This leads to a higher negative intracellular voltage and hence the retention of K⁺ ions in hepatocytes. This process requires the presence of insulin, which, in addition to stimulating NHE-1, increases the activity and number of Na-K-ATPase in the cell membrane. *Protein°*, Intracellular proteins with fewer bound H⁺ ions.

## *Clinical implications*

The infusion of L-lactic acid in fed rats and in rats with acute hyperkalemia induced by the infusion of HCl or KCl was associated with a fall in the concentration of $K^+$ ions in plasma ($P_K$) from arterial blood samples. This was due to a shift of $K^+$ ions into the liver. A shift of $K^+$ ions into the liver was also observed with the infusion of Na lactate. The administration of a relatively large dose of insulin is the mainstay of therapy in patients with emergency hyperkalemia; hypoglycemia is a frequent complication. The administration of Na lactate with a smaller dose of insulin may provide an effective means to lower $P_K$ with less risk of hypoglycemia in the emergency treatment of patients with hyperkalemia than when a higher dose of insulin alone is used. Further studies are required to examine the effectiveness of this approach.

### ACTIVATE PRE-EXISTING Na-K-ATPASE

The second mechanism for increasing flux through Na-K-ATPase is also a rapid one. It involves activation of existing Na-K-ATPase units in the cell membrane. Unphosphorylated FXYD1 (phospholemann) binds to the α-subunit of the Na-K-ATPase, which diminishes the pump activity by decreasing its affinity for $Na^+$ ions and/or its $V_{max}$. Insulin causes phosphorylation of FXYD1 via atypical protein kinase C; this disrupts the interaction of FXYD1 with the α-subunit of Na-K-ATPase, which results in an increase in the affinity of the Na-K-ATPase for $Na^+$ ions and/or its $V_{max}$ (see Figure 13-5).

β2-Adrenergic agonists activate adenylate cyclase, which leads to stimulation of the conversion of ATP to cyclic adenosine monophosphate (cAMP). This second messenger, in turn, activates protein kinase-A, which induces phosphorylation of the FXYD1, and results in an increase in the affinity of the Na-K-ATPase for intracellular $Na^+$ (Figure 13-6). The increase in export of pre-existing intracellular $Na^+$ ions out of the cells leads to a higher negative voltage in cells and hence a shift of $K^+$ ions into cells.

This effect of β2-adrenergic agonists to induce a shift of $K^+$ ions into cells is particularly important during vigorous exercise, the second major physiologic setting where there is a need to shift $K^+$ ions into cells quickly. In the fight-or-flight response, the stimulus for muscle contraction is the entry of $Na^+$ ions through the voltage-gated $Na^+$ ion channel during the depolarization phase of muscle action potential. This entry of positive charges diminishes the cell interior negative voltage, which promotes the entry of ionized $Ca^{2+}$ ions via the voltage-gated calcium channel, and therefore muscle contraction. It also causes $K^+$ ions to exit from exercising muscles during the repolarization phase of the muscle action potential. Hence, there is a danger of acute hyperkalemia (see margin note). To minimize this risk, the β2-adrenergic effect of adrenaline released in this setting is exerted on hepatocytes and possibly on resting muscle cells, which obligates them to take up much of this $K^+$ ion load and thereby prevent a dangerous rise in the $P_K$.

In conditions associated with a large surge of catecholamines, the α-adrenergic effect dominates over the β-adrenergic effect. The α-adrenergic effect causes inhibition of the release of insulin, which may lead to a shift of $K^+$ ions out of cells. Therefore, hyperkalemia may develop.

### Clinical implications

An acute shift of $K^+$ ions into cells causing hypokalemia may be seen in conditions associated with a surge of catecholamines (e.g., patients with head trauma, subarachnoid hemorrhage, myocardial infarction, an

**MECHANISMS FOR THE RELEASE OF $K^+$ IONS FROM MUSCLE CELLS DURING EXERCISE**

- $Na^+$ ions enter muscle cells via open $Na^+$ ion channels during the depolarization phase of muscle action potential; this diminishes the negative voltage in cells. $K^+$ ions exit from muscle cells during repolarization.
- Intracellular alkalinization occurs when phosphocreatine is hydrolyzed. This activates the extrusion of $HCO_3^-$ ions via the electroneutral $Cl/HCO_3^-$ anion exchanger with the entry of $Cl^-$ ions into cells. The subsequent electrogenic exit of $Cl^-$ ions from cells via $Cl^-$ ion channels diminishes the negative voltage in cells and hence $K^+$ ions exit cells (see Chapter 1 and Figure 13-5).

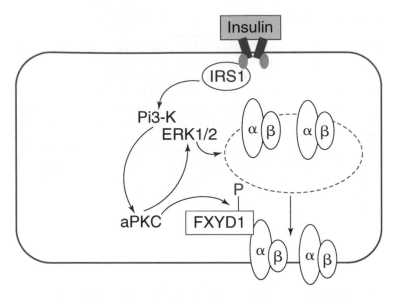

**Figure 13-5 Mechanism of the Effect of Insulin to Cause a Shift of K⁺ Ions into Cells.** The *rectangle* represents a cell membrane. In addition to its effect to activate NHE-1 and the electroneutral entry of Na⁺ ions into cells, insulin causes phosphorylation of FXYD1 (indicated by the letter *P* in the figure) via atypical protein kinase C (aPKC). Insulin also increases the expression of Na-K-ATPase in cell membranes. This effect is mediated through phospho-inositide 3-kinase (Pi3-K) and extracellular signal regulated kinases 1 and 2 (ERK1/2). ERK1/2 kinases induce phosphorylation of the α subunit of the Na-K-ATPase, which promotes the translocation of Na-K-ATPase from an intracellular pool to the cell membrane. The vertically oriented, side-by-side ovals labeled α and β represent the Na-K-ATPase. Insulin binds to its cell surface receptor. This causes activation of insulin receptor substrate (ISR-1). This in turn activates phosphoinositide 3-kinase(Pi3-K). Activated Pi3-K phosphorylates thereby activates atypical protein kinase C (aPKC). This has two effects. First, activated aPKC phosphorylates FXYD1. Second, it also acti-vates the extracellular signal regulated kinases 1 and 2 (ERK1/2) to phospho-rylate the alpha-subunit of Na-K-ATPase in the cytosol of the cell, promoting its translocation to the cell membrane. *IRS1,* Insulin receptor substrate 1.

extreme degree of anxiety). $\beta_2$-agonists may be used to shift K⁺ ions into cells in patients with an emergency associated with hyperkalemia. On the other hand, nonspecific β-blockers are being used for therapy of the sub-type of hypokalemic periodic paralysis associated with hyperthyroidism. In states with a very low effective arterial blood volume (EABV), the large α-adrenergic response leads to a shift of K⁺ ions out of cells. This shift of K⁺ ions out of cells is valuable to prevent a severe degree of hypokale-mia when the underlying disorder is also associated with a large loss of K⁺ ions (e.g., in patients with cholera or other infections causing severe secretory diarrhea). Hypokalemia becomes evident during therapy with restoration of the EABV.

## INCREASE IN THE NUMBER OF NA-K-ATPASE UNITS IN CELL MEMBRANES

### Insulin

Another effect of insulin which induces a shift of K⁺ ions into cells is by increasing the expression of Na-K-ATPase in cell membranes. This effect is mediated through phosphoinositide 3-kinase and extracellu-lar signal regulated kinases 1 and 2 (ERK1/2). ERK1/2 kinases induce

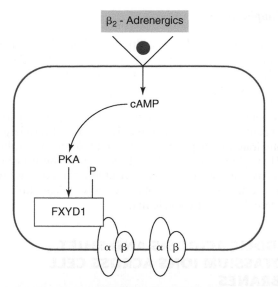

**Figure 13-6 Mechanism of the Effect of β₂-Adrenergic Agonists to Cause a Shift of K⁺ Ions into Cells.** The *rectangle* represents a cell membrane. β₂-Adrenergic agonists activate adenylate cyclase, and this leads to stimulation of the conversion of adenosine triphosphate (ATP) to cyclic adenosine monophosphate (cAMP). This second messenger, in turn, activates protein kinase-A (PKA), which induces phosphorylation of the FXYD1 (indicated by the letter *P* in the figure). This disrupts the interaction of FXD1 with the α-subunit of the Na-K-ATPase, which results in an increase in the affinity of Na-K-ATPase for Na⁺ ions and/or its $V_{max}$. The increase in export of pre-existing intracellular Na⁺ ions leads to a higher negative voltage in cells and hence a shift of K⁺ ions into cells.

phosphorylation of the α subunit of the Na-K-ATPase, which promotes the translocation of Na-K-ATPase from an intracellular pool to the cell membrane (see Figure 13-5). Notwithstanding, the glucose transporter, GLUT4, and the Na-K-ATPase do not colocalize to the same intracellular vesicles in skeletal muscle and hence the effect of insulin to shift K⁺ ions into cells is separate from its effect on glucose transport into these cells.

### Clinical implications

Because of its multiple effects to induce a shift of K⁺ ions into cells, insulin has been utilized to treat patients with an emergency caused by the adverse cardiac effects of hyperkalemia. In contrast, in patients with diabetic ketoacidosis (DKA), a lack of actions of insulin results in a shift of K⁺ ions out of cells and the development of hyperkalemia despite a total body deficit of K⁺ ions.

### Exercise training

Having more Na-K-ATPase units in the cell membrane of skeletal muscle cells is not important at rest, but it is very important during vigorous exercise. There is a strong positive correlation between the activity of this ion pump, which is essential for recovery from cell depolarization, and the maximum ability for skeletal muscle to contract during vigorous exercise.

### Thyroid hormones

Hyperthyroidism is also associated with a higher content of Na-K-ATPase units in the cell membrane.

*Clinical implications*

A severe degree of hypokalemia due to a shift of $K^+$ ions into cells is seen in patients with the thyrotoxic subtype of hypokalemic periodic paralysis. These patients can be managed effectively during their attacks with the administration of nonselective β-blockers and a small dose of KCl (see Chapter 14 for more details). Although not supported by epidemiological data, it is thought that many of these patients have attacks of acute hypokalemia and paralysis after eating a large amount of carbohydrates. Perhaps the effect of high levels of insulin to activate NHE-1, phosphorylate FXYD1, and cause the translocation of Na-K-ATPase into cell membranes, in addition to the effect of thyroid hormone to cause the synthesis of more Na-K-ATPase units, may lead to the severe degree of hypokalemia.

## METABOLIC ACIDOSIS AND SHIFT OF POTASSIUM IONS ACROSS CELL MEMBRANES

The effect of an acid load on the $P_K$ depends on whether the anions accompanying the $H^+$ ions can be transported into cells on the monocarboxylic acid cotransporter (MCT).

Monocarboxylic acids (e.g., L-lactic acid, ketoacids) can be transported into cells on the MCT. Because the transport of these acids into cells occurs in an electroneutral fashion, it does not change the magnitude of the negative voltage inside the cells and therefore does not result in a shift of $K^+$ ions. Notwithstanding, if subsequent to the entry of these acids into cells there is an increase in $H^+$ ion concentration in the submembrane area adjacent to NHE-1, this may may cause its activation. If in addition there is activation of Na-K-ATPase because of the administration of insulin in a patient with DKA or the release of $β_2$ adrenergics in a patient with L-lactic acidosis due to vigorous exercise, the voltage inside cells may become more negative and a shift of $K^+$ ions into cells may occur.

Inorganic acids (e.g., HCl) and nonmonocarboxylic organic acids (e.g., citric acid) cannot enter cells by the MCT. In addition, their $H^+$ ions cannot enter cells via NHE-1 because this exchanger can cause only the export of $H^+$ ions from, and not their entry into, cells. Hence, a different mechanism is needed to permit some of these $H^+$ ions to be titrated using $HCO_3^-$ anions in the ICF compartment. This may involve activation of the $Cl^-/HCO_3^-$ anion exchanger (perhaps because of a low $P_{HCO_3}$, but the exact mechanism is not known) with transport of $HCO_3^-$ ions out of cells and of $Cl^-$ ions into cells. Because this exchange of anions has a 1:1 stoichiometry, it is electroneutral and it does not change the magnitude of the negative voltage in these cells. Nevertheless, as a result of the combination of the higher concentration of $Cl^-$ ions in cells, the negative intracellular voltage, and the presence of open $Cl^-$ ion channels in cell membranes, $Cl^-$ ions are forced out of cells in an electrogenic fashion, and therefore the voltage in these cells becomes less negative, and $K^+$ ions exit the cells (see Figure 13-7).

### CLINICAL IMPLICATIONS

If hyperkalemia is present in a patient with metabolic acidosis caused by increased production of a monocarboxylic organic acid, causes of hyperkalemia other than the acidemia should be sought (e.g., lack of

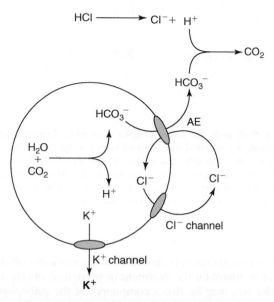

**Figure 13-7 Shift of K⁺ Ions Out of Cells in Patients with Metabolic Acidosis Caused by the Addition of Nonmonocarboxylic Acids.** The *circle* represents a cell. Inorganic acids (e.g., HCl) or nonmonocarboxylic organic acids (e.g., citric acid) cannot enter cells by the monocarboxylic acid transporter. Therefore, a mechanism is needed to permit some of these H⁺ ions to be titrated using $HCO_3^-$ anions in the intracellular fluid compartment. This may involve activation of the $Cl^-/HCO_3$ anion exchanger (AE) with transport of $HCO_3^-$ ions out of cells and of $Cl^-$ ions into cells. $Cl^-$ ions are forced out of cells in an electrogenic fashion because of the electrochemical driving force and the presence of open $Cl^-$ ion channels in cell membranes, the voltage in these cells becomes less negative, and K⁺ ions exit the cells.

insulin in patients with DKA, tissue injury or a decreased availability of ATP to drive the Na-K-ATPase in patients with L-lactic acidosis due to hypoxia).

Although acidemia because of addition of inorganic acids (addition of HCl) causes a shift of K⁺ ions out of cells, patients with chronic hyperchloremic metabolic acidosis may have a low $P_K$ because of excessive loss of K⁺ ions in the diarrheal fluid in patients with chronic diarrhea or in the urine (e.g., patients with distal renal tubular acidosis; see Chapter 4 for more discussion).

There are only small changes in the $P_K$ in patients with respiratory acid–base disorders because there is little movement of Na⁺ or Cl⁻ ions across cell membranes and hence no change in the ICF negative voltage.

## HYPERTONICITY AND SHIFT OF POTASSIUM IONS ACROSS CELL MEMBRANES

A rise in effective osmolality (i.e., tonicity) in the interstitial fluid causes the movement of water out of cells via aquaporin-1 (AQP1) water channels in cell membranes. This raises the concentration of K⁺ ions in the ICF, which provides a chemical driving force for the movement of K⁺ ions out of cells (Figure 13-8). Although some may call this osmotic drag, this is not really an appropriate description of the phenomenon because the movement of K⁺ ions out of cells is not through AQP1 but through specific K⁺ ion channels.

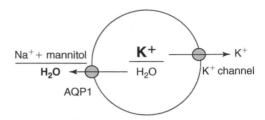

**Figure 13-8 Shift of K$^+$ Ions Out of Cells Caused by Exposure to a Hypertonic Solution.** A sustained rise in tonicity in the interstitial fluid (addition of mannitol in this example) causes the movement of water out of cells via aquaporin-1 (AQP1) water channels in cell membranes. This raises the concentration of K$^+$ ions in the cells, which provides a chemical driving force for the movement of K$^+$ ions out of cells via K$^+$ ion channels.

### CLINICAL IMPLICATIONS

Severe hyperkalemia has been described as a complication of the administration of mannitol for the treatment or prevention of cerebral edema. This mechanism may be also a component of the pathophysiology of hyperkalemia in patients with DKA and a severe degree of hyperglycemia.

# PART C
# RENAL EXCRETION OF POTASSIUM IONS

Arguably the most important immediate function of the kidney is to excrete a large K$^+$ ion load to avoid the development of hyperkalemia and the risk of a cardiac arrhythmia. Control of K$^+$ ion secretion occurs primarily in the CDN, which includes the late DCT, the connecting segment, and the CCD. Most of the secretion of K$^+$ ions occurs in the late DCT and the connecting segment; the CCD also participates in this process when the K$^+$ ion load is large.

Although the usual intake of K$^+$ ions in adults eating a typical Western diet is close to 1 mmol/kg body weight, the rate of excretion of K$^+$ ions can rise or fall by close to a factor of five to match its intake with only a minor rise or fall in the $P_K$. Although most of this K$^+$ ion intake occurs during the evening meal, its excretion typically occurs around noon the next day (see margin note).

## COMPONENTS OF THE EXCRETION OF K$^+$ IONS IN THE CORTICAL DISTAL NEPHRON

There are two components that affect the rate of excretion of K$^+$ ions: (1) the rate of net secretion of K$^+$ ions by principal cells in the CDN and (2) the flow rate in the terminal CDN (i.e., the number of liters of fluid that exit the CCD).

### SECRETION OF K$^+$ IONS IN THE CORTICAL DISTAL NEPHRON

A large quantity of K$^+$ ions is filtered daily (720 mmol in an adult; $P_K$ 4 mmol/L × 180 L glomerular filtration rate (GFR)/day). Five-sixths of this amount is reabsorbed passively in the proximal convoluted tubule (PCT). Because a similar proportion of filtered Na$^+$ ions and water are

---

**DIURNAL VARIATION IN THE EXCRETION OF K$^+$ IONS**

- The bulk of excretion of K$^+$ ions occurs close to noontime.
- This does not seem to be related to a rise in the level of aldosterone in plasma or in the delivery of Na$^+$ ions to the CDN.
- Although the mechanism is still open for debate, it is possible that it is due to an increased delivery of HCO$_3^-$ ions to the CDN during the alkaline tide.

**ABBREVIATIONS**

PCT, proximal convoluted tubule
NCC, Na-Cl cotransporter
NDCBE, sodium-dependent chloride-bicarbonate exchanger
SGK-1, serum and glucocorticoid regulated kinase-1
ANG$_{II}$, angiotensin II
SPAK, STE 20-related proline-alanine-rich-kinase
OSR1, oxidative stress response kinase type 1
K$_{CDN}$, concentration of K$^+$ ions in the cortical distal nephron

reabsorbed, the concentration of $K^+$ ions in luminal fluid in PCT remains close the value of the $P_K$. Because 30 L of fluid exit the PCT per day (see Chapter 9), 120 mmol of $K^+$ ions are delivered to the loop of Henle (4 mmol/L × 30 L/day). Although there is a large passive entry of $K^+$ ions into the lumen of the loop of Henle via ROMK, there is net reabsorption of $K^+$ ions in the loop of Henle of about 80 mmol/day (see margin note), and hence about 40 mmol of $K^+$ ions/day are delivered to the CDN, the nephron sites where $K^+$ ion secretion occurs.

Two elements are required for the process of $K^+$ ion secretion in the CDN: (1) the generation of a transepithelial lumen-negative voltage, and (2) the presence of $K^+$ channels in an open configuration in the luminal membranes of principal cells.

## Generation of a Lumen-Negative Voltage

$K^+$ ions are actively transported from the interstitium across the basolateral membrane via the Na-K-ATPase. Although $K^+$ ion channels are also present in the basolateral membrane, $K^+$ ions preferentially leave principal cells across the apical membrane because the electrochemical gradient for $K^+$ ion exit across the apical membrane is more favorable than across the basolateral membrane. This is because of the electrogenic movement of $Na^+$ ions across the apical membrane through ENaC, which depolarizes the apical membrane and creates a lumen-negative transepithelial potential.

### Electrogenic reabsorption of $Na^+$ ions in the CDN

A lumen-negative voltage is generated in the CDN by the electrogenic reabsorption of $Na^+$ ions (i.e., reabsorption of $Na^+$ ions without their accompanying anions [usually $Cl^-$ ions]). Electrogenic reabsorption of $Na^+$ ions occurs via the amiloride-sensitive epithelial $Na^+$ ion channel (ENaC) in the luminal membrane of principal cells in the CDN.

Aldosterone is the major hormone that causes an increase in the number of open ENaC units in the luminal membrane of principal cells. The driving forces for reabsorption of $Na^+$ ions via ENaC is the higher concentration of $Na^+$ ions in the lumen of the CDN than in principal cells (~10 to 15 mmol/L) and the negative cell interior voltage caused by the actions of the Na-K-ATPase at the basolateral membrane in these cells. One $Na^+$ ion must be delivered and reabsorbed without its accompanying anion (usually $Cl^-$ ions) for every $K^+$ ion secreted in the CDN. Under most circumstances, the concentration of $Na^+$ ions in luminal fluid is sufficient for the maximum rate of reabsorption of $Na^+$ ions via ENaC. Usual variations in the luminal concentration of $Na^+$ ions in the luminal fluid in the CDN do not regulate the rate of secretion of $K^+$ ions.

### Mechanism of action of aldosterone

The steps involved include binding of aldosterone to its receptor in the cytoplasm of principal cells, entry of this hormone-receptor complex into the nucleus, and then the synthesis of new proteins including the serum and glucocorticoid regulated kinase-1 (SGK-1). SGK-1 increases the expression of ENaC in the apical membrane of principal cells. The mechanism seems to be related to the effect of SGK-1 to phosphorylate and inactivate the ubiquitin ligase Nedd-4-2, which ubiquinates ENaC subunits, leading to their removal from the cell membrane and degradation in proteasomes. Therefore, inhibition of the Nedd-4-2 leads to diminished endocytosis and hence increased expression of ENaC units in the luminal membrane of principal cells

---

**REABSORPTION OF $K^+$ IONS IN THE LOOP OF HENLE**

- In micropuncture experiments in rats, the concentration of $K^+$ ions in the luminal fluid at the earliest part of the DCT is ~1.5 mmol/L. A reasonable estimate of the volume of filtrate delivered to the distal nephron in humans is ~27 L/day (see Chapter 9). Hence, ~40 mmol of $K^+$ ions are delivered to the CDN (1.5 mmol/L × 27 L/day).
- Therefore, there is net reabsorption of ~80 mmol of $K^+$ ions per day in the loop of Henle.

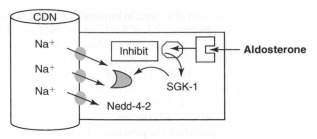

**Figure 13-9 Mechanism of Action of Aldosterone.** The *barrel-shaped structure* represents the cortical distal nephron (CDN), and the *rectangle* represents a principal cell. The *ovals* in the luminal membrane of the principal cell are epithelial Na+ ion channels (ENaC). Aldosterone binds to its receptor in the cytoplasm of principal cells; this hormone-receptor complex enters the nucleus and causes the synthesis of new proteins including the serum and glucocorticoid regulated kinase-1 (SGK-1). SGK-1 phosphorylates and inactivates the ubiquitin ligase Nedd-4-2, which leads to diminished endocytosis and hence increased expression of ENaC in the luminal membrane.

(Figure 13-9). Another mechanism by which aldosterone activates ENaC involves proteolytic cleavage of the channel by serine proteases. Aldosterone induces production of "channel activating proteases" (CAP 1-3). These proteases activate ENaC by increasing their open probability, rather than by increasing their expression at the luminal membrane.

Although the concentration of cortisol in plasma is at least hundreds of times higher than that of aldosterone, and these two hormones bind to the aldosterone receptor with near-equal avidity, cortisol does not exert mineralocorticoid actions because it is converted into an inactive form, cortisone, by the 11β-hydroxysteroid dehydrogenase 1 and 2 enzyme system (11β-HSDH); cortisone does not bind to the aldosterone receptor.

### Electroneutral reabsorption of Na+ ions in the CDN

If the reabsorption of Na+ ions in the CDN occurs via an electroneutral processes (i.e., Na+ ions and their accompanying anions, which are usually Cl− ions, are reabsorbed), a negative luminal voltage will not be generated. Hence, this component of reabsorption of Na+ ions in the CDN does not lead to the secretion of K+ ions.

The pathway(s) for the reabsorption of Cl− ions in the CDN is (are) not well defined, but it was thought that the paracellular pathway played an important role. This seems unlikely, however, because of the magnitude of the luminal negative transtubular voltage and the large concentration difference for Cl− ions between plasma and the luminal fluid that there would not be sufficient electrochemical gradient to drive the paracellular reabsorption of Cl− ions. Recently, an electroneutral, thiazide-sensitive, amiloride-resistant Na+ and Cl− ion transport mechanism was identified in the β-intercalated cells of the CCD in rats and mice. This seems to be mediated by the parallel activity of two different Cl−/HCO3− anion exchangers: (1) the Na+-dependent Cl−/HCO3− exchanger (NDCBE), which promotes the electroneutral exchange of one intracellular Cl− ion with one luminal Na+ ion and two luminal HCO3− ions, and (2) the Na+ independent Cl−/HCO3− anion exchanger (pendrin) (Figure 13-10). This transport mechanism is apparently responsible for as much as 50% of mineralocorticiod-stimulated NaCl reabsorption in the CCD of mice.

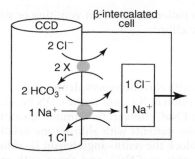

**Figure 13-10 Electroneutral Reabsorption of Na⁺ Ions in the Cortical Collecting Duct (CCD).** The *barrel-shaped structure* represents the CCD, and the *rectangles* represent a β-intercalated cell. The *top pink circle* represents pendrin. The *bottom pink circle* represents the Na⁺-dependent Cl⁻/HCO₃⁻ anion exchanger (NDCBE). The exchange of 2 Cl⁻ ions for 2 HCO₃⁻ ions via two cycles of pendrin (illustrated in the figure by the symbol 2X) with the subsequent uptake of 2 HCO₃⁻ ions and 1 Na⁺ ion in exchange for 1 Cl⁻ ion via one cycle of NDCBE results in net electroneutral transport of 1 Na⁺ ion and 1 Cl⁻ ion across the luminal membrane with the recycling of 2 HCO₃⁻ ions and 1 Cl⁻ ion.

A high concentration of HCO₃⁻ ions in the luminal fluid and/or an alkaline luminal fluid pH seems to increase the amount of K⁺ ions secreted in the CDN. It was suggested that this might be due to a decrease in the apparent permeability of Cl⁻ ions and/or an increase in the open probability of ROMK in the CDN. It is also possible that the increase in luminal HCO₃⁻ ion concentration in the CDN inhibits the Cl⁻/HCO₃⁻ anion exchanger (pendrin), and hence the NDCBE and the electroneutral NaCl reabsorption, leading to a higher rate of electrogenic reabsorption of Na⁺ ions and therefore a higher rate of K⁺ ion secretion in the CDN (see Figure 13-10).

## Clinical implications

### Hypokalemia

In a patient with chronic hypokalemia, a higher than expected rate of excretion of K⁺ ions in the urine implies that the lumen-negative voltage is abnormally more negative and that open ROMK are present in the luminal membranes of principal cells in the CDN. The greater lumen-negative voltage is due to more electrogenic versus electroneutral reabsorption of Na⁺ ions in the CDN. The primary reason is an increased number of open ENaC units in the luminal membrane of principal cells in the CDN. This could be due to two groups of disorders. Patients in the first group have a secondary increase in ENaC activity due to the release of aldosterone in response to a low EABV (e.g., due to protracted vomiting, diuretics, Bartter's syndrome, and Gitelman's syndrome). Patients in the second group have a condition that is associated with a primary increase in ENaC activity (e.g., primary hypereninemic hyperaldosteronism, primary hyperaldosteronism, disorders in which cortisol acts as a mineralocorticoid in the CDN, constitutively active ENaC in luminal membrane of principal cells in the CDN; see Chapter 14). Patients in this second group are expected to have hypertension and an EABV that is not low. In some patients, a decreased rate of electroneutral Na⁺ ion reabsorption may contribute to the increased rate of electrogenic Na⁺ ion reabsorption and hence the enhanced kaliuresis. This may be the case when Na⁺ ions are delivered to the CDN with a small amount of Cl⁻ ions (e.g., delivery of Na⁺ ions with

$HCO_3^-$ ions in a patient with recent vomiting or with an anion of a drug such as penicillin).

### Hyperkalemia

In some patients with chronic hyperkalemia, there is diminished electrogenic reabsorption of $Na^+$ ions in the CDN because of a decreased number of open ENaC units in the luminal membrane of principal cells. This includes patients with aldosterone deficiency, those who take drugs that block the renin–angiotensin II–aldosterone axis, the aldosterone receptor or ENaC, and those with molecular defects that involve the aldosterone receptor or ENaC (see Chapter 15). In another subset of patients, the site of the lesion is the early DCT, where there is enhanced electroneutral reabsorption of $Na^+$ and $Cl^-$ ions via the $Na^+$-$Cl^-$ cotransporter (NCC). Suppression of the release of aldosterone by an expanded EABV leads to a diminished number of open ENaC units in the luminal membranes of principal cells in the CDN. Examples include patients with the syndrome of hypertension and hyperkalemia, patients treated with calcineurin inhibitors, and some patients with diabetic nephropathy and hyporeninemic hypoaldosteronism. In another group of patients, the pathophysiology may be an increased electroneutral reabsorption of $Na^+$ and $Cl^-$ ions in the CCD caused by increased parallel transport activity of pendrin and NDBCE. This may be the pathophysiology for what used to be thought of as a "chloride shunt disorder"; an example may be a subset of patients with diabetic nephropathy and hyporenineic hypoaldosteronism (see Chapter 15).

### K+ ION CHANNELS

The main channel for $K^+$ ion secretion in the CDN is ROMK. The role of big $K^+$ ion conductance channel ("BK" or maxi-$K^+$ ion channel) in the physiologic regulation of renal excretion of $K^+$ ions is not clear.

### ROMK channels

Several types of $K^+$ ion channels are expressed in the apical membrane of principal cells in the CDN. ROMK ($K_{ir}1.1$) are the most important for the secretion of $K^+$ ions.

Regulation of ROMK channels is via phosphorylation/dephosphorylation-induced endocytosis/exocytosis, which involves a complicated mixture of kinases and phosphatases including the WNK kinases (see margin note), tyrosine kinases, and SGK-1. Angiotensin II ($ANG_{II}$) has been shown to inhibit ROMK activity in rats on a $K^+$ ion restricted diet but not in rats on their usual dietary $K^+$ ion intake. The effect of $ANG_{II}$ may be mediated via increasing the expression of Scr family of protein tyrosine kinases, which phosphorylates ROMK and results in its endocytosis.

WNK4 inhibits ROMK by stimulating its endocytosis. When the intake of $K^+$ ions is high, $ANG_{II}$ is suppressed but SGK-1 is increased due to the actions of aldosterone. In this setting, SGK-1 phosphorylates WNK4 and reverses its inhibition of ROMK (Figure 13-11).

Alternative promoter usage of the WNK1 gene produces a kidney-specific, truncated form of WNK1, called KS-WNK1, and a more ubiquitous long form, called L-WNK1. L-WNK1 inhibits ROMK by inducing its endocytosis, whereas the KS-WNK1 isoform inhibits this effect of L-WNK1. The relative abundance of the WNK1 isoforms is regulated by dietary $K^+$ intake. An increase in dietary $K^+$ ion intake leads to an increased ratio of KS-WNK1 to L-WNK1,

**WNK KINASES (WITH NO LYSINE KINASES)**
- K is the single-letter symbol for the amino acid lysine, which is important for catalytic actions of most kinases.
- In these kinases, lysine is near but not in the catalytic site.

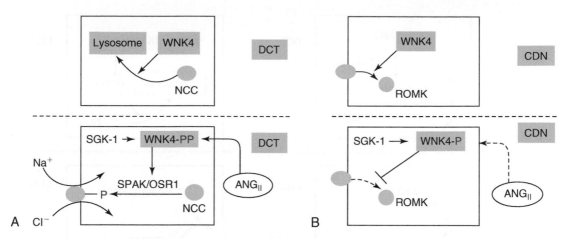

**Figure 13-11  Effects of WNK4 on the Na-Cl Contransporter (NCC) and the Renal Outer Medullary K⁺ Ion Channels (ROMK). A,** WNK4 inhibits NCC activity by reducing its abundance in luminal membranes by diverting NCC to the lysosome for degradation. Angiotensin II (ANG$_{II}$) signaling through its AT1 receptor converts WNK4 from an NCC-inhibiting kinase to an NCC-activating kinase. The activated form of WNK4 phosphorylates STE 20-related proline-alanine-rich-kinase (SPAK) and oxidative stress response kinase type 1 (OSR1). Phosphorylated SPAK/OSR1 in turn phosphorylates and activates NCC. **B,** WNK4 inhibits ROMK by stimulating its endocytosis. When ANG$_{II}$ is suppressed but serum and glucocorticoid regulated kinase-1 (SGK-1) is present, SGK-1 phosphorylates WNK4 and reverses its inhibition of ROMK. *CDN,* Cortical distal nephron; *DCT,* distal convoluted tubule; *WNK4-PP,* WNK4 phosphorylated at 2 different sites by ANG$_{II}$ and SGK-1.

so there is reduced endocytosis of ROMK; the ratio is decreased by dietary K⁺ ion restriction, which thereby leads to greater endocytosis of ROMK (Figure 13-12).

### Big conductance K⁺ ion channel (maxi K⁺ ion channel)

α-Intercalated cells in the medullary collecting duct (MCD) and the CDN in rats and mice have another K⁺ ion channel called big conductance K⁺ ion channel (BK) or maxi K⁺ ion channel. BK channels are activated (have higher opening probability) when the flow rate in the collecting ducts is high; this is mediated by an increase in the intracellular concentration of ionized calcium. The role of BK channels in physiological regulation of renal excretion of K⁺ ions is not clear. BK channel activity is increased in the CDN from rats fed a high K⁺ diet. Furthermore, in BK-α-subunit knockout mice, an increase in flow in the distal nephron failed to stimulate K⁺ ion secretion. Notwithstanding, deletion of BK-α-subunit does not affect net K⁺ ion excretion in mice fed a high K⁺ diet. It is important to recall that the role of these channels was examined in laboratory rodents, which consume 10-fold more K⁺ ions per kg body weight compared to human subjects who eat a typical Western diet. Therefore, it is possible that the BK channel may provide a way for a "speedy" K⁺ ion excretion if there is a very large intake of K⁺ ions and if flow rate through the CDN were augmented in this setting. It is interesting to note that increasing flow rate also stimulates ENaC activity and hence the electrogenic reabsorption of Na⁺ ions in the CDN. Furthermore, in addition to the electrical driving force for K⁺ ion secretion, the increase in luminal flow rate lowers the concentration of K⁺ ions in luminal fluid, and hence there is a higher concentration difference for the diffusion of K⁺ ions into the luminal fluid in CDN. BK channel activity seems to be stimulated by the purinergic system (see margin note).

BK channels likely mediate K⁺ ion secretion in patients with Bartter's syndrome that is due to a loss-of-function mutation in ROMK

**PURINERGIC SYSTEM AND K⁺ ION SECRETION**

- It has recently been proposed that β-intercalated cells, in response to high flow rate, release ATP, which sends a message via binding to purinergic receptors to cause activation of the BK channel in α-intercalated cells.
- It is interesting to note, however, that this signaling system leads also to inhibition of ENaC activity in principal cells, so we are not clear about the role of the purinergic system in causing a large increase in K⁺ ion excretion.

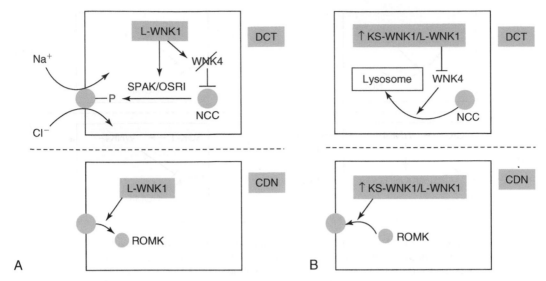

**Figure 13-12 Effects of WNK1 on Na-Cl Contransporter (NCC) and Renal Outer Medullary K⁺ Ion Channels (ROMK).** Alternative promoter usage of the WNK1 gene produces a kidney-specific, truncated form of WNK1, called KS-WNK1, and a more ubiquitous long form, called L-WNK1. **A,** L-WNK1 upregulates NCC either by blocking the inhibitory form of WNK4 or directly by phosphorylation of STE 20-related proline-alanine-rich-kinase (SPAK) and oxidative stress response kinase type 1 (OSR1). L-WNK1 inhibits ROMK by inducing its endocytosis. **B,** The KS-WNK1 isoform inhibits these effects of L-WNK1. An increase in dietary K⁺ ion intake leads to an increased ratio of KS-WNK1 to L-WNK1, so there is reduced expression of NCC in the luminal membrane of the distal convoluted tubule (DCT) and decreased endocytosis of ROMK. *CDN,* Cortical distal nephron.

(see Chapter 14). It seems that BK channels have a developmental delay, hence affected infants present initially with a severe degree of hyperkalemia during the first month of life. After this time, these channels are present in the CDN, and the clinical picture changes to one of hypokalemia.

## WNK KINASES (WITH NO LYSINE KINASES)

A complex network of WNK kinases, WNK4 and WNK1, via effects on the thiazide-sensitive Na-Cl cotransporter (NCC) in the early DCT and hence the delivery of NaCl and the rate of electrogenic reabsorption of Na⁺ ions in the CDN and effects on ROMK, seem to function as part of a switch system to change the renal response to aldosterone to either conserve Na⁺ ions or excrete K⁺ ions, depending on whether the release of aldosterone is induced by a reduction in dietary Na⁺ ion intake (low EABV) or an increase in dietary K⁺ ion intake.

## WNK4

### Effect on NCC

WNK4 is thought to inhibit NCC activity by reducing its abundance in luminal membranes by diverting post-Golgi NCC to the lysosome for degradation. ANG$_{II}$ is released in response to low EABV (or low salt intake). ANG$_{II}$ signaling through its AT1 receptor phosphorylates WNK4 and converts it from an NCC-inhibiting to an NCC-activating kinase. The activated form of WNK4 phosphorylates members of the STE 20 family of serine/threonine kinases, specifically the STE 20-related proline-alanine-rich-kinase (SPAK) and the oxidative stress response kinase type 1 (OSR1). Phosphorylated SPAK/OSR1 in turn phosphorylates and activates NCC (Figure 13-11).

### Effect on ROMK

WNK4 inhibits ROMK by stimulating endocytosis of the channel via clathrin-coated vesicles. When $ANG_{II}$ is suppressed but SGK-1 is present, as in conditions of high $K^+$ ion intake, SGK-1 phosphorylates WNK4 and reverses its inhibition of ROMK (Figure 13-11).

### WNK1

As mentioned above, alternative promoter usage of the WNK1 gene produces a kidney-specific, truncated form of WNK1, called KS-WNK1, and a more ubiquitous long form, called L-WNK1. The KS-WNK1 isoform inhibits the effects of L-WNK1. An increase in dietary $K^+$ ion intake leads to an increased ratio of KS-WNK1 to L-WNK1; this ratio is decreased by dietary $K^+$ ion restriction.

### Effect on NCC

L-WNK1 upregulates NCC either by blocking the inhibitory form of WNK4 or directly by phosphorylation of SPAK/OSR1. The KS-WNK1 isoform inhibits this effect of L-WNK1 and hence there is diminished expression of NCC in the luminal membrane in the DCT (Figure 13-12).

### Effect on ROMK

L-WNK1 inhibits ROMK by inducing its endocytosis. The KS-WNK1 isoform inhibits this effect of L-WNK1. An increase in dietary $K^+$ ion intake leads to an increased ratio of KS-WNK1 to L-WNK1, so there is reduced endocytosis of ROMK. This ratio is decreased by dietary $K^+$ ion restriction, hence there is greater endocytosis of ROMK (see Figure 13-12).

## THE ALDOSTERONE PARADOX

The paradox derives from the fact that aldosterone can be an NaCl-retaining hormone or a kaliuretic hormone. Aldosterone is released in response to separate stimuli: $ANG_{II}$ when there is a low EABV and a higher $P_K$ following a large intake of $K^+$ ions. Each of these stimuli for the release of aldosterone has an identical effect; an increase in the number of open ENaC units in the luminal membrane of principal cells. Therefore, the kidney must "know" whether the appropriate response is to reabsorb more NaCl or to secrete more $K^+$ ions when the concentration of aldosterone in plasma ($P_{Aldosterone}$) is high. WNK kinases and modulation of delivery of $HCO_3^-$ ions to the CDN may act in concert to achieve the desired effect of aldosterone. The complex interplay of these mechanisms may be better understood if analyzed from a Paleolithic perspective. The diet consumed by our ancient ancestors consisted mainly of fruit and berries, which provided small amounts of NaCl but episodic and at times large loads of $K^+$ ions. Therefore, there was a need for mechanisms to ensure renal conservation of NaCl to avoid a hemodynamic threat. To avoid the risk of dangerous hyperkalemia and cardiac arrhythmia, there was a need to have mechanisms to switch the renal response from NaCl conservation to $K^+$ ion excretion when faced with a load of $K^+$ ions. This will be discussed in more detail in Section D.

**FLOW RATE AND K⁺ ION SECRETION IN CDN**

- Increasing flow rate also increases K⁺ ion secretion in the CDN; this may be mediated via BK channels.
- Increasing flow rate stimulates ENaC activity and the electrogenic reabsorption of Na⁺ ions in the CDN.
- Increasing luminal flow rate lowers the concentration of K⁺ ions in luminal fluid. Therefore, there is a higher concentration difference for the diffusion of K⁺ ions from principal cells into the luminal fluid in the CDN.

**NUMBER OF OSMOLES IN LUMINAL FLUID IN TERMINAL CDN**

- Because there is little reabsorption or secretion of Na⁺ or K⁺ ions in the nephron segments distal to the CCD, we estimated that the number of osmoles of electrolytes that are present in luminal fluid in the terminal CCD would be approximately equal to their excretion in the urine. Therefore, in subjects eating a typical Western diet, about 500 osmoles of Na⁺ and K⁺ ions with their accompanying anions would exit the terminal CCD per day.

**LUMINAL ACCEPTORS FOR H⁺ IONS**

- Hypokalemia is associated with intracellular acidosis in cells of PCT, which enhances reabsorption of $HCO_3^-$ ions and stimulates production of ammonium ($NH_4^+$) ions. As a result, $NH_3$ rather than $HCO_3^-$ ions is the most likely H⁺ ion acceptor in the lumen of the collecting duct in this setting.
- As discussed in Part D, enhanced reabsorption of $HCO_3^-$ ions in the PCT diminishes its delivery to the CDN, which is a component of the integrated renal response to decrease net K⁺ ion secretion in the presence of K⁺ ion depletion.

## FLOW RATE IN THE CORTICAL DISTAL NEPHRON

The amount of K⁺ ions excreted by the CDN per time unit is a function of two factors: the activity of net K⁺ ion secretion in the CDN and the number of liters of fluid that exit from the CDN during that time period (see margin note).

When vasopressin acts, the late distal nephron becomes permeable to water because of the insertion of aquaporin water channel-2 (AQP2) in the luminal membrane of principal cells. The osmolality of fluid in the terminal CCD becomes equal to the plasma osmolality and hence is relatively fixed. Therefore, the number of osmoles present in luminal fluid determines the flow rate in the terminal CDN (i.e., the number of liters of fluid that exit the CCD). These osmoles are largely urea, $Na^+$, $Cl^-$, and K⁺ ions with their accompanying anions. There is little reabsorption or secretion of electrolytes in the nephron segments distal to the CDN, and hence the number of electrolyte osmoles in the terminal CDN is close to their excretion in the urine, but this is not the case for urea osmoles. A quantitative analysis of the process of intrarenal urea recycling reveals that the amount of urea delivered to the early DCT is about two-fold higher than the amount of urea that is excreted in the urine.

## INTRARENAL UREA RECYCLING

The process and the quantitative aspects of the intrarenal recycling of urea were discussed in detail in Chapter 9. We estimated that in subjects consuming a typical Western diet, ~ 600 mmol of urea per day are reabsorbed in the inner MCD and delivered back to the early DCT. Therefore, this process of urea recycling adds an extra 2 L per day to the flow rate in the terminal CDN (600 mosmol divided by a luminal fluid osmolality that is equal to that in plasma or ~300 mosmol/kg $H_2O$). A reasonable estimate of the number of liters of fluid that exit the terminal CCD per day is close to 5 L (1500 mosmol/day exit the terminal CCD [1000 mosmol/day of urea and 500 mosmol/day of electrolytes] divided by 300 mosmol/kg $H_2O$ [see margin note]). This means that, in quantitative terms, 40% of the flow rate in the terminal CDN is the result of this process of recycling of urea. The importance of this process of intrarenal recycling of urea for K⁺ ion excretion becomes evident when one considers that the second source of dietary K⁺ ions is from ingestion of animal organs (e.g., muscle). The anions that accompany this K⁺ ion load are organic phosphates or sulfate ions, which, unlike $HCO_3^-$ ions, do not augment the secretion of K⁺ ions in the CDN unless the concentration of $Cl^-$ ions in luminal fluid in the CDN is very low. Urea is produced when the amino acid constituents of protein are oxidized. By increasing the volume of fluid that exits the terminal CDN, this process of urea recycling aids the excretion of a K⁺ ion load from the ingestion of dietary proteins.

### Clinical implications

In Part D, we illustrate using quantitative analysis that urea recycling aids the excretion of K⁺ ions; this process is especially important in subjects with disorders or those who are taking drugs that lead to a less lumen-negative voltage in the CDN.

## REABSORPTION OF K⁺ IONS IN THE MEDULLARY COLLECTING DUCT

Reabsorption of K⁺ ions occurs primarily in the MCD (Figure 13-13). It is stimulated by K⁺ ion depletion, and the transporter involved is an $H^+/K^+$-ATPase. This exchange is electroneutral and requires the

**Figure 13-13 K⁺ Ion Reabsorption in the Medullary Collecting Duct (MCD).** The *barrel-shaped structure* represents the MCD. The reabsorption of K⁺ ions is stimulated by K⁺ ion depletion and is mediated by an H⁺/K⁺-ATPase. This requires the presence of H⁺ ion acceptors in the luminal fluid. Hypokalemia is associated with intracellular acidosis in cells of the proximal convoluted tubule, which enhances reabsorption of $HCO_3^-$ ions and stimulates production of $NH_4^+$ ions. As a result, $NH_3$ rather than $HCO_3^-$ ions is the H⁺ ion acceptor in the lumen of the MCD in this setting. K⁺ ion reabsorption by the H⁺/K⁺-ATPase adds $HCO_3^-$ ions to the medullary interstitial compartment, hence it becomes more alkaline, which may increase the risk for formation of Randall's plaque (see Part D). *AE*, $Cl^-/HCO_3^-$ anion exchanger; *Rhcg*, Rh C glycoprotein.

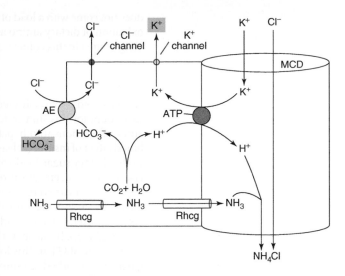

presence of H⁺ ion acceptors in the luminal fluid (i.e., $HCO_3^-$ ions and/or $NH_3$; see margin note).

# PART D
# INTEGRATIVE PHYSIOLOGY

## INTEGRATIVE PHYSIOLOGY OF THE RESPONSE TO A DIETARY K⁺ ION LOAD: A PALEOLITHIC PERSPECTIVE

Because control mechanisms that are essential for survival were likely developed in Paleolithic times, we think the physiology of K⁺ ion homeostasis can be better revealed when examined from what was required to avoid threats and achieve balance in Paleolithic times. The diet consumed by our ancient ancestors consisted mainly of fruit and berries, which provided sugar, K⁺ ions, and organic anions but little NaCl. Therefore, there was a need for mechanisms to ensure renal conservation of NaCl to avoid a hemodynamic threat. Because the intake of K⁺ ions was episodic and large at times, to avoid the risk of dangerous hyperkalemia and cardiac arrhythmia, there was a need to have mechanisms to shift ingested K⁺ ions rapidly into the liver before K⁺ ions could reach the heart and mechanisms to switch the renal response from NaCl conservation to K⁺ ion excretion. With regard to K⁺ ion shift into hepatocytes, we proposed a novel mechanism that integrates the role of L-lactic acid released from enterocytes in the process of absorption of dietary sugars. With regard to control of renal excretion of K⁺ ions, we attempt to integrate the role of WNK kinases along with modulation of delivery of $HCO_3^-$ ions to the CDN to achieve the desired renal response.

In addition, because the Paleolithic diet had very little NaCl but 1 mmol of Na⁺ ions must be reabsorbed in the CDN in electrogenic fashion to secrete 1 mmol of K⁺ ions, there must be a mechanism to increase the delivery of Na⁺ ions to the CDN when there is a large intake of K⁺ ions. We will examine the role of medullary recycling of K⁺ ions in this regard.

Finally, a different mechanism to enhance the excretion of K⁺ ions is required if its source is from the ingestion of animal organs and hence does not come with a load of $HCO_3^-$ ions. Because urea is produced from oxidation of dietary amino acids, we examine the role of intrarenal recycling of urea in this context.

## MECHANISM TO SHIFT K⁺ IONS INTO LIVER CELLS

As discussed previously (see Figure 13-3), the mechanism that is likely to account for this shift of $K^+$ ions is the activation of the electroneutral entry of $Na^+$ ions into hepatocytes on NHE-1. This is due to the combined effect of insulin (released from β-cells of the pancreas in response to the dietary sugar load with the ingestion of fruit and berries) and a rise in the concentration of $H^+$ ions in the submembrane region of hepatocytes near NHE-1 subsequent to the entry of L-lactic acid, produced by enterocytes, into hepatocytes on the monocarboxylic acid cotransporter. L-Lactic acid is produced in enterocytes during absorption of glucose because of the increased demand for ATP. This occurs because the SLGT in this location is SLGT-1. Hence, when 1 mmol of glucose is absorbed, 2 mmol of $Na^+$ ions must be absorbed. Therefore, more ATP is required to absorb a given quantity of glucose than if the stoichiometry of the transporter was the absorption of 1 mmol of $Na^+$ ions per 1 mmol of glucose. Should glycolysis occur at a faster rate than pyruvate oxidation, L-lactic acid will be formed and released into the portal vein. In addition to its activation of NHE-1, insulin also causes phosphorylation of FXYD1 and the translocation of Na-K-ATPase units to the cell surface from an intracellular pool.

## CONTROL OF THE EXCRETION OF K⁺ IONS

### Integration of the role of WNK kinases and delivery of $HCO_3^-$ ions to CDN

WNK4 and WNK1, via effects on NCC in the DCT and on ROMK in the CDN, seem to function as a switch to change the aldosterone response of the kidney to either conserve $Na^+$ ions or excrete $K^+$ ions, depending on whether the release of aldosterone is induced by a reduction in dietary $Na^+$ ion intake or an increase in dietary $K^+$ ion intake.

In addition, modulation of the delivery of $HCO_3^-$ ions to the CDN may play a role in determining the rate of electrogenic versus electroneutral $Na^+$ ion reabsorption in the CDN and hence the ability to generate a luminal negative voltage in the CDN.

### Conservation of NaCl (Figure 13-14, A)

$ANG_{II}$ is released in response to a low EABV (or low salt intake). $ANG_{II}$ signaling through its AT1 receptor converts WNK4 from an NCC-inhibiting to an NCC-activating kinase. The activated form of WNK4 phosphorylates SPAK and OSR1. Phosphorylated SPAK/OSR1 in turn phosphorylates and activates NCC, enhancing reabsorption of $Na^+$ and $Cl^-$ ions in the DCT.

$ANG_{II}$, however, also causes the release of aldosterone and SGK-1. This would tend to enhance $K^+$ ion excretion; therefore, other mechanisms are needed to make aldosterone function in the CDN as an NaCl-retaining hormone and not a kaliuretic hormone. First, $ANG_{II}$ induces endocytosis of ROMK via increasing the expression of protein tyrosine kinase. Second, $ANG_{II}$ is a potent activator of $Na^+/H^+$ exchanger-3 (NHE-3) and the reabsorption of $HCO_3^-$ ions in the cells of the PCT. This diminishes the delivery of $HCO_3^-$ ions to the CDN, which may enhance the electroneutral reabsorption of $Na^+$ ions by the parallel activity of pendrin and the NDCBE (see Figure 13-10). As a result, the rate of electrogenic reabsorption of $Na^+$ ions in CDN may be decreased, and hence the luminal negative voltage in the CDN and the secretion of $K^+$ ions may be diminished.

### Excretion of a large $K^+$ ion load (Figure 13-14, B)

In response to a large intake of $K^+$ ions, the release of $ANG_{II}$ is inhibited while the release of aldosterone and SGK-1 is stimulated. Increasing $K^+$ ion secretion requires the delivery of more NaCl to the CDN by inhibiting its reabsorption in the DCT. In the absence of sufficient $ANG_{II}$, WNK4 will be in its NCC-inhibiting form, and therefore NCC will be diverted to the lysosome for degradation and its abundance in the luminal membrane in DCT will be diminished (see margin note). An increase in dietary $K^+$ ion intake leads to an increased ratio of KS-WNK1 to L-WNK1. L-WNK1 has an inhibitory effect on WNK4, while the KS-WNK1 isoform blocks this effect of L-WNK1 on WNK4. Hence, with an increased ratio of KS-WNK1 to L-WNK1, WNK4 will be in its NCC-inhibiting form. As a result, delivery of NaCl to the CDN will be increased.

As the delivery of NaCl to the CDN is increased, two additional requirements are needed to achieve a high rate of $K^+$ ion secretion in the CDN: a high rate of electrogenic reabsorption of $Na^+$ ions in CDN, and the presence of open ROMK in the luminal membrane of principal cells in CDN.

#### A high rate of electrogenic reabsorption of $Na^+$ ions

In Paleolithic times, the major source of dietary $K^+$ ion intake was from fruit and berries. This also provided organic anions that can be metabolized to produce $HCO_3^-$ ions. This increases the filtered load of $HCO_3^-$ ions. In addition, a higher $P_K$ is associated with alkalinization of cells in the PCT, which leads to inhibition of the reabsorption of $HCO_3^-$ ions in PCT and hence the delivery of $HCO_3^-$ ions to the distal nephron is increased. The increase in luminal $HCO_3^-$ ion concentration in the CDN may inhibit the $Cl^-/HCO_3^-$ exchanger (pendrin), and hence the NDCBE and the electroneutral NaCl reabsorption, leading to a higher rate of electrogenic reabsorption of $Na^+$ ions.

#### Open ROMK in the luminal membrane of principal cells

Two processes seem to be involved to diminish endocytosis of ROMK. First, WNK4 inhibits ROMK by stimulating its endocytosis. When $ANG_{II}$ is suppressed but SGK-1 is present (as in conditions of high $K^+$ ion intake), SGK-1 phosphorylates WNK4 and reverses its inhibition of ROMK. Second, L-WNK1 inhibits ROMK by inducing its endocytosis; the KS-WNK1 isoform inhibits this effect of L-WNK1. An increase in dietary $K^+$ ion intake leads to an increased ratio of KS-WNK1 to L-WNK1, so there is reduced endocytosis of ROMK.

### Re-establishment of an NaCl-retaining state (Figure 13-14, C)

After the danger of a large $K^+$ ion load is dealt with, the NaCl retaining mode needs to be re-established. As $P_K$ returns to a lower value, the ratio of KS-WNK1 to L-WNK1 isoforms would be decreased, and L-WNK1 will exert its effect to upregulate NCC either by blocking the inhibitory form of WNK4 or directly by phosphorylation of SPAK/OSR1. Hence, reabsorption of NaCl in the DCT will be enhanced. L-WNK1 also inhibits ROMK via endocytosis. As $ANG_{II}$ is released,

**INACTIVATION OF EXISTING NCC UNITS IN LUMINAL MEMBRANE**

- WNK4 does not cause endocytosis of NCC. Rather it interferes with the forward trafficking pathway by diverting NCC to the lysosome for degradation and hence reduces its steady-state abundance in the luminal membrane in the DCT.
- A mechanism is needed, however, to inactivate the existing NCC units in the luminal membrane (perhaps via dephosphorylation) or cause their removal from the luminal membrane in response to an acute $K^+$ ion load. The mechanism(s) involved is (are) yet to be identified.

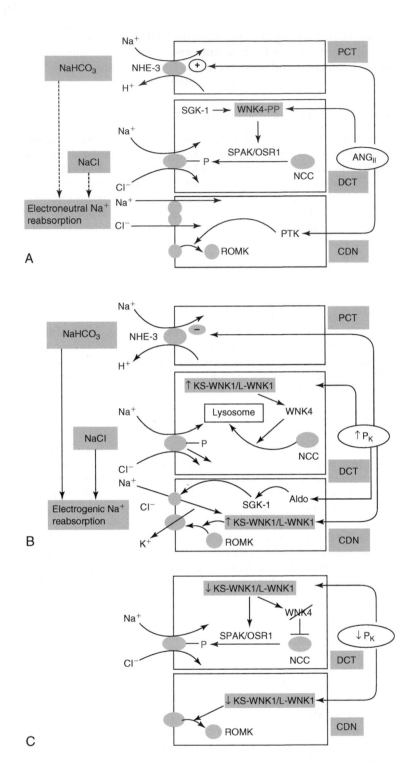

**Figure 13-14 Integration of the Role of WNK Kinases and Modulation of Delivery of HCO$_3^-$ Ions in Regulation of K$^+$ Ion Secretion in a Cortical Distal Nephron (CDN).** In **A** and **B,** the *upper rectangle* represents a proximal convoluted tubule (PCT) cell, the *middle rectangle* represents a distal convoluted tubule (DCT) cell, and the *lower rectangle* represents a CDN cell (principal cells and intercalated cells are not separated in this figure). In **C,** only a DCT cell and a CDN cell are shown. **A,** NaCl retaining state. Angiotensin II (ANG$_{II}$) phosphorylates and activates WNK4, activated WNK4 phosphorylates STE 20-related proline-alanine-rich-kinase (SPAK) and oxidative stress response kinase type 1 (OSR1), which in turn phosphorylates and activates Na-Cl contransporter (NCC). To prevent K$^+$ ion secretion, ANG$_{II}$ induces endocytosis of renal outer medullary K$^+$ ion channels (ROMK) via increasing the expression of protein tyrosine kinase (PTK). ANG$_{II}$ enhances the reabsorption of HCO$_3^-$ ions in the cells of the PCT and hence diminishes their delivery to the CDN, which may enhance the electroneutral reabsorption of Na$^+$ ions by the parallel activity of pendrin and the sodium-dependent chloride-bicarbonate exchanger (NDCBE; the two transprters are shown as two adjacent *circles* in the luminal membrane of the CDN cell) and hence diminishes the luminal-negative voltage in the CDN. **B,** Events after a K$^+$ ion load. Because of inhibition of ANG$_{II}$ release and an increase in the ratio of KS-WNK1 to L-WNK1, WNK4 will be in its NCC-inhibiting mode. Existing phosphorylated NCC in the luminal membrane will need to be deactivated or removed from the luminal membrane (mechanism involved is not known). The increased ratio of KS-WNK1 to L-WNK1 leads to more ROMK units in the luminal membrane of principal cells in the CDN. A higher P$_K$ leads to inhibition of the reabsorption of HCO$_3^-$ ions in the PCT. A higher luminal HCO$_3^-$ ion concentration may increase the rate of electrogenic reabsorption of Na$^+$ ions and the generation of luminal negative voltage in CDN. **C,** Events involved in re-establishment of the NaCl-retaining mode. Because the ratio of KS-WNK1 to L-WNK1 isoforms is decreased, L-WNK1 exerts its effects to upregulate NCC either by blocking the inhibitory form of WNK4 or directly by phosphorylation of SPAK/OSR1. L-WNK1 inhibits ROMK via endocytosis. As ANG$_{II}$ is released, WNK4 will be converted to its NCC-activating kinase form. The effects of ANG$_{II}$ to diminish the delivery of HCO$_3^-$ ions to the CDN and to inhibit ROMK will re-establish the role of aldosterone as an NaCl-retaining hormone in the CDN. *SGK-1,* Serum and glucocorticoid regulated kinase-1; *WNK4-PP,* WNK4 phosphorylated at 2 different sites by ANG$_{II}$ and SGK-1.

---

WNK4 will be converted to its NCC-activating kinase form. The effects of ANG$_{II}$ to diminish the delivery of HCO$_3^-$ ions to the CDN and to inhibit ROMK will re-establish the role of aldosterone as a NaCl-retaining hormone in CDN.

### Mechanism to increase the delivery of Na$^+$ ions to the CDN

The Paleolithic diet contained a very small amount of NaCl. Because for each 1 mmol of K$^+$ ion to be secreted in the CDN, 1 mmol of Na$^+$ ion need to be reabsorbed in an electrogenic fashion in the CDN, there should be a mechanism to cause inhibition of the reabsorption of NaCl in a nephron segment upstream to the CDN in response to an intake of a load of K$^+$ ions to increase the delivery of Na$^+$ ions to the CDN. This mechanism, however, should not allow for a large natriuresis to occur.

This issue was examined in a study in rats that was designed to mimic the intake in Paleolithic diet. In more detail, rats were fed a diet that contained small amounts of NaCl and K$^+$ ion salts for 4 days, then on the day of the experiment, they were given a large load of KCl via the intraperitoneal route. A large dose of deoxycorticosterone was administered to ensure that mineralocorticoid actions were present.

There was a large increase in the rate of excretion of K$^+$ ions, but two distinct phases were observed. In the first 2 hours, the increase in K$^+$ ion excretion was largely caused by a rise in net K$^+$ ion secretion in the CDN. This was thought to be due to the insertion of K$^+$ ion channels in the luminal membrane of principal cells in the CDN, because of a rise in the P$_K$. In the following 4 hours, there was a substantial increase in K$^+$ ion excretion. Its basis, however, was different because it was mostly accounted for by an increase in flow through the CDN. This rise in flow rate was explained by inhibition of NaCl reabsorption in the loop of Henle in response to a K$^+$ ion load because the urine flow rate and the rate of excretion of Na$^+$ plus K$^+$ ions were significantly higher, whereas the urine osmolality was significantly lower in rats given KCl compared with control rats; these are findings which mimic the effect of a loop diuretic. Of note, there was also a significant increase in the medullary interstitial K$^+$ ion concentration in rats which received a KCl load. Hence, a possible mechanism to explain this observation is that a higher K$^+$ ion concentration in the medullary interstitial compartment could inhibit the absorption of NaCl from the medullary thick ascending limb (mTAL) of the loop of Henle (Figure 13-15). A rise in medullary interstitial K$^+$ ion concentration results in a lower negative voltage across the basolateral membrane of mTAL cells, and hence a decreased exit of Cl$^-$ ions. This in turn raises the concentration of Cl$^-$ ions in mTAL cells, which slows the reabsorption of Na$^+$ and Cl$^-$ ions via the furosemide sensitive Na$^+$-K$^+$-2 Cl$^-$ cotransporter-2 (NKCC-2). The net effect is an increased delivery of Na$^+$ and Cl$^-$ ions to the CDN. The degree of inhibition of Na$^+$ and Cl$^-$ reabsorption in the mTAL is only modest in vivo but enough to increase the delivery of Na$^+$ ions and the flow

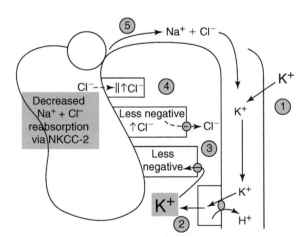

**Figure 13-15 Inhibition of the Reabsorption of NaCl in the Loop of Henle by a K$^+$ Ion Load.** The *stylized structure* represents a nephron. (1) Shortly after K$^+$ ions are ingested, there is a somewhat higher secretion of K$^+$ ions in the cortical distal nephron. (2) As a result, more K$^+$ ions are delivered to the medullary collecting duct, where some of the K$^+$ ions are reabsorbed by the H$^+$/K$^+$-ATPase, which may still be active because of the prior K$^+$ ion depletion. (3) The higher concentration of K$^+$ ions in the medullary interstitial compartment leads to a diminution in the negative voltage in cells of the medullary thick ascending limb. This negative voltage in mTAL cells provides the driving force for the exit of Cl$^-$ ions from these cells. As a result of this diminished driving force, the concentration of Cl$^-$ ions rises in cells of the mTAL. This higher intracellular concentration of Cl$^-$ ions diminishes reabsorption of NaCl via the Na$^+$, K$^+$, 2 Cl$^-$-cotransporter (NKCC-2).

rate in the CDN to augment the excretion of $K^+$ ions, without causing a large natriuresis.

### Reinterpretation of the medullary recycling of $K^+$ ions

It is known that in response to a $K^+$ ion load, there is increased reabsorption of $K^+$ ions in the inner MCD (see margin note). This medullary reabsorption of $K^+$ ions, although this seems to be paradoxical, increases the rate of excretion of $K^+$ ions in the urine. The explanation may be as discussed previously, that the increase in medullary interstitial $K^+$ ion concentration leads to inhibition of reabsorption of NaCl in mTAL of the loop of Henle, which increases the delivery of $Na^+$ ions and the flow rate in the CDN.

## INTEGRATION OF FLOW RATE IN THE TERMINAL CDN AND ACTIVITY OF $K^+$ ION SECRETION IN THE PATHOPHYSIOLOGY OF HYPERKALEMIA

Patients who develop chronic hyperkalemia have a renal defect that is characterized by an inability to generate a sufficiently large transepitheleal lumen-negative voltage in the CDN to secrete all their daily intake of $K^+$ ions while maintaining a normal $P_K$. These patients, however, will achieve a chronic steady state in which they will excrete in their urine all the $K^+$ ions they ingest and absorb. To understand how this steady state is achieved, we shall consider how a $K^+$ ion load of 70 mmol/day is handled in normal subjects and a patient who has a defect that leads to diminished ability to generate a sufficiently large transepitheleal lumen-negative voltage in the CDN. Before proceeding with this analysis, there are two points to emphasize regarding the flow rate in the terminal CDN:

1. In the presence of vasopressin actions, because the osmolality of the fluid in the terminal CCD is relatively fixed (equals $P_{Osm}$) the number of liters of fluid that exit the CCD is determined by the number of effective osmoles that are present in the luminal fluid in the terminal CCD.
2. A reasonable estimate of the number of liters of fluid that exit the terminal CCD per day is ~5 L (~1500 mosmol/day are present in the terminal CCD [~1000 mosmol/day of urea and ~500 mosmol/day of electrolytes] and a luminal fluid osmolality that is equal to $P_{Osm}$ or 300 mosmol/kg $H_2O$ for easy math).

Normal subjects have a much larger capacity to secrete $K^+$ ions in their CDN compared to the usual daily intake of $K^+$ ions. Most of the daily intake is excreted over a relatively short period of time close to noon each day. This likely reflects an increase in the lumen-negative voltage in the CDN caused by a larger delivery of $NaHCO_3$ to the CDN at the time of the alkaline tide. If a normal subject has a $P_K$ of 4 mmol/L and a transepitheleal voltage in the CDN of −61 mV, the concentration of $K^+$ ions in luminal fluid in the CDN ($K_{CDN}$) by the Nernst equation would be 10 times the $P_K$ or 40 mmol/L. If this voltage could be maintained for a period of 5 hours (flow rate in the terminal CCD would be ~1 L in this time period), 40 mmol of the daily intake of 70 mmol of $K^+$ ions would be excreted in these 5 hours. For the next 19 hours, 4 L of fluid would exit the terminal CCD, and even with a concentration of $K^+$ ions of only 7.5 mmol/L, the remaining 30 mmol of $K^+$ ions can be excreted to achieve $K^+$ ion balance.

The point to emphasize is that an appreciable degree of hyperkalemia will not occur even if there is a large reduction in the

**REABSORPTION OF $K^+$ IONS IN THE MCD**

- This may be mediated by the $H^+/K^+$-ATPase, which may be active because of the prior $K^+$ ion depletion.
- Recall that the Paleolithic diet provided a family of organic anions that can be converted to $HCO_3^-$ ions and that a rise in $P_K$ diminishes the reabsorption of $HCO_3^-$ ions in the PCT. As a result, this $H^+$ ion acceptor may be available in the luminal fluid when the $H^+/K^+$-ATPase is active.

transepitheleal lumen-negative voltage in the CDN unless there is decreased flow rate in the terminal CCD. To illustrate this point in a quantitative fashion, let us consider a subject who has a large defect that leads to a lumen-negative transepitheleal voltage in the CDN of only −29.1 mV. At this transepitheleal voltage, the $K_{CDN}/P_K$ can rise to a value of only 3 (Table 13-1). At a $P_K$ of 4.7 mmol/L, the $K_{CDN}$ will be 14 mmol/L; therefore, at the usual flow rate in the terminal CCD of 5 L/day, this patient can excrete 70 mmol of $K^+$ ions daily and maintain a normal $P_K$. If the number of liters exiting the CCD per day were to be reduced to 4 L instead of 5 L, the $K_{CDN}/P_K$ were 3, and if this patient were to continue to consume 70 mmol of $K^+$ ions/day, the $P_K$ will have to rise to 5.8 mmol/L to maintain $K^+$ ion balance and only if this maximum rate of $K^+$ ion secretion is maintained throughout the 24-hour period. If the volume of filtrate that exits the terminal CCD were only 3 L/day, at the same transepitheleal voltage in the CDN of only −29.1 mV and hence $K_{CDN}/P_K$ of only 3, the $P_K$ would have to be close to 8 mmol/L to excrete 70 mmol $K^+$ ions/day. Notwithstanding, as illustrated in Table 13-1, if the maximum transepitheleal voltage were to fall to −18.4 mV, the $K_{CDN}/P_K$ can only be raised by a factor of 2. Therefore, even with a flow rate in the terminal CCD of 5 L/day, hyperkalemia would develop unless $K^+$ ion intake were to be decreased appreciably.

This analysis shows that patients who have disorders and/or are taking drugs that significantly affect the ability to generate transepitheleal lumen-negative voltage in their CDN are dependent on maintaining a high flow rate in their terminal CDN to achieve $K^+$ ion balance without the need for an appreciably higher $P_K$. In the presence of vasopressin action, the number of osmoles in the luminal fluid determines the flow rate in the terminal CCD. Because of the process of intrarenal recycling of urea, a large fraction of the osmoles delivered to the CDN are urea osmoles. Therefore, restricting protein intake may decrease the amount of urea that recycles and hence the volume of fluid that exits the terminal CDN, and thus diminish the rate of excretion of $K^+$ ions. The other major osmoles that are present in the luminal fluid in the terminal CDN are $Na^+$ and $Cl^-$ ions. If a patient is given a diuretic and becomes intravascular volume depleted, the increase in NaCl reabsorption in the PCT will decrease the number of osmoles of $Na^+$ and $Cl^-$ ions in the luminal fluid of the terminal CDN and hence the rate of flow in the terminal CDN. Therefore, if diuretics are used to increase the rate of $K^+$ ion excretion, one must be careful to avoid intravascular volume depletion.

This analysis may also provide new insights into understanding the pathophysiology of hyperkalemia that may develop in patients on an angiotensin converting enzyme (ACE) inhibitor or an angiotensin II

TABLE 13-1  **INTERACTION BETWEEN THE TRANSEPITHELIAL VOLTAGE, THE CONCENTRATION OF $K^+$ IONS IN PLASMA, AND RATE OF FLOW ON THE RATE OF $K^+$ ION SECRETION IN THE CORTICAL DISTAL NEPHRON**

| TRANSEPITHELIAL VOLTAGE (MV) | $K_{CDN}/P_K$ | $P_K$ (mmol/L) | $K_{CDN}$ (mmol/L) | FLOW RATE $K_{CDN}$ (L/day) | $K^+$ EXCRETION (mmol/day) |
|---|---|---|---|---|---|
| −29.1 | 3 | **4.7** | 14.1 | **5** | 70 |
| −29.1 | 3 | **5.8** | 17.5 | **4** | 70 |
| −29.1 | 3 | **7.8** | 23.4 | **3** | 70 |
| −18.4 | 2 | **7.0** | 14 | **5** | 70 |

The $K_{CDN}/P_K$ is calculated from the transepithelial voltage using the Nernst equation. The numbers in bold are the required values of the plasma $K^+$ ion concentration ($P_K$) and the flow rate in the terminal CDN to achieve a rate of $K^+$ ion excretion of approximately 70 mmol/day. Even with a low transepithelial voltage of −29.1 mV, $K^+$ ion balance can be maintained without a large rise in the $P_K$ if the flow rate in the terminal CDN were at its usual value of 5 L/day. If the flow rate in the terminal CDN were to decrease to 4 L/day, the $P_K$ must rise to 5.8 mmol/L to excrete the entire daily intake of $K^+$ ions of 70 mmol and remain in $K^+$ ion balance.

receptor blocker (ARB). The usual explanation for the basis of hyperkalemia is a diminished secretion of $K^+$ ions because $ANG_{II}$ is a secretagogue for aldosterone. Nevertheless, as suggested previously, an appreciable degree of hyperkalemia will not occur even if there is a large reduction in transepitheleal voltage in the CDN unless there is a decreased flow rate in the terminal CDN. It is interesting to note that $ANG_{II}$ stimulates the transport of urea in the inner MCD in the presence of vasopressin. Furthermore, if deficiency of actions of $ANG_{II}$ were to decrease the vasoconstrictor tone of blood vessels that descend into the renal medulla, urea may be washed out of the deeper region of the outer medulla. This may cause the concentration of urea to decline in the medullary interstitial compartment, and hence the driving force for urea entry into the DtL of superficial nephrons will be diminished. Therefore, hyperkalemia may be more likely to develop in patients who are taking ACE inhibitors or ARBs if they are protein restricted because there would now be other reasons for diminished urea recycling and therefore diminished rate of $K^+$ ion excretion.

## INTEGRATION OF THE RENAL RESPONSE TO DIETARY $K^+$ ION RESTRICTION

There are three components to the renal response to dietary restriction of $K^+$ ions to diminish the rate of $K^+$ ion excretion:

1. *Decrease the rate of electrogenic $Na^+$ ion reabsorption in the CDN:*

Dietary $K^+$ ion restriction is associated with a decreased ratio of KS-WNK1/L-WNK1. This may decrease delivery of NaCl to the CDN due to its enhanced reabsorption via NCC in the DCT. Furthermore, $K^+$ ion depletion is associated with intracellular acidosis in the cells of the PCT and a rise in $ANG_{II}$, both of which stimulate the reabsorption of $HCO_3^-$ ions in the PCT and hence diminish the delivery of $HCO_3^-$ ions to the CDN. A lower luminal $HCO_3^-$ ion concentration in the CDN may augment flux through pendrin and NDCBE and thereby result in an increase in electroneutral NaCl reabsorption in the CDN.

2. *Decrease abundance of open ROMK in the luminal membrane of principal cells in the CDN:*

$ANG_{II}$ via increasing the expression of protein tyrosine kinase leads to phosphorylation of ROMK, which results in its endocytosis. The ratio of KS-WNK1 to L-WNK1 is decreased by dietary $K^+$ ion restriction, which also leads to endocytosis of ROMK.

3. *Increase reabsorption of $K^+$ ions in the MCD:*

$K^+$ ion depletion enhances the expression of $H^+/K^+$-ATPase in the luminal membrane of intercalated cells in the MCD. Nevertheless, for this to result in increased rate of reabsorption of $K^+$ ions, an acceptor of $H^+$ ions should be present in the luminal fluid. Hypokalemia is associated with intracellular acidosis in the cells of the PCT, which stimulates ammoniagensis. Therefore, $NH_3$ becomes the $H^+$ ion acceptor in the lumen of the MCD.

## $K^+$ ION DEPLETION AND HYPERTENSION

There is experimental and epidemiologic evidence to support the notion of a role of $K^+$ ion depletion in the pathogenesis of hypertension. The link may be that renal mechanisms to diminish kaliuresis may also result in expansion of the EABV.

$K^+$ ion depletion is associated with an acidified PCT cell, which increases the reabsorption of $HCO_3^-$ ions in PCT and diminishes the delivery of $HCO_3^-$ ions to the CDN. This has the advantage of diminishing an unwanted kaliuresis by promoting the electroneutral reabsorption of NaCl in the CDN, but at the expense of expansion of the EABV. $K^+$ ion depletion is associated with a decreased ratio of KS-WNK1/L-WNK1. This may have an advantage to diminish the renal excretion of $K^+$ ions because it is associated with decreased delivery of NaCl to the CDN due to its enhanced reabsorption via NCC in the DCT. Again, this also may lead to expansion of the EABV.

## $K^+$ ION DEPLETION AND THE PATHOPHYSIOLOGY OF CALCIUM KIDNEY STONES

The initial solid phase of calcium oxalate stone formation in patients with idiopathic hypercalciuria is a nidus of calcium phosphate (apatite) known as Randall's plaque, which is formed at the basolateral aspect of the thin ascending limb of the loop of Henle. This subsequently erodes into the collecting duct and provides a nidus for the deposition of calcium oxalate. $K^+$ ion depletion is associated with increased number of active $H^+/K^+$-ATPase units in the luminal membrane of the MCD. When $K^+$ ions are reabsorbed by the $H^+/K^+$-ATPase, $K^+$ and $HCO_3^-$ ions are added to the medullary interstitial compartment, hence it becomes more alkaline, which increases the risk for formation of Randall's plaque. Precipitation of apatite, however, would require a marked degree of medullary alkalinization. Notwithstanding, medullary alkalinization may lead to formation of a precipitate of calcium carbonate that may act as a nidus for the precipitation of apatite and the formation of Randall's plaque.

$K^+$ ion depletion is also associated with an acidified PCT cell pH. This enhances the reabsorption of citrate anions in the PCT leading to hypocitraturia. This results in an increase in the concentration of ionized calcium in the urine and the risk of calcium stone formation.

## DISCUSSION OF CASE 13-1

### CASE 13-1: WHY DID I BECOME SO WEAK?

**What is the most likely basis for the repeated episodes of acute hypokalemia?**

Because the time course seems to be only a matter of hours, the excretion of $K^+$ ions in the urine was low ($U_K/U_{Creatinine}$ was ~1), there was no major metabolic acid–base disorder, and the recovery was so rapid and required only a small infusion of KCl, the major cause for the hypokalemia is an acute shift of $K^+$ ions into cells.

**Was an adrenergic effect associated with the acute hypokalemia?**

It appears that the answer is yes because the patient had tachycardia, systolic hypertension, and a wide pulse pressure during each episode. Notwithstanding, there was no obvious source for the adrenergic surge. In more detail, she denied the intake of drugs that have a $\beta_2$-adrenergic effect (e.g., amphetamines, ephedrine, albuterol), or the ingestion of a large amount of caffeine. There was no evidence of a disease with a similar hormonal milieu (e.g., hyperthyroidism, pheochromocytoma). Therefore, the cause of the surge of $\beta_2$-adrenergics was not obvious.

**Are there any clues in her laboratory results to suggest what the cause of acute hypokalemia might be?**

As discussed previously, hypokalemia was due to an acute shift of $K^+$ ions into cells because of a surge in catecholamines, the reason for which is not clear. It is interesting to note that the $P_{Glucose}$ was a little higher than expected at 133 mg/dL (7.4 mmol/L). Because of this finding, we suggest that these episodes of acute hypokalemia were initiated by the release of insulin from an insulinoma, which caused a sustained period of hypoglycemia and thereby an adrenergic surge. The metabolic consequence could be hypoglycemia, which is followed by the breakdown of storage glycogen in the liver and the release of glucose into the circulation, leading to the observed higher $P_{Glucose}$ on presentation.

## DISCUSSION OF QUESTION

*13-1   Is the $K_{ATP}$ channel regulated by ATP?*

The name of this channel is incorrect because $K_{ATP}$ channels are in fact not regulated by the intracellular concentration of ATP. This is because the concentration of ATP in cells does not rise or fall sufficiently in health to modulate the flux through these channels. In fact, at the prevailing concentration of ATP in cells, this channel would be closed. Nevertheless, if one includes the effects of ADP, which open this channel, at the usual ATP concentration in cells, the channel may have a certain degree of open probability. Thus, when the concentration of ADP in cells rises, there is a higher degree of open probability of this channel; conversely, when the concentration of ADP in cells falls, this channel closes.

To understand what the change in voltage in cells is when the $K_{ATP}$ channel opens, recall that a cationic charge leaves the cell; hence, the voltage in cells becomes more negative, which may affect the gating of voltage-gated channels. The best example is the voltage-gated $Ca^{2+}$ channel, which is closed when there is a more negative voltage in cells. Conversely, when fewer $K^+$ ions leave the cell because the $K_{ATP}$ channel is closed, the voltage in cells becomes less negative. This less negative intracellular voltage opens the voltage-gated $Ca^{2+}$ channels and thereby causes a higher intracellular ionized $Ca^{2+}$ concentration. By modulating the concentration of ionized $Ca^{2+}$ in cells, many other functions are affected because ionized $Ca^{2+}$ is a major signal for the regulation of many intracellular processes.

### $K_{ATP}$ channel and the release of insulin

Closing the $K_{ATP}$ channel by a fall in the concentration of ADP plays a critical role in the release of insulin from β-cells of the pancreas. In more detail, when the $P_{Glucose}$ is high, more glucose enters β-cells because of their nonregulated glucose transporter (GLUT-2). Hence, some ADP is converted to ATP in glycolysis, and the intracellular concentration of ADP falls, which causes the $K_{ATP}$ channels to close. The voltage in cells thus becomes less negative, which increases the conductance of the voltage-gated $Ca^{2+}$ channels. The resultant rise in the intracellular ionized $Ca^{2+}$ concentration provides the final signal for the release of insulin from β-cells.

### $K_{ATP}$ channel and vasodilatation

A similar logic can be used to deduce how the blood flow to exercising muscle may be controlled using intracellular $Ca^{2+}$ as the signal.

During a sprint, L-lactic acid is released from exercising skeletal muscle cells. When L-lactic acid enters vascular smooth muscle cells, the concentrations of $H^+$ ions and L-lactate anions rise. This rise in the concentrations of $H^+$ ions and L-lactate anions in cells causes opening of the $K_{ATP}$ channel that is independent of the effect of ADP on this channel. As a result, $K^+$ ions exit and the voltage in these cells becomes more negative. This causes closure of voltage-gated $Ca^{2+}$ channels and less entry of ionized $Ca^{2+}$ into cells and hence vasodilatation.

It has been suggested that using a drug that closes the $K_{ATP}$ channels (e.g., sulfonylureas) may be a useful adjunct for therapy of patients with shock due to vasodilatation (e.g., septic shock).

# 14

# Hypokalemia

# Introduction

Hypokalemia, usually defined as a concentration of potassium ($K^+$) ions in plasma ($P_K$) of less than 3.5 mmol/L, is a common electrolyte disorder both in the outpatient and the inpatient setting. When faced with a patient with hypokalemia, the first step is to determine whether an emergency is present. The most serious emergency due to hypokalemia is a cardiac arrhythmia. The other emergency that is directly related to hypokalemia is respiratory muscle weakness. This is of particular concern in a patient with hypokalemia and metabolic acidemia (e.g., a patient with diarrhea or distal renal tubular acidosis [RTA]) because the superimposed respiratory acidosis due to hypoventilation may lead to severe acidemia. If an emergency is present, therapy to raise the $P_K$ must begin without delay.

It is important to recognize that hypokalemia may be caused by a number of disorders with diverse etiologies. The underlying disorder must be identified because this may have not only diagnostic but also therapeutic implications. The major basis of the hypokalemia may be an acute shift of $K^+$ ions into cells. This is important to recognize because there is a risk with excessive administration of $K^+$ ions (rebound hyperkalemia), and in a certain subset of patients, use of a nonselective β-blocker may lead to prompt correction of the hypokalemia with the administration of only a small dose of $K^+$ ion supplementation. Chronic hypokalemia is the result of a total body deficit of $K^+$ ions due to renal or extrarenal loss of $K^+$ ions. In a patient with chronic hypokalemia and an inappropriately high rate of excretion of $K^+$ ions in the urine, the underlying pathophysiology is a high rate of electrogenic reabsorption of sodium ($Na^+$) ions and hence a high transepithelial lumen-negative voltage in the cortical distal nephron (CDN), leading to an increased rate of net secretion of $K^+$ ions in the CDN. Clues to determining the underlying disorder can be obtained from the medical history, the acid–base status, an assessment of the effective arterial blood volume (EABV) and blood pressure (BP), and measurements of the concentration of aldosterone in plasma ($P_{Aldosterone}$) and the mass or activity of renin in plasma ($P_{Renin}$).

## OBJECTIVES

- To emphasize that hypokalemia is a common electrolyte abnormality that may be life threatening. Hypokalemia, however, is not a diagnosis, but rather the result of many different disorders.
- To provide a clinical approach to the patient with hypokalemia based on an understanding of the physiology of the distribution of $K^+$ ions between the extracellular fluid (ECF) compartment and the intracellular fluid (ICF) compartment and the physiology of the regulation of the renal excretion of $K^+$ ions.
- To provide an approach to the therapy of the patient with hypokalemia.

## CASE 14-1: HYPOKALEMIA WITH PARALYSIS

A 45-year-old man developed profound weakness in both his lower and upper extremities over the past few hours. He had two similar episodes in the preceding two months. Prior to each of these episodes, he had a very large intake of sweetened soft drinks. He was not taking any medications, including diuretics or laxatives. He has no family history of hypokalemia, periodic paralysis, or hyperthyroidism. On physical examination, he was alert and oriented. His BP was 150/70 mm Hg, his heart rate was 124 beats/min, and his respiratory rate was 18 breaths/min. The only neurologic finding was symmetrical flaccid paralysis with areflexia in all four limbs. The pH and $PCO_2$ values shown in the table below were from an arterial blood sample, whereas all other data were from a venous blood sample. The ECG showed sinus tachycardia and prominent U waves. Tests of thyroid function were normal.

|  |  | PLASMA | URINE |
|---|---|---|---|
| $Na^+$ | mmol/L | 138 | 103 |
| $K^+$ | mmol/L | 1.9 | 10 |
| $Cl^-$ | mmol/L | 102 | 112 |
| $HCO_3^-$ | mmol/L | 26 | — |
| Phosphate | mg/dL (mmol/L) | 2.0 (0.7) | 1.3 (0.4) |
| pH |  | 7.41 | — |
| $PCO_2$ | mm Hg | 36 | — |
| Glucose | mg/dL (mmol/L) | 90 (5.0) | — |
| Creatinine | mg/dL (μmol/L) | 0.6 (52) | 1 g/L (9.0 mmol/L) |

## Questions

Is there a medical emergency in this patient?
What is the basis of hypokalemia in this patient?
What is the best therapy for the hypokalemia in this patient?

## Case 14-2: Hypokalemia With a Sweet Touch

A 76-year-old Asian man became very weak this morning and was unable to walk for the past 6 hours. He denied nausea, vomiting, or diarrhea. He did not take diuretics or laxatives. Hypokalemia ($P_K$ 3.3 mmol/L) and hypertension were noted by his family physician about 1 year ago but were not investigated further. He had no previous history or family history of similar episodes. His BP was 160/96 mm Hg, and his heart rate was 70 beats/min. The only positive finding on physical examination was symmetric flaccid paralysis with areflexia. His ECG showed prominent U waves and prolonged Q-T interval. The laboratory data on admission are presented in the following table:

|  |  | PLASMA | URINE |
|---|---|---|---|
| $Na^+$ | mmol/L | 147 | 132 |
| $K^+$ | mmol/L | 1.8 | 26 |
| $Cl^-$ | mmol/L | 96 | 138 |
| $HCO_3^-$ | mmol/L | 38 | — |
| pH (arterial) |  | 7.50 | — |
| $PCO_2$ (arterial) | mm Hg | 45 | — |
| Creatinine | mg/dL (μmol/L) | 0.8 (70) | 0.6 g/dL (5 mmol/L) |

The patient was given a large quantity of KCl; his weakness improved when his $P_K$ rose to 2.5 mmol/L. Over the following 2 weeks, his $P_K$ and his BP returned to normal levels and his body weight decreased from 78 to 74 kg. When the results became available, his $P_{Renin}$ mass was low, his $P_{Aldosterone}$ was low, and the concentration of cortisol in his plasma ($P_{Cortisol}$) was in the normal range.

## Questions

Is there a medical emergency in this patient on presentation?
Is there a danger to anticipate during the initial therapy?
What is the basis for the hypokalemia in this patient?

## Case 14-3: Hypokalemia in a Newborn

A young boy, who is now 2 years of age, is the first child of a consanguineous marriage (his parents are first cousins). Pregnancy was complicated by severe polyhydramnios, for which amniocentesis was performed on two occasions early in the course of pregnancy. Delivery occurred in the 26th week; he weighed 2.2 lb (1 kg). His urine volume was very large, which resulted in a loss of more than 20% of his weight in the first 24 hours. The concentration of $Na^+$ ions in his urine ($U_{Na}$) was very high (98 mmol/L; expected, <10 mmol/L). His $P_K$ was high (5.5 mmol/L), but after aggressive infusion of isotonic saline, hypokalemia was consistently present ($P_K \sim 3.3$ mmol/L).

During the first month of life, he required a large daily fluid volume to replace his urine output (~250 mL/kg/day). There was also a huge excretion of NaCl (~12 mmol/kg/day), and he required supplements of NaCl to maintain hemodynamic stability. He was treated with a prostaglandin synthesis inhibitor (indomethacin), and his renal salt wasting largely disappeared. Notwithstanding, this seemed to have uncovered a second abnormality because he developed water diuresis with large urine volume and urine osmolality ($U_{Osm}$) of less than 100 mosmol/kg $H_2O$. In response to the administration of 1-deamino 8-D-arginine vasopressin (desmopressin [dDAVP]), his urine flow rate did not fall and his $U_{Osm}$ did not rise. The laboratory data in the following table are typical of measurements done during his first week of life:

|  |  | PLASMA | URINE |
| --- | --- | --- | --- |
| $Na^+$ | mmol/L | 133 | 89 |
| $K^+$ | mmol/L | 3.3 | 26 |
| $Cl^-$ | mmol/L | 96 | 92 |
| Osmolality | mosmol/kg $H_2O$ | 276 | 250 |
| Creatinine | mg/dL (µmol/L) | 1.1 mg/dL (90 µmol/L) | 10 mg/dL (850 µmol/L) |

### Questions

Is there a medical emergency in this patient?

What is the basis of the hypokalemia in this patient?

Why did the patient have nephrogenic diabetes insipidus?

In what nephron segment might indomethacin have acted to result in a marked decrease in renal loss of $Na^+$ ions?

# PART A
# SYNOPSIS OF K⁺ ION PHYSIOLOGY

A detailed discussion of the physiology of $K^+$ ion homeostasis is presented in Chapter 13. In this chapter, we shall provide a brief synopsis of the main points that are necessary to understand the pathophysiology of hypokalemia.

## REGULATION OF DISTRIBUTION OF K⁺ IONS BETWEEN THE EXTRACELLULAR FLUID AND THE INTRACELLULAR FLUID COMPARTMENTS

$K^+$ ions are kept inside cells because of the negative voltage in the cell interior. To shift $K^+$ ions into cells, a more negative cell voltage is required. This is generated by increasing the flux through the sodium/potassium ATPase (Na-K-ATPase) because it is an electrogenic pump, which exports three $Na^+$ ions out of the cell while importing only two $K^+$ ions into the cell (see Figure 13-1). There are three ways to acutely increase flux through the Na-K-ATPase: first, a rise in the concentration of its rate-limiting substrate—intracellular $Na^+$ ions; second, an increase in its affinity for $Na^+$ ions or its maximum velocity ($V_{max}$) of cation flux; third, an increase in the number of active Na-K-ATPase pump units in the cell membrane via recruitment of new units from an intracellular pool. For this increase in Na-K-ATPase activity to increase the negative voltage inside the cell, however, the source of $Na^+$ ions that are pumped out of the cell must be $Na^+$ ions that existed in the cell or $Na^+$ ions that entered the cell in an electroneutral fashion. In more detail, if $Na^+$ ions entered the cells in an electroneutral fashion, their subsequent electrogenic exit via the Na-K-ATPase results in a more negative cell interior voltage, and hence there is less net exit of $K^+$ ions from these cells. This occurs when $Na^+$ ions enter cells in exchange for $H^+$ ions on the sodium/hydrogen cation exchanger-1(NHE-1).

Insulin causes a shift of $K^+$ ions into cells because (1) it activates NHE-1 and hence causes an increase in the electroneutral entry of $Na^+$ ions into cells; (2) it induces phosphorylation of FXYD1(phospholemann) by atypical protein kinase C, which disrupts FXYD1 interaction with the α-subunit of Na-K-ATPase, resulting in an increase in its $V_{max}$; and (3) insulin promotes the translocation of Na-K-ATPase units from an intracellular pool, increasing their expression at the cell membrane.

$\beta_2$-adrenergic agonists via increasing intracellular cyclic adenosine monophosphate (cAMP) activate protein kinase A and induce phosphorylation of the FXYD1 and results in increased affinity of the Na-K-ATPase for intracellular $Na^+$ ions.

A chronic increase in Na-K-ATPase pump activity requires the synthesis of new pump units as occurs with chronic excess thyroid hormones.

## CLINICAL IMPLICATIONS

There are a number of clinical implications from the understanding of this physiology of the distribution of $K^+$ ions between the ECF and ICF compartments. An acute shift of $K^+$ ions into cells occurs when insulin is given to a patient with diabetic ketoacidosis (DKA). In patients with DKA who present with a $P_K$ of less than 4 mmol/L, it is suggested that the administration of insulin be delayed for 1-2 hours and aggressive therapy with the administration of intravenous KCl be promptly started to bring the $P_K$ to a value that is close to 4 mmol/L to avoid the risk of a severe degree of hypokalemia and possible cardiac arrhythmia when insulin is given. As a general rule, in patients with a severe degree of hypokalemia, KCl should not be administered in a solution that contains glucose, because even a small degree of an acute shift of $K^+$ ions into cells due to the release of insulin can be dangerous in this setting. Although not supported by data, the notion that a high carbohydrate load is a risk factor for development of an acute attack in patients with hypokalemic periodic paralysis may be explained by a spike in blood insulin level that triggers a shift of $K^+$ ions into cells.

In patients with a severe degree of hypokalemia and acidemia due to metabolic acidosis, the $P_K$ should be raised to at least 3 mmol/L before administering $NaHCO_3$, because even a small degree of an acute shift of $K^+$ ions into cells can be dangerous in this setting (see margin note).

An acute shift of $K^+$ ions into cells may occur in conditions associated with an adrenergic surge (e.g., acute myocardial infarction, acute pancreatitis, subarachnoid hemorrhage, and traumatic brain injury;

**SHIFT OF $K^+$ INTO CELLS WITH $NaHCO_3$ ADMINISTRATION**

- A major activator of NHE-1 is intracellular acidosis because not only are $H^+$ ions a substrate for NHE-1, they also bind to the modifier site that activates this cation exchanger.
- In the setting of metabolic acidemia and a rise in intracellular concentration of $H^+$ ions, resulting in activation of NHE-1, the administration of $NaHCO_3$ may decrease the concentration of $H^+$ ions in the ECF compartment and thereby may promote the electroneutral exit of $H^+$ ions and entry of $Na^+$ ions into cells via NHE-1.
- The subsequent electrogenic exit of $Na^+$ ions from the cells via the Na-K-ATPase increases the magnitude of the cell interior negative voltage, and hence more $K^+$ ions will be retained in cells.

see discussion of Case 14-1). Acute hypokalemia may also occur in patients who are given a large dose of $\beta_2$-agonists (e.g., albuterol for treatment of bronchial asthma, amphetamine for weight loss). Because large doses of caffeine result in an adrenergic surge, acute hypokalemia may be also seen in this setting. Nonselective $\beta_2$-antagonists are suggested in the treatment of patients with acute hypokalemia precipitated by an adrenergic surge.

Patients with catabolic states such as DKA have a deficit of $K^+$ ions and phosphate anions because these ions were released from cells and lost in the urine. A shift of $K^+$ ions into cells occurs when patients with DKA are treated with insulin and phosphate anions are provided from the diet. Hence, hypokalemia may develop if a sufficient amount of $K^+$ ions is not given. A similar situation arises in cachectic patients when they are treated with parenteral nutrition and in patients with pernicious anemia early in the course of therapy with vitamin $B_{12}$.

# REGULATION OF RENAL EXCRETION OF K⁺ IONS

**FLOW RATE IN THE CDN**

- A high flow rate in the CDN is not likely to be a sole cause of hypokalemia.
- Although a high flow rate may activate maxi-$K^+$ ion channels, generation of a lumen-negative voltage is required to achieve a high rate of excretion of $K^+$ ions.
- Patients with diabetes insipidus, despite having a high rate of flow in the CDN, they do not usually develop hypokalemia because vasopressin actions are required for increasing the flux of $Na^+$ ions via ENaC.

Control of $K^+$ ion secretion occurs primarily in the CDN, which includes the late distal convoluted tubule (DCT), the connecting segment, and the cortical collecting duct (CCD). Two factors influence the rate of excretion of $K^+$ ions: its net secretion by principal cells in the CDN (which raises the concentration of $K^+$ ions in the fluid in the lumen of the CDN) and the flow rate in the CDN (see margin note).

## SECRETION OF K⁺ IONS IN THE CDN

The process of secretion of $K^+$ ions by principal cells in the CDN has two elements. First, a lumen-negative transepithelial voltage must be generated by the electrogenic reabsorption of $Na^+$ ions (i.e., reabsorption of $Na^+$ ions without their accompanying anions, which are largely $Cl^-$ ions) via the epithelial sodium ion channel (ENaC). Second, open renal outer medullary $K^+$ ion (ROMK) channels must be present in the luminal membrane of principal cells.

Aldosterone actions lead to an increase in the number of open ENaC units in the luminal membrane of principal cells in the CDN and hence the rate of electrogenic reabsorption of $Na^+$ ions. Aldosterone binds to its receptor in the cytoplasm of principal cells, and the hormone–receptor complex enters the nucleus, leading to the synthesis of new proteins, including the serum and glucocorticoid regulated kinase-1 (SGK-1). SGK-1 increases the number of open ENaC in the luminal membrane of principal cells via its effect to phosphorylate and inactivate the ubiquitin ligase, Nedd 4-2 (see Chapter 13, Fig. 13-9).

The concentration of cortisol in plasma is at least a hundred times higher than that of aldosterone. Moreover, cortisol binds to the intracellular aldosterone receptor with the same avidity as aldosterone. Nevertheless, cortisol does not normally act as a mineralocorticoid because it is converted to an inactive form (cortisone) by the 11 $\beta$-hydroxy steroid dehydrogenase (11 $\beta$-HSDH) 1 and 2 enzyme system before it can reach the receptor for aldosterone (see Chapter 13). There are three circumstances, however, when cortisol acts as a mineralocorticoid: first, when 11$\beta$-HSDH is congenitally lacking (e.g., in patients with apparent mineralocorticoid excess syndrome); second, when 11$\beta$-HSDH is inhibited (e.g., by glycyrrhizinic acid in licorice); and third, when the activity of 11$\beta$-HSDH is overwhelmed by a large excess of cortisol (e.g., in a patient with an ACTH-producing tumor).

An electroneutral NaCl transport in the CCD seems to be mediated by the parallel activity of the $Na^+$-independent $Cl^-/HCO_3^-$ anion exchanger (pendrin) and the $Na^+$-dependent $Cl^-/HCO_3^-$ anion exchanger (NDCBE) (see Chapter 13, Fig. 13-10). An increase in luminal fluid concentration of $HCO_3^-$ ions and/or an alkaline luminal fluid pH seem to increase the amount of $K^+$ secreted in the CDN. An increase in luminal $HCO_3^-$ ion concentration may inhibit pendrin, and hence NDCBE, and thereby the electroneutral NaCl reabsorption. In addition, an increase in luminal fluid $HCO_3^-$ ion concentration may increase the abundance and activity of ENaC in the luminal membrane of principal cells. This may also lead to a higher rate of electrogenic reabsorption of $Na^+$ ions and hence secretion of $K^+$ ions, providing that open ROMK are present in the luminal membrane of principal cells.

In addition to control by the lumen-negative voltage, the secretory process for $K^+$ in principal cells is dependent on having a sufficient number of open ROMK channels in the luminal membrane of principal cells. Regulation of these channels is via phosphorylation/dephosphorylation-induced endocytosis/exocytosis of ROMK. This involves a complicated mixture of kinases and phosphatases including the With No Lysine (WNK) kinases, protein tyrosine kinases, and SGK-1. Angiotensin II ($ANG_{II}$), via increasing the expression of protein tyrosine kinase, leads to phosphorylation of ROMK, which results in its endocytosis. The ratio of the kidney-specific form of WNK1 (KS-WNK1) to the long form of WNK1 (L-WNK1) is decreased by dietary $K^+$ ion restriction, which leads to endocytosis of ROMK.

It seems that in humans, the number of open ROMK channels may not limit the net secretion of $K^+$ ions unless the $P_K$ falls to the range of 3.5 mmol/L. Because there is a time lag before a sufficient number of open ROMK channels are reinserted into the luminal membrane of principal cells in the CDN following chronic hypokalemia, hyperkalemia may develop with aggressive $K^+$ ion replacement therapy in this setting.

$K^+$ reabsorption occurs primarily in the medullary collecting duct (MCD) (see Chapter 13, Fig. 13-13). It is stimulated by $K^+$ ion depletion, and the transporter is an $H^+/K^+$-ATPase. This exchange is electroneutral and requires the presence of a sufficient number of $H^+$ ion acceptors in the luminal fluid (i.e., $HCO_3^-$ ions and/or $NH_3$).

## Clinical Implications

In a patient with hypokalemia, a higher than expected rate of excretion of $K^+$ ions in the urine indicates a more negative voltage in the lumen of the CDN. This greater lumen-negative voltage is due to a higher rate of electrogenic versus electroneutral $Na^+$ ion reabsorption in the CDN because of an increased number of open ENaC units in the luminal membrane of principal cells in the CDN. This could be due to one of two groups of disorders. The first is a secondary increase in ENaC activity due to the release of aldosterone in response to a low EABV. The second group of disorders consists of conditions that lead to a primary increase in ENaC activity (e.g., primary hyperreninemic hyperaldosteronism, primary hyperaldosteronism, disorders in which cortisol acts as a mineralocorticoid in the CDN, constitutively active ENaC in the luminal membrane of principal cells in the CDN).

**ABBREVIATIONS**

ENaC, epithelial sodium channel
ROMK, renal outer medullary $K^+$
SGK-1, serum and glucocorticoid regulated kinase-1
11β-HSDH, 11β-hydroxysteroid dehydrogenase
$ANG_{II}$, angiotensin II
WNK kinase, with no lysine kinase
L-WNK1, long WNK1
KS-WNK1, kidney-specific WNK1
ACTH, adrenocorticotropic hormone
MCD, medullary collecting duct
NDCBE, sodium-dependent chloride–bicarbonate exchanger
$K_{CDN}$, concentration of $K^+$ ions in the lumen of the CDN
$U_{Creatinine}$, concentration of creatinine in the urine
GFR, glomerular filtration rate
PCT, proximal convoluted tubule
TPP, thyrotoxic periodic paralysis
FPP, familial periodic paralysis
TAL, thick ascending limb
GRA, glucocorticoid remediable aldosteronism
AME, apparent mineralocorticoid excess syndrome

# PART B
# CLINICAL APPROACH

## TOOLS USED IN THE CLINICAL ASSESSMENT OF THE PATIENT WITH HYPOKALEMIA

### ASSESSMENT OF THE RATE OF EXCRETION OF K⁺ IONS IN THE URINE

A 24-hour urine collection is not necessary to assess the daily rate of excretion of $K^+$ ions. Taking advantage of the fact that creatinine is excreted at a near-constant rate throughout the day, we use the ratio of the concentration of $K^+$ ions in the urine ($U_K$) to the concentration of creatinine in the urine ($U_{Creatinine}$) (i.e., the $U_K/U_{Creatinine}$) for this purpose (see margin note). The use of $U_K/U_{Creatinine}$ to assess the rate of excretion of $K^+$ ions in the urine has advantages over 24-hour urine collection. Data needed for making decisions about therapy and diagnosis can be available in a short period of time. In addition, more relevant information can be gathered if one were to obtain a measurement of $P_K$ in the same time frame, and hence one can assess the renal response in view of the stimuli present at that time. On the other hand, it has a limitation because there is a diurnal variation in the rate of excretion of $K^+$ ions. This, however, does not affect its validity because data are interpreted in view of the presence of hypokalemia. The expected $U_K/U_{Creatinine}$ in patients with hypokalemia caused by a shift of $K^+$ ions into cells, or in those with chronic hypokalemia caused by the extrarenal loss of $K^+$ ions, is less than 15 mmol $K^+$/g creatinine (or <1.5 mmol $K^+$/mmol creatinine).

### The transtubular K concentration gradient (TTKG)

The TTKG was developed to provide a semiquantitative reflection of the driving force to secrete $K^+$ ions in the CDN. The goal in this calculation was to adjust the value of the $U_K$ for the amount of water that is reabsorbed in downstream nephron segments (i.e., the MCD) to estimate the concentration of $K^+$ ions in the luminal fluid in the terminal CDN ($K_{CDN}$). To calculate the $K_{CDN}$, we suggested dividing the $U_K$ by the ratio of urine osmolality ($U_{Osm}$) to the plasma osmolality ($P_{Osm}$) (i.e., $U_{Osm}/P_{Osm}$) because the $P_{Osm}$ should be equal to the osmolality in the luminal fluid in the terminal CDN when vasopressin acts and AQP2 are present in the luminal membrane of principal cells in the CDN.

The assumption made when using the $U_{Osm}/P_{Osm}$ ratio to adjust for the amount of water that is reabsorbed in the MCD is that the majority of the osmoles delivered to the MCD were not reabsorbed in this nephron segment. Although, in the absence of a marked degree of contraction of the EABV, the amount of electrolytes reabsorbed in the MCD should not pose a problem, this is, however, not true for urea because of the intrarenal urea recycling. It is estimated that in subjects eating a typical Western diet, close to 600 mmol of urea are reabsorbed downstream from CDN per day (see Chapter 13). Therefore, the calculated $K_{CDN}$ obtained from $U_K/(U_{Osm}/P_{Osm})$ is likely to be appreciably higher than the actual value in vivo. Therefore, we do not use the TTKG in the clinical assessment of patients with a dyskalemia; rather, we rely on the $U_K/U_{Creatinine}$ to assess the renal response in these patients.

**RATE OF EXCRETION OF CREATININE**

- The usual daily rate of excretion of creatinine is 20 mg/kg body weight or 200 μmol/kg body weight in males and 15 mg/kg body weight or 150 μmol/kg body weight in females.

## TOOLS TO ESTABLISH THE BASIS FOR THE INAPPROPRIATELY HIGH RATE OF EXCRETION OF K⁺ IONS

In a patient with hypokalemia, a higher than expected rate of excretion of $K^+$ ions implies a more negative voltage in the lumen of CDN, which drives the secretion of $K^+$ ions in the presence of open ROMK in the lumen of principal cells in the CDN. This higher lumen-negative voltage is caused by an increased rate of electrogenic versus electroneutral reabsorption of $Na^+$ ions in the CDN due to a higher number of open ENaC units in the luminal membrane of principal cells in the CDN. The clinical indices that are used to determine the basis of this increase in ENaC activity are an assessment of the EABV and the presence or absence of hypertension. The measurements of $P_{Renin}$ and $P_{Aldosterone}$ are also helpful in this differential diagnosis.

# STEPS IN THE CLINICAL APPROACH TO A PATIENT WITH HYPOKALEMIA

### DEAL WITH EMERGENCIES

The major emergencies related to hypokalemia are cardiac arrhythmias and respiratory muscle weakness leading to respiratory failure (Flow Chart 14-1). Because the administration of a large, rapid dose of $K^+$ ions is likely required, the concentration of $K^+$ ions in the administered intravenous fluid will need to be high. Therefore, $K^+$ ions may have to be administered via a large central vein; cardiac monitoring is essential in this setting.

### ANTICIPATE AND PREVENT DANGERS DUE TO THERAPY

Because one does not know in any individual patient to what degree hypokalemia is due to a shift of $K^+$ ions into cells versus a total body deficit of $K^+$ ions, in the absence of an emergency related to hypokalemia, one should not replace the deficit of $K^+$ ions rapidly because of the risk of causing acute hyperkalemia. Therapy should not contain compounds that may cause $K^+$ to shift into cells. Hence, the initial infusion should not contain glucose or $NaHCO_3$, and $\beta_2$-adrenergic

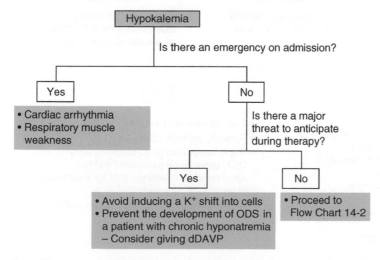

**Flow Chart 14-1 Initial Steps in the Management of a Patient With Hypokalemia.** The steps are to deal with emergencies and to anticipate and prevent dangers during therapy. *dDAVP*, Desmopressin; ODS, osmotic demyelination syndrome.

agonists should be avoided. In patients who also have hypomagnesemia, hypokalemia may be refractory to the administration of KCl until supplements of magnesium salts are given. This is particularly important in patients with a cardiac arrhythmia.

There are a number of reasons why the administration of KCl may cause a rapid or excessive rise in the $P_{Na}$ and hence the risk of osmotic demyelination in a patient with chronic hyponatremia. In terms of body tonicity, $Na^+$ ions (the main ECF cations) and $K^+$ ions (the main ICF cations) are equivalent. During the development of hypokalemia caused by the loss of $K^+$ ions, $K^+$ ions are lost mainly from the ICF compartment. Some of these $K^+$ ions in the ICF compartment are replaced by $Na^+$ ions from the ECF compartment. When $K^+$ ions are administered, $K^+$ ions enter cells, and $Na^+$ ions that entered these cells to replace the $K^+$ ions that were lost from cells will exit from these cells. Therefore, the administration of $K^+$ ions will cause a rise in body tonicity, which will be reflected by a rise in $P_{Na}$ similar to that with the administration of an equivalent amount of $Na^+$ ions, if there is no change in total body water. Furthermore, because $Na^+$ ions are retained in the ECF compartment, EABV may become expanded and a water diuresis may ensue. This is of particular concern because patients with hypokalemia are at high risk for the development of osmotic demyelination. Therefore, the administration of $K^+$ ions should be in a solution that is isotonic to the patient. For example, if the patent has a $P_{Na}$ of 120 mmol/L, a solution of half normal saline (0.45% NaCl, or 77 mmol/L) with 40 mmol of KCl/L will have a concentration of $Na^+ + K^+$ ions that is reasonably close to the patient's $P_{Na}$. Administration of dDAVP to prevent the occurrence of a water diuresis may be considered.

## DETERMINE IF THE MAJOR BASIS FOR HYPOKALEMIA IS AN ACUTE SHIFT OF $K^+$ IONS INTO CELLS (FLOW CHART 14-2)

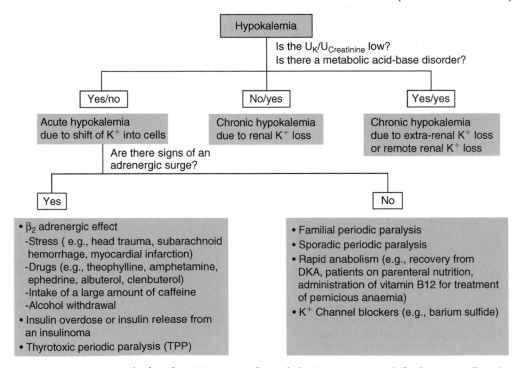

**Flow Chart 14-2 Determine Whether the Major Basis of Hypokalemia Is an Acute Shift of $K^+$ into Cells.** A low rate of excretion of $K^+$ ions in the urine and the absence of a metabolic acid–base disorder suggest that the major basis of hypokalemia is an acute shift of $K^+$ ions into cells. The causes of a shift of $K^+$ ions into cells can be separated into two groups based on the presence of signs of an adrenergic surge. *DKA*, Diabetic ketoacidosis.

A low rate of excretion of $K^+$ ions in the urine and the absence of a metabolic acid-acid base disorder provide clues to suggest that the major basis of the hypokalemia is an acute shift of $K^+$ ions into cells.

We begin by examining the rate of excretion of $K^+$ ions in the urine. The expected renal response in a patient with hypokalemia that is due to a shift of $K^+$ ions into cells is to decrease the rate of excretion of $K^+$ ions in the urine to the minimum, that is, 15 mmol/day).

We use the $U_K/U_{Creatinine}$ ratio in a spot urine sample to assess the rate of excretion of $K^+$ ions in the urine. In a patient with acute hypokalemia due solely to a shift of $K^+$ ions into cells, and assuming a usual rate of creatinine excretion of 1 g (~10 mmol/day), $U_K/U_{Creatinine}$ should be less than 15 mmol of $K^+$ ions/g creatinine or less than 1.5 mmol of $K^+$ ions/mmol creatinine.

There are possible caveats in using the $U_K/U_{Creatinine}$ to determine if the basis of hypokalemia is an acute shift of $K^+$ into cells. This ratio may be low in a patient with chronic hypokalemia due to extrarenal loss of $K^+$ ions or a renal loss of $K^+$ ions that have occurred in the recent past without an ongoing loss of $K^+$ ions in the urine. In both of these settings, however, it is likely that a metabolic acid–base disorder will be present.

If we have established that the major basis of hypokalemia is an acute shift of $K^+$ ions into cells, the next step is to determine whether an adrenergic surge is its cause. In these settings, tachychardia, a wide pulse pressure, and systolic hypertension are often present. It is very important to recognize this group of patients because the administration of nonselective β-blockers (e.g., propranolol) can lead to a rapid rise in $P_K$ without the need for a large infusion of KCl, and hence avoid the risk of development of rebound hyperkalemia when the stimulus for the shift of $K^+$ ions into cells abates.

Patients with hypokalemia due to an acute shift of $K^+$ ions into cells caused by an adrenergic surge can be divided into two groups based on whether there is an exogenous or endogenous source of the $β_2$-adrenergic effect. There are several exogenous causes of $β_2$ adrenergic effect. Amphetamines may be used to suppress appetite and induce weight loss or to increase alertness. A shift of $K^+$ ions may be provoked by the repeated use of large doses of $β_2$-agonists (e.g., albuterol) to relieve bronchospasm in a patient with bronchial asthma. Hypokalemia due to use of clenbuterol, a $β_2$-adrenergic agonist, has been reported in body builders, who use the drug as an alternative to anabolic steroids, and also in users of heroin that was adulterated with clenbuterol. The intake of a very large quantity of caffeine (e.g., coffee, caffeinated soda, cocoa, or a very large intake of chocolate) can cause a large surge of catecholamines, which may induce a shift of $K^+$ ions into cells. The source of the $β_2$-adrenergic effect may also be endogenous. For example, hypokalemia may occur in acute stress states (e.g., head trauma, subarachnoid hemorrhage, myocardial infarction, acute pancreatitis, alcohol withdrawal). Another example is thyrotoxic periodic paralysis (TPP), which is more commonly seen in young males of Asian or Hispanic descent. Other disorders with a long-acting endogenous adrenergic surge that can induce an acute shift of $K^+$ ions into cells such as hypoglycemia due to an insulin overdose, the release of insulin from an insulinoma, or a $β_2$-adrenergic effect in a patient with a pheochromocytoma.

In the absence of a high adrenergic state, suspect familial periodic paralysis, more commonly seen in Caucasians, sporadic periodic paralysis, a rapid anabolic state if a sufficient amount of $K^+$ ions is not given (e.g., patients recovering from DKA, patients who are treated with parenteral nutrition, and patients with pernicious anemia early in the course of their therapy with vitamin $B_{12}$), or the presence of a $K^+$ ion channel blocker (e.g., ingestion of barium sulfide).

### CLINICAL APPROACH TO THE PATIENTS WITH CHRONIC HYPOKALEMIA

The first step to the diagnosis of the cause of hypokalemia in the patient with chronic hypokalemia is to examine the acid–base status in plasma.

### Subgroup with metabolic acidosis

The group of patients with chronic hypokalemia and metabolic acidosis (usually hyperchloremic metabolic acidosis) can be divided into two categories by examining the rate of excretion of ammonium ($NH_4^+$) ions in the urine (Flow Chart 14-3). The rate of excretion of $NH_4^+$ ions can be estimated using the calculation of the urine osmolal gap (see Chapter 2).

### Subgroup with metabolic alkalosis

The first step in this subgroup of patients is to determine whether the site of loss of $K^+$ ions is renal or extrarenal based on assessment of the rate of excretion of $K^+$ ions in the urine. This can be done with the use of the $U_K/U_{Creatinine}$ ratio. Patients who have hypokalemia, metabolic alkalosis, and a $U_K/U_{Creatinine}$ ratio that is <15 mmol of $K^+$ ions/g of creatinine (<1.5 mmol of $K^+$ ions/mmol of creatinine) are likely to have a condition associated with the loss of $K^+$ ions via a nonrenal route, such as in sweat (e.g., patients with cystic fibrosis) or via the intestinal tract (e.g., patients with diarrhea associated with decreased activity of the colonic downregulated in adenoma [DRA] $Cl^-/HCO_3^-$ anion exchanger; see Chapter 4). Notwithstanding , the $U_K/U_{Creatinine}$ ratio may be low in patients with a remote renal loss of $K^+$ ions ( e.g., due to prior use of diuretics)

On the other hand, patients who have hypokalemia, metabolic alkalosis, and a $U_K/U_{Creatinine}$ ratio that is higher than these values

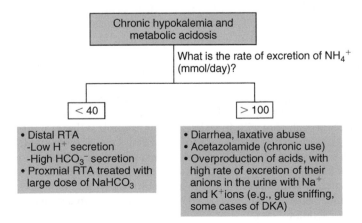

**Flow Chart 14-3 Chronic Hypokalemia and Metabolic Acidosis.** The first step in these patients is to estimate the rate of excretion of $NH_4^+$ ions in the urine using the urine osmolal gap to determine the cause of the hyperchloremic metabolic acidosis and hence the cause of hypokalemia. *DKA,* Diabetic ketoacidosis; *RTA,* renal tubular acidosis.

have a condition associated with a renal loss of K⁺ ions. The steps to take to determine the underlying pathophysiology in this group of patients are outlined in Flow Chart 14-4. In essence, we are trying to determine the cause of a higher rate of electrogenic reabsorption of Na⁺ ions in the CDN. The primary pathophysiology is an increased number of open ENaC units in the luminal membrane of principal cells in the CDN. This could be due to two groups of disorders. Patients in the first group have low EABV causing the release of aldosterone, and hence an increased number of open ENaC units in the luminal membrane of principal cells in the CDN. These patients are not likely to have high BP. The most common causes are protracted vomiting or the use of diuretic agents. In some patients, a diuretic effect may be due to an inherited disorder affecting NaCl reabsorption in the medullary thick ascending limb (TAL) of the loop of Henle (i.e., Bartter syndrome) or in the DCT (i.e., Gitelman syndrome). Ligands that occupy the calcium-sensing receptor in the medullary TAL of the loop of Henle (e.g., calcium in a patient with hypercalcemia, drugs [e.g., gentamicin, cisplatin], and possibly cationic proteins [e.g., cationic monoclonal immunoglobulins in a patient with multiple myeloma]) may result in a clinical picture that mimics Bartter syndrome. The use of urine electrolytes in the differential diagnosis of hypokalemia in a patient with a contracted EABV is summarized in Table 14-1.

Patients in the second group have conditions that are associated with a primary increase in ENaC activity. The EABV in these patients is not low, and the BP is commonly high. These disorders

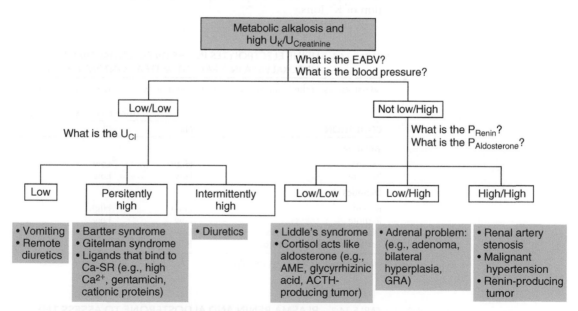

**Flow Chart 14-4 Chronic Hypokalemia With Metabolic Alkalosis and a High $U_K/U_{Creatinine}$.** The goal is to determine the cause of an increased number of open ENaC units in the luminal membrane of principal cells in the CDN. This could be due to two groups of disorders, which can be separated based on the effective arterial blood volume (EABV) and the blood pressure (BP). The first group of disorders is the patients who have secondary increase in the epithelial sodium channel (ENaC) activity due to the release of aldosterone in response to a low EABV. Therefore, these patients are not likely to have high BP. The differential diagnosis in this group of patients can be based on measurement of the concentration of Cl⁻ in the urine ($U_{Cl}$). Patients in the second group have conditions that are associated with a primary increase in ENaC activity. Their EABV is not low and their BP is high. The differential diagnosis in this group of patients is based on measurements of the $P_{Renin}$ and the $P_{Aldosterone}$. *ACTH*, Adrenocorticotropic hormone; *AME*, apparent mineralocorticoid excess syndrome; *GRA*, glucocorticoid remediable aldosteronism; *Ca-SR*, calcium ion–sensing receptor.

include primary hypereninemic hyperaldosteronism (e.g., renal artery stenosis, malignant hypertension, renin secreting tumor), primary hyperaldosteronism (e.g., adrenal adenoma, bilateral adrenal hyperplasia, glucocorticoid remediable aldosteronism [GRA]), disorders in which cortisol acts as a mineralocorticoid in CDN (e.g., apparent mineralocorticoid excess syndrome [AME], inhibition of 11β-HSDH by glycyrrhizinic acid, ACTH-producing tumor), and conditions with constitutively active ENaC in the luminal membrane of principal cells in the CDN [e.g., Liddle syndrome]). The measurement of $P_{Renin}$ and $P_{Aldosterone}$ are helpful in this differential diagnosis in this group of patients (Table 14-2).

In some patients, a decreased rate of electroneutral reabsorption of $Na^+$ ions may contribute to the increased rate of electrogenic reabsorption of $Na^+$ ions and enhanced kaliuresis. This may be the case when $Na^+$ ions are delivered to the CDN with a small amount of $Cl^-$ ions (e.g., delivery of $Na^+$ ions with $HCO_3^-$ anions in a patient with recent vomiting or with anions of a drug [e.g., penicillin]).

Magnesium ($Mg^{2+}$) deficiency is frequently associated with hypokalemia. This relationship is likely due to the underlying disorders that cause both $Mg^{2+}$ and $K^+$ ions loss (e.g., diarrhea, diuretic therapy, Gitelman syndrome). $K^+$ ion secretion in the CDN is mediated by ROMK, a process that is inhibited by intracellular $Mg^{2+}$ ions. A decrease in intracellular concentration of free $Mg^{2+}$ ions, caused by $Mg^{2+}$ ion deficiency, releases the inhibition of ROMK. $Mg^{2+}$ ion deficiency alone, however, does not necessarily cause hypokalemia, because an increase in the rate of electrogenic reabsorption of $Na^+$ ions is required to enhance the rate of secretion of $K^+$ ions.

TABLE 14-1  **URINE ELECTROLYTES IN THE DIFFERENTIAL DIAGNOSIS OF HYPOKALEMIA IN A PATIENT WITH A CONTRACTED EABV**

Adjust Values of the Urine Electrolyte Concentration When Polyuria Is Present

| CONDITION | Urine Electrolyte | |
|---|---|---|
| | **Na+** | **Cl−** |
| **Vomiting** | | |
| Recent | High | Low |
| Remote | Low | Low |
| **Diuretics** | | |
| Recent | High | High |
| Remote | Low | Low |
| **Diarrhea or laxative abuse** | Low | High |
| **Bartter or Gitelman syndrome** | High | High |

*High,* > mmol/L; *Low,* < 15 mmol/L.

TABLE 14-2  **PLASMA RENIN AND ALDOSTERONE TO ASSESS THE BASIS OF HYPOKALEMIA DUE TO A LESION WITH PRIMARY ACTIVE ENaC**

| | RENIN | ALDOSTERONE |
|---|---|---|
| Primary hyperaldosteronism | Low | High |
| Glucocorticoid remediable hyperaldosteronism | Low | High |
| Renal artery stenosis | High | High |
| Malignant hypertension | High | High |
| Renin-secreting tumor | High | High |
| Liddle syndrome | Low | Low |
| Disorders in which cortisol acts as a mineralocorticoid | Low | Low |

# PART C
# SPECIFIC CAUSES OF HYPOKALEMIA

A list of the causes of hypokalemia is provided in Table 14-3. We begin with the disorders in which acute hypokalemia is caused by a shift of K+ ions into cells and then discuss the disorders of chronic hypokalemia caused by the loss of K+ ions.

The only symptom that is attributable to hypokalemia per se is muscle weakness, but it is not present in all patients with this electrolyte disorder. Notwithstanding, it may be more prevalent in patients

---

TABLE 14-3    **CAUSES OF HYPOKALEMIA**

**A. Shift of K+ Ions into Cells**
- Associated with an adrenergic surge:
  - $\beta_2$-Adrenergics surge due to stress conditions (e.g., head trauma, subarachnoid hemorrhage, myocardial infarction), drugs (e.g., amphetamines, theophylline, albuterol, clenbuterol), large dose of caffeine, pheochromocytoma
  - High insulin levels causing hypoglycemia
  - Thyrotoxic periodic paralysis
- Not associated with an adrenergic surge:
  - Familial hypokalemic periodic paralysis, sporadic hypokalemic periodic paralysis
  - K+ ion channel blockers (e.g., barium sulfide)
  - States with rapid anabolism (e.g., recovery from diabetic ketoacidosis)

**B. Conditions With Increased K+ Ion Loss Associated With Hyperchloremic Metabolic Acidosis**
- Gastrointestinal loss of $NaHCO_3$ (e.g., diarrhea, laxative abuse, fistula, ileus, ureteral diversion into an ileal conduit)
- Overproduction of acids, with the loss of their anions in the urine with K+ ions (e.g., hippuric acid in toluene abuse, some cases of diabetic ketoacidosis)
- Reduced reabsorption of $NaHCO_3$ in PCT (e.g., proximal renal tubular acidosis treated with large amounts of $NaHCO_3$, chronic use of acetazolamide)
- Distal renal tubular acidosis
  - Low distal H+ ion secretion subtype (e.g., Sjögren syndrome)
  - High distal secretion of $HCO_3^-$ ions (e.g., Southeast Asian ovalocytosis with a second mutation involving the $Cl^-/HCO_3^-$ anion exchanger, causing it to be mistargeted to the luminal membrane of $\alpha$-intercalated cells)

**C. Conditions With Increased K+ Ion Loss Associated With Metabolic Alkalosis**
1. Extrarenal loss of K+ ions
   a. Loss of K+ ions in sweat (e.g., patients with cystic fibrosis)
   b Loss of K+ ions in diarrheal fluid (patients with diarrhea due to diminished DRA activity)
2. Renal loss of K+ ions
   a. Increased ENaC activity due to release of aldosterone caused by low EABV
      - Vomiting, diuretic use or abuse
      - Bartter syndrome, Gitelman syndrome
      - Pseudo-Bartter syndrome due to ligand binding to Ca-SR in the mTAL of the loop of Henle (e.g., $Ca^{2+}$ in patients with hypercalcemia, drugs [gentamicin, cisplatin], cationic proteins)
   b. Primary increase in ENaC activity
      - Primary hypereninemic hyperaldosteronism (e.g., renal artery stenosis, malignant hypertension, renin secreting tumor)
      - Primary hyperaldosteronism (e.g., adrenal adenoma, bilateral adrenal hyperplasia, glucocorticoid remediable aldosteronism)
      - Disorders in which cortisol acts as a mineralocorticoid (e.g., apparent mineralocorticoid excess syndrome [AME], inhibition of 11β-HSDH by glycyrrhinizic acid [e.g., in licorice], ACTH producing tumor)
      - Constitutively active ENaC (e.g., Liddle syndrome)

---

A decreased intake of K+ ions is rarely a sole cause of chronic hypokalemia unless the intake of K+ is very low for a prolonged period of time. Nevertheless, a low intake of K+ ions can lead to a more severe degree of hypokalemia if there is an ongoing K+ ion loss. *ACTH,* Adrenocorticotropic hormone; *DRA,* downregulated in adenoma; *EABV,* effective arterial blood volume; *ENaC,* epithelial sodium channel; *PCT,* proximal convoluted tubule; *Ca-SR,* calcium sensing receptor; *mTAL,* medullary thick ascending limb.

with an acute and severe degree of hypokalemia. Severe $K^+$ ion depletion can lead to rhabdomyolysis. Involvement of respiratory muscles may cause respiratory failure. Involvement of muscles of the intestinal tract may lead to decreased intestinal motility, with symptoms ranging from constipation to those caused by paralytic ileus.

Patients with hypokalemia may have paresthesias and depressed deep tendon reflexes due to delayed peripheral nerve conduction. Patients with hypokalemia and magnesium deficiency may have more severe symptoms (e.g., tetany).

There is a large variability among patients in the $P_K$ that is associated with ECG changes or arrhythmia. Hypokalemia-associated ECG changes include flat T waves, ST segment depression, and prominent U waves. A variety of arrhythmias may be seen in patients with hypokalemia including premature atrial and ventricular beats, sinus bradycardia, paroxysmal atrial or junctional tachycardia, atrioventricular block, and ventricular tachycardia or fibrillation.

It is well documented that chronic hypokalemia can predispose to the development or worsening of hypertension that may be due to the retention of NaCl (see Chapter 13).

Chronic hypokalemia may lead to carbohydrate intolerance and possibly overt diabetes mellitus. This effect may be an important factor in the pathophysiology of the observed association between the use of thiazide diuretics and the development of new onset diabetes mellitus.

Chronic $K^+$ ions depletion is associated with changes in renal function. Chronic hypokalemia has been associated with chronic tubulointerstitial kidney disease with interstitial fibrosis, tubular atrophy cyst formation, and renal insufficiency (hypokalemic nephropathy). One possible explanation for this observation is that hypokalemia is associated with intracellular acidosis in the cells of the PCT, which results in increased rate of production of $NH_4^+$ ions, and accumulation in the medullary interstitial compartment. It is thought that $NH_4^+$ ions may activate complement components by amidation, leading to tubulointerstitial injury. Hypokalemia is often listed as a cause of nephrogenic diabetes insipidus. The defect in renal concentrating ability, however, may reflect the lower osmolality in the medullary interstitial compartment due to chronic medullary interstitial disease, rather than a defect in the renal response to vasopressin with failure to insert a sufficient number of AQP2 channels in the luminal membrane of principal cells in the collecting ducts (discussed in more detail in Chapter 11). Chronic hypokalemia is associated with metabolic alkalosis. Hypokalemia is associated with intracellular acidosis in PCT cells. This, in addition to stimulating the production of $NH_4^+$ ions and the generation of new $HCO_3^-$ ions, enhances the rate of reabsorption of $HCO_3^-$ ions in the PCT, and hence, a higher $P_{HCO_3}$ is maintained. Chronic $K^+$ ion depletion is also associated with calcium stone formation and nephrocalcinosis (see Chapter 13).

## HYPOKALEMIC PERIODIC PARALYSIS

Acute hypokalemia with paralysis could be caused by a genetic disorder or acquired causes that provoke a prolonged adrenergic surge and hence induce a sustained shift of $K^+$ ions into cells (e.g., ingestion of amphetamines, excessive intake of caffeine, use of a large dose of $\beta_2$-adrenergics to treat bronchial asthma). The genetic group of disorders includes two entities: thyrotoxic periodic paralysis and familial periodic paralysis.

Thyrotoxic periodic paralysis is more common in Asian and Hispanic males, with the first attack usually occurring between the ages of 20 to 50 years old. Familial periodic paralysis is more common in Caucasian males, with the first attack usually occurring under the age of 20 years old. Although it is said that attacks are commonly provoked by a large carbohydrate meal (release of insulin) or develop during the period of rest after strenuous exercise ($\beta_2$-adrenergic surge), most patients do not have clear precipitating factors for their attacks.

## PATHOPHYSIOLOGY

An increased Na-K-ATPase activity due to excess thyroid hormones, which can lead to a greater shift of $K^+$ ions into cells in the presence of a stimulus that would not cause acute hypokalemia in normal subjects, has been implicated in the pathogenesis of thyrotoxic periodic paralysis (TPP). Recent studies have shown that susceptibility to TPP can be conferred by loss-of-function mutations in the skeletal muscle–specific inward rectifying $K^+$ ion (Kir) channel, Kir2.1. The dual hits of increased intracellular $K^+$ ion influx because of increased numbers of activated Na-K-ATPase units and decreased $K^+$ ion efflux because of defective Kir channels lead to hypokalemia with decreased muscle excitability in these patients.

Familial periodic paralysis is inherited as an autosomal dominant disorder. Genetic analyses in patients with familial periodic paralysis have suggested that the abnormality in many of these patients is linked to the gene that encodes for the $\alpha$-subunit of the dihydropyridine-sensitive calcium ion channel in skeletal muscles; it is not clear how this leads to periodic hypokalemia and paralysis.

## CLINICAL PICTURE

The dominant finding is recurrent, transient episodes of muscle weakness that may progress to paralysis in association with a severe degree of hypokalemia ($P_K$ is often <2.0 mmol/L). In Asian and Hispanic populations, it is commonly associated with thyrotoxicosis, although signs and symptoms of thyrotoxicosis are often subtle.

## DIAGNOSIS

The first step is to determine if the hypokalemia is acute (caused by a shift of $K^+$ ions into cells) or chronic (caused by a total body deficit of $K^+$ ions). A low rate of excretion of $K^+$ ions in the urine as assessed by the $U_K/U_{Creatinine}$ ratio and the absence of a metabolic acid-acid base disorder provide clues to suggest that the major basis of the hypokalemia is an acute shift of $K^+$ ions into cells. The presence of tachycardia (systolic hypertension with wide pulse pressure) suggest that the basis of the acute shift of $K^+$ ions into cells is an acute adrenergic surge or hyperthyroidism. Hypophosphatemia is usually present in both the thyrotoxic and the familial forms of hypokalemic periodic paralysis. The signs of hyperthyroidism may be present in patients with thyrotoxic periodic paralysis but more often are subtle; the diagnosis is made by finding elevated levels of thyroid hormones in plasma.

## DIFFERENTIAL DIAGNOSIS

The clinical and laboratory findings help to differentiate patients with hypokalemic periodic paralysis from patients with chronic hypokalemia due to $K^+$ ion loss who may also have a component of their hypokalemia due to an acute shift of $K^+$ ions into cells. One other point helps in the differential diagnosis. Patients with hypokalemic periodic paralysis usually need far less KCl supplementation to bring their $P_K$ to a safe level (~3 mmol/L) than do patients who have chronic hypokalemia with total body $K^+$ ion deficit (~1 vs. >3 mmol of KCl/kg body weight).

### THERAPY

During an acute attack, patients are treated with the administration of KCl. The rate of administration of KCl should not exceed about 10 mmol/hr unless there is a cardiac arrhythmia. There is, however, the risk of development of rebound hyperkalemia as $K^+$ ions move back into the ECF compartment. In retrospective case-controlled studies, rebound hyperkalemia ($P_K$>5.0 mmol/L) was observed in 30% to 70% of patients with thyrotoxic hypokalemic periodic paralysis if more than 90 mmol of KCl were given in a 24 hour period or at a rate higher than 10 mmol/hr. Patients with thyrotoxic hypokalemic periodic paralysis have been successfully treated with the administration of a nonselective β-blocker (propranolol, 3 mg/kg orally) without the administration of KCl resulting in rapid reversal of weakness and hypokalemia and without the development of rebound hyperkalemia. The administration of a nonselective β-blocker may also be useful to treat other conditions of acute hypokalemia that are associated with a high adrenergic surge (e.g., intake of amphetamines or large doses of caffeine). Hyperthyroidism, if present, is treated in the usual fashion. To prevent recurrence of attacks, patients are usually advised to avoid carbohydrate-rich meals and vigorous exercise. In the longer term, administration of nonselective β-blockers may reduce the number of the attacks of paralysis but seems to have little effect on the degree of fall in the $P_K$ during an attack. Acetazolamide (250 to 750 mg/day) has been used successfully to reduce the number of attacks in some patients with familial hypokalemic periodic paralysis. The mechanism of the beneficial effect of this carbonic anhydrase inhibitor in this condition is not clear.

## DISTAL RENAL TUBULAR ACIDOSIS

### PATHOPHYSIOLOGY

Hypokalemia, which can be severe at times, is commonly seen in patients with distal renal tubular acidosis that is due to a low net rate of secretion of $H^+$ ions. This low rate of net $H^+$ ion secretion could be caused of a defect affecting the $H^+$-ATPase in the distal nephron (e.g., an inherited disorder, an acquired defect in a number of autoimmune disorders, or dysproteinemias), or a defect resulting in the secretion of $HCO_3^-$ ions in the distal nephron (e.g., in patients with Southeast Asian ovalocytosis and a second mutation affecting the $Cl^-/HCO_3^-$ anion exchanger, causing it to be mistargeted to the luminal membrane of α-intercalated cells) (see Chapter 4 for more discussion of this topic). The accelerated secretion of $K^+$ ions could be due to an effect of $HCO_3^-$ in the lumen of the CDN to diminish the electroneutral NaCl transport via pendrin/NDCBE, which may lead to an increase in the rate of electrogenic reabsorption of $Na^+$ ions and the magnitude of the lumen-negative voltage in the CDN.

### DIAGNOSIS

The clinical features include the presence of hypokalemia, metabolic acidemia with a normal value of the anion gap in plasma ($P_{Anion\ gap}$),

**ABBREVIATIONS**

$P_{Anion\ gap}$, anion gap in plasma
NKCC-2, $Na^+$, $K^+$, 2 $Cl^-$ cotransporter 2
NCC, $Na^+$, $Cl^-$ cotransporter
ClC-Kb, $Cl^-$ ion channel
mTAL, medullary thick ascending limb

a low rate of excretion of $NH_4^+$ ions, and a high value of the urine pH (~7.0). Many patients with this disorder present with recurrent calcium phosphate stones or nephrocalcinosis.

### THERAPY

$K^+$ ions should be given as a KCl preparation if the patient has a significant degree of hypokalemia. $NaHCO_3$ must not be administered until the $P_K$ is raised to a safe level (i.e., >3 mmol/L) because its administration may induce a shift of $K^+$ ions into cells, and hence a more severe degree of hypokalemia may develop. The administration of $K^+$ ions with a precursor of $HCO_3^-$ ions (e.g., citrate anions) seems rational to correct both the hypokalemia and metabolic acidemia. This therapy, however, may lead to a further increase in urine pH and hence in the fraction of the total amount of phosphate in the urine that is in the form of divalent phosphate, which may increase the risk of precipitation of calcium phosphate stones. Nevertheless, the incremental increase in the concentration of divalent phosphate with further rise in the urine pH above a value of 7.0 is small (see Chapter 4, Table 4-8). This risk may be outweighed by the possible benefit from increasing the rate of excretion of citrate anions in the urine, as a result of correcting the acidemia and hypokalemia, resulting in decreasing the concentration of ionized calcium in the urine.

## GLUE SNIFFING

### PATHOPHYSIOLOGY

Metabolism of toluene leads to the production of hippuric acid (see Figure 3-2). The excretion of hippurate anions in the urine at a rate that exceeds that of $NH_4^+$ ions leads to loss of $Na^+$ ions and contraction of the EABV. Hpokalemia results from excessive loss of $K^+$ ions in the urine because of a high rate of secretion of $K^+$ ions in the CDN as a result of a more negative lumen voltage in the CDN. This higher lumen-negative voltage is caused by a higher rate of electrogenic reabsorption of $Na^+$ ions in the CDN. This is because of the presence of more numbers of open ENaC units in the luminal membrane of principal cells in the CDN due to the actions of aldosterone released in response to low EABV and the delivery of $Na^+$ ions with hippurate anions, which are not reabsorbed in the CDN.

### DIAGNOSIS

Diagnosis is based on the presence of hypokalemia, metabolic acidosis with a normal $P_{Anion\ gap}$, and a high rate of excretion of $NH_4^+$ ions in the urine with anions other than $Cl^-$. One can deduce that the anions excreted in the urine with $NH_4^+$ ions are hippurate anions from their high fractional excretion rate because hippurate anions are freely filtered and are also secreted in the PCT.

### THERAPY

If the patient presents with a significant degree of hypokalemia, $K^+$ ions must be given as a KCl preparation. The administration of $NaHCO_3$ should be delayed until the $P_K$ is raised to a safe level (i.e., >3 mmol/L).

# DIARRHEA

There are two groups of patients who have diarrhea and may develop hypokalemia:

## PATIENTS WITH SECRETORY DIARRHEA

### Pathophysiology

The prototype of this type of disorder is the patient with cholera. This type of diarrhea has an explosive onset and a huge loss of $Na^+$, $Cl^-$, and $HCO_3^-$ ions in the diarrheal fluid. The major pathophysiology is due to the effect of the cholera toxin to increase the formation intracellular cyclic adenosine monophosphate (cAMP), which activates protein kinase A, and leads to the insertion of the CFTR $Cl^-$ channels in the luminal membrane of crypt cells of the early small intestine. This causes a large delivery of $Na^+$ and $Cl^-$ ions to the colon, substantially more than can be absorbed in this segment of the bowel (see Chapter 4 for more discussion). Therefore, these patients develop a very large deficit of $Na^+$ and $Cl^-$ ions that is often close to half of their content in the ECF compartment.

These patients have large losses of $K^+$ ions in their diarrheal fluid (~15 mmol/L). In addition to the large volume of diarrhea, the rise in cAMP stimulates the secretion of $K^+$ ions via the maxi-$K^+$ ion channel in the colon. The α-adrenergic response to the very severe degree of contraction of the EABV, however, leads to inhibition of the release of insulin. As a result, there is a shift of $K^+$ ions out of cells. Therefore, the $P_K$ is commonly in the higher end of the normal range, despite a large total body deficit of $K^+$ ions. With the infusion of a large volume of saline, the α-adrenergic effects may be suppressed. If the $β_2$-adrenergic response persists, the $P_K$ may fall to dangerously low values.

Therefore, these patients will need a large quantity of KCl after the first few liters of intravenous saline are given, and one must monitor the $P_K$ closely to plan further therapy with $K^+$ ions. These patients also have a very large deficit of $HCO_3^-$ ions in the ECF compartment due to the loss of $NaHCO_3$ in diarrheal fluid. Notwithstanding, the $P_{HCO_3}$ may be close to the normal range because the ECF volume may be reduced by more than 50% (see Chapter 2 for more details). Therefore, with the infusion of a large volume of saline, a severe degree of acidemia will develop. In fact, some of these patients develop pulmonary edema if $NaHCO_3$ is not given (see Chapter 3 for explanation of the mechanism). Therefore, these patients should be given enough $NaHCO_3$ (or $Na^+$ ions with anions that can be metabolized to produce $HCO_3^-$ ions [e.g., lactate anions in Ringer solution]) to prevent the development of a severe degree of acidemia. This is an exception to the rule that patients with metabolic acidemia and hypokalemia should not be treated with $NaHCO_3$, because it is being given to prevent the development of a more severe degree of acidemia (recall that the diarrheal fluid has a high concentration of $HCO_3^-$ [~40 to 45 mmol/L]). We think it should be reasonably safe in terms of avoiding the danger of inducing a shift of $K^+$ ions into cells as long as the $P_{HCO_3}$ does not rise appreciably. Accordingly, the concentration of $HCO_3^-$ ions in the administered intravenous fluid should be close to the $P_{HCO_3}$ if the goal is to re-expand the EABV, whereas the concentration of $HCO_3^-$ ions in the administered intravenous fluid should be close to the concentration of $HCO_3^-$ ions in diarrheal fluid when the goal is to replace ongoing losses.

## PATIENTS WITH DIARRHEA DUE TO DIMINISHED REABSORPTION OF Na⁺ AND Cl⁻ IONS IN THE COLON

These patients do not have a large increase in the delivery of $Na^+$ and $Cl^-$ ions to the colon. Therefore, the volume of diarrheal fluid and the electrolyte deficits are much smaller than in patients with the secretory subtype of diarrhea.

The pathophysiology in these patients is a diminished activity of the downregulated in adenoma $Cl^-/HCO_3^-$ anion exchanger (AE) in the luminal membrane of colonic cells (see Chapter 4).

These patients have a modest loss of $K^+$ ions in diarrheal fluid; hypokalemia may develop if their dietary intake of $K^+$ is poor. $\beta_2$-Adrenergic release in response to a mild degree of contraction of the EABV may induce a shift of $K^+$ ions into cells, hence these patients may present with a more severe degree of hypokalemia.

### Diagnosis

A history of diarrhea may be obtained; abuse of laxatives, however, may be denied. If suspected, measurement of the urine electrolytes may provide helpful clues (see Table 14-2). The $U_{Na}$ is low if the EABV is contracted, but the $U_{Cl}$ may be high if the rate of excretion of $NH_4^+$ ions in the urine is high due to the effect of metabolic acidemia to stimulate ammoniagenesis.

In patients with diarrhea due to a reabsorptive defect in the colon, intravenous saline may be required to re-expand the EABV. Therapy for hypokalemia is discussed in detail in Part D of this chapter.

## DIURETICS

### PATHOPHYSIOLOGY

The increased secretion of $K^+$ ions in the CDN in patients taking diuretics is due to increased lumen-negative voltage in the CDN caused by an enhanced rate of electrogenic reabsorption of $Na^+$ ions via ENaC as a result of the effects of aldosterone released in response to a contracted EABV.

### CLINICAL PICTURE

The hypokalemia is usually modest in degree if there is the usual dietary intake of $K^+$ ions. A $P_K$ that is less than 3 mmol/L is observed in less than 10% of patients taking thiazide diuretics for treatment of hypertension, and is usually present within the first 2 weeks of starting therapy.

### DIAGNOSIS

This diagnosis is usually evident. Abuse of diuretics, however, may be denied. Measurements of $U_{Na}$ and $U_{Cl}$ in multiple spot urine samples is helpful to separate patients with Bartter syndrome or Gitelman syndome (persistently high $U_{Na}$ and $U_{Cl}$) from those who are abusing diuretics (intermittently high $U_{Na}$ and $U_{Cl}$). Abuse of diuretics may be confirmed by a urine assay for diuretics. The assay should be performed on urine samples that contain an appreciable amount of $Na^+$ and $Cl^-$, which may reflect the effect of a diuretic. Examining $U_{Na}$ and $U_{Cl}$ can also provide clues to distinguish between patients with hypokalemia caused by abuse of diuretics from those with hypokalemia caused by "occult" vomiting or the abuse of laxatives (see Table 14-1).

### THERAPY

Patients with ischemic heart disease or left ventricular hypertrophy and those receiving digitalis may be at increased risk for cardiac arrhythmias in the presence of hypokalemia. Therefore, even a modest degree of hypokalemia should be avoided in these patients. Of note, in patients with hypertension treated with thiazides, $K^+$ ion depletion may cause a rise in BP by 5 to 7 mm Hg, thus diminishing the antihypertensive effect of the diuretic (see Chapter 13).

Other effects of chronic $K^+$ ion depletion include the development of nephropathy with interstitial fibrosis. In addition, reabsorption of citrate in the PCT cells is increased in patients with hypokalemia because of the associated intracellular acidosis. Hypocitraturia may develop, which may diminish the beneficial effect of thiazide diuretics to prevent the recurrence of calcium stones.

There are several ways to minimize the degree of diuretic-induced hypokalemia. First, because the risk of hypokalemia is dose dependent, the lowest effective dose of the diuretic should be used. In most patients with primary hypertension, a dose of 12.5 to 25 mg of hydrochlorothiazide produces as great a fall in BP as higher doses of the drug. Second, the intake of $K^+$ ions should not be low. Salt substitutes such as Co-Salt (which contains 14 mmol of $K^+$ ions/g) are an inexpensive way to provide $K^+$ ions while decreasing the intake of $Na^+$ ions. Third, lowering the rate of $K^+$ ion excretion can minimize the degree of hypokalemia. This may be achieved in part by limiting the intake and thereby the excretion of NaCl to less than 100 mmol/day. The renal loss of $K^+$ ions can also be reduced with the use of potassium-sparing diuretics. We do not favor the use of tablets that combine a thiazide or a loop diuretic plus a diuretic that blocks ENaC (e.g., amiloride) in one preparation. This is because a higher distal flow rate due to the actions of a thiazide or loop diuretic lowers the luminal concentration of the blockers of ENaC, which makes them less effective.

## HYPOMAGNESEMIA

There is an important clinical association between hypomagnesemia and hypokalemia. Nevertheless, it is not clear whether $Mg^{2+}$ ion depletion per se leads to renal $K^+$ ion wasting and hypokalemia or whether both the hypomagnesemia and the hypokalemia are caused by the same underlying disorder (e.g., diarrhea, diuretic therapy, Gitelman syndrome). Regardless, it is important to keep in mind that patients with cardiac arrythmias associated with hypokalemia may not respond to therapy with the administration of KCl until their deficit of $Mg^{2+}$ ions is corrected.

## VOMITING

### PATHOPHYSIOLOGY

Balance data from experimental, gastric drainage studies in human volunteers have revealed that, at the end of the postdrainage period, there was a cumulative negative balance for both $Cl^-$ and $K^+$ ions, which were of similar magnitude (see Chapter 7 for more discussion). Because the concentration of $K^+$ ions in gastric fluid is less than 15 mmol/L, hypokalemia in patients with vomiting or nasogastric suction results primarily from a large loss of $K^+$ ions in the urine. Renal wasting of $K^+$ ions results from increased electrogenic reabsorption of $Na^+$ ions in the CDN because of an increased number of open ENaC in the CDN due to the effects of aldosterone, which is released in response to the low EABV. An increase in the concentration of $HCO_3^-$

anions in the fluid in the lumen of the CDN, as may occur during an acute bout of vomiting, may inhibit pendrin, and hence NDCBE and the electroneutral NaCl reabsorption, which may also lead to a higher rate of electrogenic reabsorption of $Na^+$ ions in the CDN. A higher net secretion of $K^+$ is also due to the delivery of $Na^+$ ions to the CDN with nonabsorbable anions (i.e., $SO_4^{2-}$ anions from the oxidation of sulfur-containing amino acids and/or organic anions).

## CLINICAL PICTURE

Key elements in the clinical picture are a history of vomiting (or nasogastric suction), hypokalemia, metabolic alkalosis, and a very low $U_{Cl}$. In a patient with a recent bout of vomiting, $U_{Na}$ may not be low despite the presence of EABV contraction because the excretion of $HCO_3^-$ ions in the urine obligates the excretion of $Na^+$ ions.

The patient may deny vomiting. There are some helpful clues to suggest the diagnosis—the patient is particularly concerned with body image, has a profession where weight control is important (e.g., ballet dancer, fashion model), has an eating disorder, and/or has a psychiatric disorder that might lead to self-induced vomiting. The physical examination may also provide some helpful clues, including a calloused lesion on the back of the finger or knuckles, which are often inserted into the mouth to induce vomiting, and erosion of dental enamel from repeated exposure to HCl.

The use of $U_{Na}$ and $U_{Cl}$ in the differential diagnosis in the patients with hypokalemia and a low EABV is shown in Table 14-1.

## THERAPY

Therapy is directed toward the underlying cause of vomiting and the administration of $K^+$ ions to correct the hypokalemia. These patients also have a deficit of $Cl^-$ ions; therefore, KCl should be administered.

# BARTTER SYNDROME

## PATHOPHYSIOLOGY

Patients with Bartter syndrome have a genetic defect affecting one of the transporters involved in NaCl reabsorption in the medullary thick ascending limb (mTAL) of the loop of Henle, leading to renal salt wasting. Renal wasting of $K^+$ ions results primarily from increased electrogenic reabsorption of $Na^+$ ions in the CDN because of an increased number of open ENaC in the CDN due to the effects of aldosterone, which is released in response to the low EABV. Two other functions of the mTAL of the loop of Henle are compromised in patients with Bartter syndrome. First, because this nephron segment is responsible for the generation of a high effective osmolality in the medullary interstitial compartment by the addition of $Na^+$ and $Cl^+$ ions, these patients have a urinary concentrating defect and, in response to the administration of dDAVP, their urine effective osmolality is lower than expected (see Chapter 11). Second, because a large amount of filtered calcium ions is reabsorbed in the mTAL of the loop of Henle, if this reabsorption is diminished, the distal delivery of calcium ions can readily exceed the capacity for its reabsorption in downstream nephron segments. Accordingly, hypercalciuria is a common finding in these patients. In contrast, although a considerable amount of magnesium ions is reabsorbed in the mTAL of the loop of Henle, hypomagnesemia is not a common finding in patients with Bartter syndrome. This is because reabsorption of magnesium ions in the late DCT may be upregulated in these patients;

this diminishes the loss of magnesium ions in the urine and therefore prevents the development of hypomagnesemia.

## MOLECULAR BASIS

Mutations that cause Bartter syndrome have been identified in five separate genes (Figure 14-1). The first two abnormalities lead to antenatal Bartter syndrome and include mutations in the gene encoding the $Na^+$, $K^+$, 2 $Cl^-$ cotransporter (NKCC-2) and the gene encoding the ROMK channel. A third lesion involves the basolateral $Cl^-$ channel (ClC-Kb). Because the channel is also expressed in the basolateral membrane of cells in the DCT, this lesion may also affect NaCl reabsorption in the DCT. Mutations in the gene that encodes for an essential β-subunit of this $Cl^-$ channel, called Barttin, have been reported in patients with Bartter syndrome and sensory-neural deafness, which suggests that Barttin is also involved in the function of the $Cl^-$ channels in the inner ear. Patients with Bartter syndrome and hypocalcemia have been reported; the basis of this disorder is an activating mutation in the gene encoding the calcium ion–sensing receptor (Ca-SR).

## CLINICAL PICTURE

These patients usually present early in life. There is often a positive family history and/or consanguinity. The clinical picture is characterized by EABV contraction with renal salt wasting, hypokalemia, and metabolic alkalosis. Hypercalciuria is common but hypomagnesemia is not. Patients with Bartter syndrome due to a defective $Cl^-$ channel (ClC-Kb) may have a more severe clinical disorder or a phenotype that resembles Gitelman syndrome (e.g., hypocalciuria, hypomagnesemia) because ClC-Kb is also expressed in the DCT.

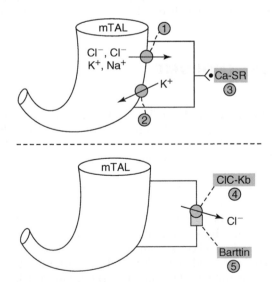

**Figure 14-1 Possible Molecular Basis of Bartter Syndrome.** The possible lesions that may diminish the reabsorption of $Na^+$ and $Cl^-$ ions in the medullary thick ascending limb ( mTAL) of the loop of Henle (the stylized structure in the figure) and hence cause Bartter syndrome are illustrated in this figure. The figure is divided into two parts for clarity, but all the lesions occur in a single cell type. The lesions shown in the *upper portion of the figure* are those that involve the luminal $Na^+$, $K^+$, 2 $Cl^-$ cotransporter 2 (NKCC-2; *site 1*); the renal outer medullary potassium ion (ROMK) channel (*site 2*); or the calcium-sensing receptor (Ca-SR; *site 3*). In the *lower portion of the figure*, lesions affecting the basolateral $Cl^-$ ion channel (ClC-Kb) (*site 4*) or its β-subunit protein, Barttin (*site 5*), are shown.

A gain of function mutation in the Ca-SR in the parathyroid gland results in downward resetting of the receptor. These patients may have hypocalcemia because the release of parathyroid hormone is inhibited at a lower level of ionized calcium in plasma (autosomal dominant hypoparathyroidism).

There are also acquired disorders that may lead to loop diuretic-like effects and hence a Bartter-like clinical picture (pesudo-Bartter syndrome). Examples include hypercalcemia and cationic drugs that bind to the Ca-SR (e.g., gentamicin, cisplatin). It is also possible that cationic proteins may bind to the Ca-SR and lead to a Bartter-like clinical picture, as may be the case in a patient with multiple myeloma or in some autoimmune disorders.

### THERAPY

This is discussed in the section on Gitelman syndrome.

### ANTENATAL BARTTER SYNDROME

Antenatal Bartter syndrome results from a loss of function mutation in the gene encoding NKCC-2 or the gene encoding ROMK. The pregnancy is usually complicated by polyhydramnios and premature delivery.

This is a very serious illness because the newborn has a large degree of renal wasting of NaCl. To put this in a quantitative perspective, we estimated that 2640 mmol of $Na^+$ ions per day in an adult human subject are reabsorbed in the loop of Henle with its medullary and cortical portions (see Chapter 9). This amount is appreciably larger than the amount of $Na^+$ ions in the ECF compartment in an adult 70 kg subject (ECF volume 15 L $\times$ $P_{Na}$ 150 mmol/L = 2250 mmol). Because patients with antenatal Bartter syndrome survive, there must be mechanisms that decrease the loss of $Na^+$ and $Cl^-$ ions.

1. *Decrease the delivery of $Na^+$ and $Cl^-$ ions to the loop of Henle*: There is an initial large loss of $Na^+$ and $Cl^-$ ions, which results in a marked degree of contraction of the EABV. As a result, there is both a large reduction in the GFR and a marked increase in the reabsorption of $Na^+$ and $Cl^-$ ions in the PCT.
2. *Enhanced reabsorption of $Na^+$ and $Cl^-$ ions in nephron sites downstream to the LOH*: This response, however, seems to be limited by prostaglandins. Hence, inhibiting prostaglandin synthesis with cyclooxygenase inhibitors leads to an enhanced reabsorption of $Na^+$ and $Cl^-$ in the late distal nephron, which makes these drugs effective in decreasing renal salt wasting in patients with antenatal Bartter syndrome (see the discussion of Case 14-4 for more information).

Patients with an inactivation mutation in ROMK causing antenatal Bartter syndrome present initially with hyperkalemia and not hypokalemia. In the first weeks of life, maxi-$K^+$ ion channels are not yet expressed in the CDN. Hence, these patients have hyperkalemia, marked renal NaCl wasting, a very contracted EABV, and high aldosterone levels, and hence they are diagnosed with pesudohypoaldosteronism. A few weeks later, maxi-$K^+$ ion channels appear to be present in the luminal membrane of the CDN. As a result, there is abundant $K^+$ ion secretion and the clinical picture changes to hypokalemia.

## GITELMAN SYNDROME

### PATHOPHYSIOLOGY

Patients with this disorder have a genetic defect involving the transport of $Na^+$ and $Cl^-$ ions in the DCT leading to renal salt wasting and EABV contraction. Renal wasting of $K^+$ ions and hypokalemia result primarily from increased electrogenic reabsorption of Na$^+$ ions in the CDN because of an increased number of open ENaC units in the CDN caused by the effects of aldosterone, which is released in response to the low EABV.

Because the function of the loop of Henle is not affected, these patients do not have a urinay concentring defect. Hypocalciuria with a very low urine calcium-to-urine creatinine ratio and hypomagnesemia due to renal Mg$^{2+}$ wasting are common findings in patients with Gitelman syndrome (Figure 14-2).

### Hypocalciuria

The likely explanation for hypocalciuria in patients with Gitelman syndrome is enhanced reabsorption of calcium (Ca$^{2+}$) ions in the PCT secondary to the contracted EABV (see Figure 14-2). The reabsorption of calcium ions might also be upregulated in nephron segments downstream to the DCT. In fact, the connecting segment has all the components needed for the reabsorption of Ca$^{2+}$ ions. This enhanced reabsorption of calcium ions in the connecting segment might diminish the degree of hypercalciuria in patients with Bartter syndrome and cause a very low rate of excretion of Ca$^{2+}$ ions in patients with Gitelman syndrome. It is intriguing to consider how Ca$^{2+}$ ion balance is maintained in the face of the marked and long-standing hypocalciuria in patients with Gitelman syndrome.

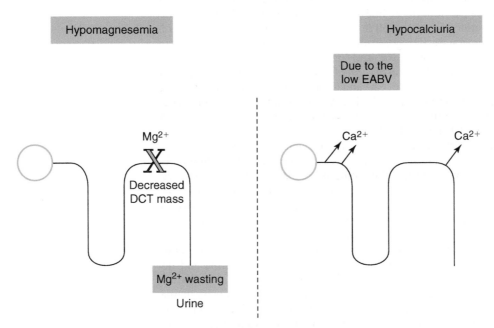

**Figure 14-2 Hypothesis to Explain the Hypomagnesemia and the Hypocalciuria in Patients With Gitelman Syndrome.** The *structure* represents a nephron. The *portion on the left* depicts the mechanism to explain the high excretion of magnesium (Mg$^{2+}$) ions in patients with Gitelman syndrome. The most likely basis of the renal Mg$^{2+}$ ion wasting resulting in hypomagnesemia is progressive atrophy or apoptosis of cells of the late distal convoluted tubule. This leads to Mg$^{2+}$ wasting because this nephron segment is the last major nephron segment that reabsorbs Mg$^{2+}$ ions. The *portion of the figure to the right* depicts the mechanism to explain hypocalciuria in these patients. The major reason for the low excretion of Ca$^{2+}$ ions is enhanced reabsorption of Ca$^{2+}$ ions in the proximal convoluted tubule owing to the contracted effective arterial blood volume (EABV). Perhaps there may also be upregulated Ca$^{2+}$ ions reabsorption in the connecting segment of the cortical distal nephron.

## Hypomagnesemia

Although the bulk of filtered load of $Mg^{2+}$ ions (60% to 70%) is reabsorbed in the TAL of the loop of Henle, with only a small fraction (5% to 10%) reabsorbed in the DCT, hypomagnesemia is much more common in patients with Gitelman syndrome than in patients with Bartter syndrome. It is not clear why patients with Gitelman syndrome have renal wasting of $Mg^+$ ions and hypomagnesemia. Our preferred explanation for the renal $Mg^{2+}$ ion wasting in these patients is that although a small fraction of the reabsorption of $Mg^{2+}$ ions occurs in the DCT, it is the critical, final site at which reabsorption of $Mg^{2+}$ ions takes place (see Figure 14-2). It has been shown in rats that inhibition of reabsorption of $Na^+$ and $Cl^-$ ions in DCT for a prolonged period of time with the administration of thiazide diuretics leads to apoptosis and a decrease in cell mass in this nephron segment. Hence, renal wasting of $Mg^{2+}$ ions may occur, leading to hypomagnesemia.

### MOLECULAR BASIS

The vast majority of patients with Gitelman syndrome have mutations in the gene encoding the $Na^+$-$Cl^-$ cotransporter (NCC) in the early DCT (Figure 14-3). Mutations in the gene encoding for the basolateral $Cl^-$ channel (ClC-Kb) usually cause a clinical picture of Bartter syndrome. In some patients, the phenotype resembles Gitelman syndrome.

### CLINICAL PICTURE

For the most part, Gitelman syndrome is a disease of young adults. In contrast, patients with a $Cl^-$ channel (ClC-Kb) defect often present earlier in life, and the findings resemble those in a patient with Bartter syndrome. There is often a positive family history and/or consanguinity. The main clinical symptoms are cramps in arms and legs, which may be at times severe and present as tetany. Polyuria and nocturia/enuresis are also common. The major clinical findings are a low EABV. The major laboratory abnormalities are hypokalemia, hypomagnesemia, metabolic alkalosis, and renal wasting of $Na^+$, $Cl^-$, $K^+$, and $Mg^2$ ions and a low urine calcium-to-urine creatinine ratio.

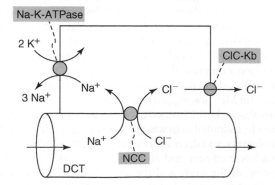

**Figure 14-3 Possible Molecular Basis for Gitelman Syndrome.** The most common defect causing Gitelman syndrome is a mutation involving the $Na^+$-$Cl^-$ cotransporter (NCC) in the distal convoluted tubule (DCT). Mutations in the gene encoding for the basolateral $Cl^-$ channel (ClCN-Kb) usually causes a clinical picture of Bartter syndrome. In some patients, the phenotype, however, resembles Gitelman syndrome. NA-K-ATPase, sodium–potassium ATPase.

## Diagnosis

The typical clinical findings often leave little doubt as to the diagnosis. Nevertheless, there can be three possible difficulties in differentiating Gitelman syndrome from Bartter syndrome on clinical grounds. First, the $U_{Osm}$ may not be as high as expected if there is renal medullary damage due to the chronic hypokalemia or if the patient has an osmotic diuresis due to the very high excretion of electrolytes. Second, a low urine calcium-to-creatinine ratio may develop later in the course of the disease; early on, this may be observed only in more concentrated urine samples. Third, hypomagnesemia may develop later in the course of the disease.

The differential diagnosis of hypokalemia with a low EABV is the same as discussed in the section on Bartter syndrome.

## Therapy

The following issues in therapy apply to patients with Bartter syndrome or Gitelman syndrome.

Correction of hypokalemia is extremely difficult in these patients, even with large supplements of $K^+$ ions. Hypomagnesemia may be an important factor in the enhanced kaliuresis in some patients with Gitelman syndrome. Correction of hypomagnesemia with oral magnesium supplements is usually limited by gastrointestinal side effects. Angiotensin-converting enzyme inhibitors have been tried in some patients with variable success, but hypotension is a major concern. We have reservations about the prolonged use of nonsteroidal anti-inflammatory drugs because of the potential for chronic renal dysfunction. Potassium-sparing diuretics (e.g., amiloride, spironolactone, or eplerenone) may help conserve $K^+$ ions, but they may also exacerbate renal salt wasting. A common clinical observation is that even high doses of amiloride may fail to curtail the excessive kaliuresis in patients with Bartter syndrome or Gitelman syndrome. Part of the explanation for this diminished effect could be related to lower concentrations of these drugs in the lumen of the CDN. In more detail, lesions that inhibit the reabsorption of $Na^+$ and $Cl^-$ ions in the loop of Henle or in the DCT should increase the distal delivery of NaCl osmoles and thereby the volume of fluid in the CDN. This higher luminal fluid volume lowers the concentration of ENaC blockers by dilution. Therefore, to be effective, a large dose of amiloride must be given. Also, a potential concern of using these agents in patients with Bartter syndrome or Gitelman syndrome is that the wasting of $Na^+$ ions in these patients might become a major problem, especially if dietary NaCl intake declines and/or if the patient develops diarrhea that leads to nonrenal loss of NaCl.

A recent open-label, randomized, crossover study with blind endpoint evaluation examined the efficacy on $P_K$ and the safety of 6-week treatments with indomethacin, eplerenone, or amiloride added to constant $K^+$ ion and $Mg^{2+}$ ion supplementation. $P_K$ increased by 0.38 mmol/L with indomethacin, by 0.15 mmol/L with eplerenone, and by 0.19 mmol/L with amiloride. Indomethacin was the most effective but caused gastrointestinal intolerance and decreased estimated GFR. Amiloride and eplerenone had a lower efficacy and also exacerbated $Na^+$ ion depletion. The short duration of the study and the high incidence of side effects even within the short time period of the study make it difficult to determine the possible benefit versus harm from long-term use of these medications. It is also not determined whether the benefits from these drugs, which were rather modest with eplerenone and amiloride, would be sustained over a long period of time.

An interesting clinical observation in patients with Bartter syndrome or Gitelman syndrome is that hypokalemia persists despite large oral KCl supplements. Hence, the rate of excretion of $K^+$ ions must rise appreciably when K$^+$ ion supplements are given. We offer the following speculation that focuses on modulation of the number of open ROMK channels in the luminal membranes of principal cells in the CDN. When the degree of hypokalemia becomes more severe, the number of open luminal ROMK channels in the CDN may be down-regulated; this could diminish the rate of net secretion of K$^+$ ions in the CDN. When the P$_K$ rises with KCl supplementation, the number of open ROMK channels in the luminal membranes of the CDN may increase. Accordingly, the usual negative lumen voltage in the CDN could now augment the rate of secretion of K$^+$ ions as long as the P$_K$ remains in this somewhat higher range. Therefore, giving K$^+$ supplements in small, divided doses may be more effective in keeping the P$_K$ near the normal range.

## CATIONIC DRUGS THAT BIND TO THE Ca-SR

### PATHOPHYSIOLOGY

Gentamicin and tobramycin are cationic antibiotics that bind to the Ca-SR on the basolateral aspect of cells of the mTAL of the loop of Henle (Figure 14-4). This leads to inhibition of ROMK and thus to a "loop diuretic-like" effect. A similar mechanism might apply for other cationic drugs that might bind to the Ca-SR, such as cisplatin.

### CLINICAL PICTURE

This disorder is often accompanied by the presence of a low EABV due to renal salt wasting, hypokalemia, hypomagnesemia, hypercalciuria, and metabolic alkalosis. After discontinuation of the drug, there may be a considerable lag time before its effects disappear because the covalent binding of gentamicin or cisplatin to the Ca-SR may persist for a long period of time. Supportive therapy with Na$^+$, K$^+$, and Mg$^{2+}$ ion supplementation should be given as needed.

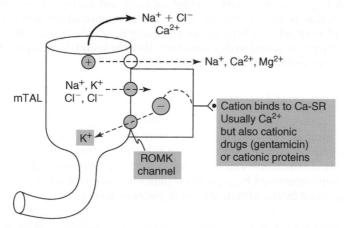

**Figure 14-4 Hypokalemia due to Drugs that Bind to the Calcium-Sensing Receptor (Ca-SR).** When ionized calcium (Ca$^{2+}$) ions or cationic drugs such as gentamicin bind to the Ca-SR in the basolateral membrane of cells of the medullary thick ascending limb (mTAL) of the loop of Henle, renal outer medullary potassium (ROMK) channels are inhibited. Reentry of K$^+$ ions into the lumen of the mTAL of the loop of Henle is diminished, and hence the flux through the Na$^+$, K$^+$, 2 Cl$^-$ cotransporter is decreased and the lumen voltage becomes less positive. As a result, there is less reabsorption of Na$^+$, Cl$^-$, and ionized Ca$^{2+}$ ions in the loop of Henle. This could lead to findings akin to actions of a loop diuretic with wasting of Na$^+$, Cl$^-$, K$^+$, and Ca$^{2+}$ ions in the urine, and the development of metabolic alkalosis.

# PRIMARY HYPERALDOSTERONISM

## PATHOPHYSIOLOGY

Patients with primary hyperaldosteronism have a high rate of secretion of aldosterone due to the presence of an adrenal adenoma or bilateral adrenal hyperplasia.

## MOLECULAR BASIS

Point mutations in the gene encoding for the $K^+$ ion channel KCNJ5 have been identified in about 40% of patients with aldosterone-producing adenoma. These mutations, which are in or near the selectivity filter of the channel, lead to an increased conductance and entry of $Na^+$ ions into the glomerulosa cells of the adrenal gland. This results in cell depolarization with increased entry of $Ca^{2+}$ ions, which signals the release of aldosterone and induces cell proliferation.

## CLINICAL PICTURE

This diagnosis should be suspected in patients with hypertension and unexplained hypokalemia with renal potassium wasting. Nevertheless, a large proportion of these patients do not have hypokalemia; the reason for this is not clear. Primary hyperaldosteronism should also be suspected in patients who are taking drugs that may decrease the rate of $K^+$ ion excretion (e.g., angiotensin converting enzyme inhibitors, angiotensin II receptor blockers) if their $P_K$ is toward the lower end of the normal range.

## DIAGNOSIS

The diagnosis hinges on the finding of an elevated $P_{Aldosterone}$ and a very low $P_{Renin}$ (see Table 14-2). A high $P_{Aldosterone}$:$P_{Renin}$ ratio in a random blood sample is usually a sufficient screening test. Primary hyperaldosteronism must be confirmed by finding a nonsuppressible high $P_{Aldosterone}$ or urinary aldosterone excretion during salt loading. A CT scan is the best imaging test to detect an adrenal adenoma versus bilateral adrenal hyperplasia. If surgery is an option, adrenal vein sampling is required to determine whether the lesion detected on the CT scan is a functioning adenoma.

## DIFFERENTIAL DIAGNOSIS

The finding of very low $P_{Renin}$ with high $P_{Aldosterone}$ separates patients with primary hyperaldosteronism from those with other causes of hypertension and hypokalemia (see Table 14-2). Patients with glucocorticoid remediable aldosteronism (GRA) also have elevated $P_{Aldosterone}$ with suppressed $P_{Renin}$. In these patients, however, the $P_{Aldosterone}$ is suppressed by the administration of glucocorticoids.

## THERAPY

Laparoscopic unilateral adrenalectomy is generally the preferred treatment in a patient with an adrenal adenoma. If successful, reduction in aldosterone secretion, a fall in BP, and correction of the hypokalemia are expected. Notwithstanding, hypertension persists in a large number of patients after unilateral adrenalectomy, especially in those with a family history of hypertension and those who were taking two or more antihypertensive medications prior to surgery.

In patients with bilateral adrenal hyperplasia, or in those with an adrenal adenoma who are not candidates for surgery, medical therapy is the preferred treatment. The goals of therapy, however, are not only to control BP and to correct the hypokalemia but also to reverse the unwanted effects of hyperaldosteronism on the heart. Hence, the administration of a mineralocorticoid receptor antagonist (spironolactone or eplerenone) is preferred. Amiloride is an alternative in patients who are intolerant of these drugs. The issue about the need for a low intake of NaCl to decrease the flow rate in the CDN that was discussed earlier in the Therapy section under Gitelman Syndrome applies in this setting.

# GLUCOCORTICOID REMEDIABLE ALDOSTERONISM

## PATHOPHYSIOLOGY

This condition is a rare form of bilateral adrenal hyperplasia in which adrenocorticotropic hormone (ACTH) is the exclusive regulator of the secretion of aldosterone. There is also marked overproduction of C-18 oxidation products of cortisol, 18-hydroxycortisol and 18-oxocortisol.

## MOLECULAR BASIS

The genetic basis for this disorder is a chimeric gene in which the regulatory region of the gene encoding for the enzyme required for the synthesis of cortisol in the zona fasciculata is linked to the coding sequence of the gene for the enzyme aldosterone synthase, which is required for the synthesis of aldosterone. Hence, ACTH regulates the secretion of aldosterone. Also, because of an apparent expression of this enzyme in the zona fasciculata, cortisol (a C-17 hydroxylated steroid) becomes hydroxylated at the C-18 position, leading to the production of cortisol–aldosterone hybrid compounds.

## CLINICAL PICTURE

This disease is inherited as an autosomal dominant disorder. The onset of severe hypertension usually occurs in early adulthood. There is often a strong family history of hypertension and early onset of cardiovascular and cerebrovascular diseases. Interestingly, hypokalemia is not present in a significant number of these patients.

## DIAGNOSIS

The diagnosis hinges on demonstrating suppression of aldosterone with the administration of glucocorticoids (dexamethasone or prednisone), detection of very high levels of C-18 oxidation products of cortisol in the urine, and, ultimately, genetic testing to detect the chimeric gene.

## DIFFERENTIAL DIAGNOSIS

Other causes of hypertension and unexplained hypokalemia must be ruled out.

## THERAPY

Administration of glucocorticoids (dexamethasone or prednisone) corrects the hypersecretion of aldosterone by suppressing ACTH.

# ADRENOCORTICOTROPIC HORMONE-PRODUCING TUMOR OR SEVERE CUSHING SYNDROME

## PATHOPHYSIOLOGY

The clinical picture is similar to that of primary hyperaldosteronism, but the $P_{Aldosterone}$ is low. Because of an overabundance of cortisol, the activity of the enzyme 11β-HSDH is insufficient to inactivate all the cortisol that enters principal cells in the CDN. Very high levels of ACTH may also inhibit 11β-HSDH. As a result, cortisol binds to the mineralocorticoid receptor and exerts mineralocorticoid actions.

## CLINICAL PICTURE

ACTH overproduction is commonly seen in patients with small cell carcinoma of the lung. In patients with ACTH-producing tumors, overt signs of glucocorticoid excess may not be evident at the time of diagnosis. The $P_K$ is often very low.

## DIAGNOSIS

The $P_{Aldosterone}$ and $P_{Renin}$ are both suppressed (see Table 14-2). Cortisol levels in plasma are high. Plasma ACTH levels are high if there is an ACTH-producing tumor and are markedly suppressed in patients with Cushing syndrome due to overproduction of cortisol by an adrenal adenoma.

## DIFFERENTIAL DIAGNOSIS

Other causes of hypertension and hypokalemia must be ruled out (see Table 14-2).

## THERAPY

Therapy is directed at the primary disease. For treatment of hypokalemia, large supplements of KCl and drugs that block the aldosterone receptor or ENaC are often necessary.

# SYNDROME OF APPARENT MINERALOCORTICOID EXCESS

## PATHOPHYSIOLOGY

The clinical picture is similar to that in patients with primary hyperaldosteronism, but the $P_{Aldosterone}$ is very low. Because of decreased activity of the enzyme 11β-HSDH, cortisol binds to the mineralocorticoid receptors and exerts mineralocorticoid actions.

## MOLECULAR BASIS

Several mutations in the gene that encodes for the kidney isoform of the enzyme 11β-HSDH-2 have been identified. These mutations result in decreased enzyme activity and therefore impaired inactivation of cortisol.

## CLINICAL PICTURE

This syndrome is inherited as an autosomal recessive disorder. It is characterized by juvenile onset of hypertension and hypokalemia.

## Diagnosis

The $P_{Aldosterone}$ and $P_{Renin}$ are both suppressed (see Table 14-2). The diagnosis is confirmed by the finding of an elevated cortisol-to-cortisone ratio in a 24-hour urine collection.

## Differential Diagnosis

A similar clinical picture is seen in patients with chronic ingestion of licorice or other compounds that contain glycyrrhizinic acid, which inhibits the enzyme 11β-HSDH. Other possible inhibitors of 11β-HSDH include a large dose of flavonoids and bile acids.

## Therapy

Patients respond well to the administration of blockers of the aldosterone receptor or of ENaC (e.g., amiloride or triamterene; salt intake must be restricted as discussed earlier).

# LIDDLE SYNDROME

## Pathophysiology

The pathophysiology of Liddle syndrome is a constitutively active ENaC in the CDN.

## Molecular Basis

Several mutations in the genes encoding for the β- or γ-subunits of ENaC have been described in patients with this syndrome. Some of these mutations result in truncation of the cytoplasmic regions of the β- or γ-subunits of the ENaC complex. Others are missense mutations involving a proline-rich region (PxYY motif) of these subunits. These regions are critical in the interaction between ENaC and intracellular ubiquitin ligases proteins such as Nedd4-2. When Nedd4-2 binds to the β- or γ-subunit of ENaC, not only is ENaC removed from the luminal membrane by endocytosis, but Nedd4-2 also ligate ubiquitin to ENaC, which results in its targeting to the proteasome for destruction. Therefore, these mutations compromise the removal of ENaC and lead to an increased number of open ENaC units in the luminal membrane of principal cells in the CDN.

## Clinical Picture

This syndrome is an autosomal dominant inherited disorder that is characterized by early onset of severe hypertension and hypokalemia. Interestingly, a number of patients do not have hypokalemia.

## Diagnosis

A positive family history of early-onset hypertension and hypokalemia as well as very low $P_{Aldosterone}$ and $P_{Renin}$ are key elements in the diagnosis (see Table 14-2). There is no excess secretion of cortisol, and the urine cortisol-to-cortisone ratio is not elevated. While aldosterone receptor blockers are effective in patients with apparent mineralocorticoid excess syndrome, they are not effective in patients with Liddle syndrome. Diagnosis can be confirmed with genetic testing.

## Differential Diagnosis

Other causes of hypertension and hypokalemia must be ruled out (see Table 14-2).

### THERAPY

Control of hypertension and correction of hypokalemia can be achieved with the administration of large doses of ENaC blockers (amiloride or triamterene) but not with aldosterone receptor blockers (e.g., spironolactone). The effect of ENaC blockers is more evident in patients who are on a salt-restricted diet.

## AMPHOTERICIN B-INDUCED HYPOKALEMIA

### PATHOPHYSIOLOGY

Amphotericin B-induced hypokalemia can be thought of as a disorder in which there are artificial ENaC-like channels that are permanently in an open configuration in the luminal membrane in the CDN.

### CLINICAL PICTURE

The clinical picture is predominantly that of the underlying illness that necessitated the administration of amphotericin B. Hypokalemia is usually associated with an expanded ECF volume.

### THERAPY

In addition to the administration of a sufficient amount of KCl to raise the $P_K$ to the normal range, the infusion of a large volume of saline with the administration of amphotericin B should be avoided to prevent having a very large flow rate in the CDN when amphotericin B acts, which may increase the loss of $K^+$ ions in the urine.

---

# PART D
# THERAPY OF HYPOKALEMIA

## MEDICAL EMERGENCIES

There are two potentially life-threatening complications related to hypokalemia that require aggressive therapy. The most common is a cardiac arrhythmia, and the other is extreme weakness involving the respiratory muscles, especially when metabolic acidemia is present (e.g., patients with distal renal tubular acidosis, or patients with severe diarrhea). Having decided that hypokalemia requires urgent therapy, enough $K^+$ ions must be given to raise the $P_K$ quickly and to a high enough value (~3.0 mmol/L) to avert these dangers. The total $K^+$ ion deficit should be replaced much more slowly. Because a large dose of $K^+$ ions may need to be given over a short period of time, a solution with a high concentration of $K^+$ ions will be needed, and therefore $K^+$ ions should be administered via a central vein and under cardiac rhythm monitoring. In an emergency situation, a large peripheral vein may be temporarily used until a central venous access is established. As a rule, the infusion should not contain glucose (which may cause the release of insulin) or $HCO_3^-$ ions because this may lead to a shift of $K^+$ ions into cells, which would aggravate an already severe degree of hypokalemia. We provide the following as a rough guideline as to how much $K^+$ ions to administer in an emergency situation. Consider this example of a patient who has a $P_K$ of 2 mmol/L and a life-threatening cardiac arrhythmia. The immediate aim of therapy is to rapidly raise the concentration of $K^+$ ions in the interstitial fluid bathing his cardiac myocytes (which is really what is needed to deal with the cardiac arrhythmia) by 1 mmol/L up to 3 mmol/L. Because the blood volume in a 70 kg adult subject is 5 L, the cardiac output is 5 L/min, and 60% of the blood volume is plasma (i.e., 3 L), we would infuse 3 mmol of $K^+$ ions/min for the first 5 minutes. Following this initial bolus, we would reduce the rate of infusion of $K^+$ ions to 1 mmol /min for 5 minutes. We would then measure the $P_K$ (stopping the infusion for at least 1 minute to avoid a spuriously high $P_K$ value). If the cardiac arrhythmia persists, we would repeat the procedure. If the cardiac arrhythmia disappears, but $P_K$ remains appreciably <3 mmol/L, we would administer 20 mmol of $K^+$ ions over 1 hour to bring the $P_K$ close to 3 mmol/L.

# NONMEDICAL EMERGENCIES

The specific issues in therapy of patients with hypokalemia depend on its cause and were discussed previously. In this section, we provide general comments about replacing a large deficit of $K^+$ ions.

## GENERAL ISSUES IN TREATMENT OF THE PATIENT WITH HYPOKALEMIA

### Magnitude of the potassium ion deficit

It is commonly suggested that there is a $K^+$ ion deficit of 100 to 400 mmol if the $P_K$ is reduced from 4.0 to 3.0 mmol/L and that a $P_K$ of 2 mmol/L indicates that there is a much larger deficit of $K^+$ ions (as high as 800 mmol in a 70-kg adult). In our view, there is no useful quantitative relationship between the $P_K$ and the total body $K^+$ ion deficit in the individual patient. This is because a component of the hypokalemia of variable magnitude is the result of a shift of $K^+$ ions into cells. Hence, careful monitoring of the $P_K$ during replacement of the $K^+$ deficit is mandatory.

## ROUTE OF POTASSIUM ADMINISTRATION

The oral route is preferred. Certain factors may necessitate using the intravenous route, including the urgency of therapy, the level of consciousness, and the presence of gastrointestinal problems. As a rule, the concentration of $K^+$ ions in the intravenous fluid should not be greater than 40 mmol/L if infused via a peripheral vein because higher concentrations of $K^+$ ions may cause phlebitis. The rate of administration of $K^+$ ions should not exceed 60 mmol/hr in most settings.

## POTASSIUM PREPARATIONS

Most preparations in tablet form release $K^+$ ions slowly. Although these are usually well tolerated, they occasionally cause ulcerative and ultimately stenotic lesions in the gastrointestinal tract because of a high local $K^+$ ion concentration. Oral KCl can also be given in a crystalline form (e.g., salt substitutes, such as Co-Salt, which provide 14 mmol of $K^+$ ions per g); this is generally well tolerated and is an inexpensive form of potassium supplementation.

For electroneutrality, a deficit of $K^+$ ions must be accompanied by the loss of $Cl^-$ or $HCO_3^-$ ions or by a gain of $Na^+$ ions. With a KCl deficit (e.g., because of chronic vomiting or diuretic use), KCl is needed. In contrast, with a $KHCO_3$ deficit (e.g., because of diarrhea), $K^+$ ion should be replaced with $HCO_3^-$ anions or anions that can be metabolized to produce $HCO_3^-$ anions (e.g., citrate anions). A note of caution is necessary: the administration of $HCO_3^-$ ions may cause a shift of $K^+$ ions into cells in certain settings. Therefore, in a patient who is markedly hypokalemic and acidemic, KCl should be given initially; alkali in the form of $NaHCO_3$ may then be administered after the $P_K$ approaches a safer level (~3 mmol/L). In conditions in which part of the loss of $K^+$ ions was accompanied by the gain of $Na^+$ ions (e.g., in a patient with primary hyperaldosteronism), $K^+$ ions are usually given as KCl while measures are taken to ensure that NaCl is excreted (e.g., administration of $K^+$ ion sparing diuretics such as the ENaC blocker amiloride or the aldosterone receptor blocker spironolactone). The need for $K^+$ ion replacement as its phosphate salt is most evident when there is rapid anabolism; examples include patients on nutritional support or those in the acute recovery phase of a catabolic disorder such as DKA. If given, phosphate should not be administered at a rate that exceeds 50 mmol in 8 hours because a large phosphate load has the danger of inducing metastatic calcification and hypocalcemia. Notwithstanding, we give $K^+$ ions as KCl in the treatment of patients with DKA and rely on the patient's diet to supply the phosphate needed for the anabolic phase of the illness, which occurs later. Although it is commonly advised, increasing the intake of foods that contain $K^+$ ions (e.g., bananas, fruit juice) is not an effective or ideal way to replace a $K^+$ ion deficit (see margin note).

### ADJUNCTS TO THERAPY

Administering potassium-sparing diuretics to patients with chronic hypokalemia can diminish renal loss of $K^+$ ions. Amiloride and triamterene are better tolerated than spironolactone because they lack the gastrointestinal and hormonal complications of spironolactone (amenorrhea, gynecomastia, decreased libido). Eplerenone is a highly selective mineralocorticoid receptor antagonist that is associated with a lower incidence of these endocrine side effects, but it is also significantly more expensive than spironolactone. When using the ENaC blockers, amiloride or triamterene, the patient should have a low intake of NaCl because this leads to a lower flow rate in the CDN. With a lower flow rate, the concentration of these drugs in luminal fluid in the CDN will be higher, and hence they become more effective blockers of ENaC. There is an important note of caution: hyperkalemia may develop when $K^+$ ion supplements are given along with potassium-sparing diuretics, especially if other conditions that may compromise potassium excretion are present.

### RISKS OF THERAPY

With prolonged hypokalemia, the CDN may become hyporesponsive to the kaliuretic effect of aldosterone. This may be due to the presence of fewer ROMK in the luminal membrane of principal cells in the CDN. The ratio of KS-WNK1 to L-WNK1 is decreased by dietary $K^+$ ion restriction, which leads to endocytosis of ROMK. This allows aldosterone to continue to be a NaCl-retaining hormone while diminishing its kaliuretic effect. Hence, it is important to monitor the $P_K$ frequently during the treatment of hypokalemia.

Patients with renal failure and diabetes mellitus, especially if they are taking drugs that block the renin–angiotensin–aldosterone system, β-blockers, or nonsteroidal anti-inflammatory drugs, may be at risk for development of hyperkalemia with chronic $K^+$ ion supplementation. These patients should have their $P_K$ monitored closely.

**EATING BANANAS TO REPLACE A DEFICIT OF $K^+$ IONS**

- The ratio of $K^+$ ions to calories in bananas is very low. Hence, to supply a large $K^+$ ion load in this form, the excessive caloric intake can cause a large weight gain.
- The caloric gain from eating bananas to provide 50 mmol of $K^+$ ions/day for 1 year could lead to more than 50 lb of weight gain if there was no change in diet or physical activity.

# PART E
# DISCUSSION OF CASES

## CASE 14-1: HYPOKALEMIA WITH PARALYSIS

### IS THERE A MEDICAL EMERGENCY IN THIS PATIENT?

The major dangers related to hypokalemia are cardiac arrhythmias and weakness of the respiratory muscles, especially if there is a need for increased ventilation (e.g., in a patient with metabolic acidemia). There were no emergencies demanding urgent therapy in this patient. Because the major cause of hypokalemia in this patient, as will be discussed later, is a shift of $K^+$ ions into cells, the major danger to anticipate is rebound hyperkalemia if a large dose of KCl is administered.

### WHAT IS THE BASIS OF THE HYPOKALEMIA IN THIS PATIENT?

The short time period over which symptoms developed suggests that the basis of hypokalemia in this patient was an acute shift of $K^+$ ions into cells. Moreover, the low rate of $K^+$ ion excretion as assessed by the $U_K/U_{Creatinine}$ ratio (10 mmol $K^+$/g creatinine or 1 mmol $K^+$/ mmol creatinine) and the absence of a metabolic acid–base disorder are in keeping with an acute shift of $K^+$ ions into cells as the primary cause of hypokalemia. Because he had a rapid pulse rate, systolic hypertension, and a wide pulse pressure, it was thought that the major basis for this shift of $K^+$ ions was an adrenergic surge. There were no abnormalities in the thyroid function tests. Because he had a very large intake of caffeine from the soda (5 L of soda; see margin note), this was suggested to be the cause of the adrenergic surge. Perhaps insulin release because of the large intake of sugar with these sweetened soda drinks has also contributed to the acute shift of $K^+$ ions into cells.

As shown in Figure 14-5, a high intake of caffeine can lead to a surge of catecholamines through blocking the binding of adenosine

**CAFFEINE CONTENT IN BEVERAGES OR FOOD**
- Coffee: ~60 mg/100 mL
- Soda: ~12 mg/100 mL
- Chocolate: 1 to 35 mg/oz

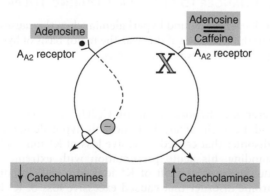

**Figure 14-5 Relationship Between Caffeine and an Adrenergic Surge.** The *circle* represents a cell membrane in the central nervous system. The receptor of interest is an adenosine $A_{A2}$ receptor. When adenosine binds to this receptor (shown on the *left*), there is a diminished release of catecholamines. In contrast, in the presence of caffeine (shown on the *right*), adenosine cannot bind to this receptor (*bold double lines*). As a result, there is no longer the inhibitory effect of adenosine and the net effect is a surge in release of catecholamines.

to its $A_2$ receptors. A $\beta_2$-adrenergic effect causes a shift of $K^+$ ions into cells by activating the Na-K-ATPase and may also diminish the open probability of $K_{ATP}$ channels which may cause an even greater trapping of $K^+$ ions in cells.

Caffeine is metabolized by one of the cytochrome $P_{450}$ enzymes. Although the affinity of this enzyme for caffeine is high, its maximum velocity is not large. Therefore, low doses of caffeine should be removed quickly, but high doses should be removed slowly because more half-lives are needed to remove a certain amount of caffeine when its concentration is much greater than the concentration, which causes the half-maximal rate ($K_m$) catalyzed by the enzyme. Therefore, the very large intake of caffeine could explain its effect to cause a prolonged surge of catecholamines and hypokalemia.

### WHAT IS THE BEST THERAPY FOR ACUTE HYPOKALEMIA IN THIS PATIENT?

There is a danger of rebound hyperkalemia if large doses of KCl are given. The patient was given a nonselective β-blocker, propranolol, and a small amount of KCl. He had rapid biochemical and clinical response to this therapy. The patient had no further episodes since he discontinued his caffeine intake. Nevertheless, we cannot rule out that he has an underlying mild form of sporadic hypokalemic paralysis, which makes him more susceptible to these attacks in the presence of a strong stimulus that causes a shift of $K^+$ ions into cells.

## CASE 14-2: HYPOKALEMIA WITH A SWEET TOUCH

### IS THERE A MEDICAL EMERGENCY IN THIS PATIENT?

Although the $P_K$ is very low, there were no changes in his electrocardiogram. Hence, there was no cardiac emergency. Despite the paralysis, he did not have a high arterial $PCO_2$. Therefore, his respiratory muscles were not involved and ventilation was not compromised.

### IS THERE A DANGER TO ANTICIPATE DURING THERAPY?

The major danger is rebound hyperkalemia when the cause of shift of $K^+$ ions into the cell abates if this was the major basis of hypokalemia and a large dose of KCl was administered.

### WHAT IS THE BASIS OF THE HYPOKALEMIA IN THIS PATIENT?

In the presence of hypokalemia, his $U_K/U_{Creatinine}$ was 5. In addition, he had metabolic alkalosis; hence, his hypokalemia was largely due to a disorder that caused excessive loss of $K^+$ ions in his urine. Notwithstanding, his acute presentation with extreme weakness is likely due to an acute shift of $K^+$ ions into cells in conjunction with a chronic disorder that caused excessive loss of $K^+$ ions. This component of an acute shift of $K^+$ ions into cells could have been induced by vigorous exercise ($\beta_2$-adrenergic effect) and a large carbohydrate intake during breakfast (insulin release) prior to the onset of symptoms.

On clinical assessment, his EABV was not contracted and he had hypertension. Therefore, the increased electrogenic reabsorption of $Na^+$ ions in his CDN was due to a primary increase in ENaC activity.

The differential diagnosis is guided by measurements of the $P_{Renin}$ and $P_{Aldosterone}$ (see Table 14-2). Because both his $P_{Aldosterone}$ and his $P_{Renin}$ were suppressed, the differential diagnosis was between disorders in which cortisol acts as mineralocorticoid and those with a constitutively active ENaC in the luminal membrane of principal cells in the CDN. Inherited disorders in which ENaC is constitutively active (Liddle syndrome) seemed unlikely considering the patient's age. Plasma cortisol levels were not elevated. A CT scan of his chest did not reveal a lung mass. While the patient denied consuming licorice or chewing tobacco, it turned out that he used a herbal preparation that contained large amounts of glycyrrhizinic acid (the active ingredient in licorice) to sweeten his tea.

## CASE 14-3: HYPOKALEMIA IN A NEWBORN

### IS THERE A MEDICAL EMERGENCY IN THIS PATIENT?

There is always a concern that the patient may develop a medical emergency as a result of the excessive loss of $Na^+$ and $Cl^-$ ions in his urine because he has a molecular defect that gives him lifelong complete absence of NKCC-2 and therefore an inability to reabsorb NaCl in his loop of Henle. Factors that may bring on this emergency are a sudden decrease in his ability to consume and/or absorb dietary NaCl and/or a large nonrenal loss of NaCl (e.g., diarrhea).

### WHAT IS THE BASIS OF THE HYPOKALEMIA IN THIS PATIENT?

The basis for the hypokalemia is excessive renal excretion of $K^+$ ions due to increased electrogenic reabsorption of $Na^+$ ions in the CDN, which is caused by an increased number of open ENaC units in the CDN from the effects of aldosterone, which is released in response to the low EABV.

### WHY DID THE PATIENT HAVE NEPHROGENIC DIABETES INSIPIDUS?

The nephrogenic diabetes insipidus represents the usual physiology in the newborn (see Chapter 11 for more discussion of this topic). In the absence of actions of vasopressin, however, the $U_{Osm}$ depends primarily on the osmole excretion rate. Although the patient had nephrogenic diabetes insipidus, his $U_{Osm}$ was not very low because of a high rate of excretion of electrolytes. The decline in his $U_{Osm}$ after the administration of indomethacin does not indicate the development of a new defect (because his urine flow rate did not increase) but rather a fall in the rate of excretion of osmoles, namely, the excretion of NaCl.

### IN WHAT NEPHRON SEGMENT MIGHT INDOMETHACIN HAVE ACTED TO CAUSE A MARKED DECREASE IN RENAL LOSS OF $Na^+$ IONS?

To decrease the excretion of $Na^+$ ions without a decrease in the urine flow rate, the site of action of indomethacin must be after the water-permeable PCT. Because there is a molecular defect in the TAL of the loop of Henle, which leads to a near-complete absence of NKCC-2, it is unlikely that indomethacin has caused an increase of reabsorption of $Na^+$ ions in the loop of Henle (Figure 14-6). Therefore, the most likely site is the distal nephron, including its cortical and medullary segments.

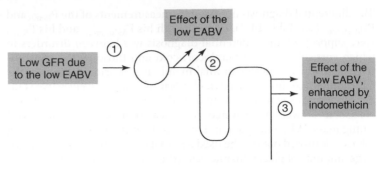

**Figure 14-6 Mechanisms for Decreasing the Rates of Excretion of Na⁺ and Cl⁻ Ions in Patients with Antenatal Bartter Syndrome.** The *stylized structure* represents a nephron, and the *circle* represents its glomerulus. In patients with antenatal Bartter syndrome, there is a contracted effective arterial blood volume (EABV). Hence, there are three major effects that lead to a reduced rate of excretion of Na⁺ ions. As shown in *site 1*, there is a marked reduction in the glomerular filtration rate (GFR) and thereby in the filtered load of Na⁺ ions. As shown in *site 2*, the marked reduction in the EABV markedly augments Na⁺ and Cl⁻ ion reabsorption in the proximal convoluted tubule. As shown in *site 3*, there is upregulation of the reabsorption of Na⁺ and Cl⁻ ions in the late distal convoluted tubule and the collecting ducts. It appears that indomethacin enhances the reabsorption of Na⁺ and Cl⁻ ions in *site 3*.

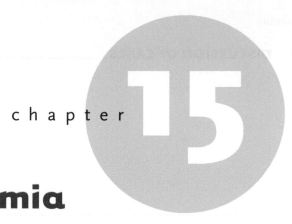

chapter **15**

# Hyperkalemia

# Introduction

Hyperkalemia is usually defined as a concentration of potassium ions ($K^+$) in plasma ($P_K$) that is greater than 5 mmol/L. Hyperkalemia is a common electrolyte disorder that may be present in a number of disease states. Hyperkalemia may have detrimental effects, the most serious of which is a cardiac arrhythmia. Therefore, the first step in the clinical approach to the patient with hyperkalemia is to determine whether an emergency is present (i.e., changes in the electrocardiogram [ECG] due to hyperkalemia). If so, therapy must be instituted promptly, with measures to antagonize the cardiac effect of hyperkalemia and measures to induce a shift of $K^+$ ions into cells. Notwithstanding, there is large variability among patients in the absolute value of the $P_K$, which leads to ECG changes and cardiac toxicity.

If the time course for the development of hyperkalemia is short and/or if there has been little intake of $K^+$ ions, the basis for the hyperkalemia is likely an acute shift of $K^+$ ions out of cells or pseudohyperkalemia. Conversely, chronic hyperkalemia implies that there is a defect in the regulation of the excretion of $K^+$ ions by the kidney. Steps should be taken to identify why the net secretion of $K^+$ ions in the cortical distal nephron (CDN) is low. Even in patients with a large defect in their ability to generate a lumen-negative voltage in the CDN, an appreciable degree of hyperkalemia is not likely to develop with the usual intake of $K^+$ ions unless there is decreased flow rate in the terminal CDN. Therefore, one should also determine whether there is a cause for a low flow rate in the terminal CDN. Based on this analysis, one can determine where leverage can be exerted for therapy to increase the rate of excretion of $K^+$ ions by the kidney in the individual patient with chronic hyperkalemia. There are growing concerns about both the safety and efficacy of using the cation exchange resin sodium polysterene sulfonate (Kexeylate), to achieve loss of $K^+$ ions via the gastrointestinal tract. There are data to suggest effectiveness and good tolerability of two new oral polymers, patiromer and sodium zirconium, in lowering $P_K$ and maintaining normokalemia in patients with chronic kidney disease who have diabetes or congestive heart failure and who are receiving drugs that block the renin-angiotensin-aldosterone axis.

## OBJECTIVES

- To emphasize that hyperkalemia is a common electrolyte abnormality that may pose a major threat to the patient because of the risk of cardiac arrhythmia.
- To emphasize that hyperkalemia is not a diagnostic category but a disorder that may be present in a number of disease states; its basis must be defined in each patient.

■ To provide a clinical approach to the patient with hyperkalemia based on an understanding of the physiology of the shift of $K^+$ ions into cells and the physiology of the renal regulation of the excretion of $K^+$ ions.

■ To provide an approach to the therapy of the patient with hyperkalemia.

## CASE 15-1: MIGHT THIS PATIENT HAVE PSEUDOHYPERKALEMIA?

A 5-year-old male had neurosurgery to remove a tumor in the frontal lobe of his brain. There were no complications during surgery, and his course while in the intensive care unit was uneventful. At the time of his transfer to the ward, his $P_K$ was 4.0 mmol/L. The next morning, however, his $P_K$ was 6.0 mmol/L. There was no hemolysis or any reason to suspect a laboratory problem in the measurement of the $P_K$. In addition, hyperkalemia was present in repeated blood testing. He was not given any medications that might cause a shift of $K^+$ ions out of cells, and his intake of $K^+$ ions was low. He did not have a family history of hyperkalemia. His ECG did not show signs of hyperkalemia. The concentration of $K^+$ ions in his urine ($U_K$) was only 10 mmol/L, and he was not polyuric. A clinical decision was made to treat him with mineralocorticoids. Several days later, his $P_K$ returned to the normal range. The suspicion of hypoaldosteronism was thought to be confirmed as the concentration of aldosterone in his plasma ($P_{Aldosterone}$), when results became available several days later, was found to be very low.

### Questions

Why did hyperkalemia develop so soon after he left the intensive care unit?

What could be the basis for the high $P_K$ that was only noted after the patient was transferred to the ward?

## CASE 15-2: HYPERKALEMIA IN A PATIENT TREATED WITH TRIMETHOPRIM

A 23-year-old man had a long history of acquired human immunodeficiency syndrome. He now developed pneumonia due to *Pneumocystis jiroveci*. His dietary intake has been poor and he appeared malnourished. On admission, he was febrile, his effective arterial blood volume (EABV) did not seem to be contracted, and the electrolyte values in his plasma were all in the normal range. Three days after receiving treatment with sulfamethoxazole and trimethoprim, his blood pressure was low, his pulse rate was high, and his jugular venous pressure was low. Of note, his $P_K$ was 6.8 mmol/L. His ECG showed tall, peaked T waves. His laboratory data in plasma and urine samples that were obtained on that day are summarized in the following table. His urine volume was 0.8 L/day.

| | | PLASMA | URINE |
|---|---|---|---|
| Na$^+$ | mmol/L | 130 | 60 |
| K$^+$ | mmol/L | 6.8 | 14 |
| Cl$^-$ | mmol/L | 105 | 43 |
| BUN (urea) | mg/dL (mmol/L) | 14 (5) | 100 mmol/L |
| Creatinine | mg/dL (μmol/L) | 0.9 (100) | 7 mmol/L |
| Osmolality | mosmol/kg H$_2$O | 272 | 280 |

### ABBREVIATIONS

$P_K$, concentration of potassium ($K^+$) ions in plasma

$U_K$, concentration of $K^+$ ions in the urine

$P_{Na}$, concentration of sodium ($Na^+$) ions in plasma

$U_{Na}$, concentration of $Na^+$ ions in the urine

$P_{Cl}$, concentration of chloride ($Cl^-$) ions in plasma

$U_{Cl}$, concentration of $Cl^-$ ions in urine

$P_{HCO_3}$, concentration of bicarbonate ($HCO_3^-$) ions in plasma

$P_{Osm}$, osmolality in plasma

$U_{osm}$, osmolality in the urine

$P_{Albumin}$, concentration of albumin in plasma

BUN, blood urea nitrogen

$P_{Aldosterone}$, concentration of aldosterone in plasma

$P_{Renin}$, mass or activity of renin in plasma

CDN, cortical distal nephron, which includes the late distal convoluted tubule, the connecting segment, and the cortical collecting duct

CCD, cortical collecting duct

DCT, distal convoluted tubule

$K_{CDN}$, concentration of $K^+$ ions in the lumen of the CDN

NHE-1, sodium-hydrogen cation exchanger-1

AE, $Cl^-/HCO_3^-$ anion exchanger

EABV, effective arterial blood volume

ENaC, epithelial sodium ion channel

**Questions**

What is the cause of the hyperkalemia in this patient

What are the major issues for the treatment of the hyperkalemia in this patient?

If trimethoprim must be continued, what measures can be taken to minimize its ability to block the epithelial sodium channel (ENaC) in the CDN?

### CASE 15-3: CHRONIC HYPERKALEMIA IN A PATIENT WITH TYPE 2 DIABETES MELLITUS

A 50-year-old male with a 5-year history of type 2 diabetes mellitus was referred for investigations of hyperkalemia. His $P_K$ ranged from 5.5 to 6 mmol/L in a number of measurements that were done over the last several weeks. He was on an angiotensin converting enzyme (ACE) inhibitor for treatment of hypertension, but hyperkalemia persisted after this medication was discontinued. He was noted to have micro-albuminuria, but no other history of macrovascular or microvascular disease related to diabetes mellitus. He is currently on amlodipine 10 mg once a day. On physical examination, his blood pressure was 160/90 mm Hg, his jugular venous pressure was about 2 cm above the level of the sternal angle, and he had pitting edema around his ankles. Results of laboratory investigations are shown in the following table:

| | | | | | |
|---|---|---|---|---|---|
| $P_{Na}$ | mmol/L | 140 | $P_{HCO_3}$ | mmol/L | 19 |
| $P_K$ | mmol/L | 5.7 | $P_{Albumin}$ | mg/dL (g/L) | 4.0 (40) |
| $P_{Cl}$ | mmol/L | 108 | $P_{Creatinine}$ | mg/dL (umol/L) | 1.2 (100) |
| $P_{Renin}$ | ng/L | 4.50 (Normal range 9.30-43.4 ng/L) | | | |
| $P_{Aldosterone}$ | pmol/L | 321 (Normal range 111-860 pmol/L) | | | |

**Questions**

What is the cause for the hyperkalemia in this patient?

# PART A
# SYNOPSIS OF THE PHYSIOLOGY OF K⁺ ION HOMEOSTASIS

A detailed discussion of the physiology of K⁺ ion homeostasis is presented in Chapter 13. In this chapter, we only provide a brief synopsis of the main points that are necessary to understand the pathophysiology of hyperkalemia.

## REGULATION OF DISTRIBUTION OF K⁺ IONS BETWEEN THE EXTRACELLULAR FLUID AND THE INTRACELLULAR FLUID COMPARTMENTS

K⁺ ions are kept inside cells by the negative voltage in the cell interior caused by the net negative charge on intracellular organic phosphates. To shift K⁺ ions into cells, a more negative cell voltage is required. A more negative cell voltage is generated by increasing the flux through the sodium/potassium ATPase (Na-K-ATPase) pump. This is because the Na-K-ATPase is an electrogenic pump; it exports three $Na^+$ ions out of the cell while importing only two $K^+$ ions into the cell. There are three ways to acutely increase ion pumping by the Na-K-ATPase: first, a rise in the concentration of its rate-limiting substrate—intracellular $Na^+$ ions; second, an increase in its affinity for $Na^+$ ions or its maximum velocity ($V_{max}$) of cation flux; and third, an increase in the number of active Na-K-ATPase pump units in the cell membrane via recruitment of new units from an intracellular pool.

The impact of this increase in Na-K-ATPase activity on cell voltage, however, depends on whether the $Na^+$ ions that are pumped out of the cell had entered the cell in an electrogenic or electroneutral fashion.

*Electrogenic entry of $Na^+$ ions into cells*: When the $Na^+$ ion channel in cell membranes is open, three cationic charges enter the cell per three $Na^+$ ions that enter the cell. The subsequent exit of the three $Na^+$ ions out of the cell via the Na-K-ATPase results in the net export of only one cationic charge out of the cell because two cationic charges enter the cell (two $K^+$ ions are imported into the cell). Hence, the magnitude of the intracellular negative voltage diminishes, and as a result, $K^+$ ions exit the cell.

There are a number of clinical implications of this physiology. During muscle contraction, depolarization is followed quickly by repolarization. In the repolarization phase, $Na^+$ ions that entered cells during depolarization are pumped out of cells by the Na-K-ATPase. This permits most of the $K^+$ ions that were released during depolarization to return to cells. To make this process efficient in skeletal muscle, the $K^+$ ions released during depolarization are largely trapped in a local area (T-tubular region), which prevents the development of a severe degree of hyperkalemia when muscles contract. Hyperkalemia may develop during exhausting exercise, after seizures, or in patients with status epilepticus. Patients who are cachectic may not have an efficient trapping of $K^+$ ions in the T-tubular region during muscle contraction. Therefore, they may have pseudohyperkalemia because of repeated fist clenching in preparation for brachial venipuncture. Patients with hyperkalemic periodic paralysis have defective $Na^+$ ion channels that fail to close when the resting membrane potential approaches $-50\,mV$ during depolarization. This leads to the persistent $Na^+$ ion influx into muscle cells, which drives an outward flux of $K^+$ ions into the ECF compartment, causing hyperkalemia.

*Electroneutral entry of $Na^+$ ions into cells*: If $Na^+$ ions enter the cell in an electroneutral fashion, their subsequent electrogenic exit via the Na-K-ATPase results in a more negative cell interior voltage, and hence the retention of $K^+$ ions in these cells. This occurs when $Na^+$ ions enter cells in exchange for $H^+$ ions on the sodium-hydrogen cation exchanger-1 (NHE-1). Although the NHE-1 is normally inactive in cell membranes, it may become activated if there is a sudden rise in insulin levels in the extracellular fluid (ECF) compartment or in the presence of a higher concentration of $H^+$ ions in the intracellular fluid (ICF) compartment.

## HORMONES THAT AFFECT THE DISTRIBUTION OF $K^+$ IONS BETWEEN THE ECF AND ICF COMPARTMENTS

### Catecholamines

As discussed in Chapter 13, unphosphorylated FXYD1 (phospholemman) binds to the α-subunit of the Na-K-ATPase and inhibits its pump activity by decreasing its affinity for $Na^+$ ions and/or its $V_{max}$. $\beta_2$-Adrenergic agonists, via increasing intracellular levels of cyclic adenosine monophosphate (cAMP), activate protein kinase A and induce phosphorylation of FXYD1, which disrupts its interaction with the α subunit of Na-K-ATPase. The increase in export of pre-existing intracellular

Na$^+$ ions out of cells via the Na-K-ATPase pump results in an increase in the negative voltage in cells and the retention of K$^+$ ions in cells.

### Clinical implications

The use of β$_2$-agonists is suggested in the management of patients with emergency hyperkalemia to induce a shift of K$^+$ ions into cells. As discussed later, we do not consider these agents as a first line treatment in this setting.

### Insulin

Insulin causes a shift of K$^+$ ions into cells because (1) it activates NHE-1 and hence causes an increase in the electroneutral entry of Na$^+$ ions into cells; (2) it induces phosphorylation of FXYD1 by atypical protein kinase C, which disrupts FXYD1 interaction with the α-subunit of the Na-K-ATPase, resulting in an increase in its V$_{max}$; and (3) it promotes the translocation of Na-K-ATPase units from an intracellular pool, and hence increase their abundance at the cell membrane.

### Clinical implications

Insulin has been utilized clinically in the treatment of patients with emergency hyperkalemia. A lack of actions of insulin in patients with diabetic ketoacidosis results in a shift of K$^+$ ions out of cells and the development of hyperkalemia despite a total body deficit of K$^+$ ions.

### EFFECT OF METABOLIC ACIDOSIS ON THE DISTRIBUTION OF K$^+$ IONS BETWEEN THE ECF AND THE ICF COMPARTMENTS

Transport of monocarboxylic acids (e.g., ketoacids or L-lactic acid) into cells on the monocarboxylic acid transporter (MCT) is an electroneutral process and hence it does not have a direct effect on a transcellular shift of K$^+$ ions. Nevertheless, entry of organic acids into cells may have an indirect effect that promotes the shift of K$^+$ ions into cells. In more detail, when L-lactic acid produced during vigorous exercise, for example, enter nonexercising cells (e.g., hepatocytes) on the MCT, the release of H$^+$ ions inside the cells may create a high local concentration of H$^+$ ions at the inner aspect of the cell membrane in the vicinity of NHE-1, which may activate NHE-1 and increase the electroneutral entry of Na$^+$ ions into these cells. The export of Na$^+$ ions by the Na-K-ATPase causes a more negative voltage in cells and thereby the retention of K$^+$ ions in cells.

Conversely, acids that cannot enter cells via the MCT (e.g., HCl, citric acid) may cause a shift of K$^+$ ions out of cells, resulting in hyperkalemia (see Chapter 13, Figure 13-7).

### Clinical implications

1. In a patient with ketoacidosis or L-lactic acidosis, the cause of hyperkalemia is not the acidemia but rather the lack of insulin in patients with DKA, or diminished availability of ATP to permit cation flux via the Na-K-ATPase in patients with L-lactic acidosis due to hypoxia.
2. The infusion of L-lactic acid in fed rats, and in rats with acute hyperkalemia induced by the infusion of HCl or KCl, was associated with a fall in the arterial P$_K$ due to the shift of K$^+$ ions into liver cells. This effect was also observed with the infusion of Na-L-lactate. The administration of a relatively large dose of insulin is the mainstay of therapy in patients with emergency hyperkalemia; hypoglycemia is

a frequent complication. The administration of Na-L-lactate with a smaller dose of insulin in this setting may provide an effective means to lower the $P_K$ with less risk of hypoglycemia than when a larger dose of insulin alone is used. Studies in humans are required to examine the effectiveness of this approach.

3. Although the addition of nonmonocarboxylic acids may cause a shift of $K^+$ ions out of cells, patients with chronic hyperchloremic metabolic acidosis may have hypokalemia. This occurs if they also have excessive loss of $K^+$ ions in diarrheal fluid in patients with chronic diarrhea or in the urine (e.g., in patients with distal renal tubular acidosis due to a defect in net $H^+$ ion secretion in the distal nephron).

## HYPERKALEMIA IN PATIENTS WITH TISSUE CATABOLISM

Hyperkalemia may be seen in patients with a crush injury or tumor lysis syndrome. In these patients, factors that compromise the renal excretion of $K^+$ ions are usually present as well. In patients with DKA, there is a total body deficit of $K^+$ ions because both $K^+$ ions and phosphate anions, released from cells in this catabolic state, are lost in the urine. Despite this deficit of $K^+$ ions, hyperkalemia is commonly present as a result of a shift of $K^+$ ions out of cells secondary to lack of actions of insulin. The corollary is that during therapy for DKA, complete replacement of the deficit of $K^+$ ions must wait for the provision of intracellular constituents (e.g., phosphate, essential amino acids, magnesium) and the presence of anabolic signals.

## HYPERTONICITY AND SHIFT OF $K^+$ IONS OUT OF CELLS

A rise in effective osmolality (i.e., tonicity) in the interstitial fluid causes the movement of water out of cells via aquaporin-1 (AQP1) water channels in cell membranes. This raises the concentration of $K^+$ ions in the ICF, which provides a chemical driving force for the movement of $K^+$ ions out of cells. Although some may call this osmotic drag, this is not the correct description of this process, because the movement of $K^+$ ions out of cells is not through AQP1 but through specific $K^+$ ion channels (see Chapter 13, Figure 13-8).

### Clinical implications

Severe hyperkalemia has been described as a complication of the administration of mannitol for the treatment or the prevention of cerebral edema. This mechanism may be also a component of the pathophysiology of hyperkalemia in patients with DKA and a severe degree of hyperglycemia.

## REGULATION OF RENAL EXCRETION OF $K^+$ IONS

Control of $K^+$ ion secretion occurs primarily in the CDN, which includes the late distal convoluted tubule (DCT), the connecting segment, and the cortical collecting duct (CCD). Most of the secretion of $K^+$ ions occurs in the late DCT and the connecting segment; nevertheless, $K^+$ ions are also secreted in the CCD if the $K^+$ ion load is large. Two factors influence the rate of excretion of $K^+$ ions in the CDN: (1) the net secretion of $K^+$ ions by principal cells in the CDN (which raises the concentration of $K^+$ ions in the fluid in the lumen of the CDN) and (2) the flow rate in the terminal CDN (i.e., the number of liters of fluid that exit from the CDN).

**ABBREVIATIONS**

ENaC, epithelial sodium channel
ROMK, renal outer medullary $K^+$ ion channels
SGK-1, serum and glucocorticoid regulated kinase-1
ANG$_{II}$, angiotensin II
WNK kinase, with No lysine kinase
L-WNK1, long WNK1
KS-WNK1, kidney-specific WNK1
NCC, $Na^+/Cl^-$ cotransporter
NDBCE, sodium-dependent bicarbonate-chloride exchanger
PCT, proximal convoluted tubule
MCD, medullary collecting duct

## K$^+$ Ion Secretion in the CDN

The process of secretion of K$^+$ ions by principal cells in the CDN has two elements. First, a lumen-negative transepithelial voltage must be generated by the electrogenic reabsorption of Na$^+$ ions (i.e., reabsorption of Na$^+$ ions without their accompanying anions, which are largely Cl$^-$ ions) via the epithelial sodium ion channel (ENaC) in the luminal membrane of principal cells in the CDN. Second, the presence of a sufficient number of open renal outer medullary K$^+$ ion channels (ROMK) in the luminal membrane of principal cells.

Aldosterone actions lead to an increase in the number of open ENaC units in the luminal membrane of principal cells in the CDN and hence the rate of electrogenic reabsorption of Na$^+$ ions. Aldosterone binds to its receptor in the cytoplasm of principal cells and the hormone–receptor complex enters the nucleus, leading to the synthesis of new proteins, including the serum and glucocorticoid regulated kinase-1 (SGK-1). SGK-1 increases the number of open ENaC in the apical membrane of principal cells via its effect to phosphorylate and inactivate the ubiquitin ligase, Nedd 4-2 (see Chapter 13, Figure 13-9).

An electroneutral NaCl transport process in CDN seems to be mediated by the parallel activity of the Na$^+$ ion-independent Cl$^-$/HCO$_3^-$ anion exchanger (called pendrin) and the Na$^+$ ion-dependent Cl$^-$/HCO$_3^-$ anion exchanger (NDCBE) (see Chapter 13, Fig. 13-10). Increased electroneutral NaCl reabsorption diminishes the luminal-negative voltage and hence the rate of secretion of K$^+$ ions. An increase in the concentration of HCO$_3^-$ ions and/or an alkaline luminal fluid pH seem to increase the amount of K$^+$ ions secreted in the CDN. An increase in the concentration of HCO$_3^-$ ions in the fluid in the lumen of the CDN may inhibit pendrin and hence NDCBE and the electroneutral NaCl reabsorption. This may result in an increased rate of electrogenic reabsorption of Na$^+$ ions and a higher negative-lumen voltage in CDN. In addition, an increase in the luminal fluid HCO$_3^-$ concentration may increase the abundance and activity of ENaC in the luminal membrane of principal cells in CDN.

A complex network of "With No Lysine" (WNK) kinases, WNK4 and WNK1, through effects on the Na$^+$/Cl$^-$ ion cotransporter (NCC) in the DCT and ROMK in the CDN, may function as a switch to change the aldosterone response of the kidney to either conserve Na$^+$ ions or excrete K$^+$ ions.

WNK4 is thought to inhibit NCC activity by reducing its abundance in luminal membranes by diverting post-Golgi NCC to the lysosome for degradation. Angiotensin II (ANG$_{II}$) signaling through its AT1 receptor converts WNK4 from an NCC-inhibiting to an NCC-activating kinase. The activated form of WNK4 phosphorylates members of the STE-20 family of serine/threonine kinases, specifically SPAK and OSR1. Phosphorylated SPAK/OSR1 in turn phosphorylate and activate NCC. Alternative promoter usage of the *WNK1* gene produces a kidney-specific, truncated form of WNK1, called KS-WNK1, and a more ubiquitous long form, called L-WNK1. L-WNK1 upregulates NCC either by blocking the inhibitory form of WNK4 or directly by phosphorylation of SPAK/OSR1. An increase in the rate of reabsorption of NaCl in the DCT decreases its delivery to the CDN. Therefore, the rate of electrogenic reabsorption of Na$^+$ ions in CDN is decreased and the negative-lumen voltage is diminished.

In addition to control by the lumen-negative voltage, the process for secretion of K$^+$ ions in principal cells is dependent on having a sufficient number of open ROMK channels in the luminal membrane of principal cells. Regulation of these channels is via phosphorylation/dephosphorylation-induced endocytosis/exocytosis, which involves a complicated mixture of kinases and phosphatases, including WNK kinases, tyrosine kinases, and SGK-1. L-WNK1 inhibits ROMK by inducing its endocytosis; the KS-WNK1 isoform inhibits this effect of L-WNK1. An increase in dietary intake of K$^+$ ions leads to an increased ratio of KS-WNK1 to L-WNK1, so there is reduced endocytosis of ROMK and increased rate of secretion of K$^+$ ions, if a large enough negative-lumen voltage can be generated. On the other hand, this ratio is decreased by dietary K$^+$ ion restriction, which leads to greater endocytosis of ROMK and hence less secretion of K$^+$ ions.

### Clinical implications

Chronic hyperkalemia implies that there is a defect in renal excretion of K$^+$ ions due to diminished ability to generate a large enough lumen-negative voltage in the CDN. This may be due to diminished reabsorption of Na$^+$ ions via ENaC in the CDN caused by the presence of a smaller number of open ENaC units in the luminal membrane of principal cells in the CDN. This group of patients includes patients who have aldosterone deficiency, those who are taking drugs that block the renin–angiotensin II–aldosterone axis, the aldosterone receptor or ENaC, and those with molecular defects that involve the aldosterone receptor or ENaC. In another subset of patients, the site of the lesion is the early DCT, where there is enhanced electroneutral reabsorption of Na$^+$ and Cl$^-$ ions via NCC. The increase in NCC activity may be caused by an increase in the NCC activating form of WNK4 or an increase in L-WNK1. The enhanced reabsorption of NaCl causes EABV expansion, which suppresses the release of aldosterone and leads to a diminished number of open ENaC units in the luminal membranes of principal cells in the CDN. These kinases also cause the endocytosis of ROMK from the luminal membrane of principal cells in the CDN. Examples of this pathophysiology include patients with the syndrome of hypertension and hyperkalemia, patients taking calcinuerin inhibitors, and some patients with diabetic nephropathy and hyporeninemic hypoaldosteronism. In another group of patients, the pathophysiology may be an increased electroneutral reabsorption of Na$^+$ ions in the CCD caused by increased parallel transport activity of pendrin and NDBCE. This may be the pathophysiology for what used to be thought of as a "chloride shunt disorder." Examples of this pathophysiology may include a subset of patients with diabetic nephropathy and hyporeninemic hypoaldosteronism.

## FLOW RATE IN THE TERMINAL CDN

When vasopressin acts, the CDN becomes permeable to water because of the insertion of AQP2 water channels in the luminal membrane of its principal cells. The osmolality of fluid in the terminal CDN becomes equal to the plasma osmolality and therefore is relatively fixed. Therefore, the flow rate in the terminal CDN (i.e., the number of liters that exit the CDN) is determined by the number of effective osmoles present in the luminal fluid. These osmoles are largely urea, and Na$^+$ and K$^+$ ions with their accompanying anions. Because of the process of intrarenal urea recycling, most of the osmoles delivered to the terminal CDN are urea osmoles. In subjects eating a typical Western diet, the amount of urea that recycles would be approximately 600 mmol per day. This process of urea recycling adds an extra 2 L to the flow rate in the terminal CCD (600 mosmol divided by a luminal fluid osmolality that is equal to plasma osmolality, i.e., ~300 mosmol/kg H$_2$O).

### Clinical implications

A quantitative analysis shows that even in patients with a large defect in their ability to generate a lumen-negative voltage in the CDN, an appreciable degree of hyperkalemia is not likely to develop while consuming the usual dietary intake of $K^+$ ions unless there is decreased flow rate in the terminal CDN (see Chapter 13). Because urea accounts for most of the osmoles delivered to the terminal CDN, restricting protein intake may decrease the amount of urea that recycles and hence the rate of flow in the terminal CDN. $ANG_{II}$ stimulates the transport of urea in the inner medullary collecting duct (MCD) in the presence of vasopressin. Hence, hyperkalemia may be more likely to develop in patients who are taking angiotensin converting enzyme (ACE) inhibitors or angiotensin receptor blockers if they were to consume a protein-restricted diet because there would now be another reason for diminished intrarenal urea recycling and therefore a decreased rate of flow in the terminal CDN.

Diuretics may be used in patients with chronic hyperkalemia to increase the rate of excretion of $K^+$ ions by increasing the delivery of NaCl and hence the rate of flow in the terminal CDN. Nevertheless, if the patient becomes EABV depleted, the increase in NaCl reabsorption in the proximal convoluted tubule (PCT) will decrease the number of osmoles of $Na^+$ and $Cl^-$ ions in the lumen of the terminal CDN, and hence the number of liters of fluid that exit the CDN, and therefore decreases the rate of excretion of $K^+$ ions.

A decreased rate of flow in the CDN may cause an increase in the concentrations of drugs such as trimethoprim and amiloride in the luminal fluid; therefore, they become more effective blockers of ENaC.

# PART B
# STEPS IN THE CLINICAL APPROACH TO THE PATIENT WITH HYPERKALEMIA

The first step in the clinical approach to the patient with hyperkalemia is to determine if an emergency is present because dealing with the emergency must take precedence over making a diagnosis of the cause of hyperkalemia.

## STEP 1: ADDRESS EMERGENCIES

Hyperkalemia constitutes a medical emergency, primarily due to its effect on the heart. Therapy should be instituted promptly because even mild ECG changes due to hyperkalemia may deteriorate rapidly into a serious arrhythmia (Flow Chart 15-1).

The effects of hyperkalemia on the heart can be divided into those that are due to rapid repolarization and those that are due to slow depolarization. To understand the effects of hyperkalemia on cardiac myocytes, we start from phase 4 of the action potential, the resting phase (the phase associated with diastole). Because the cell membrane is most permeable to $K^+$ ions and relatively impermeable to other ions during this phase of the action potential, the resting membrane potential (RMP) is determined by the $K^+$ ion equilibrium potential across the cell membrane. During hyperkalemia, the ratio of the concentration of $K^+$ ions inside the cell ($K_{in}$) to the concentration of $K^+$ ions outside the cell ($K_{out}$) will be reduced; therefore, the RMP will become less negative.

Stage 0 of the action potential is the rapid depolarization phase. This phase is due to opening of the fast $Na^+$ ion channels, which causes a rapid influx of $Na^+$ ions into cells. The magnitude of $Na^+$ ion inward

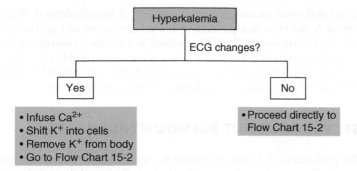

**Flow Chart 15-1  Initial Treatment of the Patient with Hyperkalemia.** If there are ECG changes related to hyperkalemia, intravenous $Ca^{2+}$ must be given and therapy to shift $K^+$ ions into cells and to remove $K^+$ ions from the body is instituted.

current determines the rate of rise of the action potential upstroke (also called $V_{max}$), which determines the speed of impulse propagation. The ability of the cell to open the fast $Na^+$ ion channels during phase 0 is related to the membrane potential at the onset of depolarization. If the RMP is less negative, fewer $Na^+$ ion channels become activated during depolarization, thus the magnitude of the inward $Na^+$ ion current and the $V_{max}$ of the action potential are diminished. The decrease in $V_{max}$ results in a reduction in myocardial conduction with progressive prolongation of the P wave, PR interval, and widening QRS complex.

The rapid delayed rectifier $K^+$ ion channel ($I_{Kr}$) is mostly responsible for the efflux of $K^+$ ions, which occurs during phase 3 of the cardiac action potential: the rapid repolarization phase. The $I_{Kr}$ current is sensitive to extracellular $K^+$ ion concentration. For reasons that are not well understood, as extracellular concentration of $K^+$ ions rises, conductance of $K^+$ ions through these channels increases so that more $K^+$ ions leave the myocytes in a given time period. This leads to shortening of the repolarization time, which is thought to be responsible for some of the electrocardiographic manifestations observed with a modest degree of hyperkalemia, such as ST segment depression, peaked T waves, and QT shortening.

The earliest ECG manifestations of hyperkalemia include the appearance of narrow-based, peaked, tent-shaped symmetrical T waves. These T waves are of relatively short duration, which help distinguish them from the broad T waves typically seen in patients with myocardial infarction or intracerebral hemorrhage. Peaked T waves are generally only seen when the $P_K$ is >5.5 mmol/L.

As the $P_K$ increases to greater than 6.5 mmol/L, the manifestations of slow cardiac conduction become apparent: broad, flat P wave (delayed sinoatrial conduction), prolonged PR interval (delayed atrioventricular conduction), and wide QRS complexes (delayed intraventricular conduction). The QRS complex may take the appearance of right or left bundle branch block.

As the $P_K$ reaches 8 to 9 mmol/L, P waves may be absent, indicating atrial arrest. The QRS complex continues to widen and eventually blends with the T wave, producing the classical sine wave pattern. As hyperkalemia worsens and the $P_K$ reaches 10 mmol/L, sinoventricular conduction no longer occurs, and ventricular fibrillation and asystole are likely to develop.

It is important to note that this correlation between the absolute level of $P_K$ and the ECG changes is based largely on experiments in animals with the acute infusion of $K^+$ ions. There is large variability among patients in the absolute $P_K$ leading to ECG changes and the cardiac toxicity of hyperkalemia. Variables include the rapidity of the onset of hyperkalemia, underlying cardiac disease, and the presence of hypocalcemia, acidemia, and/or hyponatremia (all seem to be associated with increased cardiac toxicity of hyperkalemia). There-fore, it is our view that patients with a severe degree of hyperkalemia (i.e., $P_K > 7.0$ mmol/L) should be treated as a medical emergency with maneuvers to induce a shift of $K^+$ ions into cells, even in the absence of ECG changes, and perhaps at even lower $P_K$ (e.g., >6.5 mmol/L) in the presence of hypocalcemia, acidemia, and/or hyponatremia.

## STEP 2: RULE OUT PSEUDOHYPERKALEMIA

The presence of ECG changes related to hyperkalemia rules out pseudo-hyperkalemia as the major cause for the high $P_K$. Pseudohyperkalemia is caused by the release of $K^+$ ions during or after venipuncture (see margin note). Excessive fist clenching during blood sampling may increase the release of $K^+$ ions from contracting muscles and thus raise the measured $P_K$. Pseudohyperkalemia can be present in cachectic patients because the normal T-tubule architecture in skeletal muscle may be disturbed. Mechanical trauma to red blood cells during venipuncture can result in their hemolysis and the release of $K^+$ ions in the test tube. $K^+$ ions are normally released from platelets during blood clotting; therefore, pseu-dohyperkalemia may be noted in patients with thrombocytosis (espe-cially megakaryocytosis). Pseudohyperkalemia may also be present in patients with leukocytosis (especially due to fragile leukemia cells) because of breakdown of white blood cells during venipuncture. Cool-ing of blood prior to the separation of cells from plasma is a recognized cause of pseudohyperkalemia. There are several hereditary subtypes of pseudohyperkalemia, caused by increase in passive $K^+$ ion permeability of erythrocytes. This leak of $K^+$ ions increases in blood samples from these patients if left for a period of time at room temperature.

## STEP 3: DETERMINE IF THE CAUSE OF THE HYPERKALEMIA IS AN ACUTE SHIFT OF $K^+$ IONS OUT OF CELLS

If hyperkalemia developed over a short period of time, or over a period of time during which the intake of $K^+$ ions has been low, the cause of hyper-kalemia is likely to be an acute shift of $K^+$ ions out of cells in the body (see Flow Chart 15-2). $K^+$ ions are released from cells if they are broken down (e.g., crush injury, rhabdomyolysis, tumor lysis syndrome), or in conditions in which there is a less negative voltage in cells. A less negative voltage inside cells may be due to hypoxia causing lack of adenosine tri-phosphate (ATP) for the function of the Na-K-ATPase pump (e.g., condi-tions causing hypoxic L-lactic acidosis, exhausting exercise, after seizures, status epilepticus), lack of a stimulus for the Na-K-ATPase (e.g., lack of insulin in patients with DKA, inhibition of the release of insulin by an α-adrenergic surge due to, for example, marked EABV contraction, $\beta_2$-adrenergic blockade), or the presence of an inhibitor of the Na-K-ATPase (e.g., digoxin overdose). Bufadienolide, a structurally similar glycoside to digoxin, is present in high concentration in the skin and venom gland of the toad *Bufo marinus*. The ingestion of such toads or their extracts can result in fatal hyperkalemia. Several cases of hyperkalemia have been reported after the ingestion of certain herbal aphrodisiac pills containing large amounts of toad venom. The stems, leaves, flowers, and roots of yel-low oleander contain a high concentration of cardiac glycosides; ingestion of yellow oleander for attempting suicide has been noted with increasing frequency in South Asia.

A shift of $K^+$ ions out of cells may also occur in conditions with met-abolic acidosis due to nonmonocarboxylic acids (i.e., acids that cannot

**A CLINICAL CLUE TO THE PRESENCE OF PSEUDOHYPER-KALEMIA**

- Hyperkalemia is associated with alkalosis in the cells of the PCT and hence inhibition of ammoniagenesis.
- True hyperkalemia is commonly accompanied by hyperchloremic metabolic acidosis.

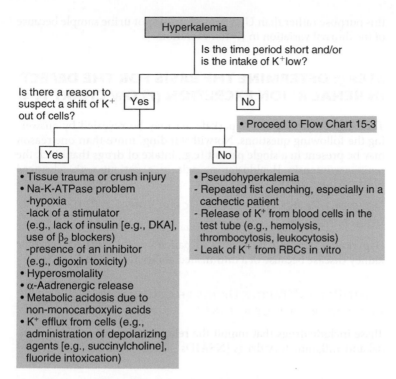

**Flow Chart 15-2 Determine If the Cause of Hyperkalemia Is a Shift of K⁺ Ions Out of Cells.** If hyperkalemia developed over a short period and/or there was little intake of K⁺ ions, its basis is likely a shift of K⁺ out of cells or peudohyperkalemia. Red blood cells; white blood cells; *DKA,* diabetic ketoacidosis.

be transported on the monocarboxylic acid cotransporter (e.g., metabolic acidosis due to a gain of HCl acid because of loss of $NaHCO_3$ in a patient with diarrhea, ingestion of citric acid). Severe hyperkalemia has been described as a complication of the administration of mannitol for the treatment or prevention of cerebral edema. Succinylcholine depolarizes muscle cells, resulting in the efflux of K⁺ ions through acetylcholine receptors in conditions that may lead to upregulation of these receptors (e.g., burn patients, patients with neuromuscular injury, disuse atrophy, or prolonged immobilization). Fluoride can open the calcium-sensitive K⁺ ion channels, and as a result, fluoride intoxication can lead to fatal hyperkalemia. A positive family history for acute hyperkalemia suggests that there may be a molecular basis for the acute shift of K⁺ ions out of cells (e.g., hyperkalemic periodic paralysis).

## STEP 4: IS THE RATE OF EXCRETION OF K⁺ IONS HIGH ENOUGH IN A PATIENT WITH CHRONIC HYPERKALEMIA?

In a patient with chronic hyperkalemia, pseudohyperkalemia should be first ruled out.

Normal subjects who are given a load of K⁺ ions can augment the rate of excretion of K⁺ ions in the urine to greater than 200 mmol/day with only a minor increase in the $P_K$. Therefore, patients with chronic hyperkalemia have a defect in the excretion of K⁺ ions by the kidneys. In a steady state, they excrete the K⁺ ions what they ingest (minus the amount of K⁺ ions lost in stool) but at the expense of a higher $P_K$. Therefore, the value of examining the rate of K⁺ ion excretion in these patients is to assess the contribution of K⁺ ion intake to the degree of hyperkalemia. A 24-hour urine collection is necessary for this purpose rather than $U_K/U_{Creatinine}$ on a spot urine sample because of the diurnal variation in $K^+$ ion excretion.

## STEP 5: DETERMINE THE BASIS FOR THE DEFECT IN RENAL K⁺ ION EXCRETION (FLOW CHART 15-3)

The basis of the chronic hyperkalemia may be revealed by answering the following questions. Notwithstanding, more than one reason may be present in a single patient (e.g., intake of drugs that block the renin–angiotensin II–aldosterone axis in a patient with advanced renal dysfunction).

### DOES THE PATIENT HAVE ADVANCED CHRONIC RENAL INSUFFICIENCY?

Hyperkalemia occurs frequently in patients with advanced, chronic kidney disease because of a diminished ability to excrete $K^+$ ions.

### IS THE PATIENT TAKING DRUGS THAT INTERFERE WITH THE RENAL EXCRETION OF K⁺ IONS?

These include drugs that inhibit the release of renin (e.g., nonsteroidal anti-inflammatory drugs [NSAIDs], direct renin blockers), drugs

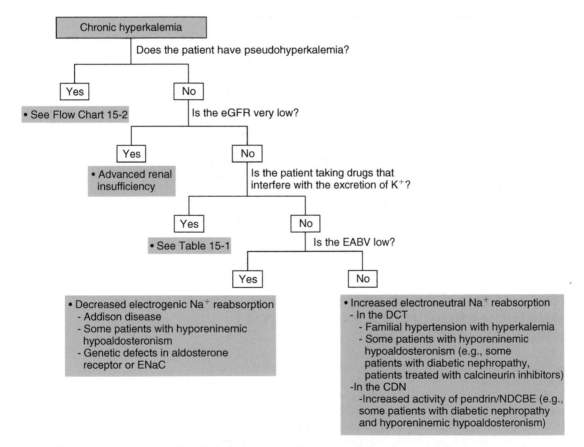

**Flow Chart 15-3  Steps in the Clinical Diagnosis of the Cause of Chronic Hyperkalemia.** See text for details. More than one cause of hyperkalemia may be present in the same patients. *CDN,* Cortical distal nephron; *DCT,* distal convoluted tubule; *EABV,* effective arterial blood volume; *eGFR,* estimated glomerular filtration rate; *ENaC,* epithelial sodium ion channel; *NDCBE,* sodium-dependant chloride/bicarbonate exchanger.

that interfere with the renin–angiotensin II–aldosterone axis (e.g., ACE inhibitors and angiotensin II receptor blockers [ARBs]), drugs that inhibit the synthesis of aldosterone (e.g., heparin, ketoconazole), aldosterone receptor blockers (e.g., spironolactone), and drugs that block ENaC in the CDN (e.g., amiloride, trimethoprim). Other examples include drugs that increase electroneutral reabsorption of $Na^+$ and $Cl^-$ ions via NCC in the early DCT (e.g., calcineurin inhibitors).

## DOES THE PATIENT HAVE A DISORDER THAT LEADS TO DIMINISHED REABSORPTION OF Na⁺ IONS VIA ENaC IN THE CDN?

There are a number of subgroups of patients who may have a decreased rate of $K^+$ ion excretion caused by an inability to generate a large enough lumen-negative voltage in the CDN due to diminished electrogenic reabsorption of $Na^+$ ions via ENaC. The first subgroup consists of patients who have a very low delivery of $Na^+$ to the CDN, due to a marked decrease in their EABV. The second subgroup consists of patients who have lesions that lead to a diminished number of open ENaC units in the luminal membrane of principal cells in the CDN. This includes patients who have low aldosterone actions (e.g., adrenal insufficiency) and those with molecular defects that involve the aldosterone receptor or ENaC. Patients in this subgroup have a low EABV, a higher than expected rate of excretion of $Na^+$ and $Cl^-$ ions in the urine in a setting of low EABV, and a high $P_{Renin}$. The $P_{Aldosterone}$ is helpful to determine the reason for this diminished $Na^+$ ion reabsorption via ENaC in the CDN.

A subset of patients has a low EABV, a low $P_{Aldosterone}$, and a low $P_{Renin}$. Their lesion may be destruction of, or a biosynthetic defect in, the juxtaglomerular apparatus, which leads to a low $P_{Renin}$ and thereby a low $P_{Aldosterone}$. Patients with this subtype of the syndrome of hyporeninemic hypoaldosteronism (see the following) are expected to have a significant rise in their rate of excretion of $K^+$ ions with the administration of exogenous mineralocorticoids.

## DOES THE PATIENT HAVE A DISORDER THAT INCREASES ELECTRONEUTRAL REABSORPTION OF Na⁺ IONS IN THE DCT?

In this group of patients, the site of the lesion is the early DCT, where there is enhanced electroneutral reabsorption of $Na^+$ and $Cl^-$ ions via NCC because of an increase in the NCC activating form of WNK4 or an increase in L-WNK1. Suppression of release of aldosterone by an expanded EABV leads to a diminished number of open ENaC units in the luminal membranes of principal cells in the CDN. These kinases also cause the endocytosis of ROMK from the luminal membrane of principal cells in the CDN. These patients will tend to have an expanded EABV, hypertension, and suppressed $P_{Renin}$ and $P_{Aldosterone}$ (hyporeninemic hypoaldosteronism). Patients with this pathophysiology are expected to have a good response in terms of their hypertension and hyperkalemia to the administration of thiazide diuretics.

Patients with the syndrome of familial hyperkalemia with hypertension (also known as pseudohypoaldosteronism type II or Gordon's syndrome) behave as if they have a gain-of-function in the thiazide-sensitive NCC. A similar set of clinical findings to those in patients with familial hyperkalemia with hypertension may occur in other patients, most commonly those with diabetic nephropathy. Another example of this pathophysiology is the hyperkalemia in patients who are treated with calcineurin inhibitors.

### DOES THE PATIENT HAVE A DISORDER THAT INCREASES ELECTRONEUTRAL REABSORPTION OF Na$^+$ IONS IN THE CDN?

The pathophysiology in these patients may be an increase in parallel transport activity of pendrin and NDBCE. This may be the pathophysiology for what used to be thought of as a "chloride shunt disorder." These patients will also have an expanded EABV and suppressed $P_{Renin}$ and $P_{Aldosterone}$ (hyporeninemic hypoaldosteronism). Patients with this disorder are expected to have an increase in K$^+$ ion excretion with increasing the delivery of HCO$_3^-$ ions to the CDN with the administration of the carbonic anhydrase inhibitor, acetazolamide. Examples of this pathophysiology may include some patients with diabetic nephropathy and hyporeninemic hypoaldosteronism.

### IS A LOW FLOW RATE IN THE TERMINAL CDN CONTRIBUTING TO HYPERKALEMIA?

Because of the process of intrarenal urea recycling, a large fraction of the osmoles delivered to the terminal CDN are urea osmoles. A low protein intake may lead to a decrease in the amount of urea that recycles and hence the rate of flow in the terminal CDN. The usual rate of excretion of urea in subjects consuming a typical Western diet is about 400 mmol/day. If the rate of excretion of urea is appreciably lower than that, a low flow rate in the terminal CDN may be a contributing factor to the degree of hyperkalemia. A low flow rate in the terminal CDN may be caused by diminished delivery of NaCl because of decreased EABV, the use of diuretics, or the extrarenal loss of NaCl (e.g., due to diarrhea).

---

# PART C
# SPECIFIC CAUSES OF HYPERKALEMIA

A list of the causes of hyperkalemia based on their possible underlying pathophysiology is provided in Table 15-1.

## CHRONIC RENAL INSUFFICIENCY

Hyperkalemia occurs frequently in patients with advanced chronic kidney disease. It has been suggested that at least in some patients, the pathophysiology that leads to decreased K$^+$ ion secretion resembles a "chloride shunt disorder." In this setting, diminished K$^+$ ion secretion may be due to an enhanced rate of electroneutral NaCl reabsorption in the DCT or in the CDN. In addition, decreased flow rate in the terminal CDN may be a contributing factor to diminished rate of K$^+$ ion excretion. In more detail, when vasopressin acts, flow rate in the terminal CDN is directly related to the number of effective osmoles in the lumen in the terminal CDN. The major effective osmoles are urea and Na$^+$ + Cl$^-$ ions. The number of osmoles of Na$^+$ + Cl$^-$ ions in the terminal CDN may be diminished because of dietary salt restriction and/or the use of diuretics that may decrease the EABV. The number of urea osmoles in the terminal CDN may be decreased because of dietary protein restriction and diminished intrarenal urea recycling because of medullary interstitial disease involving the inner MCD. In addition, some patients may be taking drugs that compromise the ability to excrete K$^+$ ions. Prominent on the list are drugs that diminish the secretion of aldosterone (e.g., ACE-inhibitors or angiotensin II receptor blockers

TABLE 15-1  **CAUSES OF HYPERKALEMIA**

**High Intake of K+ Ions**
- Only if there is also a disorder leading to a low rate of excretion of K+ ions

**Shift of K+ Ions Out of Cells**
- Tissue breakdown (e.g., crush trauma, rhabdomyolysis, tumor lysis), exhausting exercise, after seizures, status epilepticus
- Na/K-ATPase problem
  - Tissue hypoxia
  - Lack of a stimulus (e.g., lack of insulin [e.g., patients with DKA], inhibition of insulin release by α-adrenergic surge, use of nonselective β-blockers)
  - Inhibition of Na/K-ATPase (e.g., by drugs, e.g., digoxin)
- α-Adrenergic surge (causing inhibition of the release of insulin or a direct effect to cause a shift of K+ ions out of cells)
- Hyperosmolality (e.g., administration of mannitol)
- Metabolic acidosis due to acids that cannot be transported on the monocarboxylic acid cotransporter (e.g., HCl, citric acid)
- Increase K+ efflux from cells (administration of succinylcholine, fluoride intoxication)
- Hereditary causes (e.g., hyperkalemic periodic paralysis)

**Diminished K+ Ion Loss in the Urine**
- *Advanced chronic renal insufficiency*
- *Drugs that interfere with renal K+ ion excretion*
  - Drugs that cause acute renal failure or acute interstitial nephritis
  - Drugs that interfere with the renin–angiotensin–aldosterone axis (e.g., nonsteroidal anti-inflammatory drugs, direct renin blockers, ACE inhibitors, angiotensin receptor blockers)
  - Drugs that inhibit aldosterone synthesis (e.g., heparin, ketoconazole)
  - Aldosterone receptor blockers (e.g., spironolactone, eplerenone)
  - Drugs that block ENaC in the CDN (e.g., amiloride, trimethoprim)
  - Drugs the interfere with activation of ENaC via proteolytic cleavage (e.g., nafamostat mesylate)
- *Diminished electrogenic reabsorption of Na+ ions in the CDN*
  - Very low delivery of Na+ ions to the CDN
  - Some patients with hyporeninemic hypoaldosteronism
  - Low levels of aldosterone (e.g., Addison's disease)
  - Genetic disorders involving the aldosterone receptor or ENaC (type I pesudohypoaldosteronism)
- *Increased electroneutral reabsorption of Na+ ions in DCT or CDN*
  - Increased reabsorption of Na+ and Cl- ions in the DCT (e.g., familial hypertension with hyperkalemia [WNK 4 or WNK1 mutations]), drugs (e.g., calcineurin inhibitors), and some patients with diabetic nephropathy and hyporeninemic hypoalosteronism
  - Increased electroneutral reabsorption of Na+ and Cl- ions in the CDN due to increased parallel activity of pendrin and NDCBE (e.g., some patients with hyporeninemic hypoalosteronism)

*ACE*, angiotensin converting enzyme; *DKA*, diabetic ketoacidosis; *CDN*, cortical distal nephron; *DCT*, distal convoluted tubule; *ENaC*, epithelial sodium ion channel; *NDCBE*, sodium-dependent chloride/bicarbonate exchanger.

[ARBs]) and aldosterone receptor blockers (e.g., spironolactone). The degree of hyperkalemia will obviously be more severe if the intake of K+ ions is particularly high, due to, for example, the intake of salt substitutes that contain KCl or the ingestion of a large volume of fruit juice.

## ADDISON'S DISEASE

The most common cause of this disorder used to be bilateral adrenal destruction due to tuberculosis, but now autoimmune disease, either as an isolated disorder or as part of polyglandular endocrinopathy, accounts for the majority of cases. Human immunodeficiency virus is now the most important infectious cause of adrenal insufficiency, with cytomegalovirus infection being the most likely cause in this setting. Additional causes of Addison's disease include adrenal infiltration by amyloidosis, metastatic carcinoma or lymphoma, adrenal hemorrhage or infarction (as may occur in patients with the antiphospholipid antibody syndrome), and drugs that impair the synthesis of aldosterone (e.g., heparin, ketoconazole, and possibly fluconazole).

Patients with chronic primary adrenal insufficiency may present with chronic malaise, fatigue, anorexia, generalized weakness, and weight loss. Salt craving is a distinctive feature in some patients. Hyperpigmentation is evident in nearly all patients. In most patients, the blood pressure is low and postural symptoms of dizziness and syncope are common. The $P_K$ is usually close to 5.5 mmol/L, unless a significant degree of intravascular volume depletion diminishes the flow rate in the CDN, leading to a more severe degree of hyperkalemia. Nevertheless, hyperkalemia is not seen on presentation in approximately one-third of the cases. The absence of hyperkalemia in such a large percentage of patients is probably due to a low dietary intake of $K^+$ ions. Other abnormal laboratory findings include hyponatremia, hyperchloremic metabolic acidosis, hypoglycemia, and eosinophilia. Some patients may present with acute adrenal crisis and shock.

The diagnosis can be established by finding a low $P_{Aldosterone}$ and plasma cortisol ($P_{Cortisol}$), high $P_{Renin}$, and a blunted cortisol response to the administration of adrenocorticotropic hormone.

Adrenal crisis is an emergency that requires immediate restoration of the intravascular volume with the administration of intravenous saline and correction of the cortisol deficiency with the administration of dexamethasone or hydrocortisone. Beware of raising the $P_{Na}$ too rapidly if hyponatremia is present because of the increased risk of osmotic demyelination in these catabolic patients. The administration of cortisol can lead to a fall in the circulating level of vasopressin (see Chapter 10). We prefer to give dDAVP at the outset of therapy to avoid a large water diuresis that could result in a sudden and excessive rise in the $P_{Na}$.

Patients with chronic adrenal insufficiency should receive replacement therapy with glucocorticoids and, in most patients, a mineralocorticoid. For glucocorticoid replacement, a short acting glucocorticoid, such as hydrocortisone, 15-25 mg/day in two or three divided doses is usually given. For mineralocorticoid replacement, fludrocortisone in a single dose of 50 to 200 μg is usually used. Dose adjustments are made based on the patient's symptoms, EABV status, blood pressure, and $P_K$.

## HYPERKALEMIA DUE TO INHERITED DISORDERS OF ALDOSTERONE SYNTHESIS

The inherited deficiencies in the enzymes involved in aldosterone synthesis include 21-hydroxylase, 3-hydroxysteroid dehydrogenase, cholesterol desmolase, and aldosterone-synthetase. Except for aldosterone-synthetase deficiency, patients with the other three disorders (also called congenital adrenal hyperplasia) have also glucocorticoid deficiency because cortisol synthesis is also affected. Among these disorders, 21-hydrolyase deficiency is the most common and more easily recognized in affected females who usually have masculine-type genitalia at birth due to excess secretion of fetal adrenal androgen. Salt wasting, hyponatremia, hyperkalemia, and hypotension are common features.

## PSEUDOHYPOALDOSTERONISM TYPE I

The underlying pathophysiology in patients with pseudohypoaldosteronism type I (PHA-I) resembles "closed" ENaC in the luminal membrane of principal cells in the CDN. There are two different forms of this disorder with two different modes of inheritance.

### AUTOSOMAL DOMINANT DISORDER

This disorder results from loss of function mutations involving the mineralocorticoid receptor. The clinical picture is usually mild and often remits with time. Patients with this disorder have markedly elevated $P_{Aldosterone}$ and $P_{Renin}$, and fail to respond to the administration of exogenous mineralocorticoids. Treatment includes supplementation with NaCl and inducing the loss of $K^+$ ions through the gastrointestinal (GI) tract. Dialysis may be required for treatment of life-threatening hyperkalemia.

## AUTOSOMAL RECESSIVE FORM

This disorder results from various mutations involving one of the three subunits of ENaC. Unlike the autosomal dominant form of PHA-I, the disease is permanent and does not improve in adulthood. Patients usually present in the neonatal period with renal salt wasting, hyperkalemia, metabolic acidosis, failure to thrive, and weight loss. ENaC activity in the lungs is also impaired, and this leads to excessive airway fluid accumulation and recurrent lower respiratory tract infections.

# SYNDROME OF HYPORENINEMIC HYPOALDOSTERONISM

Although patients with this syndrome all have a common feature, hypereninemia and hypoaldosteronism, they represent a heterogeneous group with regard to the pathophysiology of their disorder.

1. *Group with low capability of producing renin*: The pathophysiology in this group of patients is destruction of, or a biosynthetic defect in, the juxtaglomerular apparatus, which leads to a low $P_{Renin}$ and therefore a low $P_{Aldosterone}$. Accordingly, there is a less negative luminal voltage in the CDN due to less ENaC activity and hence a lower rate of electrogenic reabsorption of $Na^+$ ions in the CDN. These patients tend to have low EABV with renal salt wasting, and are expected to have a significant rise in their rate of excretion of $K^+$ ions with the administration of exogenous mineralocorticoids.

2. *Group with low stimulus to produce renin*: A subset of this group of patients is those with "familial hyperkalemia with hypertension" (also known as pseudohypoaldosteronism type II [PHA-II] or Gordon syndrome). Patients with this disorder behave as if they have a gain-of-function in the thiazide-sensitive NCC with enhanced reabsorption of $Na^+$ and $Cl^-$ ions in the DCT (the molecular defects leading to this disorder are discussed in the following). This enhanced reabsorption of $Na^+$ and $Cl^-$ ions in the DCT results in a low delivery of $Na^+$ and $Cl^-$ ions to the CDN, with diminished rate of electrogenic reabsorption of $Na^+$ ions and hence decreased capacity to generate luminal-negative voltage in the CDN. Alterations in WNK kinases in this disorder may also lead to decreased abundance of ROMK in luminal membranes of principal cells in the CDN. This, however, does not seem to be rate limiting for the secretion of $K^+$ ions because thiazide diuretics are effective in the treatment of hyperkalemia in these patients. EABV expansion is a hallmark of the pathophysiology and results in a low $P_{Renin}$, and therefore a lower than expected $P_{Aldosterone}$, given the presence of hyperkalemia. Accordingly, these patients are not expected to have an appreciable rise in their rate of excretion of $K^+$ ions with the administration of exogenous mineralocorticoids. Hyperkalemia resolves in these patients, however, with the administration of thiazide diuretics. The explanation for this is that the effect of thiazide diuretics to inhibit NCC leads to increased delivery of $Na^+$ and $Cl^-$ ions to the CDN. This may result in a high rate of electrogenic reabsorption of $Na^+$ ions in the CDN and hence a greater negative-lumen voltage if there is an increase in the number of open ENaC units in the luminal membrane of principal cells in the CDN. The latter may occur because of the effect of thiazide diuretics to cause natriuresis, and hence a rise in $P_{Renin}$ and $P_{Aldosterone}$ as the EABV becomes less expanded. The effect of thiazide diuretics may

also be due to the inhibition of the electroneutral NaCl transport, mediated by the parallel activity of pendrin and NDCBE because thiazide diuretics have been shown to inhibit this process, although the mechanism is not understood.

A similar set of clinical findings to those described previously may be observed in other patients, most commonly patients with diabetic nephropathy. Support to the hypothesis that suppression of renin release in at least some patients with diabetic nephrothy, hyperkalemia, and hyporeninemic hypoaldosteronism is the result of EABV expansion are the findings of elevated levels of circulating atrial natriuretic peptide, and a rise in $P_{Renin}$ with restriction of dietary NaCl intake or administration of furosemide. A similar pathophysiology (i.e., that suppression of renin release is due to EABV expansion) has been suggested in patients with chronic renal failure and patients with lupus nephritis with hyperkalemia and hyporeninemic hypoaldosteronism. The basis of the disorder remains to be established. It is possible, however, that the reabsorption of $Na^+$ and $Cl^-$ ions in the DCT may be augmented akin to patients with "familial hyperkalemia with hypertension."

It is also possible that EABV expansion and hyperkalemia in these patients may reflect an increased electroneutral NaCl reabsorption in the CDN due possibly to increased electroneutral reabsorption of NaCl by the parallel activity of pendrin and NDCBE. Patients with this pathophysiology of enhanced electroneutral reabsorption of NaCl in the CDN are expected to have a rise in their rate of excretion of $K^+$ ions with increasing the delivery of $HCO_3^-$ ions to the CDN (e.g., with administration of acetazolamide).

Differentiation between these two groups of patients with hyporeninemic hypoaldosteronism has implications for therapy. The use of exogenous mineralocorticoids ($9\alpha$-fludrocortisone) is of benefit for the first group of patients because it results in both a kaliuresis and re-expansion of the EABV due to retention of $Na^+$ ions. Diuretic therapy would pose a threat to these patients because it would cause a more severe degree of EABV depletion. In contrast, mineralocorticoids may increase the degree of hypertension in those who have excessive reabsorption of $Na^+$ and $Cl^-$ ions in the DCT. In this group of patients, the administration of a thiazide diuretic to inhibit the NCC is effective therapy for both the hypertension and the hyperkalemia. Increasing the delivery of $HCO_3^-$ ions to the CDN (e.g., with the administration of acetazolamide) if this were to decrease the rate of electroneutral reabsorbtion of $Na^+$ ions in the CDN via pendrin/NDCBE, resulting in a higher rate of electrogenic reabsorption. The administration of diuretics to patients with enhanced electroneutral $Na^+$ and $Cl^-$ ion reabsorption in the CDN may increase their rate of excretion of $K^+$ ions by increasing the flow rate in the CDN. The secretion of $K^+$ ions may be also increased with increased delivery of $HCO_3^-$ ions to the CDN (e.g., with the administration of acetazolamide). The loss of $HCO_3^-$ ions may have to be replaced to avoid the development of metabolic acidemia.

## FAMILIAL HYPERKALEMIA WITH HYPERTENSION

The term pseudohypoaldosteronism type II (PHA-II) is misleading from a physiologic perspective because patients with this syndrome have salt retention and hypertension, findings associated with more rather than with less aldosterone effect.

Patients with the syndrome of familial hyperkalemia with hypertension (also known as pseudohypoaldosteronism type II or Gordon syndrome) behave as if they have a gain-of-function in the thiazide-sensitive NCC. The cause for increased reabsorption of $Na^+$ and $Cl^-$ ions in the DCT in this disorder has been clarified. Major deletions in the gene encoding for *WNK1* and missense mutations in the gene encoding for *WNK4* were found in these patients. When activated by $ANG_{II}$, WNK4 phosphorylates SPAK/OSR1, which then phosphorylate and activate NCC. Mutations in WNK4 in patients with this syndrome result in WNK4 being constitutively active, causing phosphorylation and activation of NCC via SPAK/OSR1, with no further increase in its activity by $ANG_{II}$.

The molecular defect in WNK1 is deletion of intron 1, resulting in a gain of function. Since L-WNK1 has an antagonistic effect on the inhibitory form of WNK4, and it can also activate the SPAK/OSR1-NCC signaling pathway, this defect results in increased NCC activity in DCT.

Thiazide diuretics are particularly effective in lowering the blood pressure in these patients and also their $P_K$.

## HYPERKALEMIC PERIODIC PARALYSIS

This syndrome has an autosomal dominant inheritance and is the result of a mutation in the gene encoding for the $\alpha$-subunit of the tetrodotoxin-sensitive $Na^+$ ion channel in skeletal muscle. When the muscle is stimulated to contract, $Na^+$ ion influx depolarizes the skeletal muscle cell. As the resting membrane potential approaches $-50\,mV$, normal $Na^+$ ion channels close. In patients with hyperkalemic periodic paralysis, these defective $Na^+$ ion channels fail to close. The persistent influx of $Na^+$ ions leads to membrane depolarization, which drives the outward efflux of $K^+$ ions into the ECF compartment, thus causing hyperkalemia. Muscle symptoms vary from myotonia to paralysis, depending on the severity of the defect and the resulting change in muscle cell voltage. Attacks seem to be trigged by a number of factors, including rest after exercise, consumption of foods that are rich in $K^+$ ions, cold environment, emotional stress, and fasting.

Acute attacks of hyperkalemic periodic paralysis are treated by inducing a shift of $K^+$ ions into cells with administration of $\beta_2$-adrenergics. Inducing a large loss of $K^+$ ions should be avoided, as these patients do not have a total body excess of $K^+$ ions. Acetozolamide seems to be effective in prevention of recurrence of attacks, although its mechanism of action is not clear.

## DRUGS ASSOCIATED WITH HYPERKALEMIA

Drugs that cause hyperkalemia can be classified into drugs that affect the shift of $K^+$ ions into cells and those that impair the renal excretion of $K^+$ ions.

### DRUGS THAT AFFECT CELLULAR REDISTRIBUTION OF $K^+$ IONS

Nonselective $\beta$-adrenergic blockers may diminish the $\beta_2$-adrenergic-mediated shift of $K^+$ ions into cells. In general, only a minor rise in the $P_K$ is observed. Nevertheless, more significant degrees of hyperkalemia may develop after vigorous exercise or the intake of drugs that may impair the excretion of $K^+$ by the kidneys.

Digitalis overdose may be accompanied by hyperkalemia as a result of the inhibition of the Na-K-ATPase pump.

The use of depolarizing agents such as succinylcholine during anesthesia may cause a shift of $K^+$ ions out of cells and hyperkalemia. This effect of succinylcholine is more pronounced in patients with conditions that may lead to upregulation of acetylcholine receptors in skeletal muscles, such as neuromuscular injury (upper or lower motor neuron lesion), immobilization, muscle inflammation, muscle trauma, or burn injury.

Arginine hydrochloride used in the treatment of hepatic coma and severe metabolic alkalosis, and epsilon-aminocaproic acid, a synthetic amino acid that is structurally similar to arginine and used to treat severe hemorrhage, may cause an efflux of $K^+$ ions from cells, resulting in life-threatening hyperkalemia, especially in patients with impaired renal function.

Hyperkalemia may also result from inhibition of insulin secretion by the somatostatin agonist octreotide.

## DRUGS THAT INTERFERE WITH RENAL EXCRETION OF $K^+$ IONS

### Drugs that inhibit the release of renin: Nonsteroidal antiinflammatory drugs (NSAIDs) and COX-2 inhibitors

Secretion of renin by cells in the afferent glomerular arterioles and by cells of the macula densa in the early DCT appears to be mediated in part by prostaglandins produced locally from arachidonic acid in the pathway catalyzed by the enzyme cyclooxygenase-2 (COX-2). As a result, prostaglandin synthesis inhibition can lead to low $P_{Renin}$ and low $P_{Aldosterone}$. NSAIDs also blunt the adrenal response to hyperkalemia, which is at least partially dependent on prostaglandins. The rise in the $P_K$ is usually small in normal subjects, but a significant degree of hyperkalemia may develop in the presence of diseases (e.g., chronic renal dysfunction, diabetic nephropathy) or with the intake of drugs (e.g., ACE inhibitors, ARBs, spironolactone) that may impair the renal excretion of $K^+$ ions.

### Drugs that interfere with the renin–angiotensin–aldosterone axis: Direct renin blockers, ACE inhibitors, and ARBs

The two major stimuli for the release of aldosterone are $ANG_{II}$ and an increase in the $P_K$. Hyperkalemia and $ANG_{II}$ that is generated locally within the adrenal glomerulosa act synergistically to stimulate the release of aldosterone. Therefore, blocking the renin–angiotensin–aldosterone axis is expected to reduce aldosterone secretion and therefore impair the renal excretion of $K^+$ ions. Of note, however, aldosterone blood levels are not fully suppressed in patients on chronic therapy with ACE inhibitors. Furthermore, there are no reported studies that examined the effect of the administration of exogenous mineralocorticoids on the renal excretion of $K^+$ ions in patients who develop hyperkalemia while on drugs that block the renin–angiotensin–aldosterone system (RAAS).

Notwithstanding, an appreciable degree of hyperkalemia is not likely to occur, even if there is a large reduction in the lumen-negative voltage in the CDN, unless there is decreased flow rate in the terminal CDN. A deficiency of actions of $ANG_{II}$ may diminish intrarenal urea recycling because $ANG_{II}$ stimulates the transport of urea in the inner MCD in the presence of vasopressin. Hence, hyperkalemia seen in some patients on ACE inhibitors or ARBs may be due to a combination of diminished electrical driving force for the net secretion of $K^+$ in the CDN and a diminished rate of flow in the terminal CDN due to a decrease in urea recycling, perhaps especially in those patients who are protein restricted.

In patients with hypertension without risk factors for hyperkalemia, the incidence of hyperkalemia with RAAS inhibitor monotherapy is low (<2%), whereas rates are higher with dual RAAS blockade (5%). The incidence of hyperkalemia is also increased in patients with congestive heart failure or chronic kidney disease (5% to 10%). Of note, these estimates are based on data from patients in a study setting and hence may not reflect the incidence of hyperkalemia in an outpatient setting. The rise in the $P_K$ is less than 0.5 mmol/L in patients with relatively normal renal function. In contrast, a more severe degree of hyperkalemia may be seen in patients with chronic kidney disease, with concurrent use of drugs that impairs renal $K^+$ ion excretion such as a $K^+$ ion-sparing diuretics or NSAIDs, or among the elderly.

### Drugs that inhibit aldosterone synthesis: heparin

Aldosterone synthesis is selectively reduced in patients who are treated with heparin. This seems to be due to an effect of heparin that leads to a reduction in the number and affinity of adrenal $ANG_{II}$ receptors. It has been estimated that a greater than normal $P_K$ occurs in about 7% of patients receiving heparin. Both unfractionated and low-molecular weight heparin preparations can cause hyperkalemia. Hyperkalemia due to prophylactic subcutaneous unfractionated heparin (5000 units twice daily) has also been reported. Notwithstanding, the observed degree of decrease in the $P_{Aldosterone}$ may not be of sufficient magnitude to affect the renal excretion of $K^+$ in many patients who receive heparin. Severe hyperkalemia occurs only if the patient has another disorder that impairs the excretion of $K^+$ ions (e.g., chronic renal insufficiency) or is taking an ACE inhibitor or an ARB, NSAIDs, or a $K^+$ ion-sparing diuretic.

### Aldosterone receptor antagonists: spironolactone and eplerenone

Hyperkalemia is of particular concern in patients on the nonspecific mineralocorticoid receptor antagonist spironolactone or the selective mineralocorticoid receptor antagonist eplerenone, because of the increasing indications to use a combination of spironolactone or eplerenone with an ACE inhibitor and/or an ARB in patients with congestive heart failure and reduced ejection fraction. The prevalence of hyperkalemia with the combined use of a mineralocorticoid receptor antagonist and an ACE inhibitor/an ARB appears to be much higher in clinical practice (~10%) than what has been reported in large clinical trials. This may in part due to the use of higher than recommended doses. The incidence of hyperkalemia associated with the use of the aldosterone receptor antagonists is dose dependent, with detectable effects even at doses of 25 mg spironolactone per day; the risk of severe hyperkalemia increases with the use of higher dose. A population-based study of computerized drug prescription records and hospitalizations in Ontario, Canada, examined the correlation between the rate of spironolactone prescription for patients with heart failure on ACE inhibitors with hyperkalemia and associated morbidity, following the publication of "The Randomized Aldactone Evaluation Study" (RALES). The study found that the frequency with which spironolactone was prescribed to patients with heart failure who were taking an ACE inhibitor rose significantly after the publication of RALES. Over the same time interval, there were significant increases in the rates of hospital admissions for hyperkalemia and of in-hospital death from hyperkalemia among these patients. Notwithstanding, a study from the United Kingdom found a similar increase in spironolactone use after the publication of RALES, but no increase in hyperkalemia or hyperkalemia-associated admissions to hospital.

### Drugs that block ENaC: amiloride, triamterene, trimethoprim, and pentamidine

Amiloride and triameterne are cationic drugs that block ENaC and diminish the lumen-negative voltage in the CDN.

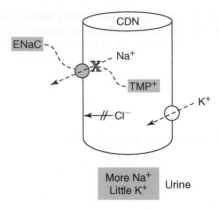

**Figure 15-1 Mechanism of Impaired Excretion of K⁺ Ions in Patients on Trimethoprim (TMP).** The *cylindrical structure* represents the cortical distal nephron (CDN). When TMP is in its cationic form (TMP⁺) in the lumen of the CDN, it blocks the epithelial Na⁺ ion channel (ENaC) (*X symbol*). As a result, there is renal salt wasting and diminished negative voltage in the lumen of the CDN, leading to decreased rate of excretion of K⁺ ions in the urine.

The cationic form of the antibiotics trimethoprim and pentamidine are structurally similar to amiloride and cause hyperkalemia and renal salt wasting by blocking ENaC (Figure 15-1). Hyperkalemia frequently develops in patients with HIV and *pneumocystis jiroveci* pneumonia who are treated with trimethoprim. Although this was attributed to the use of high doses of trimethoprim in these patients, trimethoprim may cause a rise in $P_K$ even when used in conventional doses in patients with renal insufficiency, hyporeninemic hypoaldosteronism, and concomitant use of ACE inhibitors or ARBs.

Another factor that may explain the observed high incidence of hyperkalemia in patients with HIV and *pneumocystis jiroveci* pneumonia treated with trimethoprim is perhaps a low flow rate in the CDN because of poor dietary intake and therefore diminished number of osmoles in the luminal fluid in the terminal CDN. In addition to its effect to diminish the rate of excretion of K⁺ ions, a low flow rate in the CDN may also increase the concentration of trimethoprim in the lumen of the CDN for a given amount of this drug (the same quantity of trimethoprim is in a smaller volume). Therefore, the ability of trimethoprim to block ENaC in principal cells in the CDN will be enhanced.

Issues in therapy are discussed under the discussion of Case 15-2.

### Drugs that increase electroneutral NaCl reabsorption in the DCT: calcineurine inhibitors (cyclosporin, tacrolimus)

Hyperkalemia develops in some patients receiving the calcineurine inhibitors cyclosporin or tacrolimus following organ transplantation. The pathophysiology of hyperkalemia and the clinical findings in these patients resembles that of "familial hyperkalemia with hypertension." Mice that were given tacrolimus developed salt-sensitive hypertension and increased the abundance of phosphorylated NCC and the NCC-regulatory kinases WNK3, WNK4, and SPAK. They also developed hyperkalemia when placed on a chow with a high content of K⁺ ions.

### Drugs that interfere with activation of ENaC via proteolytic cleavage: nafamostat mesylate

The activation of ENaC by aldosterone involves proteolytic cleavage of the channel by serine proteases such as channel-activating protease, CAP1. These proteases activate ENaC by increasing the open probability of the channels rather than by increasing their expression at the cell surface. Nafamostat mesylate is a potent serine protease inhibitor that has been widely used in Japan for the treatment of acute pancreatitis, disseminated intravascular coagulation, and also as an anticoagulant in patients on hemodialysis. It can cause hyperkalemia primarily as metabolites of nafamostat inhibit these aldosterone-inducible, channel-activating proteases.

# PART D
# THERAPY OF HYPERKALEMIA
## EMERGENCY HYPERKALEMIA

The major danger of hyperkalemia is the development of a life-threatening cardiac arrhythmia. Because even mild ECG changes may progress rapidly to a dangerous arrhythmia, any patient with an ECG abnormality related to hyperkalemia should be treated as a medical emergency.

Because some patients may develop cardiac arrhythmia or even cardiac arrest even in the absence of changes associated with hyperkalemia in the initial ECG, it is our view that severe hyperkalemia (i.e., $P_K > 7.0$ mmol/L) should be treated as an emergency with maneuvers to induce a shift of $K^+$ ions into cells even in the absence of ECG changes, and perhaps at even lower $P_K$ (i.e., >6.5 mmol/L) in the presence of hypocalcemia, acidemia, and/or hyponatremia. Notwithstanding, some patients on chronic hemodialysis, for example, seem to tolerate even more severe degrees of hyperkalemia without adverse effects.

### ANTAGONIZE THE CARDIAC EFFECTS OF HYPERKALEMIA

In cells in which the rate of rise of action potential upstroke ($V_{max}$) is dependent on the inward $Na^+$ ion current, administration of calcium ions alters the relation between the $V_{max}$ and the RMP at the onset of depolarization such that the $V_{max}$ is greater at a less negative RMP, and hence conduction velocity is increased.

Both calcium chloride and calcium gluconate can be used. Although a 10 mL of a 10% solution of calcium chloride contains about three times the amount of elemental calcium compared to 10 mL of 10% solution of calcium gluconate. Calcium gluconate is preferred because there is less risk of tissue necrosis if it extravasates from the vein during infusion. The usual dose of calcium gluconate is 1000 mg (10 mL of a 10% solution) infused over 2 to 3 minutes. The effect of intravenous calcium occurs in 1 to 3 minutes but lasts for only 30 to 60 minutes. This dose can be repeated in 5 minutes if ECG changes persist or if they recur. Caution should be exercised in patients on digitalis because hypercalcemia may aggravate digitalis toxicity. It is recommended that calcium be given in hyperkalemic patients on digitalis only if there is loss of P wave, or a wide QRS complex. In this case, calcium gluconate should be diluted in 100 mL of $D_5W$ and infused over 20 to 30 minutes to avoid acute hypercalcemia. The administration of digoxin-specific antibody fragments is the preferred therapy in these patients.

### INDUCE A SHIFT OF $K^+$ IONS INTO THE ICF

#### Insulin

Administration of insulin is the most reliable therapy to induce a shift of $K^+$ ions into cells that has been shown to be effective in lowering $P_K$

in a number of studies. The effect of insulin on the $P_K$ is independent of its hypoglycemic effect, which may be impaired in patients with end-stage renal disease. There is no consensus, however, on the optimal dose and method of administration of intravenous insulin (bolus or infusion) in the management of emergency hyperkalemia. A recent systematic review of the available data in the literature (11 studies) found no statistically significant difference in the fall in $P_K$ among the 6 studies in which 10 units of regular insulin were given as an intravenous bolus ($0.78 \pm 0.25$ mmol/L), the 2 studies in which 10 units of regular insulin were given as an infusion over 15-30 minutes ($0.39 \pm 0.09$ mmol/L), and the 3 studies in which ~20 units of regular insulin were given as an infusion over 60 minutes ($0.79 \pm 0.25$ mmol/L). Careful analysis of the data from these studies (the majority of which had serious or high risk of bias), however, suggested that an infusion of 20 units of regular insulin over 60 minutes may be a more reliable method in inducing the desired fall in $P_K$. Furthermore, the levels of plasma insulin that are required to achieve maximal shift of $K^+$ ions, based on data from studies using insulin clamp technique, were more likely to be achieved and maintained with the infusion of 20 units of regular insulin over 60 minutes. It was suggested to use the regimen of 20 units of regular insulin over 60 minutes in patients with severe degree of hyperkalemia (i.e., $P_K > 6.5$ mmol/L) and in those with marked ECG changes related to hyperkalemia (e.g., prolonged PR interval, wide QRS complex). Hypoglycemia is clearly a major concern with the administration of such large doses of insulin. Sufficient amount of glucose (60 g of glucose when 20 units of insulin are given and 50 g of glucose when 10 units are given) should be administered to prevent the occurrence of hypoglycemia; plasma glucose should be monitored frequently.

Although some suggest treating nondiabetic, hyperkalemic patients with a bolus of glucose without exogenous insulin, we do not favor this approach, considering that one is dealing with a life-threatening emergency. The high levels of insulin required to induce an adequate shift of $K^+$ ions into cells may not be achieved without an infusion of insulin. Moreover, hypertonic glucose may cause $K^+$ ions to shift out of cells in patients with inadequate insulin reserves, leading to an unwanted rise in the $P_K$.

### $\beta_2$-Adrenergic agonists

Although a number of studies suggest that $\beta_2$-adrenergic agonists (e.g., 20 mg of nebulized albuterol) are effective to lower the $P_K$ rapidly, we do not use these agents as first-line treatment of emergency hyperkalemia for two reasons. First, they are not effective in a significant proportion of patients. In a number of studies, 20% to 40% of patients who received these agents had a decline in $P_K$ of less than 0.5 mmol/L. It is unclear why certain patients do not exhibit a fall in $P_K$ following the administration of $\beta_2$-agonists, and it is not possible to predict which patients will not respond. Second, we are concerned about the safety of the doses that are needed to treat patients with hyperkalemia, which are four to eight times those prescribed for the treatment of acute asthma. Although no severe adverse events were reported in studies examining the use of these agents in patients with hyperkalemia, most of these studies have been performed in stable patients with a mild degree of hyperkalemia prior to their regular hemodialysis session. Moreover, a number of these studies excluded patients taking $\beta$-blockers and selected those with no significant history of coronary heart disease or unstable heart rhythms. Therefore, the safety of these agents was determined in a group of patients that may not resemble the general population with end-stage renal disease that has a high prevalence of cardiac disease. It is not clear whether $\beta_2$-agonists have an additive effect to the administration of 20 units of regular insulin.

## NaHCO$_3$

A number of studies have shown that the administration of hypertonic or isotonic NaHCO$_3$ does not lower the $P_K$ acutely. Understanding the possible mechanism of the effect of NaHCO$_3$ to induce a shift of K$^+$ ions into cells may provide an explanation as to why NaHCO$_3$ was found to be ineffective and under what conditions it may be useful in the therapy of emergency hyperkalemia. The first step in the proposed mechanism of NaHCO$_3$ is to decrease the concentration of H$^+$ ions in the ECF compartment and therefore promote the electroneutral exit of H$^+$ ions and the entry of Na$^+$ ions into cells via NHE-1. The increase in intracellular concentration of Na$^+$ ions activates the Na-K-ATPase, and the subsequent exit of Na$^+$ ions will make the cell interior more negative; therefore, K$^+$ ions will be retained inside cells. Notwithstanding, only if the NHE-1 is in active mode would the administration of NaHCO$_3$ have the potential to lower the $P_K$. One major activator of NHE-1 is a higher intracellular concentration of H$^+$ ions near NHE-1 because not only are H$^+$ ions a substrate for NHE-1, but they also bind to the modifier site that activates it.

Of note, many of the studies that evaluated the role of NaHCO$_3$ to lower the $P_K$ were carried out in stable hemodialysis patients who did not have a significant degree of acidemia. In other words, these studies examined the effect of NaHCO$_3$ when the NHE-1 was presumably in an inactive mode. The question remains as to whether NaHCO$_3$ would be effective in patients with a more significant degree of acidemia when the NHE-1 may become activated.

We use NaHCO$_3$ in patients with a significant degree of acidemia, but *not* as the only emergency therapy. Excessive administration of NaHCO$_3$ should be avoided because of the risk of inducing hypernatremia, ECF volume expansion, carbon dioxide retention, and also a fall in the concentration of ionized calcium in plasma, which may aggravate the cardiac effects of hyperkalemia. Studies that examined the combined use of NaHCO$_3$ with insulin have yielded conflicting results.

## REMOVE K$^+$ IONS FROM THE BODY

It is important to appreciate that to raise the $P_K$ from 5 mmol/L to 6 mmol/L requires an appreciably larger positive balance of K$^+$ ions than that required to raise the $P_K$ from 6 mmol/L to 7 mmol/L. This is because most of the K$^+$ ions are retained in the ICF compartment, largely in exchange for intracellular Na$^+$ ions. As the amount of Na$^+$ ions in the ICF declines appreciably, more of a K$^+$ ion load will accumulate in the ECF compartment. Therefore, a severe degree of hyperkalemia may develop with the retention of an additional relatively small load of K$^+$ ions (see Figure 15-2). The corollary is that during therapy, inducing a small loss of K$^+$ ions may cause a large fall in the $P_K$ in patients with severe hyperkalemia. In patients in whom the major basis of hyperkalemia is a shift of K$^+$ ions out of cells, one should avoid inducing a large loss of K$^+$ ions because this may lead to the development of hypokalemia because these patients do not have a total body surplus of K$^+$ ions. Maneuvers to induce a loss of K$^+$ ions and their limitations are discussed in the following paragraphs.

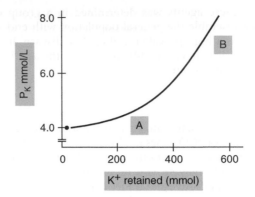

**Figure 15-2 Rise in $P_K$ With the Retention of a Load of $K^+$ Ions.** The numbers used in the figure are for illustrative purposes. The retention of a relatively large quantity of $K^+$ results in only a modest rise in the $P_K$ (to close to 5.0 mmol/L) because cells still have enough intracellular $Na^+$ ions to exchange with $K^+$ ions, and almost all the $K^+$ ion load is retained in the ICF compartment (*part A of the curve*). Once the quantity of intracellular $Na^+$ ions is diminished appreciably, a small additional $K^+$ ion load causes a larger rise in the $P_K$ (part *B* of the curve). The corollary in therapy of hyperkalemia is that even a small $K^+$ ion loss can cause a relatively large fall in $P_K$ in a patient with a severe degree of hyperkalemia.

## NONEMERGENCY HYPERKALEMIA

### REMOVAL OF $K^+$ IONS FROM THE BODY

### Enhancing the excretion of $K^+$ ions in the urine

Although a number of maneuvers may be suggested to increase the excretion of $K^+$ in the urine, there are no data to support their efficacy, particularly in an acute setting. The administration of a loop diuretic may induce kaliuresis by increasing the flow rate in the terminal CDN. One should avoid inducing intravascular volume depletion because this may lead to the opposite effect of decreasing the flow rate in the terminal CDN. Kaliuresis may be also enhanced by giving a synthetic mineralocorticoid (e.g., 100 to 300 µg 9α-fludrocortisone) and possibly by increasing the delivery of $HCO_3^-$ ions to the CDN by inhibiting the reabsorption of $NaHCO_3$ in the PCT with the administration of a carbonic anhydrase inhibitor (e.g., acetazolamide). $NaHCO_3$ may need to be given to replace the $HCO_3^-$ ions lost in the urine to avoid the development of metabolic acidemia.

### Enhancing the removal of $K^+$ ions via the gastrointestinal tract

**SPS**

Although "SPS" is often used as an abbreviation for sodium polystyrene sulfonate, SPS® is actually a brand name for sodium polystyrene sulfonate in sorbitol.

Sodium polysterene sulfonate (SPS; see margin note) is a cross-linked polymer to which reactive sulfonic groups are attached and preloaded with cations: $Na^+$ ions. When SPS is placed in a solution, its reactive sulfonate group exchanges its bound $Na^+$ ions for cations in the solution. SPS has long been used by clinicians for the treatment of hyperkalemia with the assumption that it exchanges most of its bound $Na^+$ ions with $K^+$ ions in the lumen of the GI tract and hence causes the loss of $K^+$ ions in the stool.

SPS contains 4 mEq of $Na^+$ ions per gram, which could be available for exchange for $K^+$ ions in the lumen of the GI tract. Based on the affinity of SPS for $Na^+$ and $K^+$ ions, and if one considers the measured concentrations of $Na^+$ and $K^+$ ions at different sites in the lumen of the GI tract, it seems that the only favorable site for this exchange to take place is in the lumen of the rectum (or perhaps in the entire colon).

Notwithstanding, other cations such as $NH_4^+$, $Ca^{2+}$, and $Mg^{2+}$ ions will compete with $K^+$ ions for exchange with $Na^+$ ions. Even if the exchange of $Na^+$ ions for $K^+$ ions were to occur in the colon, there is only a small amount of $K^+$ ions in the lumen of the colon to bind the resin. The amount of $K^+$ ions excreted via the GI tract in normal subjects is about 9 mmol/day. It has been suggested that patients with end stage renal disease have an enhanced colonic excretion of $K^+$ ions. Balance data are conflicting and the bulk of evidence would suggest that patients with end stage renal disease excrete only a few extra mmol of $K^+$ ions than normal subjects in their stool.

One possible theoretical benefit when using cation exchange resins is if they were to lower the concentration of $K^+$ in stool water by binding $K^+$ ions, which may enhance the net secretion of $K^+$ ions by the rectosigmoid colon, where secretion of $K^+$ ions occurs. But even if more $K^+$ ions were secreted into the lumen, the low stool volume would limit the total loss of $K^+$ ions (*see margin note*). It has been shown that the administration of SPS does not result in acute lowering of $P_K$. Moreover, the addition of resin did not result in a significant loss of $K^+$ ions in the stool over and above that achieved with the use of cathartics alone.

An increasing concern with the use of SPS in sorbitol is the development of intestinal necrosis, which usually involves the ileum and the colon. Although the incidence of this complication is not exactly known and is likely to be rather low considering the frequency with which SPS is used, it is, however, frequently fatal. The Food and Drug Administration has issued a warning against the "concomitant use of sorbitol" with Kayexalate® powder because of concerns about the risk of colonic necrosis and other GI side effects. This warning did not apply to premixed sodium polystyrene sulfonate in 33% sorbitol. There is concern, however, that at least some of the more recent reports of colonic necrosis followed use of premixed preparation containing 33% sorbitol.

In patients with life-threatening hyperkalemia, there is no role for the use of resins or attempting to induce loss of $K^+$ ions via the intestinal tract. In a patient with moderately severe hyperkalemia in whom the decision is made not to start dialysis, to induce $K^+$ loss in stool, the goal of therapy should be to induce diarrhea. The addition of SPS adds little in terms of $K^+$ ion loss to the induction of diarrhea alone. Because there is concern about the use of sorbitol 33%, the role of other cathartics, particularly those that induce secretory diarrhea (e.g., bisacodyl), is worth exploring. These diphenolic laxatives, by increasing cAMP in colonic mucosal cells, may not only increase stool volume but also stimulate $K^+$ ion secretion via the big conductance $K^+$ ion channels. Addition of SPS to cathartics, which induce secretory diarrhea, may increase the rate of excretion of $K^+$; however, the effect is modest compared to that of inducing diarrhea. With regard to patients with mild-to-moderate chronic hyperkalemia due to, for example, the use of RAAS blockers or patients with chronic kidney disease who do not yet require dialysis but need to have control of hyperkalemia, there are no studies that have examined the efficacy, safety, and tolerability of the long-term use of SPS. Furthermore, inducing a state of chronic diarrhea may not be possible or acceptable.

There are data to suggest effectiveness and good tolerability of two new oral polymers, patiromer and sodium zirconium silicate (ZS-9), in lowering $P_K$ and maintaining normokalemia in patients with chronic kidney disease who have diabetes or congestive heart failure and are receiving RAAS blockers. These drugs have not yet been approved by the FDA for the treatment of hyperkalemia. Patiromer is a spherical, nonabsorbable organic polymer; its active groups are composed of α-flouroacrylate pre-loaded with $Ca^{2+}$ ions, and it is

**$K^+$ ION LOSS VIA GI TRACT**

- If the lumen-negative transepithelial voltage in the colon were as high as –90 mV and the $P_K$ is 5 mmol/L, the concentration of $K^+$ ions in stool water would be ~100 mmol/L.
- With a usual stool volume of 125 mL, of which 75% is water, only 10 mmol of $K^+$ ions would be lost by this route.

thought to exchange $Ca^{2+}$ ions for $K^+$ ions in the lumen of the colon. ZS-9 is a nonabsorbable inorganic compound. It is not a polymer but a crystal that selectively captures $K^+$ ions, presumably by mimicking the actions of physiologic $K^+$ ion channels, and is thought to trap $K^+$ ions through the intestinal tract. Although this may decrease the net absorption of $K^+$ ions from the gastrointestinal tract, it is not clear how a large net negative balance of $K^+$ ions is achieved to lower $P_K$ because balance data are largely lacking.

### Dialysis

Hemodialysis is more effective than peritoneal dialysis for removal of $K^+$ ions. In the first hour of hemodialysis, approximately 35 mmol of $K^+$ ions can be removed with a concentration of $K^+$ ion in the bath of 1 to 2 mmol/L. Because the $P_K$ is lower in subsequent periods of dialysis, a smaller amount of $K^+$ ions is removed per hour. A glucose-free dialysate is preferable to avoid the glucose-induced release of insulin and thereby the subsequent shift of $K^+$ ions into cells, which could decrease the removal of $K^+$ ions. Notwithstanding, there is danger of inducing hypoglycemia if the patient received a bolus of insulin during emergency treatment of hyperkalemia.

# PART E
# DISCUSSION OF CASES

## CASE 15-1: MIGHT THIS PATIENT HAVE PSEUDOHYPERKALEMIA?

### WHY DID HYPERKALEMIA DEVELOP SO SOON AFTER HE LEFT THE INTENSIVE CARE UNIT?

Hyperkalemia that develops over a short period of time or during an intake of $K^+$ ions is likely to be a shift of $K^+$ ions out of cells or is pesudohyperkalemia. There was no obvious reason to suspect a shift of $K^+$ ions out of cells in vivo in this patient. With regard to pesudohyperkalemia, there was no hemolysis noted in blood samples, and the patient did not have leukocytosis or thrombocytosis. Because hyperkalemia was noted only after the patient was transferred to the ward, it was thought that pesudohyperkalemia might be due to leak of $K^+$ ions from red blood cells in the test tube if blood were left for several hours before analysis was performed or because of cooling of blood samples. Hyperkalemia, however, was still present in blood samples that were analyzed without delay after blood was drawn and without cooling of the blood samples.

A possible cause for pesudohyperkalemia is a shift of $K^+$ ions out of muscle cells locally into capillaries drained by the site of venipuncture. In fact, in the intensive care unit, blood was drawn using a T-tube connector in a vein on the dorsum of his wrist. Thus, there was no muscle contraction and the drainage bed had few muscle cells. In contrast, the child struggled vigorously and was restrained to have blood drawn from his brachial vein; furthermore, blood was drawn from an area that has a larger muscle mass. When $P_K$ was measured in blood samples drawn with the same technique used in the intensive care unit, it was 3.4 mmol/L. Therefore, the low $P_{Aldosterone}$ was likely due to hypokalemia rather than a cause of true hyperkalemia.

## CASE 15-2: HYPERKALEMIA IN A PATIENT TREATED WITH TRIMETHOPRIM

### What Is the Cause of Hyperkalemia in This Patient

Although an element of pseudohyperkalemia could be present in this cachectic patient, the presence of ECG changes indicated that he has true hyperkalemia.

Because his $U_K$ was 14 mmol/L and his urine volume was 0.8 L/day, his rate of excretion of $K^+$ ions was extremely low in the presence of hyperkalemia; therefore, one may conclude that the major basis for the hyperkalemia is a disorder causing impaired renal excretion of $K^+$ ions. This severe degree of hyperkalemia, however, developed over a relatively short period of time and while the patient had a very low intake of $K^+$ ions. Therefore, a shift of $K^+$ ions from cells rather than a large positive external balance for $K^+$ ions should be the major cause of his hyperkalemia. The cause of this shift of $K^+$ ions out of cells could be inhibition of the release of insulin due to the $\alpha$-adrenergic effect of catecholamines released in response to the low EABV. Nevertheless, the patient also had a large defect in renal excretion of $K^+$ ions. Because he had a low EABV and a $U_{Na}$ and $U_{Cl}$ that were inappropriately high in the presence of a contracted EABV, his low rate of $K^+$ ion secretion was likely due to diminished electrogenic reabsorption of $Na^+$ ions via ENaC in the CDN. The presumptive diagnosis was adrenal insufficiency due to an infection in a patient with the human immune deficiency syndrome. His $P_{Cortisol}$, however, was appropriately high and furthermore, when he was given a mineralocorticoid, there was no increase in the rate of excretion of $K^+$ ions in the urine. If a lack of aldosterone was the cause of the underlying defect in urinary excretion of $K^+$ ions, one would have expected a significant increase in urinary excretion of $K^+$ ions in response to the administration of a mineralocorticoid. It was thought that his diminished electrogenic $Na^+$ ion reabsorption in the CDN may be due to inhibition of ENaC by trimethoprim that was used to treat his *Pneumocystis jiroveci* pneumonia. Both his $P_{Renin}$ and $P_{Aldosterone}$ (which became available later) were high as expected in this setting.

*Interpretation*: Blockade of ENaC by trimethoprim caused renal salt wasting, which led to the development of EABV contraction. As a result, there was a shift of $K^+$ ions out of cells, leading to hyperkalemia because of inhibition of insulin release by $\alpha$-adrenergics.

This patient also has a very low flow rate in his CDN as suggested by his low rate of excretion of osmoles ($0.8$ L/day $\times$ 270 mosmol/kg $H_2O = 224$ mosmol/day). The low protein intake caused a low rate of delivery of urea to the CDN; the low salt intake, together with renal salt wasting, caused low EABV and thereby a low rate of delivery of $Na^+$ and $Cl^-$ ions to the CDN due to the increase in their reabsorption in the PCT. This reduced flow rate in the CDN does not only diminish the rate of excretion of $K^+$ ions but also increases the concentration of trimethoprim in the lumen of the CDN for a given amount of this drug. Hence, trimethoprim could become a more effective blocker of ENaC.

### What are the Implications for the Treatment of Hyperkalemia in this Patient?

Because the major basis of hyperkalemia in this patient is a shift of $K^+$ ions out of cells, it would be an error to induce a large loss of $K^+$ ions when it is unlikely that this patient has a total body surplus of $K^+$ ions. The appropriate treatment is to re-expand his EABV with an infusion

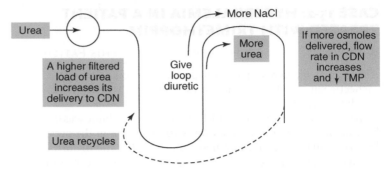

**Figure 15-3 Methods to Lower the Concentration of Trimethoprim (TMP) in the Cortical Distal Nephron (CDN).** The concentration of TMP falls in the lumen of the CDN when the number of osmoles delivered to this nephron segment rises. To achieve this aim, one could increase the excretion of urea (*red shading*) or inhibit the reabsorption of Na+ and Cl− ions in the thick ascending limb of the loop of Henle. To avoid further contraction of the effective arterial blood volume, the patient must receive more NaCl than is excreted in the urine. *CDN*, Cortical distal nephron.

of saline to suppress the α-adrenergic response; as insulin is released, it will cause the shift of K+ ions back into cells.

The question arose as to whether trimethoprim should be discontinued. Because the drug was needed to treat his *Pneumocystis jiroveci* pneumonia, means to remove its renal ENaC-blocking effect were sought (Figure 15-3). The concentration of trimethoprim in the lumen of the CDN falls if flow rate in the CDN were to increase. This can be achieved by increasing the number of osmoles delivered to this nephron segment. One could increase the delivery of urea to the CDN by increasing the intake of protein and hence the amount of urea that recycles. One could also increase the delivery of Na+ and Cl− ions to the CDN by inhibiting their reabsorption in the thick ascending loop of Henle with the administration of a loop diuretic. If the latter maneuver is used, enough NaCl should be given to avoid EABV contraction. Because it is the cationic form of trimethoprim that blocks ENaC, increasing the delivery of $HCO_3^-$ ions to the CDN could also be considered to lower the concentration of H+ ions in the luminal fluid in the CDN and thereby the concentration of the cationic, ENaC blocking form of the drug.

## CASE 15-3: CHRONIC HYPERKALEMIA IN A PATIENT WITH TYPE 2 DIABETES MELLITUS

### WHAT IS THE CAUSE FOR HYPERKALEMIA IN THIS PATIENT?

The first step is to rule out pseudohyperkalemia. The presence of hyperchloremic metabolic acidosis suggests true hyperkalemia. Hyperkalemia is associated with an alkaline PCT cell pH, which leads to inhibition of ammoniagenesis. K+ ions compete with ammonium ($NH_4^+$) ions for transport on the 2 Cl−, 1 Na+, 1 K+ cotransporter in the thick ascending limb of the loop of Henle, which leads to decreased medullary interstitial availability of $NH_3$. Both effects will result in a low rate of excretion of $NH_4^+$ ions (see Chapter 1).

The patient does not have advanced renal dysfunction and is not currently taking drugs that may interfere with renal excretion of K+ ions. The $P_{Renin}$ was decreased and his $P_{Aldosterone}$ was also suppressed, considering the presence of hyperkalemia. He was therefore thought to have hyporeninemic hypoaldosteronism, commonly labeled as type IV renal tubular acidosis. This is traditionally thought to be the result of destruction of, or a biosynthetic defect in, the juxtaglomerular apparatus, which leads to low $P_{Renin}$ and thereby to low $P_{Aldosterone}$. If that were the case, one would expect the patient to have renal salt wasting with decreased EABV and the absence of hypertension, which is not the clinical picture in many patients with this disorder. Another hypothesis is that the suppression of renin release in these patients is the result of EABV expansion. The basis of the disorder remains to be established. It is possible that the reabsorption of $Na^+$ and $Cl^-$ ions may be augmented in the DCT akin to patients with "familial hyperkalemia with hypertension." Of interest in this regard with respect to patients with type 2 diabetes mellitus who may have hyperinsulinemia and the metabolic syndrome is that chronic insulin infusion in rats is associated with the retention of NaCl due to its enhanced reabsorption in different nephron segments including the DCT and also with less WNK4 expression in the renal cortex. It has also been shown that phosphatidylinositol 3-kinase/Akt signaling pathway activates the WNK-OSR1/SPAK-NCC phosphorylation cascade in hyperinsulinemic db/db mice.

Differentiation between these two groups of patients with hyporeninemic hypoaldosteronism has implications for therapy. The use of exogenous mineralocorticoids (9α-fludrocortisone) is of benefit for the group of patients with destruction of, or a biosynthetic defect in, the juxtaglomerular apparatus because it results in both a kaliuresis and re-expansion of the EABV due to retention of $Na^+$ ions. Diuretic therapy would pose a threat to these patients because it would cause a more severe degree of EABV contraction. In contrast, mineralocorticoids may aggravate the hypertension in those who have excessive reabsorption of $Na^+$ and $Cl^-$ ions in the DCT. In this group of patients, the administration of thiazide diuretics to inhibit NCC is likely to be effective in lowering the blood pressure and correcting the hyperkalemia.

# section four
# Integrative Physiology

# Hyperglycemia

# Introduction

Because hyperglycemia due to poorly controlled diabetes mellitus is a common disorder associated with a number of disturbances in fluid and electrolyte balances, we thought it would be useful to have a separate chapter on hyperglycemia to address these different issues.

We begin this chapter with a brief description of the quantitative aspects of glucose metabolism, which illustrates that, although a relative lack of insulin is required to develop hyperglycemia, a marked reduction in glomerular filtration rate (GFR) and/or a very large intake of glucose causes the degree of hyperglycemia to become severe. This is followed by a section that examines the renal handling of glucose and the impact of hyperglycemia on volume and composition of body fluid compartments. In the clinical section, we discuss the clinical approach to the patient with a severe degree of hyperglycemia to determine its cause and design the appropriate treatment to restore the volume and composition of the extracellular fluid (ECF) and intracellular fluid (ICF). We also emphasize how to minimize the risk of developing cerebral edema, a complication that may arise during therapy, particularly in children with diabetic ketoacidosis (DKA).

---

## OBJECTIVES

- To illustrate that to develop a severe degree of hyperglycemia, a marked reduction in GFR and/or a very large intake of glucose is/are required.
- To examine the implications of hyperglycemia for salt and water balance, and discuss the clinical approach to the management of hyperglycemia with an emphasis on strategies to minimize the risk of development of cerebral edema, especially in children with DKA.

---

# PART A
# BACKGROUND

### CASE 16-1: AND I THOUGHT WATER WAS GOOD FOR ME!

A 50-kg, 14-year-old female has a long history of poorly controlled type 1 diabetes mellitus because she does not take her insulin regularly. In the past 48 hours, she felt thirsty and drank large volumes of fruit juice. She noted that her urine volume was very high. While in the Emergency Department, because she did not have access to fruit juice and continued to feel very thirsty, she drank large volumes of tap water. On physical examination, her blood pressure was 105/66 mm Hg, her heart rate was 80 beats/min, there were no significant postural changes in her blood pressure or in her heart rate, and her jugular venous pressure was not low. Her urine flow rate was 10 mL/min over the first 100-minute period of observation in the Emergency Department, and remained in the same level during the following 100-minute period. The following table shows measurements of the concentration of glucose in her plasma ($P_{Glucose}$), the concentration of sodium ($Na^+$) ions in her plasma ($P_{Na}$), the osmolality in her plasma, and the hematocrit from venous blood samples obtained at admission, 100 minutes later, and 200 minutes later. The concentrations of glucose and $Na^+$ ions and osmolality in her urine at these time periods are shown in the table. The arterial blood pH on admission was 7.33. Other laboratory data from measurements in a venous blood sample include the concentration of bicarbonate ($HCO_3^-$) ions in plasma ($P_{HCO3}$), 28 mmol/L; the anion gap in plasma ($P_{Anion\ gap}$), 16 mEq/L; the concentration of potassium ($K^+$) ions in plasma ($P_K$), 4.8 mmol/L; the concentration of creatinine in plasma ($P_{Creatinine}$), 1.0 mg/dL (88 μmol/L) (her usual $P_{Creatinine}$ was 0.7 mg/dL [60 μmol/L]); blood urea nitrogen (BUN), 22 mg/dL (concentration of urea in plasma ($P_{Urea}$) 8 mmol/L).

|  |  | ADMISSION | | AT 100 MIN | | AT 200 MIN | |
|---|---|---|---|---|---|---|---|
|  |  | Plasma | Urine | Plasma | Urine | Plasma | Urine |
| Glucose | mg/dL | 1260 | 6300 | 1260 | 6300 | 630 | 6300 |
| Glucose | mmol/L | 70 | 350 | 70 | 350 | 35 | 350 |
| Na⁺ | mmol/L | 125 | 500 | 125 | 500 | 123 | 500 |
| Osmolality | mosmol/kg H₂O | 320 | 500 | 320 | 500 | 281 | 500 |
| Hematocrit |  | 0.45 | – | 0.45 | – | 0.45 | – |

## Questions

What is the basis of the polyuria in this patient?

In what way might a severe degree of hyperglycemia have "helped" this patient?

How can the effective arterial blood volume (EABV) and plasma effective osmolality ($P_{Effective\ osm}$) be defended during therapy as the $P_{Glucose}$ falls?

Why did her $P_{Glucose}$ fail to fall in the first 100 minutes despite the large loss of glucose in the urine?

Why did the $P_{Glucose}$ and the $P_{Effective\ osm}$ fall in the second 100 minutes?

## REVIEW OF GLUCOSE METABOLISM

A more comprehensive discussion of principles of metabolic control was provided in Chapter 5. The following points summarize the normal metabolism of glucose.

1. *Brain fuels:* Glucose is the principal fuel oxidized by the brain in the fed state (Figure 16-1). In a state of a lack of insulin or a resistance to its actions (see margin note), fatty acids become almost the only fuel available for oxidation in the brain. Notwithstanding, fatty acids cannot cross the blood–brain barrier at a rapid enough rate—hence, they are not an important fuel for the brain. To provide a fat-derived fuel for the brain, fatty acids must be converted in the liver into water-soluble compounds—ketoacids.

The brain oxidizes ketoacids in preference to glucose if both are present, even if the $P_{Glucose}$ is high. The basis for this hierarchy of fuel oxidation is explained in the following paragraphs.

2. *Hierarchy of fuel oxidation:* To conserve glucose for the brain, fatty acids and/or ketoacids must be oxidized first when available.

To state it broadly, absolute control of the rate of glucose oxidation is mediated by the availability of nicotinamide adenine dinucleotide ($NAD^+$). Oxidation of fuels converts $NAD^+$ to its reduced form, $NADH,H^+$. Because $NAD^+$ is present in only tiny concentrations in both the cytosol and the mitochondria, $NADH,H^+$ must be converted back to $NAD^+$. This occurs during coupled oxidative phosphorylation, in which adenosine triphosphate (ATP) is regenerated from adenosine diphosphate (ADP) plus inorganic phosphate (Pi). In turn, ADP is formed from hydrolysis of ATP when biological work is performed. Hence, the rate of performing biologic work sets a limit on

**RELATIVE LACK OF INSULIN**

This term describes the combination of low levels of insulin and high levels of hormones with actions that oppose the actions of insulin (i.e., glucagon, cortisol, adrenaline, and the pituitary hormones—adrenocorticotropic hormone (ACTH) and growth hormone).

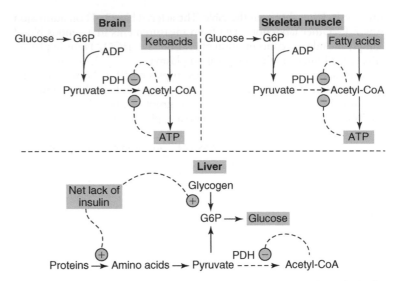

**Figure 16-1 Hyperglycemia Caused by Limited Metabolism of Glucose.** The metabolic control that sets a hierarchy of fuel oxidation is illustrated in the *upper portion* of the figure. To conserve glucose for the brain, fatty acids and/or ketoacids must be oxidized first when available. The activity of pyruvate dehydrogenase (PDH), the enzyme that controls the complete oxidation of glucose, is diminished when one or more of the following ratios are increased as a result of oxidation of fatty acids or ketoacids: ATP/ADP, NADH, $H^+$/$NAD^+$, and acetyl CoA/CoA. The metabolic events in the liver under conditions of relative lack of insulin are illustrated in the *lower portion* of the figure. Glucagon activates the enzymatic pathways for the breakdown of glycogen in the liver to produce glucose as well as the pathways involved in the conversion of amino acids to glucose (gluconeogenesis). Inhibition of PDH by the products of fat oxidation ensures that the flux of carbon proceeds toward the synthesis of glucose. *ADP,* Adenosine diphosphate; *G6P,* glucose-6-phosphate.

the rate of coupled oxidative phosphorylation (see Chapter 6). Oxidation of glucose is diminished when ketoacids in the brain or fatty acids in skeletal muscle are oxidized because their oxidation "steals $NAD^+$ and/or ADP," making them unavailable for the oxidation of glucose.

This hierarchy of fuel oxidation is the result of controls exerted at the level of two key enzymes in glucose metabolism: pyruvate dehydrogenase (PDH) and phosphofructokinase-1 (PFK-1). PDH is tightly regulated by its own specific kinase and phosphatase, inhibiting and activating it, respectively. PDH is inhibited when one or more of the following ratios are increased as a result of oxidation of fatty acids or ketoacids: ATP/ADP, $NADH,H^+$/$NAD^+$, and acetyl CoA/CoA (see Figure 16-1).

PFK-1 is a key regulatory enzyme in glycolysis in skeletal muscle and in brain cells. PFK-1 catalyzes an important "committed" step in glycolysis, the conversion of fructose 6-phosphate and ATP to fructose 1,6-bisphosphate and ADP. An increase in the concentration of ATP (or more precisely a decrease in the concentration of adenosine monophosphate [AMP]), as a result of oxidation of fat-derived fuels, diminishes the activity of PFK-1 and hence the flux in glycolysis (see Chapter 6).

## QUANTITATIVE ANALYSIS OF GLUCOSE METABOLISM

To understand why the concentration of a metabolite is abnormal requires an analysis of its rate of input and its rate of output. The daily

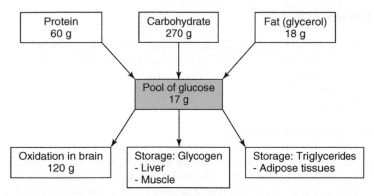

**Figure 16-2 Glucose Content in the Body Versus Turnover of Glucose on a Typical Western Diet.** The pool of glucose in the body is very small (`17 g or 95 mmol) relative to the input of glucose each day (~350 g or 1955 mmol). Glucose is the principal fuel oxidized by the brain in the fed state. The brain oxidizes close to 120 g (or 666 mmol) of glucose per day. Glucose is converted into glycogen to replenish its stores in the liver and muscle. Although some glucose may be oxidized in muscle, fatty acids are the major fuel consumed by muscle. Excess glucose is then converted in the liver into fat (triglycerides), which is stored in adipose tissues.

input of glucose typically exceeds the pool size of glucose by close to 20-fold (Figure 16-2). Therefore, extremely sensitive control mechanisms are needed to maintain such a tiny pool of glucose in the body. If these control mechanisms do not operate properly, hyperglycemia will develop, and this may occur rapidly.

## POOL OF GLUCOSE IN THE BODY

Most of the glucose in the body is in the extracellular fluid (ECF) compartment. Glucose is also present in cells of organs that do not require the effect of insulin to transport glucose across their cell membranes. These include most organs other than skeletal muscle. The ICF volume of these organs is ~5 L. Hence, in a 70-kg adult, the volume of distribution of glucose under conditions of a relative lack of insulin actions is ~19 L (14 L ECF + 5 L ICF), $P_{Glucose}$ is 5 mmol/L (90 mg/dL), and the pool of glucose in the body is 95 mmol (17 g).

## INPUT OF GLUCOSE

### From the diet

The daily intake of carbohydrates in an adult subject consuming a typical Western diet is about 270 g (~1500 mmol) (see Figure 16-2). Some glucose may also be synthesized during the metabolism of ingested proteins (60% of the daily protein intake of 100 g can be made into glucose [60 g (333 mmol)]) and some glucose is also synthesized from the metabolism of the glycerol portion of dietary triglycerides (about 18 g [100 mmol]). To put it in quantitative perspective, the quantity of the daily input of glucose (270 g + 60 g + 18 g = 348 g/day) is 20-fold larger than the entire pool of glucose in the body.

### From glycogen stores

Glycogen is stored primarily in the liver and in skeletal muscle.

### Glycogen in the liver

The size of the pool of glycogen in the liver is only about 100 g (560 mmol). The major function of glycogen in the liver is to supply the brain with glucose when the $P_{Glucose}$ declines (e.g., between meals). The breakdown of glycogen in the liver is stimulated by low insulin/high glucagon levels.

### Glycogen in skeletal muscle

Large amounts of glucose are stored as glycogen in skeletal muscles (about 450 g [~2500 mmol]). The major function of glycogen in skeletal muscle is to enable the regeneration of ATP at the fastest possible rate during vigorous exercise. This storage fuel is "reserved" because it permitted our starved ancestors to sprint and obtain food for survival. The major stimulus for the breakdown of glycogen in exercising muscle is a high adrenergic release. The first step in glycogen breakdown is catalyzed by the enzyme glycogen phosphorylase, and the product is glucose-1-phosphate. Because muscles lack the enzyme glucose-6-phosphatase, breakdown of this storage of glycogen does not result in the release of glucose into the circulation. L-Lactic acid is released when glycogenolysis is rapid—i.e., during a sprint—and lactate anions can be converted to glucose primarily in the liver and to a lesser extent in the kidneys.

## Conversion of protein to glucose

The liver is the only organ where this pathway occurs, because it contains all the enzymes required for the metabolism of all 20 different amino acids in proteins. In the fed state, dietary proteins are metabolized initially in the liver. Oxidation of 100 g of protein in the liver would yield 400 kcal (4 kcal/g), whereas the liver needs only ~300 kcal/day for the performance of its biological work. Hence, conversion of protein to glucose is an obligatory pathway in the fed state; but usually glycogen rather than glucose is the final carbon product in the fed state.

It is important to recognize when protein is being converted to glucose at an accelerated rate because this will signify a catabolic event or the loss of blood in the gastrointestinal tract. Approximately only 60% of the weight of proteins can be converted to glucose because some of the amino acids cannot be metabolized in this pathway (i.e., ketogenic amino acids such as leucine and lysine) and other amino acids must be partially oxidized in the citric acid cycle to be made into the gluconeogenic precursor pyruvate (e.g., the five-carbon skeleton in glutamine, the most abundant amino acids in proteins, is first converted to pyruvate, a three carbon compound). This process of conversion of the carbon skeleton in amino acids to pyruvate is obligatorily linked to the conversion of their nitrogen to urea (Figure 16-3). Therefore, the rate of appearance of urea provides a clue to the rate of endogenous production of glucose from protein. The stoichiometry of the process of the conversion of 100 g of protein to glucose and urea results in the production of 60 g (333 mmol) of glucose and 16 g of nitrogen (close to 600 mmol) of urea (see Chapter 12).

## REMOVAL OF GLUCOSE

Metabolic removal of glucose occurs via its oxidation or its conversion to storage compounds. During insulin deficiency, metabolic pathways for the removal of glucose are inhibited. Accordingly, renal excretion becomes the only major pathway for the removal of glucose.

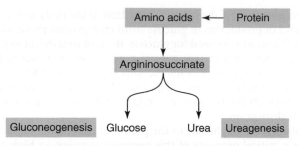

**Figure 16-3 Linkage Between the Synthesis of Glucose and Urea During Amino Acid Oxidation.** It is inaccurate to describe gluconeogenesis and ureagenesis as two separate metabolic pathways because both pathways are linked in the process of protein oxidation; in fact, they share a common intermediate, argininosuccinate, near the end of this pathway.

### Removal of glucose via metabolism

There are two major metabolic pathways for the removal of glucose: oxidation to regenerate ATP in the brain and conversion to storage forms of energy. Glucose is converted into glycogen to replenish its stores in the liver and muscle. Although some glucose may be oxidized in muscle, fatty acids are the major fuel consumed by muscle. Excess glucose is then converted in the liver into fat (triglycerides), which is stored in adipose tissues.

#### Oxidation of glucose

Glucose is the principal fuel oxidized by the brain in the fed state. The brain oxidizes close to 120 g (666 mmol) of glucose per day. Oxidation of glucose in the brain is markedly curtailed if ketoacids are present (see margin note).

#### Conversion to storage fuels

The pathway for conversion of glucose to glycogen requires the hormonal setting of sustained high net insulin actions, which leads to induction/synthesis of the enzymes required for conversion of glucose to glycogen in the liver. In addition, there must be a high $P_{Glucose}$ to drive the conversion of glucose by glucokinase to glucose-6-phosphate (G6P), the substrate for hepatic glycogen synthesis. Conversely, there is virtually no conversion of glucose to glycogen when net insulin actions are low; said another way, a high $P_{Glucose}$ is not a sufficient stimulus on its own to drive glycogen synthesis. Similarly, the conversion of glucose to fatty acids is much slower in this hormonal milieu because the key enzyme, acetyl-CoA carboxylase (ACC), which catalyzes the conversion of acetyl-CoA to malonyl-CoA (the first committed step in fatty acids synthesis), is inhibited by a low concentration of insulin in blood delivered to the liver and/or a high level of $\beta_2$-adrenergics (see Figure 5-4, Chapter 5).

Thus, removal of glucose via metabolic means is slow initially when insulin is given to a patient with hyperglycemia. The fall in the $P_{Glucose}$ during therapy is largely caused by expansion of the ECF volume with the administration of intravenous saline. This lowers the $P_{Glucose}$ by dilution, and, importantly, by the excretion of glucose as the GFR increases.

#### Excretion of glucose in the urine

Because only a small quantity of glucose is stored in the body, the excretion of glucose in the urine must be avoided to prevent the loss

**HYPEROSMOLAR HYPERGLYCEMIC STATE**
- This is usually described as a nonketotic state because these patients do not have an appreciable degree of ketoacidosis. They usually, however, have sufficient circulating ketoacids for regeneration of ATP in the brain, which may markedly decrease the need for glucose and hence lead to the development of a more severe degree of hyperglycemia.

### PRODUCTION OF GLUCOSE FROM PROTEIN CATABOLISM

- In an adult, catabolism of 1 kg of lean body mass can supply the brain with its need for glucose for less than 24 hours:
  - The brain oxidizes ~120 g of glucose per day.
  - Since only 60% of the weight of protein can be converted to glucose, catabolism of 200 g of protein is required to provide this amount of glucose. Because 80% of the weight of muscle is water, the amount of protein contained in 1 kg of muscle is close to 180 g.

of a precious fuel for the brain. In addition, if the body has to rely on high rates of production of glucose from endogenous proteins to provide the brain with its need for glucose, the cost in terms of loss of lean body mass will be high (see margin note). Further, if excreted in the urine, glucose will "drag" valuable ions (e.g., $Na^+$ and $K^+$) and water during an osmotic diuresis. Therefore, glucose is not excreted in the urine unless its filtered load exceeds the tubular maximum capacity for its reabsorption.

Reabsorption of glucose in the proximal convoluted tubule (PCT) reflects a critical property of this nephron segment—a high capacity relative to the normal filtered load of glucose (Figure 16-4). Quantitatively, the maximal reabsorption of glucose is usually 10 mmol (1.8 g) of glucose per liter of GFR (i.e., 1800 mmol [325 g]/day with a usual GFR in a 70-kg adult of 180 L/day).

The sodium-linked glucose cotransporter gene family includes six members, namely SLGT1 to SLGT6. SLGT1 is a low-capacity, high affinity sodium and glucose cotransporter and is expressed mainly in the small intestine. In contrast, SLGT2 is a high-capacity, low affinity sodium and glucose cotransporter, localized almost exclusively in the apical membranes of PCT cells. Unlike SLGT1, which mediates the sodium and glucose cotransport in a 2:1 ratio, SLGT2 mediates the sodium and glucose cotransport in a 1:1 ratio. SLGT2 inhibitors have been recently used to inhibit glucose reabsorption by the PCT and therefore to lower the $P_{Glucose}$ in patients with type 2 diabetes.

The exit of glucose from PCT cells is via a glucose transporter (GLUT2) on the basolateral membrane, which is independent of $Na^+$ ion transport.

Under conditions of relative lack of insulin, metabolic pathways for the removal of glucose are inhibited. Accordingly, renal excretion becomes the only major pathway for the removal of glucose. If the filtered load of glucose exceeds the capacity for glucose reabsorption by the PCT, glucosuria ensues. The excretion of glucose in the urine diminishes when the GFR falls. The GFR falls as a result of a significantly decreased EABV because of the glucose-induced

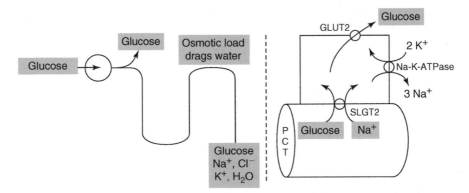

**Figure 16-4 Reabsorption of Glucose by the Proximal Convoluted Tubule.** As shown on the *left*, reabsorption of glucose occurs in the proximal convoluted tubule (PCT). The maximal reabsorption of glucose is usually 10 mmol (1.8 g) of glucose per liter of glomerular filtration rate (GFR). When too much glucose is filtered (>10 mmol/L GFR), the extra glucose is delivered distally, where it cannot be reabsorbed. As a result, an osmotic diuresis occurs. As shown on the *right*, the sodium-linked glucose transporter (SLGT) that carries out the bulk of the glucose reabsorption in the luminal membrane, SLGT2, is located in the early portion of the PCT. SGLT2 transports 1 $Na^+$ ion and 1 glucose molecule. The $Na^+$ ions reabsorbed are pumped out of cells by the Na-K-ATPase, which lowers the concentration of $Na^+$ ions in PCT cells; this provides the driving force to absorb $Na^+$ ions and glucose from the fluid in the lumen. The exit of glucose from cells of the PCT is via a glucose transporter 2 (GLUT2) on the basolateral membrane, which is independent of $Na^+$ ion transport.

osmotic natriuresis and diuresis. Expansion of the ECF volume with the administration of intravenous saline lowers the $P_{Glucose}$ by dilution, and, importantly, as the EABV is restored, the GFR rises, and excretion of glucose in the urine increases.

To maintain a severe degree of hyperglycemia in the absence of a marked reduction of GFR requires the intake of a large amount of glucose (e.g., ingestion of large volumes of fruit juice or sweetened soft drinks). Stomach emptying is usually very slow in a patient with hyperglycemia, and hence a large amount of glucose may be retained in the stomach. A sudden increase in stomach emptying and the absorption of glucose in the small intestine may result in a sudden large rise in the $P_{Glucose}$ because the volume of distribution of glucose is relatively small under conditions of relative lack of insulin.

# PART B
# RENAL ASPECTS OF HYPERGLYCEMIA
## GLUCOSE-INDUCED OSMOTIC DIURESIS

There are two factors that determine the urine flow rate during an osmotic diuresis: the rate of excretion of effective osmoles in the urine and the effective osmolality of the interstitial compartment of the renal medulla. The major effective osmole in the lumen of the inner MCD in a patient with hyperglycemia is glucose (~300 to 350 mmol/L). Although there is also a number of other effective osmoles in the urine ($Na^+$, $K^+$, and $NH_4^+$ ions, plus their attending anions) (Table 16-1) their quantity is relatively small. During an osmotic diuresis, the effective osmolality of the interstitial compartment of the renal medulla falls because of medullary washout because there is more water reabsorption in the medullary collecting duct (MCD) during an osmotic diuresis than during antidiuresis (see Chapter 12).

Osmoles that are readily transported across the luminal membrane of the terminal portion of the nephron are not effective urinary osmoles and hence do not obligate the excretion of water. Urea is not usually an effective osmole because vasopressin causes the insertion of urea transporters in the luminal membrane of cells in the inner MCD. Therefore, there is no appreciable difference in the concentration of urea in the luminal fluid and its concentration in the medullary interstitial compartment. Therefore, urea does not cause an osmotic diuresis unless the load of urea delivered to the inner MCD is so high that the transport capacity of the urea transporter is exceeded and hence the concentration of urea is higher in the luminal fluid than its concentration in the medullary interstitial compartment.

TABLE 16-1    **COMPOSITION OF 1 L OF GLUCOSE-INDUCED OSMOTIC DIURESIS**

| GLUCOSE (mmol/L) | UREA (mmol/L) | $Na^+$ (mmol/L) | $K^+$ (mmol/L) | $U_{Effective\ osm}$ (mosmol/kg $H_2O$) |
|---|---|---|---|---|
| 300-350 | 100-200 | 50 | 20 | ~450 |

The values serve as reasonable approximations.

# IMPACT OF HYPERGLYCEMIA ON BODY COMPARTMENT VOLUMES

Hyperglycemia has two major influences on the ECF and ICF volumes. First, hyperglycemia may cause a shift of water from the ICF to the ECF compartment if glucose was added to the ECF compartment as a hyperosmolal solution. Second, water and electrolytes will be lost in the urine because hyperglycemia induces an osmotic diuresis.

## HYPERGLYCEMIA AND THE SHIFT OF WATER ACROSS CELL MEMBRANES

There are two classes of particles to consider with respect to causing a shift of water across cell membranes.

1. *Particles that do not cause a shift of water:* Particles that are transported across cell membranes and hence can achieve near equal concentrations in the ECF and ICF compartments cause a rise in the osmolality in plasma ($P_{Osm}$) but do not cause a water shift—examples include urea and ethanol.
2. *Particles that cause a shift of water:* Particles that are largely restricted to one or the other compartment (e.g., $Na^+$ ions in the ECF compartment, $K^+$ ions in the ICF compartment) will cause water to shift out of or into that compartment when their concentrations in that compartment fall or rise, respectively (see margin note).

    With regard to glucose, it may be an effective osmole for some cells in the body but not for others, depending on whether insulin actions are required for the transport of glucose into these cells or not.
3. *Skeletal muscle cells:* The concentration of glucose is always much higher outside skeletal muscle cells because they depend on insulin for the transport of glucose, and thus glucose molecules are effective osmoles for these cells. Hence, if hyperglycemia is associated with a rise in the effective osmolality in plasma ($P_{Effective\ osm}$) (see Equation 1), water will shift out of skeletal muscle cells.

$$P_{Effective\ osm} = 2 \times P_{Na} + P_{Glucose} \tag{1}$$

4. *Hepatocytes:* Glucose is not an effective osmole for hepatocytes because its transport in these cells is independent of insulin actions. As a result, concentration is equal in both the ECF and the ICF compartments in the liver. Hence, hyperglycemia per se does not cause a shift of water out of liver cells. If hyponatremia is present, however, water will shift from the ECF compartment into hepatocytes, and hence they will swell.
5. *Brain cells:* Because of the brain cell heterogeneity, it is hard to be certain about whether overall brain volume falls or not in the presence of hyperglycemia and hyperosmolarity. Because glucose appears to be an effective osmole for only some brain cells, the fall in brain volume due to hyperglycemia may not be as large as one might expect. Furthermore, in experimental animals there appears to be volume regulation such that overall brain volume is close to normal in the setting of chronic hyperglycemia. If the situation in humans is comparable, this means that a sudden fall in $P_{Effective\ osm}$ can lead to a dangerous rise in brain cell volume and cerebral edema.

## QUANTITATIVE RELATIONSHIP BETWEEN RISE IN THE $P_{GLUCOSE}$ AND THE FALL IN THE $P_{Na}$

To be succinct, there is no reliable quantitative relationship between the rise in the $P_{Glucose}$ and the fall in the $P_{Na}$ in the patient with

**IMPACT OF LOSS OF $K^+$ IONS FROM THE ICF COMPARTMENT ON ICF VOLUME**

- If $K^+$ ions were to exit from cells and $H^+$ ions were to enter these cells, there will be a loss of effective osmoles from these cells because the $H^+$ ions will bind to intracellular proteins or remove $HCO_3^-$ ions; therefore, the cell volume will decline.
- If $K^+$ ions were to exit cells and $Na^+$ ions were to enter these cells in a 1:1 stoichiometry, there will be no change in the number of effective osmoles in these cells and therefore no change in their volume.
- In a catabolic state, such as in patients with diabetes mellitus in poor control, there is loss of both $K^+$ ions and organic phosphate anions from the ICF compartment. Therefore, the ICF volume will decrease.

hyperglycemia. This relationship is based on theoretical calculations of the amount of water that would shift from the ICF compartment to the ECF compartment for a certain rise in the concentration of glucose in the ECF compartment, thereby diluting its content of $Na^+$ ions and resulting in a fall in the $P_{Na}$, and different correction factors were proposed based on assumptions made about the ECF volume and the volume of distribution of glucose in the absence of insulin actions. This water shift, however, would occur only if the addition of glucose to the body is as part of a hyperosmolar solution. When glucose is added as part of an iso- or a hypo-osmolar solution, water does not exit cells. The following example illustrates the difference in the $P_{Na}$ if the same amount of glucose is added to the ECF compartment as an iso-osmolar solution or as a hyperosmolar solution.

*Example:* This patient weighs 50 kg, his ECF volume is 10 L, and his ICF volume is 20 L. Before he developed hyperglycemia, his ECF compartment contained 1400 mmol of $Na^+$ ions ($P_{Na}$ 140 mmol/L × 10 L) and 50 mmol of glucose ($P_{Glucose}$ 5 mmol/L × 10 L). His $P_{Effective\ osm}$ was 285 mosmol/kg $H_2O$, the total number of effective osmoles in his ECF compartment was 2850 mosmoles (285 mosmol/L × 10 L), and the total number of effective osmoles in his body was 8450 mosmol (285 mosmol/L × 30 L). The $P_{Glucose}$ will be raised in steady state using two different protocols. For simplicity, we shall only consider the ICF compartment of skeletal muscle (15 L) in each example.

1. *Glucose is added as an iso-osmolar solution:* Because there is no change in the effective osmolality in the ECF compartment, water will not shift across the membrane of skeletal muscle cells. Hence, the $P_{Glucose}$ will rise and the $P_{Na}$ will fall because $Na^+$-free water is retained in the ECF compartment.

   *Quantities:* A 2 L solution that has 285 mmol of glucose/L (total of 570 mmol of glucose) will be added. Because this solution has the same effective osmolality as the ECF compartment, all the water will be retained in the ECF compartment and the new ECF volume will be 12 L. Because all the glucose will be retained in the ECF compartment, the new $P_{Glucose}$ will be 51.7 mmol/L (570 + 50/12). Therefore, the rise in $P_{Glucose}$ is 46.7 mmol/L (51.7 mmol/L – 5 mmol/L). The new $P_{Na}$ would be 117 mmol/L (1400 mmol/12 L). Thus, the fall in the $P_{Na}$ is 23 mmol/L and the rise in the $P_{Glucose}$ is 47.5 mmol/L. Therefore, the ratio of the fall in the $P_{Na}$ to the rise in the $P_{Glucose}$ is close to 0.5.

2. *Glucose is added as a hyperosmolar solution:* The same amount of glucose as above, 570 mmol, will be added to the ECF compartment, but without water. Because this will cause a rise in the effective osmolality in the ECF compartment, water will shift from muscle cells to the ECF compartment.

   *Quantities:* The volume of water that will shift from the ICF compartment of muscle into the ECF compartment will depend on the rise in the effective osmolality and the fact that all of the added glucose will be retained in the ECF compartment.

   *Calculation of the new effective osmolality:* Before the addition of glucose, the patient had a total of 7125 mosmol: 25 L ([10 L ECF volume + 15 L ICF volume of skeletal muscle] × 285 mosmol/kg $H_2O$). Because 570 mmol of glucose were added, the total number of osmoles now is 7695 mosmol. Because there was no water added, the new effective osmolality is 308 mosmol/kg $H_2O$.

   *Calculation of the new ICF volume of skeletal muscle:* Because all the added glucose is retained in the ECF compartment, the number of osmoles in the ICF of skeletal muscle has not changed (15 L × 285 mosmol/kg $H_2O$ = 4275 mosmol) but is now at an effective osmolality of 308 mosmol/kg $H_2O$. Hence, the new ICF volume of skeletal muscle is 13.9 L (4275 mosmol/308 mosmol/kg $H_2O$). Therefore, 1.1 L of water has shifted from the ICF of skeletal muscle into the ECF compartment. *Calculation of the new $P_{Glucose}$ and $P_{Na}$:* Because 1.1 L of water has shifted into the ECF compartment, the new ECF volume is 11.1 L. Because all the glucose is retained in the ECF compartment, the rise in the $P_{Glucose}$ is 51.4 mmol/L (570 mmol/11.1 L). Because there was no change in the content of $Na^+$ ions in the ECF compartment, the $P_{Na}$ will fall to 126 mmol/L (1400 mmol/11.1 L). Hence, the ratio of the fall in the $P_{Na}$ (14 mmol/L) and the rise in the $P_{Glucose}$ (51.4) is 0.27, a value that is almost two-fold lower than that from the addition of the same amount of glucose but as an iso-osmolar solution.

*Conclusion:* Because patients with hyperglycemia have variable fluid intake and also variable loss of water and of $Na^+$ ions in the urine because of glucose-induced osmotic diuresis and natriuresis, one cannot assume a fixed relationship between the rise in the $P_{Glucose}$ and the fall in the $P_{Na}$. Importantly, it is incorrect to assume that will be a predictable rise and the $P_{Na}$ for a fall in $P_{Glucose}$, and administer hypotonic saline to avoid the development of hypernatremia because this may increase the risk for the development of cerebral edema.

## THE IMPACT OF AN OSMOTIC DIURESIS ON BODY FLUID COMPOSITION

The major losses in a glucose-induced osmotic diuresis are glucose, $Na^+$, $K^+$, and $Cl^-$ ions, and water. The total deficits of $Na^+$ and $K^+$ ions, and water have been estimated in balance studies in patients with diabetes mellitus who had insulin therapy withheld and from retrospective studies using the average amounts of $Na^+$ and $K^+$ ions, and water that were retained during therapy of patients with DKA. These estimates, however, are not accurate. For example, based on these estimates, more $Na^+$ ions are usually infused than the actual deficit of $Na^+$ ions, so that some patients develop edema. Moreover, these approximations are not really helpful to determine the deficits in an individual patient.

## SODIUM IONS

We describe how to estimate the deficit of $Na^+$ ions in an individual patient with a severe degree of hyperglycemia prior to instituting therapy. While one knows the $P_{Na}$, one needs a quantitative estimate of the ECF volume to calculate the deficit of $Na^+$ ions. This can be obtained using the hematocrit on presentation (in the absence of prior anemia or polycythemia) (see Chapter 2 for more discussion).

*Example:* A 70-kg patient presented to hospital with DKA; the $P_{Glucose}$ was 900 mg/dL (50 mmol/L), the $P_{Na}$ was 120 mmol/L, and the hematocrit was 0.50. Prior to the illness, this patient had a $P_{Na}$ of 140 mmol/L and an ECF volume of 14 L, and hence the ECF volume contained 1960 mmol of $Na^+$ ions.

Normal blood volume is ~70 mL/kg/body weight in adults, and is somewhat higher in the pediatric population. Therefore, a 70 kg adult has a blood volume of about 5 L. When the hematocrit is 0.40, the RBC volume is 2 L and the plasma volume is 3 L. When the hematocrit is 0.50, if RBC volume remains 2 L, the total blood volume is 4 L (0.50 = 2 L RBC volume/blood volume, blood volume = 4 L), and hence the plasma volume is now only 2 L (two-thirds of normal). Accordingly, the ECF volume is two-thirds of its normal value (~9.3 L). Multiplying the ECF volume by the $P_{Na}$ (120 mmol/L) yields the present content of $Na^+$ ions in the ECF compartment

(~1116 mmol). Therefore, the deficit of $Na^+$ ions in this patient is ~844 mmol. This provides an estimate of the total negative balance for $Na^+$ ions in the ECF compartment. This calculation, however, overestimates the loss of $Na^+$ ions from the body because a component of this $Na^+$ deficit in the ECF is the result of a shift of $Na^+$ ions into the cells to replace $K^+$ ions that were lost from cells without phosphate anions. This component of the $Na^+$ deficit in the ECF is corrected with the administration of KCl.

### POTASSIUM IONS

The total loss of $K^+$ ions in patients who present with hyperglycemia and DKA is said to be ~5 mmol/kg of body weight. The magnitude of the deficit of $K^+$ ions is likely to be variable among patients because some patients consume large volumes of fruit juice which is rich in $K^+$ ions (close to 50 mmol of $K^+$/L) to quench their thirst. A large component of the $K^+$ ion loss in the urine is accompanied with the loss of phosphate anions as a result of tissue catabolism. A component of the loss of $K^+$ ions from the ICF compartment occurs in exchange with $Na^+$ ions in the ECF compartment, with the subsequent loss of $K^+$ ions with $Cl^-$ ions in the urine.

## IMPACT OF THE INGESTION OF FRUIT JUICE

A liter of fruit juice typically contains ~750 mmol of sugar, ~ 50 mEq of $K^+$ ions, and ~50 mEq of organic anions, but little $Na^+$ and $Cl^-$ ions.

### $Na^+$ AND $Cl^-$ IONS

The presence of a large osmotic diuresis causes an appreciable loss of $Na^+$ ions in the urine (see margin note). Because dietary intake of $Na^+$ ions is usually low, a deficit of $Na^+$ ions develops, leading to EABV contraction. This fall in EABV causes the release of angiotensin II, which stimulates thirst. If the patient were to quench the feeling of thirst by drinking fruit juice or sugar-containing drinks, a more severe degree of hyperglycemia will develop, leading to further osmotic diuresis and natriuresis; therefore, a vicious cycle is created.

### WATER

While patients may ingest fruit juice to quench thirst, this will actually lead to a larger water deficit. Ingestion of 1 L of orange juice will provide 1 L of water. The excretion of this glucose load in the urine, however, will lead to the loss of more than 2 L of urine (750 mmol of glucose at a concentration of 350 mmol/L).

### POTASSIUM IONS

One liter of fruit juice typically contains ~50 mmol of $K^+$ ions. Thus, patients who consume large volumes of fruit juice are expected to have a higher $P_K$ on presentation.

### ORGANIC ANIONS

The major anions that accompany $K^+$ ions in fruit juice are organic anions (e.g., citrate anions in orange juice) that can be metabolized in the liver to produce $HCO_3^-$ ions. Therefore, the degree of acidemia may be less severe in patients with DKA who consumed a large volume of fruit juice.

**LOSS OF $Na^+$ IONS WHEN 1 L OF FRUIT JUICE IS INGESTED AND ITS SUGAR IS EXCRETED IN THE URINE**

- One liter of fruit juice contains ~750 mmol of sugar and no $Na^+$ ions.
- If all this ingested sugar is excreted in the urine at a concentration of 350 mmol of glucose per liter, the urine volume will be ~2 L.
- During a glucose-induced osmotic diuresis, the concentration of $Na^+$ ions in the urine is ~50 mmol/L. Thus, there will be a loss of ~100 mmol of $Na^+$ ions, which is equivalent to the quantity of $Na^+$ in 2/3 L of ECF volume.

# PART C
# CLINICAL APPROACH

## CLASSIFICATION OF HYPERGLYCEMIA

Hyperglycemia develops in conditions in which there is low net insulin actions. A severe degree of hyperglycemia may develop in these conditions if there is in addition a marked reduction in the GFR and/or a large intake of glucose. A large change in the $P_{Glucose}$ can occur quickly because the pool of glucose in the body is relatively small. The natural history of a hyperglycemic state begins with a polyuric phase. The major cause of the hyperglycemia at this stage is a large intake of glucose in a setting where the rate of metabolic removal of glucose is very low. Because the ECF volume and the GFR have not yet declined appreciably, there is a large excretion of glucose in the urine. Because of the glucose-induced osmotic natriuresis and diuresis, the EABV becomes contracted and the GFR falls. At this stage, the urine flow rate declines and a greater degree of hyperglycemia develops if there is a continuing input of glucose that exceeds its rate of excretion. We call the polyuric phase the "drinker" stage and the oliguric phase the "prune" stage of hyperglycemia. The clinical approach to determine the major cause of hyperglycemia is illustrated in Flow Chart 16-1.

## PATIENTS WITH HYPERGLYCEMIA AND POLYURIA

*High sugar intake (the drinker):* A very large input of glucose can overwhelm, for a period of time, the ability of the kidneys to excrete glucose, which may lead to a severe degree of hyperglycemia. Given the very large capacity to excrete glucose, a degree of reduction in GFR is also required to maintain a severe degree of hyperglycemia for a longer period. Most commonly, the source of glucose is the ingestion of large quantities of fruit juices or sweetened soft drinks to quench thirst.

In a patient with hyperglycemia, a sudden increase in the $P_{Glucose}$ may occur because of rapid absorption of glucose, which was retained in the stomach. This may be suspected if the fall in the $P_{Glucose}$ during therapy is less than what is expected from dilution caused by the reexpansion of the ECF volume and the loss of glucose in the urine with the rise in GFR as the EABV is restored (see discussion of Case 16-1).

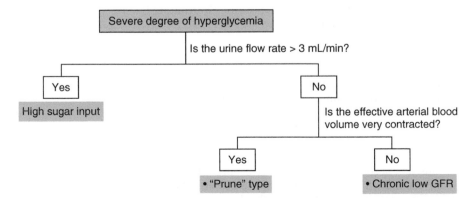

**Flow Chart 16-1 Diagnostic Approach to the Patient With a Severe Degree of Hyperglycemia.** The steps to follow are outlined in the flow chart. The final diagnostic categories appear after the *bullets* at the bottom of each column. We have selected a urine flow rate of 3 mL/min, but this is admittedly an arbitrary value. *GFR,* Glomerular filtration rate.

*High protein catabolism:* This alone cannot be the sole cause of a sustained and severe degree of hyperglycemia. This is because the breakdown of 100 g of protein provides the carbon skeleton for the synthesis of only ~333 mmol of glucose (the content of glucose in 1 L of osmotic diuresis) (see Table 16-1). Nevertheless, an increased endogenous input of glucose can result transiently from the breakdown of a large quantity of protein (e.g., with increased protein absorption from a major gastrointestinal bleed). This may be suspected if the fall in the $P_{Glucose}$ during therapy is less than what is expected and if the $P_{Urea}$ is higher than expected from the rise in $P_{Creatinine}$ (breakdown of 100 g of protein provides 16 g of nitrogen for the synthesis of ~600 mmol of urea).

## PATIENTS WITH HYPERGLYCEMIA AND OLIGURIA

*Prerenal failure:* As shown in Table 16-2, the excretion of glucose in the urine diminishes when the GFR falls. The GFR falls as a result of decreased EABV because of the glucose-induced osmotic natriuresis and diuresis. Hyperglycemia becomes more severe if the input of glucose exceeds its rate of excretion.

*Chronic renal failure:* The excretion of glucose is low in patients with advanced chronic renal disease. Because of the relatively small body pool of glucose, a severe degree of hyperglycemia develops under conditions of net lack of insulin, even without a substantially large load of glucose. Because these patients cannot produce an osmotic diuresis, the ECF volume will be expanded if the $P_{Effective\ osm}$ is high because water will be drawn into the ECF compartment primarily from skeletal muscle cells, which contain almost one-half of total body water. Also, because of the absence of osmotic natriuresis, these patients will not develop a negative balance for $Na^+$ ions.

## THERAPY FOR THE PATIENT WITH HYPERGLYCEMIA

### FLUID THERAPY

Cerebral edema is the major cause of morbidity and mortality in children with DKA. This does not seem to be a risk in most adult patients with a severe degree of hyperglycemia. Nevertheless, because similar

TABLE 16-2 **EFFECT OF HYPERGLYCEMIA AND THE GLOMERULAR FILTRATION RATE (GFR) ON THE RATE OF EXCRETION OF GLUCOSE**

| $P_{Glucose}$ (mg/dL) | GFR (L/day) | | | |
|---|---|---|---|---|
| | 180 | 100 | 50 | 25 |
| | GLUCOSE EXCRETED (g/day) | | | |
| 250 | 125 | 70 | 35 | 0 |
| **500** | 575 | 320 | **160** | 0 |
| 1000 | 1475 | 820 | 410 | 205 |

Excretion of glucose (g/day) equals the amount of filtered glucose (g/day) minus the amount of glucose that is reabsorbed in the PCT (g/day). The amount of filtered glucose (g/day) equals $P_{Glucose}$ (g/L) times GFR (L/day). Because the tubular maximum for glucose reabsorption in the PCT is 10 mmol (1.8 g)/L GFR, the amount of glucose that is reabsorbed in PCT (g/day) equals 1.8 g times GFR (L/day). With the usual daily intake of glucose (270 g) minus the amount that can be oxidized in the brain (~100 g/day), there is a net input of 170 g/day in a patient with a relative lack of insulin. Thus, to develop a steady state hyperglycemia with $P_{Glucose}$ of 500 mg/dL with the usual dietary intake of glucose requires a GFR that is less than 50 L/day (*shown in bold type*). A large intake of glucose will be required to maintain the same degree of hyperglycemia at higher values of GFR. Notwithstanding, because of the glucose induced osmotic diuresis and natriuresis and the resultant EABV contraction, the GFR will fall.

risk factors for brain swelling are present, we recommend that caution be exerted in all patients with severe chronic hyperglycemia to minimize the risk for development of brain swelling. The approach to therapy was discussed in detail in Chapter 5. Therefore, only a brief summary will be provided here.

### Treat a hemodynamic emergency if present

Enough $Na^+$ ions should be given initially to restore hemodynamic stability. A large bolus of saline should be given only if there is a hemodynamic emergency because it may be a risk factor for the development of cerebral edema. In a patient with metabolic acidemia, infuse saline, but not at a rapid rate, to lower the brachial venous $PCO_2$ to a value that is no more than 6 mm Hg above the arterial $PCO_2$. This ensures effective buffering of $H^+$ ions by the bicarbonate buffer system in muscle, and hence there will be less $H^+$ ion binding to intracellular proteins in vital organs (e.g., the brain and heart; see Chapter 1).

### Avoid a large fall in the $P_{Effective\ osm}$

Because the largest component of brain volume is its ICF volume, the major cause of development of cerebral edema is likely to be brain cell swelling. Water moves rapidly across cell membranes to achieve equal concentrations of effective osmoles in the ICF and ECF compartments. There are two major factors that could cause the ICF volume to expand: a rise in the number of effective osmoles in the ICF compartment and/or a fall in the concentration of effective osmoles in the ECF compartment (i.e., a fall in the $P_{Effective\ osm}$) (see Eqn 1; urea is not included in this calculation because urea is not an effective osmole).

Hence, an important objective during therapy is to prevent a large fall in the $P_{Effective\ osm}$ in the first 15 hours because this is the timeframe during which most cases of cerebral edema occurred in children with DKA.

The most common cause of a large fall in the $P_{Effective\ osm}$ is a large decrease in the $P_{Glucose}$. This occurs with the reexpansion of the EABV and the rise in the GFR. Therefore, the design of therapy should be to achieve a rise in the $P_{Na}$ by an amount that is one-half of the fall in the $P_{Glucose}$. This is because both $Na^+$ ions and their accompanying anions contribute to the $P_{Effective\ osm}$. For example, if $P_{Glucose}$ were to fall by 30 mmol/L, the goal of therapy should be for the $P_{Na}$ to rise by 15 mmol/L. To prevent a fall in the $P_{Effective\ osm}$, the effective osmolality of the infusate should be equal to or greater than that of the urine in this polyuric state. When $K^+$ ion infusion is needed, this goal can be achieved if KCl is added to 0.9% saline at a concentration of 30 to 40 mmol of KCl per liter. This solution has an effective osmolality that is reasonably close to the effective osmolality of the urine during a glucose-induced osmotic diuresis (see Table 16-1). Although one may be tempted to switch to hypotonic saline to treat the hyperosmolar state, it is our view that this may increase the risk of developing cerebral edema. As discussed previously, one should not adjust the $P_{Na}$ for the degree of hyperglycemia.

The usual water deficit on presentation is said to be 2 to 3 L in the adult with severe hyperglycemia. This deficit will be quite variable depending on what the intake of water was during the illness. Notwithstanding, defense of the $P_{Effective\ osm}$ should dominate decision-making for therapy.

Patients with hyperglycemia often consume large volumes of fluid to quench thirst. This ingested fluid may be retained temporarily in the stomach because hyperglycemia slows stomach emptying. This, however, will represent a gain of water when absorbed, if water has been ingested or after glucose is metabolized if fruit juice or sugar-containing soft drinks had been consumed. Rapid absorption of a large volume of water may result in an appreciable fall in the arterial $P_{Effective\ osm}$, to which the brain is exposed. This large fall in the $P_{Effective\ osm}$ in arterial blood may not be detected early on by measurements done in brachial venous blood. The clinician should take a detailed history of ingested fluids. The $P_{Effective\ osm}$ in arterial blood should be monitored if there is a history of a large intake of water. Infusion of hypertonic saline may be needed if there is a large fall in $P_{Effective\ osm}$ in arterial blood, particularly if symptoms such as headache, nausea, or obtundation develop, which may suggest an increase in intracranial pressure.

### Replace the deficit of Na+ ions

Having defined the safe rate and the tonicity of the fluid to infuse, the issue now is to define what is a reasonable total volume of saline to infuse. Enough Na+ ions should be given initially to restore hemodynamic stability and achieve a brachial venous $PCO_2$ that is no more than 6 mm Hg > arterial $PCO_2$ in a patient with metabolic acidemia. The entire Na+ deficit should not be replaced rapidly but rather over several hours, to minimize the risk of development of cerebral edema.

The deficit of Na+ on presentation can be estimated from the $P_{Na}$ and a quantitative estimate of the ECF volume using the hematocrit. This avoids the overzealous administration of saline and excessive expansion of the ECF volume. Not all of that Na+ ion loss from the ECF compartment was excreted; some Na+ ions entered cells when K+ ions exited from these cells without phosphate anions.

Ongoing losses of Na+ ions in the urine must also be replaced. Because glucose in the ECF compartment helped maintain its volume when the $P_{Glucose}$ was very high, its loss in the urine should be replaced by giving different effective osmoles for the ECF compartment, NaCl (see Discussion of Case 16-1).

### K+ ion therapy

A large component of the K+ ion loss in the urine is with phosphate anions due to tissue catabolism. The remaining component of the K+ ion loss from the ICF compartment was in exchange for Na+ ions from the ECF and the excretion of K+ ions with Cl− ions in the urine. This later portion of the K+ deficit is replaced early in therapy with the administration of KCl. Replacement of the K+ phosphate deficit occurs over days with the intake of phosphate in the diet and requires the presence of anabolic signals (e.g., actions of insulin).

Although patients may have large deficits of phosphate anions and the plasma phosphate levels may decline markedly with the administration of insulin, there are no compelling data to suggest that administration of phosphate alters the course of recovery. Notwithstanding, if a decision is made to give phosphate ions, the maximum dose is about 6 mmol/hr to avoid the danger of development of hypocalcemia because of precipitation of ionized calcium in plasma with phosphate anions.

### Insulin

The fall in the $P_{Glucose}$ during therapy is largely because of reexpansion of the ECF volume with the administration of intravenous saline, which lowers the $P_{Glucose}$ by dilution, and, importantly, the urinary excretion of glucose when the GFR increases. Removal of glucose via metabolic means is slow when insulin is given to a patient with hyperglycemia because oxidation of glucose does not occur at an appreciable rate until the circulating levels of fatty acids and ketoacids decline markedly. Furthermore, conversion of glucose to storage fuels (glycogen and/or fat) is a slow process that requires sustained insulin actions. A bolus of intravenous insulin should not be given because it is not needed, and it may activate the sodium–hydrogen exchanger-1 in brain cell membranes, which may lead to an increase in the number of effective osmoles in brain cells and the risk for developing cerebral edema (see Chapter 5).

## QUESTIONS

16-1  *A 50-kg patient has 30 L of total body water (ECF volume = 10 L, ICF volume = 20 L). She becomes very hyperglycemic ($P_{Glucose}$ 900 mg/dL, 50 mmol/L) and because the glucose induces osmotic diuresis and natriuresis, her ECF volume decreased to 7 L. How many liters of osmotic diuresis do you anticipate with therapy (assume that glucose was retained only in the ECF compartment and there will be no oxidation of glucose or synthesis of glycogen)?*

16-2  *How many liters of osmotic diuresis would have occurred if a 50-kg patient had a 600-mmol deficit of $Na^+$ ions?*

16-3  *If a patient has a gastrointestinal bleed and digests and absorbs all the protein in 1 L of blood, how many mmol of extra glucose and urea will be produced?*

# PART D
# DISCUSSION OF CASES

### CASE 16-1: AND I THOUGHT WATER WAS GOOD FOR ME!

**What is the basis of the polyuria in this patient?**

The $U_{Osm}$ of 450 mosmol/kg $H_2O$ indicates that this is an osmotic diuresis. Because her $P_{Glucose}$ was 1260 mg/dL (70 mmol/L), this is glucose-induced osmotic diuresis. This was confirmed by measurement of the concentration of glucose in her urine, which was 320 mmol/L.

**QUANTITATIVE ASSESSMENT OF THE ECF VOLUME**

- Normal blood volume in this patient is close to 3.5 L (70 mL/kg body weight × 50 kg).
- When the hematocrit is 40%, her RBC volume is close to 1.5 L and her plasma volume is close to 2 L.
- When her hematocrit is 45%, and if her RBC volume has not changed, her plasma volume has decreased by 25% to 1.5 L.
- By extrapolation, her ECF volume has decreased by 25% from 10 L to 7.5 L.

**In what way might a severe degree of hyperglycemia have "helped" this patient?**

A quantitative assessment of her ECF volume is needed to illustrate this point. Since her hematocrit was 45%, her ECF volume has decreased by approximately 25% from its normal value of 10 L to 7.5 L (see margin note). With an ECF volume of 7.5 L, she had about 488 extra mmol of glucose in her ECF compartment ([70 – 5 mmol/L] × 7.5 L). With a $P_{Effective\ osm}$ of 320 mosmol/kg $H_2O$, this degree of hyperglycemia would be responsible for maintaining close to 1.5 L (out of 7.5 L) in her ECF compartment (488 mosmol/320 mosmol/kg $H_2O$). Beware: the loss of this amount of glucose in the urine represents the loss of ECF volume. To maintain hemodynamic stability, this loss of glucose in the urine must be replaced with a solution that contains other effective ECF osmoles (i.e., NaCl).

## How can the EABV and the $P_{Effective\ osm}$ be defended during therapy?

### EABV

She has a deficit of $Na^+$ in her ECF that can be estimated from her $P_{Na}$ and a quantitative estimate of the ECF volume using the hematocrit. If her normal ECF volume was 10 L and her normal $P_{Na}$ was 140 mmol/L, the content of $Na^+$ ions in her ECF compartment was 1400 mmol. Because her ECF volume now is 7.5 L and her $P_{Na}$ is 120 mmol/L, the content of $Na^+$ ions in her ECF compartment is down to 900 mmol. Therefore, she has a deficit of $Na^+$ ions in her ECF compartment of 500 mmol. Not all of this deficit of $Na^+$ ions, however, must be replaced, because there may have been a shift of $Na^+$ ions into her ICF compartment to replace some of the $K^+$ ions that were lost from cells without phosphate anions. These $K^+$ ions were subsequently lost in the urine with $Cl^-$ ions. Therefore, administration of KCl restores this component of the deficit of $Na^+$ ions in the ECF compartment.

To avoid hemodynamic instability, ongoing losses of $Na^+$ ions in the urine must be replaced. As discussed previously, the loss of the extra glucose currently present in the ECF compartment will cause a loss of ECF volume. Therefore, this amount of glucose should be replaced with an equal amount of NaCl.

### $P_{Effective\ osm}$

The goal is to prevent a fall in the $P_{Effective\ osm}$ in the first 15 hours to avoid inducing brain cell swelling. To achieve this, the effective osmolality of the infusate should be equal to that of the urine in a polyuric state. Be aware that a fall in the $P_{Effective\ osm}$ may occur if a large volume of hypotonic fluid is absorbed from the gastrointestinal tract.

## Why did her $P_{Glucose}$ fail to fall in the first 100 minutes despite the large loss of glucose in the urine?

To answer this question, one needs to consider both the output and input of glucose.

### Output

The major output of glucose in a patient with a very high $P_{Glucose}$ and a reasonable GFR is its loss in the urine. Conversion of glucose to its metabolic products, glycogen and $CO_2$, should be very low in this setting. Because her urine volume during this time period was 1 L, and the concentration of glucose in her urine was 350 mmol/L, the output of glucose was 350 mmol; this loss of glucose is equal to the amount of glucose in 5 L of her ECF volume. Yet, there was no fall in her $P_{Glucose}$; therefore, she must have had a large input of glucose.

### Input

Although the input of glucose can be from endogenous sources, these can be dismissed in this case because of the low rate of gluconeogenesis (as deduced from the low rate of appearance of urea) and that there was likely a small quantity of glycogen remaining in her liver. Although there is a large quantity of glycogen in skeletal muscle (~450 g in a 70-kg adult), it cannot be released as glucose because skeletal muscles lack the enzyme glucose-6-phosphatase. The second source of glucose is glucose that was stored in her stomach, and this amount can be very large. Therefore, our best guess is that this patient had gastric emptying and, fortuitously, the amount of glucose absorbed from her intestinal tract was similar to the quantity of glucose lost in her urine. Because there was no change in the $P_{Na}$, there was probably an input of close to 1 L of water along with this amount of glucose, and this replaced the 1 L of water that was excreted in the urine.

### Why did the $P_{Glucose}$ and the $P_{Effective\ osm}$ fall in the second 100 minutes?

The first step is to examine the balance for water. The patient was given 1 L of water with 150 mmol NaCl (isotonic saline) and excreted 1 L of urine. Thus, there appears to be external balance for water. The fall in the $P_{Glucose}$ was consistent with the amount of glucose excreted in the urine, and this suggests that there was little glucose absorbed from the gastrointestinal tract in the second 100 minutes. Notwithstanding, the $P_{Na}$ should have risen because there was a positive balance of 100 mmol of $Na^+$ ions (input of 150 mmol minus output of 50 mmol in the urine) and zero balance for water. The $P_{Na}$ actually fell by 2 mmol/L, and hence there must be a gain of water that prevented the rise in the $P_{Na}$. Recall that the patient changed her intake from fruit juice to water in the emergency department.

#### *Implications for the risk of developing cerebral edema*

The volume of the ICF compartment rises if the $P_{Effective\ osm}$ declines while the number of effective osmoles in the ICF compartment remains largely unchanged. In the second 100 minutes, her calculated $P_{Effective\ osm}$ fell from 320 to 281 mosmol/kg $H_2O$ ($2 \times P_{Na}$ of 123 mmol/L + $P_{Glucose}$ 35 mmol/L) because she changed her intake from fruit juice, which contained the effective osmole glucose, to water and continued to have loss of glucose in her urine. Hence, brain cell swelling is now a threat to the patient. There is also the concern of a further fall in her $P_{Effective\ osm}$ because her $P_{Glucose}$ continues to fall and there may be absorption of an unknown amount of water that may have been retained in her stomach. We would administer hypertonic 3% saline in an amount sufficient to return the effective osmolality in her ECF and hence her $P_{Effective\ osm}$ to close to its previous value of 320 mosmol/kg $H_2O$. Because her ECF volume is estimated to be 7.5 L, and hypertonic 3% saline has an osmolality close to 1000 mosmol/kg $H_2O$, we would give this patient 300 mL of hypertonic 3% saline over 2 to 3 hours, and even more rapidly if the patient shows signs to suggest increased intracranial pressure (e.g., altered mental status, headache, nausea, or vomiting).

### DISCUSSION OF QUESTIONS

*16-1  A 50-kg patient has 30 L of total body water (ECF volume = 10 L, ICF volume = 20 L). She becomes very hyperglycemic ($P_{Glucose}$ 900 mg/dL, 50 mmol/L) and because of glucose-induced osmotic diuresis and natriuresis, her ECF volume has decreased to 7 L. How many liters of osmotic diuresis do you anticipate with therapy (assume that glucose was retained only in the ECF compartment and there will be no oxidation of glucose or synthesis of glycogen)?*

The concentration of the glucose in the urine during a glucose-induced osmotic diuresis is 300 to 350 mmol/L (see Table 16-1). When her $P_{Glucose}$ is 50 mmol/L, there will be 350 mmol of glucose in her

ECF compartment (7 L × 50 mmol/L). Hence, all of this glucose can be excreted in 1 L of urine.

*16-2  How many liters of osmotic diuresis would have occurred if a 50-kg patient had a 600-mmol deficit of Na⁺ ions?*

The concentration Na⁺ ions in the urine during an osmotic diuresis is close to 50 mmol/L (see Table 16-1). Therefore, if there were no intake of Na⁺ ions and trivial loss of Na⁺ ions in sweat, the urine volume would have been 12 L (600 mmol/50 mmol/L). Moreover, the excretion of glucose (12 L × 300 mmol/L = 36,000 mmol) is so large that its source has to be predominantly exogenous (drinking 6 L of fruit juice would provide ~42,000 mmol of glucose).

*16-3  If a patient has a gastrointestinal bleed and digests and absorbs all the protein in 1 L of blood, how many mmol of glucose and urea will be produced?*

One liter of blood has 140 g of hemoglobin in RBCs and about 40 g of protein in plasma (if the hematocrit is 40%, the plasma volume in 1 L of blood is 600 mL, and the concentration of total protein is 70 g/L), and hence there is a total of 180 g of protein in 1 L of blood. Approximately 60% of the weight of protein can be converted to glucose; thus out of 180 g of protein, 120 g can be converted to glucose. Because the molecular weight of glucose is 180, 666 mmol of glucose will be formed. This can drive the excretion of about 2 L of glucose-induced osmotic diuresis.

Because one-sixth of the weight of protein is nitrogen, 180 g of protein contains 30 g of nitrogen. Each mmol of urea has 28 mg of nitrogen. Therefore, about 1070 mmol of urea will be formed.

# Index

---

*Note:* Page numbers followed by *f* indicate figures, *t* indicate tables and *b* indicate boxes.

Printed and bound by CPI Group (UK) Ltd, Croydon, CR0 4YY

03/10/2024

01040305-0006

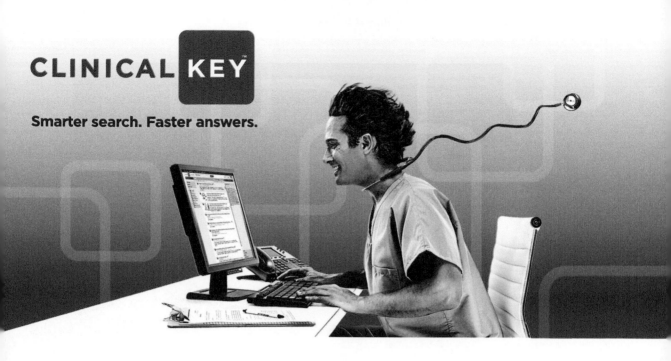